RHEUMATOLOGY

Diagnosis and Therapeutics

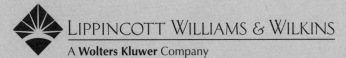
LIPPINCOTT WILLIAMS & WILKINS
A **Wolters Kluwer** Company

Philadelphia · Baltimore · New York · London
Buenos Aires · Hong Kong · Sydney · Tokyo

RHEUMATOLOGY
Diagnosis and Therapeutics

John J. Cush, MD
Clinical Associate Professor of Internal Medicine
The University of Texas Southwestern Medical Center
Chief, Division of Rheumatology and Clinical Immunology
Medical Director, Arthritis Consultation Center
Presbyterian Hospital of Dallas
Dallas, Texas

Arthur F. Kavanaugh, MD
Associate Professor of Internal Medicine
The University of Texas Southwestern Medical Center
Chief of Rheumatology
Dallas Department of Veterans Affairs Medical Center
Dallas, Texas

Nancy J. Olsen, MD
Associate Professor of Medicine
Vanderbilt University School of
  Medicine
Nashville, Tennessee

Salahuddin Kazi, MBBS
Assistant Professor of Internal Medicine
University of Texas Southwestern Medical
  Center
Dallas, Texas

C. Michael Stein, MBChB, MRCP(UK)
Assistant Professor of Medicine and
  Pharmacology
Division of Rheumatology and Clinical
  Pharmacology
Vanderbilt University School of
  Medicine
Nashville, Tennessee

Kenneth G. Saag, MD, MSc
Assistant Professor of Internal Medicine
Division of Rheumatology
University of Iowa College of Medicine
Iowa City, Iowa

Illustrations by Kathryn Born, MA

Editor: Jonathan W. Pine, Jr.
Managing Editor: Leah Ann Kiehne Hayes
Marketing Manager: Diane Harnish
Project Editor: Jennifer D. Weir

351 West Camden Street
Baltimore, Maryland 21201-2436 USA

Rose Tree Corporate Center
1400 North Providence Road
Building II, Suite 5025
Media, Pennsylvania 19063-2043 USA

Printed in the United States of America

Library of Congress Cataloging-in-Publication Data

    Rheumatology : diagnosis and therapeutics / John J. Cush . . . [et al.] ; illustrations by Kathryn Born. — 1st ed.
       p.   cm.
    Includes bibliographical references and index.
    ISBN 0-683-30014-8
    1. Rheumatism. 2. Arthritis. I. Cush, John J.
    [DNLM: 1. Rheumatic Diseases—diagnosis. 2. Rheumatic Diseases—therapy.
    WE 544 R4717 1998]
    RC927.R4835   1998
    616.7'23—dc21
    DNLM/DLC
    for Library of Congress   97-42809
                                                    CIP

The publishers have made every effort to trace the copyright holders for borrowed material. If they have inadvertently overlooked any, they will be pleased to make the necessary arrangements at the first opportunity.

To purchase additional copies of this book, call our customer service department at **(800) 638-0672** or fax orders to **(800) 447-8438.** For other book services, including chapter reprints and large quantity sales, ask for the Special Sales department.

Canadian customers should call **(800) 665-1148,** or fax **(800) 665-0103.** For all other calls originating outside of the United States, please call **(410) 528-4223** or fax us at **(410) 528-8550.**

Visit *Williams & Wilkins* on the *Internet*: http://www.wwilkins.com or contact our customer service department at **custserv@wwilkins.com.** Williams & Wilkins customer service representatives are available from 8:30 am to 6:00 pm, EST, Monday through Friday, for telephone access.

99 00 01 02
2 3 4 5 6 7 8 9 10

Dedication

This textbook is dedicated to our patients, who teach us daily.

Foreword

When I entered the field of rheumatology in 1950, clinical practice in this budding area of specialization was relatively straightforward, but at the same time it had its difficulties. Take rheumatoid arthritis as an example. The diagnosis was made essentially on the basis of the history, physical examination, and sedimentation rate. Sensitized sheep cell agglutination tests for rheumatoid factor were being done, but practitioners sneered at them, proclaiming that in those patients in whom the test was positive, they could make the diagnosis from the history and physical alone. The difficult part of treating the patient with rheumatoid arthritis came at the end of the examination. One had two drugs to offer—aspirin and gold salts. Gold salts were thought to be toxic and to be reserved for people with severe disease. So, one faced the inevitable embarrassment of telling the patient to take aspirin. Thus, a patient visit that started with a bang ended with a whimper. This period of limited treatment options has dramatically changed in the last half century.

When I started in rheumatology in 1950, laboratory investigation was centered on the composition of the connective tissue and how it became abnormal in disease. This was a natural consequence of the state of knowledge at the time. Investigation of connective tissue biochemistry had made good progress: the amino acid composition of collagen had been worked out, and the proteoglycan constituents, hyaluronic acid and chondroitin sulfate, had been isolated and characterized by Karl Meyer. A phenomenon called "fibrinoid degeneration" occupied people's minds. It was supposed to be so characteristic of the rheumatic diseases that Robert Good used to call them the "fibrinoid diseases." Observing the diffuse deposition of fibrinoid in the collagen of the connective tissue in systemic lupus erythematosus, Klemperer and coworkers in 1942 coined the name "collagen diseases." However, the rediscovery of the rheumatoid factor by Rose and Ragan and the discovery of the L.E. cell factor by Hargraves in 1948 sparked an explosion of research on the role of the immune response in the etiology and pathogenesis of this group of diseases. This, in turn, has lead to a massive growth in our knowledge of these diseases and, consequently, the number of outlets for dissemination of this knowledge.

There are journals of rheumatology in every major country, three large textbooks of rheumatology, and, inevitably, a half-dozen "condensed" texts. The present book, *Rheumatology: Diagnosis and Therapeutics* is unique among these condensed texts. Its uniqueness lies in the fact that it is essentially a compendium of the rheumatic diseases helpfully organized into three sections: (1) tests and procedures utilized in the diagnosis of the rheumatic diseases; (2) clinical information about the individual diseases, including their diagnosis and treatment; and (3) drugs used in treatment, with pertinent information about each drug. This format makes it possible for the reader to focus rapidly on the information he or she needs. In each of the three sections, the amount of information provided for each item listed is substantial.

As mentioned above, a vast amount of knowledge has accumulated in the field of rheumatology in the last fifty years. The amount of information has grown sufficiently large for the health professional to profit from having this "compendium" readily at hand.

Morris Ziff, PhD, MD
Ashbel Smith Professor Emeritus of Internal Medicine
Morris Ziff Professor of Rheumatology
The University of Texas Southwestern Medical Center
Dallas, Texas

Preface

Musculoskeletal diseases affect over 40 million Americans, 17 million of whom are limited in their daily activities because of their affliction. One-third of patients who present to primary care providers have musculoskeletal complaints, and over $150 billion is spent each year in caring for these patients. The magnitude of this problem demands both diagnostic accuracy and effective therapy. Unfortunately, formal education in the diagnosis and management of musculoskeletal disorders is limited and insufficient for most clinicians.

The primary intent of this text is to provide a succinct, but complete, reference to aid the busy clinician who cares for patients with musculoskeletal complaints. There are a number of major textbooks in rheumatology that aim to educate rheumatologists or serve as an authoritative resource on common and uncommon rheumatic conditions. Unfortunately, such texts are often too large, too expensive, and too lengthy to be useful to the clinician or trainee who wishes to expand his or her rheumatic diseases knowledge base. Instead, most physicians prefer a text that will readily fill informational gaps or clarify specific diagnostic and management issues. This text was largely written to meet the needs of clinicians in training, primary care physicians, and other medical providers who may be involved in the care of patients with musculoskeletal disorders.

This text is organized into three main sections: *Diagnosis, Rheumatic Diseases,* and a *Pharmacopeia.* Each of these sections is organized alphabetically to facilitate information access. The first section, *Diagnosis,* includes a discussion of patient evaluation, the approach to regional and systemic presentations, arthrocentesis and synovial fluid analysis, and lastly, an alphabetical listing of nearly 50 common diagnostic tests and procedures (e.g., antinuclear antibodies, electromyogram, and HLA-B27). The middle and largest section of the book is devoted to specific *Rheumatic Diseases.* Nearly 120 individual disorders are organized alphabetically, and each topic presents useful and factual information, using templates to facilitate retrieval of information. The third section of the text, the *Pharmacopeia,* is an abridged drug guide that covers over 80 of the drugs most commonly used in the treatment of musculoskeletal conditions. The user should seek specific diagnostic, disease, or treatment information by referring to the appropriate section. Throughout the book, the user may be directed to other sections for supplemental and related information. For instance, while reading about Sjögren's syndrome, the reader is referred to specific diagnostic tests (e.g., Schirmer's test and labial salivary gland biopsy) and therapies (i.e., artificial tears). Furthermore, certain drugs (e.g., NSAIDs, DMARDs, antidepressants) and diseases (e.g., septic arthritis, crystal arthritis, vasculitis) are compared in comprehensive tables found in the appendices.

The authors believe that this textbook can significantly enhance a physician's diagnostic accuracy, clinical acumen, and management of patients with musculoskeletal disorders. The concept, layout, and content of this text was influenced by feedback (from residents, fellows, and colleagues) received while teaching others. Thus, we welcome your comments and suggestions to enhance future editions of *Rheumatology: Diagnosis and Therapeutics.*

Lastly, this project is the net result of a cooperative effort between a distinguished group of rheumatologists and a talented publishing team. The authors wish to acknowledge our very talented publishing team that developed our concept of a "handbook" in rheumatology and delivered an informative, well-designed, and appealing textbook of medicine. We commend the excellence and professionalism of our team at Williams & Wilkins and are grateful for the wisdom and guidance of Jonathan Pine, the diligence and support of Leah Hayes, and the exceptional medical illustrations of Kathryn Born.

John J. Cush, MD
Arthur F. Kavanaugh, MD
Nancy J. Olsen, MD
C. Michael Stein, MBChB, MRCP (UK)
Salahuddin Kazi, MBBS
Kenneth G. Saag, MD, MSc

Abbreviations

$	see key on page 390
α	alpha
β	beta
γ	gamma
AAU	acute anterior uveitis
Ab	antibody
AC	acromioclavicular
ACD	anemia chronic disease
ACE	angiotensin converting enzyme
ACH	acetylcholine
ACL	anticardiolipin
ACR	American College of Rheumatology
AIDS	acquired immunodeficiency syndrome
AIMS	arthritis impact measurement scale
AL	amyloidosis
ALD	aldolase
ALT	alanine aminotransferase
AMA	antimitochondrial antibody
ANA	antinuclear antibodies
ANCA	antineutrophil cytoplasmic antibody
AOSD	adult-onset Still's disease
APL	antiphospholipid
APS	anti-phospholipid syndrome
ARF	acute rheumatic fever
AS	ankylosing spondylitis
ASA	acetylsalicylic acid (aspirin)
ASMA	anti–smooth muscle antibody
ASO	anti-streptolysin-O
AST	aspartate aminotransferase
ATLL	adult T cell lymphoma
AVN	avascular necrosis (osteonecrosis)
AZA	azathioprine
AZT	zidovudine
BAL	bronchoalveolar lavage
BCP	basic calcium phosphate crystals
BFP-STS	biologic false-positive serologic tests for syphilis
BM	bone marrow
BMD	bone mineral density
C	cervical
C3, C4	complement
CAH	chronic active hepatitis

CBC	complete blood count
CDC	Center for Disease Control
CHF	congestive heart failure
CK	creatine kinase
CLL	chronic lymphocytic leukemia
CMC	carpometacarpal
CML	chronic myelogenous leukemia
CMV	cytomegalovirus
CNS	central nervous system
COPD	chronic obstructive pulmonary disease
COX	cyclooxygenase
CPK	creatine kinase
CPPD	calcium pyrophosphate dihydrate
CREST	calcinosis, Raynaud's, esophageal dysmotility, sclerodactyly, telangiectasias
CRP	C-reactive protein
CSF	cerebrospinal fluid
CT	computerized tomography
CTS	carpal tunnel syndrome
CTX	cyclophosphamide
CVID	common variable immunodeficiency
CXR	chest x-ray
CYA	cyclosporine
DEXA	dual-energy x-ray absorptiometry
DFA	direct fluorescent antibody
DIC	disseminated intravascular coagulation
DIL	drug-induced lupus
DILS	diffuse infiltrative lymphocytosis syndrome
DIP	distal interphalangeal
DISH	diffuse idiopathic skeletal hyperostosis
DJD	degenerative joint disease
DLE	discoid lupus erythematosus
DM	dermatomyositis
DMARD	disease-modifying antirheumatic drug
DNA	deoxyribonucleic acid
DRVVT	dilute Russell viper venom time
dsDNA	double-stranded DNA
DU	duodenal ulcer
EA	early antigen
EBNA	Epstein-Barr
EBV	Epstein-Barr virus
ECHO	echocardiogram
ECM	erythema chronicum migrans
EDTA	ethylenediaminetetraacetic acid
EEG	electroencephalogram
EIA	enzyme immunoassay

ELISA	enzyme-linked immunosorbent assay
EM	electron microscopy
EMG	electromyography
EMS	eosinophil myalgia syndrome
ENA	extractable nuclear antigen
ESR	erythrocyte sedimentation rate
ESRD	end-stage renal disease
FDA	Food and Drug Administration
FMF	familial Mediterranean fever
G6PD	glucose-6-phosphate dehydrogenase
GBM	glomerular basement membrane
GC	gonococcus
GCA	giant cell arteritis
GCSF	granulocyte colony-stimulating factor
GI	gastrointestinal
GU	genitourinary
GU	gastric ulcer
GYN	gynecologic
h	hair
HAQ	health assessment questionnaire
HAV	hepatitis A virus
HBV	hepatitis B virus
HCQ	hydroxychloroquine
HCT	hematocrit
HCV	hepatitis C virus
Hgb	hemoglobin
HIV	human immunodeficiency virus
HLA	human leukocyte antigen
HSP	Henoch-Schönlein purpura
HTLV	human T-lymphotropic virus
IA	intraarticular
IBD	inflammatory bowel disease
IBM	inclusion body myositis
IC	immune complex
IDA	iron deficiency anemia
IEP	immunoelectrophoresis
IFA	immune fluorescent assay
IFN	interferon
Ig	immunoglobulin
IIF	indirect immunofluorescence
IIM	idiopathic inflammatory myopathy
IL	interleukin
ILD	interstitial lung disease
IM	infectious mononucleosis
ITP	idiopathic thrombocytopenic purpura
IU	international unit

IV	intravenous
IVDA	intravenous drug abuse
JA	juvenile arthritis
JRA	juvenile rheumatoid arthritis
KCS	keratoconjunctivitis sicca
KOH	potassium hydroxide
L	lumbar
LAC	lupus anticoagulant
LD	Lyme disease
LDH	lactate dehydrogenase
LE	lupus erythematosus
LFT	liver function test
LGL	large granular lymphocytes
LS	lumbosacral
LSD	lysergic acid diethylamide
MCP	metacarpophalangeal
MCTD	mixed connective tissue disease
MCV	mean corpuscular volume
MG	myasthenia gravis
MHC	major histocompatibility complex
MPA	microscopic polyangiitis
MPO	myeloperoxidase
MRA	magnetic resonance angiography
MRH	multicentric reticulohistiocytosis
MRI	magnetic resonance imaging
MS	multiple sclerosis
MSA	myositis-specific antibodies
MSU	monosodium urate
MTP	metatarsophalangeal
MTX	methotrexate
NA	not applicable (not available)
NCV	nerve conduction velocity
NMR	nuclear magnetic resonance
NPO	nothing by mouth
NSAID	nonsteroidal antiinflammatory drug
OA	osteoarthritis
OSHA	Occupational Safety and Health Administration
PAN	polyarteritis nodosa
PAS	periodic acid–Schiff
PBC	primary biliary cirrhosis
PCM	penicillamine
PCR	polymerase chain reaction
PIP	proximal interphalangeal
PM	polymyositis
PM/DM	polymyositis/dermatomyositis
PMR	polymyalgia rheumatica

PNS	peripheral nervous system
PR3	proteinase 3
PSA	psoriatic arthritis
PSS	progressive systemic sclerosis
PT	prothrombin time
PTT	partial thromboplastin time
PUD	peptic ulcer disease
PVNS	pigmented villonodular synovitis
RA	rheumatoid arthritis
RAST	radioallergosorbent test
RBC	red blood cell
RDW	red cell distribution width
RF	rheumatoid factor
RHD	rheumatic heart disease
RIA	radioimmunoassay
RNA	ribonucleic acid
ROM	range of motion
ROS	review of systems
RPGN	rapidly progressive glomerulonephritis
RPR	rapid plasma reagin test
RSD	reflex sympathetic dystrophy
S	sacral
SAA	serum amyloid A
SAARD	slow-acting antirheumatic drug
SAPHO	synovitis, acne, pustular lesions, hyperostosis, osteitis
SC	sternoclavicular
SCAT	sheep cell agglutination test
SCID	severe combined immunodeficiency
SCLE	subacute cutaneous lupus
SF	synovial fluid
SF36	short form 36
SI	sacroiliac
SIEP	serum immunoelectrophoresis
SLAM	systemic lupus activity measure
SLE	systemic lupus erythematosus
SLEDAI	SLE disease activity index
SPA	spondyloarthropathy
SPEP	serum protein electrophoresis
SRP	signal-recognition particle
SSZ	sulfasalazine
STS	soft tissue swelling
T4	thyroxine
TA	temporal arteritis
TB	tuberculosis
TIBC	total iron-binding capacity
TMJ	temporomandibular joint

TNF	tumor necrosis factor
TSH	thyroid-stimulating hormone
TTP	thrombotic thrombocytopenic purpura
UCTD	undifferentiated connective tissue disease
UPEP	urine protein electrophoresis
VCA	viral capsid antigen
WBC	white blood cell
XRAY	radiograph

Contents

SECTION 3. PHARMACOPEIA FOR RHEUMATIC DISEASES / 389

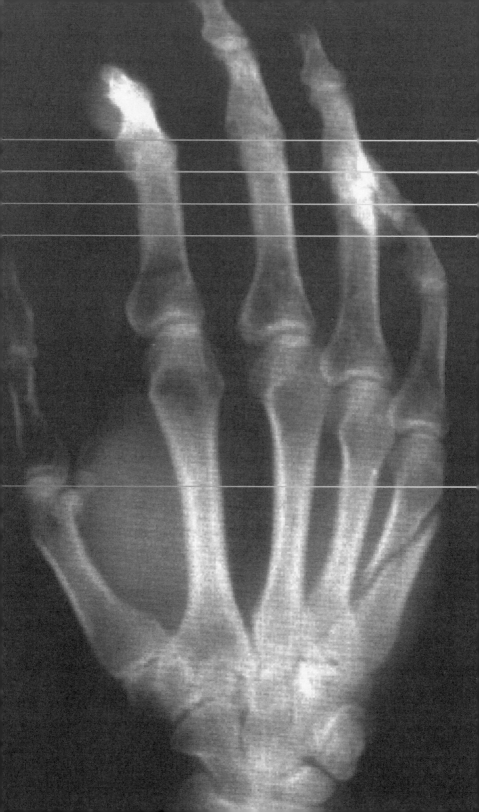

DIAGNOSIS

Diagnosis: A User's Guide

The first section of this guide focuses on the diagnosis of rheumatic complaints. An accurate diagnosis is obtained with the aid of a skillful clinical history and physical examination, with or without the aid of synovial fluid analysis, diagnostic tests, or musculoskeletal imaging. This section is divided into four chapters: 1, "Evaluation of Musculoskeletal Complaints"; 2, "Common Regional and Systemic Presentations"; 3, "Arthrocentesis and Synovial Fluid Analysis"; and 4, "Diagnostic Testing."

Evaluation of Musculoskeletal Complaints

This chapter presents the essential elements of clinical history and musculoskeletal examination. Proper categorization of the patient's complaints will aid in formulating a differential diagnosis. A detailed rheumatic review of symptoms is listed along with their associated rheumatic diagnoses. The musculoskeletal examination, demonstrating with specific maneuvers and signs, will refine the diagnosis and identify the patient's functional capacities.

Common Regional and Systemic Rheumatic Presentations

This chapter reviews the approach and diagnostic considerations in patients with specific regional and systemic presentations and emphasizes the underlying anatomic considerations, potential etiologies, key historical points, approach to evaluation, disease associations, distinctive physical findings or specific maneuvers, and the intelligent use of diagnostic tests or imaging helpful in formulating a differential diagnosis. Topics covered include evaluation of regional pain affecting the neck, shoulder, hand and wrist, low back, hip, and knee. A rational approach is offered for those patients presenting with the "hurts all over" syndrome, weakness, fever-rash-arthritis, or arthritis associated with disorders of the central nervous system, kidney, liver, neoplasia, pulmonary-renal syndromes, and pregnancy.

Synovial Fluid Analysis, Arthrocentesis, and Joint Injection Techniques

This chapter focuses on arthrocentesis and synovial fluid analysis and details the methods used in arthrocentesis, indications, contraindications, precautions, procedures, and techniques used on the most commonly aspirated and injected joints. The interpretation of synovial fluid findings is also reviewed.

Diagnostic Tests

This chapter alphabetically catalogs a variety of laboratory tests, diagnostic procedures, imaging methods, and disease assessment tools commonly used to evaluate patients with musculoskeletal conditions. Each topic describes the diagnostic test or procedure, methodology, background information, interpretation of results, guidelines for appropriate use, and information on confounding factors. Information is organized by a template of headings that may include "Synonyms," "Description," "Method," "Normal Values," "Abnormal Values," "Increased In," "Decreased In," "Interpretation," "Confounding Factors," "Complications," "Indications," Contraindications," Alternative Procedures," "Cost," and "Comment." The range of cost for select tests or procedures is based on 1997 costs gathered from several sources in the United States of America. The actual cost may very according to method, availabilty, and geographic site.

EVALUATION OF MUSCULOSKELETAL COMPLAINTS

Musculoskeletal complaints account for more than one-third of all adult outpatient evaluations in the primary care setting. A focused rheumatologic evaluation should be considered for those who manifest physical and functional limitations, focal or widespread musculoskeletal complaints, multisystem findings with rheumatic features, or (possibly) those found to have abnormal laboratory or imaging results suggesting a rheumatic disorder. Although an accurate and timely diagnosis is pivotal, many musculoskeletal complaints and conditions are self-limited and may only require symptomatic therapy. Others may take several visits and observation over time before the clinical features necessary to establish a firm diagnosis are fully manifested.

General Approach

Evaluation of musculoskeletal complaints should include a comprehensive medical history and physical examination, with particular emphasis on features that might indicate a rheumatologic process. The primary goals of the patient's evaluation are to discern if the complaint is

- Inflammatory or noninflammatory
- Articular or periarticular in origin
- Acute or chronic
- Mono/oligoarticular or polyarticular

By answering these four questions the clinician can categorize the complaint (e.g., "acute inflammatory monarthritis" or "chronic noninflammatory polyarthritis") and begin to establish a differential diagnosis (Table 1). Identification of other distinctive articular and extraarticular features (see "Essential Clinical History," below) often provides the necessary clues to make a timely and accurate diagnosis. *Only a few rheumatologic disorders are urgent and require a prompt diagnosis* and therapeutic intervention to minimize serious morbid sequelae. Such *urgent conditions* include fracture, septic arthritis/bursitis, and crystal-induced arthritis. These conditions often present as acute monarthritis.

Inflammatory versus Noninflammatory

Musculoskeletal disorders are often classified as having inflammatory or noninflammatory symptoms or signs that reflect the nature of the underlying pathologic process. *Inflammatory disorders* include a variety of infectious (e.g., tuberculosis), crystal-induced (e.g., gout), immunologic (e.g., systemic lupus erythematosus

Table 1
Differential Diagnosis of Musculoskeletal Complaints

DURATION	Articular Mono/Oligoarticular		Periarticular Focal	
	Inflammatory	Noninflammatory	Inflammatory	Noninflammatory
ACUTE	Septic arthritis Gout Pseudogout Viral arthritis[a] Reiter's syndrome Lyme disease Acute rheumatic fever Hemarthrosis Palindromic rheumatism	Fracture Trauma Mechanical derangement Sickle cell crisis	Bursitis Septic bursitis Tendinitis Tenosynovitis Costochondritis Enthesitis Periostitis	Carpal tunnel syndrome Sickle cell crisis Reflex sympathetic dystrophy
CHRONIC	Tuberculous arthritis Fungal arthritis Psoriatic arthritis Spondyloarthropathy Pseudogout Sarcoidosis Juvenile arthritis	Osteoarthritis Osteonecrosis Neuropathic arthritis Hemarthrosis Pigmented villonodular synovitis Foreign body synovitis	Tendinitis Costochondritis Enthesitis Periostitis	Carpal tunnel syndrome Myofascial pain syndrome Raynaud's phenomenon Osteoid osteoma

	Polyarticular		Widespread	
ACUTE	Viral arthritis[a] Septic arthritis Acute rheumatic fever Serum sickness Reiter's syndrome	Sickle cell crisis	Enthesitis Polymyalgia rheumatica Relapsing polychondritis	Sickle cell crisis
CHRONIC	Rheumatoid arthritis Psoriatic arthritis Enteropathic arthritis Crystal-induced arthritis Juvenile arthritis Lyme disease SLE Scleroderma MCTD	Osteoarthritis Hemochromatosis Hypertrophy osteoarthropathy	Polymyalgia rheumatica Polymyositis Myasthenis gravis Eosinophilic fasciitis Enthesitis	Fibromyalgia Chronic fatigue syndrome Myxedema Osteoporosis Paget's disease Psychogenic rheumatism

[a]Viral arthrits includes EBV, parvovirus B19, hepatitis B or C, Rubella, HIV.

(SLE)), and reactive (e.g., Reiter's syndrome) disorders. *Noninflammatory disorders* may be traumatic (e.g., fracture), degenerative (e.g., osteoarthritis), neoplastic (e.g., osteoid osteoma), or functional (e.g., psychogenic) in origin.

Inflammatory and noninflammatory features can be identified during the history and physical examination and may be supported by laboratory data (Table 2). The cardinal signs of inflammation—*erythema, warmth, pain, or swelling,* should be sought. Inflammatory pain is often maximal in the morning, improved by activity and time, and almost always associated with prolonged morning stiffness (>1 h) or systemic symptoms. Swelling of soft tissue (i.e., synovium or tenosynovium) with or without synovial effusion should suggest an inflammatory process. Laboratory evidence of inflammation (i.e., elevated erythrocyte sedimentation rate (ESR), C-reactive protein (CRP), or thrombocytosis) may be seen with inflammation and should not be elevated in uncomplicated noninflammatory disorders.

Articular *stiffness* commonly accompanies musculoskeletal disorders. Morning stiffness is ascertained by asking, "upon arising from a nights sleep, how long (minutes or hours) does it take for your stiffness to go away or get as good as it is going to get?" Rheumatologists often emphasize the importance of morning stiffness in distinguishing inflammatory and noninflammatory states. Unfortunately, the specificity of this feature is poor, as such common noninflammatory diseases as fibromyalgia and osteoarthritis (OA) may also be accompanied by more than 1 hour of morning stiffness. Stiffness brought on by brief periods of rest, lasting minutes rather than hours, is called *gel* phenomenon. Gel phenomenon is common with noninflammatory conditions such as osteoarthritis, adhesive capsulitis, and fibromyalgia.

Noninflammatory disorders are typically worsened by activity. Thus, patients typically complain of maximal pain in the evening or at night. Bony

Table 2
Distinguishing Inflammatory and Noninflammatory Findings

Feature	Inflammatory	Noninflammatory
Pain (worse when?)	Yes (morning)	Yes (night)
Swelling	Soft tissue (± effusion)	Bony
Erythema	Sometimes present	Absent
Warmth	Sometimes present	Absent
Morning stiffness	Prominent (>1 h)	Minor (<45 min)
Systemic features[a]	Sometimes present	Absent
Elevated ESR or CRP[b]	Frequent	Uncommon
Synovial fluid WBC	WBC > 2000/mm^3	WBC < 2000/mm^3
Examples	Septic arthritis, RA, gout, polymyalgia rheumatica	Osteoarthritis, adhesive capsulitis, osteonecrosis

[a]Fever, rash, weight loss, anorexia, anemia.
[b]ESR, erythrocyte sedimentation rate; CRP, C-reactive protein.

swelling and a lack of systemic features are characteristic of noninflammatory conditions.

Articular versus Periarticular

During the musculoskeletal evaluation the examiner must determine whether the complaint originates from articular or periarticular structures, as the two are commonly confused. A careful history and examination using a knowledge of local anatomy and specific maneuvers are necessary to distinguish between the two. Articular structures include the synovium, synovial fluid, articular cartilage, and joint capsule. The extent of articular involvement is defined as *monarticular* (1 joint), *oligoarticular* or pauciarticular (2–4 joints), or *polyarticular* (>4 joints). The differential etiologies of monarticular and oligoarticular complaints are similar, and they are typically considered together (i.e., mono/oligoarticular).

Periarticular structures include tendon, bursa, ligament, muscle, bone, fascia, nerve, or overlying skin. Periarticular complaints may be described as focal or widespread. Arthralgia (complaint of joint pain) may actually arise from articular or periarticular sites. Periarticular complaints are often misconstrued as articular pain because of their proximity. Table 3 details several distinguishing features useful in discriminating between articular and periarticular joint pain. The approach to evaluating articular and periarticular pain involving the hand, shoulder, neck, low back, hip, or knee is also discussed elsewhere (see pp. 17–36).

Essential Clinical History

The differential diagnosis may be narrowed further by reviewing key historical information. Because some types of arthritis may affect one population more than others, important diagnostic clues can be obtained from basic demographic information such as *sex, race,* and *family history* (Table 4). Certain disorders preferentially affect certain racial groups; polymyalgia rheumatica, giant cell arteritis, and Wegener's granulomatosis are most common in Caucasians, while sarcoid and SLE are commonly seen in African Americans.

Table 3
Distinguishing Articular and Periarticular Joint Pain

Clinical Feature	Articular	Periarticular
Anatomic structures	Synovium, synovial fluid, articular cartilage, joint capsule	Tendon, bursa, ligament, muscle, bone, fascia, nerve, skin
Painful site	Diffuse, deep tenderness	Focal or "point" tenderness
Pain on movement	Pain on active and passive motion in all planes	Pain on active motion in few, specific planes
Swelling	Common (bony or soft tissue)	Uncommon

Table 4
Clinical Associations Based on History and Physical Examination

Age
    Young (<25 years): JRA, SLE, Reiter's syndrome, gonococcal arthritis
    Middle (25–65 years): Fibromyalgia, tendinitis, bursitis, low back pain, RA
    Elderly (>65 years): OA, crystal arthritis, polymyalgia rheumatica, septic arthritis,
      osteoporosis
Sex
    Males: Gout, ankylosing spondylitis, Reiter's syndrome
    Females: Fibrositis, RA, SLE, osteoarthritis
Race
    Caucasian: PMR, giant cell arteritis and Wegener's granulomatosis
    African American: SLE, sarcoidosis
    Asian: RA, SLE, Takayasu's arteritis, Behçet's
    Mediterranean: Familial Mediterranean fever, Takayasu's arteritis
Family history
    Ankylosing spondylitis, gout, Heberden's nodes of osteoarthritis
Onset and chronology
    Acute: Fracture, septic arthritis, gout, rheumatic fever, Reiter's syndrome
    Chronic: OA, RA, SLE, psoriatic arthritis, fibromyalgia
    Intermittent: gout, pseudogout, Lyme, palindromic rheumatism, Behçet's, FMF
    Additive: OA, RA, Reiter's syndrome, psoriatic arthritis
    Migratory: Viral arthritis (hepatitis B), rheumatic fever, SLE, gonococcal arthritis
Number of joints involved
    Monarthritis (1 joint): Septic arthritis, gout, pseudogout, fracture, OA, osteonecrosis,
      Reiter's syndrome
    Oligoarthritis (2–4): OA, psoriatic, Reiter's, pseudogout, gout, Lyme, sarcoid
    Polyarthritis (>4): RA, SLE, OA, viral arthritis, psoriatic
Joint distribution (disorders to consider based on particular site(s) of involvement)
    Symmetric: RA, OA, psoriasis, tophaceous gout, viral arthritis
    Asymmetric: OA, Reiter's, psoriasis, early gout, sarcoid
    Axial: OA, ankylosing spondylitis, fibromyalgia, spinal stenosis
    Lower extremity: Reiter's, gout, sarcoid, OA, diabetes (Charcot)
    Upper extremity: RA, OA, psoriatic arthritis
    Sternoclavicular: Septic arthritis (especially in IVDA), RA, trauma
    DIP: OA (Heberden's node), psoriatic arthritis, swan-neck deformity
    PIP: RA, OA (Bouchard node), psoriatic, SLE, viral arthritis, boutonnière deformity
    MCP: RA, pseudogout, hemochromatosis, psoriatic
    Wrist: RA, psoriatic arthritis, septic (e.g., gonococcal) arthritis, De Quervain's
      tenosynovitis, carpal tunnel syndrome, ganglion cyst
    Elbow: RA, gout, olecranon bursitis, septic arthritis or bursitis, epicondylitis
    Shoulder: Rotator cuff tear, subacromial bursitis, bicipital tendinitis, OA,
      osteonecrosis, septic arthritis
    Hip: OA, RA, osteonecrosis, osteoid osteoma, fracture, iliopsoas bursitis, trochanteric
      bursitis
    Knee: OA, RA, pseudogout, gout, septic arthritis, sarcoid, Lyme, popliteal cyst,
      anserine bursitis, meniscal tear, chondromalacia patella, hemophilia, sickle cell,
      osteonecrosis
    Ankle/tarsus: Gout, septic arthritis, RA, sarcoid, hemophilia, diabetes
    MTP: RA, OA, gout, Reiter's syndrome
    Toes: RA, psoriatic arthritis, Reiter's, trauma

continued

Table 4 (continued)
Clinical Associations Based on History and Physical Examination

Drug-induced syndromes
   Arthralgias: Quinidine, amphotericin B, cimetidine, quinolones, chronic acyclovir,
      interferon, IL-2, nicardipine, vaccines
   Myalgias/myopathy: Steroids, penicillamine, hydroxychloroquine, AZT, lovastatin,
      clofibrate, interferon, IL-2, alcohol, cocaine, taxol, colchicine, tryptophan
   Gout: Diuretics, ASA, cytotoxics, cyclosporine, alcohol, moonshine, ethambutol
   Drug-induced lupus: hydralazine, procainamide, quinidine, methyldopa, phenytoin,
      isoniazid, chlorpromazine, lithium, penicillamine
   Osteonecrosis: Steroids, alcohol, radiation therapy
   Osteopenia: Steroids, chronic heparin, phenytoin, methotrexate
   Scleroderma/tight skin: Vinyl chloride, bleomycin, pentazocine, solvents, carbidopa,
      tryptophan, rapeseed oil
   Vasculitis: Allopurinol, amphetamines, cocaine, thiazide, penicillamine,
      propylthiouracil

Upon presentation, the clinician should determine if the complaint is acute or chronic, based on whether the complaint has been present 6 weeks or less (*acute*) or longer than 6 weeks (*chronic*). The presentation of fracture, gonococcal arthritis, and gout are typically acute; fibromyalgia, osteoarthritis, and rheumatoid arthritis (RA) are chronic by history. Other aspects of the *onset and chronology* often provide useful clues (Table 4). For example, *intermittent* complaints (with disease-free intervals) may indicate a crystal-induced arthropathy (e.g., gout, pseudogout). Incremental involvement of new joints describes an *additive* pattern characteristic of OA and RA. *Migratory* arthritis is defined as a rapidly changing pattern in which new joint complaints appear, resolve in days, and reappear at another site(s). A migratory pattern may be seen in rheumatic fever, viral (i.e., hepatitis B), or gonococcal arthritis. The *number and distribution* of involved joints also provide useful information (Table 4). Complaints may be described as *monarticular, oligoarticular (or pauciarticular), polyarticular, focal,* or *widespread* (Table 1). *Symmetric* joint involvement in the upper extremity is typical of RA, whereas OA, Reiter's syndrome, and gout often demonstrate *asymmetric,* lower extremity disease. *Axial (spinal) involvement* is common in OA and ankylosing spondylitis. Finally, the clinician should be aware that *drug-induced* musculoskeletal side effects or rheumatic disorders are a common and often overlooked cause of musculoskeletal complaints (Table 4).

A comprehensive *rheumatic review of systems* (ROS) may disclose extraarticular features indicating particular rheumatic disorders. Table 5 details a suggested ROS and possible clinical associations. For example, the examiner may narrow the diagnostic possibilities by questioning about the presence of fever (suggesting SLE, septic arthritis, or gout), ocular inflammation (Reiter's syndrome, sarcoid, Behçet's disease), rash (dermatomyositis, SLE, psoriatic arthritis), mucosal ulceration (Behçet's, drug induced), nail abnormalities (psoriasis,

Table 5
Rheumatic Review of Symptoms

Symptom	Clinical Associations
Fever	Septic arthritis, gout, pseudogout, SLE, viral arthritis, MCTD, Reiter's, RA, vasculitis, rheumatic fever, adult Still's disease, drug-fever, Sweet's syndrome, osteomyelitis, *Brucella*, enteropathic arthritis, Behçet's
Weight loss	Uncontrolled inflammatory disorders (SLE, RA, polymyalgia rheumatica), vasculitis (temporal arteritis, polyarteritis), NSAID-induced peptic ulcer disease, enteropathic arthritis
Morning stiffness >1 h	RA, polymyalgia rheumatica, psoriatic arthritis, ankylosing spondylitis, Reiter's, fibromyalgia
Ocular involvement	Sjögren's syndrome, Behçet's, Reiter's, spondyloarthropathies, juvenile arthritis, sarcoid, RA, Wegener's granulomatosis, Kawasaki syndrome, enteropathic arthritis, temporal arteritis, relapsing polychondritis, hydroxychloroquine therapy
Oral ulcers (painful?)	SLE (−), Reiter's (−), enteropathic arthritis (−), lues (−), Behçet's (+), herpes (+), methotrexate (+), gold (+)
Genital lesions (pain?)	Gonococcal infection (+), Behçet's (+), Reiter's (−), psoriasis (−), Lues (−)
Rash	SLE, psoriasis, dermatomyositis, vasculitis, cryoglobulinemia, Lyme disease, viral arthritis, rheumatic fever, adult Still's disease, Sweet's syndrome, sarcoid, erythema nodosum
Tight skin	Scleroderma, CREST, morphea, MCTD, eosinophilic fasciitis, eosinophilia myalgia syndrome, calcinosis, pseudosclerodactyly (e.g., diabetes, hypothyroidism), drugs (bleomycin, vinyl chloride)
Nail abnormalities	Psoriasis, Reiter's, onychomycosis, vasculitis, endocarditis, hypertrophic osteoarthropathy
Periungual erythema	Dermatomyositis, SLE, scleroderma, MCTD, psoriasis, Reiter's syndrome
Raynaud's	Scleroderma, MCTD, SLE, RA, inflammatory myositis, Buerger's disease, vasculitis, antiphospholipid syndrome, primary Raynaud's
Sausage digits (dactylitis)	Reiter's, MCTD, scleroderma, psoriasis, juvenile arthritis, sarcoid, sickle cell disease
Myalgias	Fibromyalgia, polymyositis, rhabdomyolysis, vasculitis, SLE, drug-induced lupus, RA, serum sickness, adult Still's, hypothyroidism, viral syndromes, drugs (lipid lowering agents)
Spinal pain	Lumbosacral strain, degenerative disc disease, spondylitis (AS, psoriatic, enteropathic, Reiter's), OA, DISH, fibromyalgia, septic disciitis, vertebral compression fracture, osteomyelitis, metastases, spinal stenosis, tuberculosis, brucellosis
Heel pain	Spondyloarthropathies (AS, Reiter's, psoriatic, enteropathic), osteoarthritis, plantar fasciitis, Achilles tendinitis, calcaneal fracture, fluorosis, retinoid therapy

continued

Table 5 (continued)
Rheumatic Review of Symptoms

Symptom	Clinical Associations
Subcutaneous nodules	RA, gout (tophi), rheumatic fever, hyperlipidemia (xanthomas), panniculitis, erythema nodosum, sarcoid, MCTD, polyarteritis, calcinosis, leprosy, multicentric reticulohistiocytosis, ganglion
Dysphagia	Lower (esophageal): scleroderma, CREST, MCTD, Crohn's disease Upper (pharyngeal): inflammatory myositis, Sjögren's syndrome (due to xerostomia)
Gastrointestinal involvement	Scleroderma, MCTD, enteropathic arthritis, vasculitis, Behçet's, Whipple's disease, SLE, hepatitis, FMF, intestinal bypass syndrome, primary biliary cirrhosis, cryoglobulinemia
Serositis	SLE, RA, MCTD, drug-induced lupus, rheumatic fever, adult Still's disease, FMF, Whipple's
Pulmonary involvement	Wegener's, Churg-Strauss angiitis, polymyositis, SLE, scleroderma, MCTD, Sjögren's, sarcoid, RA, ankylosing spondylitis, Goodpasture's syndrome, drug-induced lupus
Neuropathy	Carpal or tarsal tunnel syndrome, SLE, vasculitis, Lyme disease, RA, amyloidosis, cryoglobulinemia, amyloidosis, drug-induced
Sleep disturbance	Fibromyalgia, osteoarthritis, rotator cuff dysfunction, AS, steroid therapy, depression

Reiter's), myalgias (myositis, fibromyalgia, viral arthritis), heel pain (HLA-B27 spondyloarthropathies, fasciitis), nodules (RA, gout, hyperlipidemia), dysphagia (scleroderma, myositis, Sjögren's syndrome), paresthesias (carpal tunnel syndrome, vasculitis, Lyme disease), and sleep disturbance (fibromyalgia, rotator cuff dysfunction).

Physical Examination

The physical examination should confirm or expand upon the differential diagnosis established during the medical history. In addition, the physical examination will further establish whether the complaint is articular or periarticular, inflammatory or noninflammatory, focal or widespread, monarticular or polyarticular, or associated with systemic findings. Demonstration of certain physical signs and a knowledge of anatomy will distinguish articular from periarticular conditions (Table 3). After a general physical examination, the musculoskeletal examination can be performed through careful inspection, palpation, and a variety of physical maneuvers to elicit diagnostic findings.

In each patient, specific aspects of the musculoskeletal examination should be addressed (Table 6). Examination of involved and uninvolved joints should reveal

Table 6
Musculoskeletal Examination Checklist

The examiner should assess for
- Signs of inflammation
- Articular or periarticular structures involved
- Joint swelling
- Range of motion
- Crepitus
- Contracture or deformity
- Joint stability, subluxation, dislocation
- Muscle strength
- Extraarticular manifestations

the extent or presence of inflammation, indicated by *warmth, erythema,* or *swelling.* Joints should be examined from all sides and the range of motion passively assessed in all planes. The examination should discern whether the joint complaint involves articular or periarticular structures. *Joint swelling* may be caused by a synovial effusion, proliferation of the synovial membrane ("synovitis"), or bony hypertrophy and can be identified by palpation and specific maneuvers. Synovial fluid often produces fluctuant or ballottable soft tissue enlargement. In large joints such as the knee, a synovial effusion may be suggested by a "bulge sign" or ballottable patella (Table 7). Proliferation of synovial tissue can be felt as a supple, compressible, "squishy" soft tissue enlargement within the margins of the joint capsule. Bursitis (i.e., olecranon, prepatellar) may manifest as a localized, well-defined, fluctuant, subcutaneous effusion occurring over bony extensor surfaces and lying adjacent to the joint capsule. Swelling may also be caused by bony hypertrophy that may accompany OA, neuropathic arthritis, or trauma. Such hypertrophied joints often present as asymmetric, bony-hard enlargements of juxtaarticular bone that may or may not be painful.

Range of motion should be assessed with active (patient-initiated) and passive (examiner-assisted) movement in all planes and be quantified using "goniometer" or contralateral comparison. Range of motion may include flexion, extension, rotation, abduction, adduction, lateral bending, inversion, eversion, supination, pronation, and ulnar or radial deviation. The expected range of motion for individual joints is shown in Table 8. Findings may be recorded as either the arc of movement (in degrees) or that which is lacking (e.g., the shoulder lacked 30° of full abduction).

Joint *crepitus* may be felt during these maneuvers. Whereas "fine" crepitus is common and insignificant in most large joints, "coarse" crepitus indicates advanced cartilaginous and degenerative changes. Joint motion may be limited by effusion, pain, deformity, or contracture.

Contractures often indicate antecedent synovial inflammation or trauma. Joint *deformity* suggests chronic joint pathology that may result from ligamentous

Table 7
Physical Examination: Specific Signs and Maneuvers

Sign/Maneuver	Joint	Use and Description
Bulge sign	Knee	Identifies a small-to-moderate synovial effusion; the examiner should manually push or "milk" joint fluid downward and laterally from the suprapatellar pouch; a visible "bulge" (or shift in fluid) may be seen medially after applying pressure lateral to the patella
Drawer sign (Lachman's test)	Knee	Identifies joint instability and possible anterior cruciate tear; with the patient supine, leg extended, and knee at 90° angle, the examiner pulls the proximal tibia forward; excessive laxity or forward excursion may indicate an anterior cruciate tear
McMurray test	Knee	Identifies meniscal cartilage tear; with the patient supine, hip and knee flexed and internally rotated, the limb is extended while maintaining internal torque to detect a palpable or audible snap or "pop" or intraarticular pain; the procedure should be repeated in external rotation and torque
Patrick's test (Fabere test)	Hip/sacroiliac	Identifies hip and sacroiliac abnormalities (Fabere stands for *f*lexion, *ab*duction, *e*xternal *r*otation, and *e*xtension); with the patient lying supine, place the foot on the contralateral knee and externally rotate at the hip by moving the knee down and out; pain in the inguinal region may indicate hip disease; the sacroiliac (SI) joint may be compressed by simultaneously pushing the flexed ipsilateral knee and contralateral superior iliac crest downward
Straight leg raising test	Lumbar/ sciatic nerve	Identifies abnormalities of the lumbar nerve roots and/or sciatic nerve; with the patient lying supine and leg straight, elevate (flex) the limb upward by grabbing the heel; normally, the leg can be raised to an angle >80° before discomfort is noted; if pain is noted before this point, lower slightly and dorsiflex the foot to put stretch on the sciatic nerve; dorsiflexion-induced pain suggests sciatic nerve or lumbar nerve root abnormalities; if dorsiflexion of the foot does not cause pain, then limitation of motion may be from tight hamstring muscles

continued

Table 7 (continued)
Physical Examination: Specific Signs and Maneuvers

Sign/Maneuver	Joint	Use and Description
Schober test	SI/lumbar	Identifies limited motion in the SI or lumbar spine; with the patient standing upright, place pen marks at L5 and 10 cm above; ask the patient to bend as far forward as possible (without flexing the knees) and measure the distance between marks; normally the distance between marks will increase by more than 5 cm; changes less than 5 cm may indicate limited sacroiliac and lumbar mobility
Drop arm test	Rotator cuff	Identifies complete tear of the rotator cuff; with the patient standing or sitting upright, abduct the arm fully (90°); ask the patient to slowly lower the arm to his or her side; those with a complete tear of the rotator cuff will suddenly "drop" the arm down in pain or will be unable to lower the arm smoothly
Finkelstein's sign	Wrist	Identifies De Quervain's tenosynovitis (involving the abductor pollicis longus and extensor pollicis brevis); place the flexed thumb inside a clenched fist; ulnar deviation of the wrist will produce pain over involved tendons on the radial aspect of the joint (positive test)
Tinel's sign	Wrist, ankle	Identifies carpal tunnel syndrome (median nerve entrapment) by repetitively tapping (thumping) the volar aspect of the wrist to produce "electric-like" sensation or numbness in the first 3½ digits; tarsal tunnel syndrome may be diagnosed if symptoms are elicited by thumping over the flexor retinaculum (posterior to the medial malleolus) of the ankle

destruction, soft tissue contracture, bony enlargement, ankylosis, erosive disease, or subluxation.

Joint stability can be assessed by palpation and by application of manual stress, and maneuvers such as the "drawer sign" may be used to diagnose cruciate ligament damage (Table 7). *Subluxation or dislocation* can be assessed by inspection and palpation.

The *muscle examination* will document strength and the presence of atrophy and also will elicit pain or spasm. Muscle strength testing should assess the

Table 8
Joint Range of Motion

Joint	Flexion	Extension	Other
Neck	45°	>50°	Lateral bend 45°, rotation > 60°
Shoulder	180°	>40°	Abduction 90°, rotation 90°
Elbow	>150°	0–5°	Pronation 80°, supination 90°
Wrist	>80°	>60°	Ulnar[a] 60°, radial[a] 25°
MCP	>80°	>25°	
PIP	>110°	0°	
DIP	>75°	0°	
Lumbosacral	90°	30°	Lateral bend 40°, rotation 45°
Hip	120°	>15°	Abduction > 45°, IR/ER[b] > 45°
Knee	>135°	0–15°	
Ankle	Plantar > 45°	Dorsiflexion > 20°	Inversion 30°, eversion 20°
MTP	30°	80°	

[a]Refers to radial or ulnar deviation.
[b]IR/ER, inversion and eversion.

Table 9
Grading Muscle Strength

0 = No movement
1 = Trace (flicker) movement
2 = Able to move with gravity eliminated
3 = Able to move against gravity, but not resistance
4 = Able to oppose gravity and resistance
5 = Normal strength

musculature of the neck, trunk, and distal and proximal extremities and be quantified using the Medical Council of Great Britain scale (Table 9).

The examiner should carefully seek periarticular involvement, especially when articular complaints are not supported by objective findings referable to the joint capsule. Identification of periarticular pain helps prevent unwarranted and often expensive additional evaluations. Examples of periarticular abnormalities include olecranon bursitis, epicondylitis (i.e., tennis elbow), enthesitis (i.e., Achilles tendinitis), and trigger points associated with fibromyalgia. In selected instances, specific maneuvers may be used (Table 7) to identify extraarticular abnormalities, such as a carpal tunnel syndrome (identified by Tinel's sign).

Further Investigations

The vast majority of rheumatic conditions can be easily diagnosed by a complete history and physical examination. Further investigations are infrequently required to establish the correct diagnosis. The clinician should avoid the temptation to use screening tests or broad batteries ("rheumatic panels") of tests as an aid to diagnosis. Indiscriminate testing is expensive and often yields results with low predictive value. The utility and predictive value of "rheumatic tests" are disappointingly low when the pretest probability of a specific diagnosis is low. Primary indications for further testing include any monarticular presentation (consider arthrocentesis), systemic features (e.g., fever, rash), neurologic manifestations, antecedent trauma (consider radiographs, imaging), or chronic symptoms that are undiagnosed after an appropriate evaluation, symptomatic therapy, and observation over time (>6 weeks).

Any history of recent trauma should prompt a careful examination and consideration of an appropriate imaging procedure. If necessary, laboratory investigations may include a complete blood count, selected chemistries, an acute-phase reactant (e.g., ESR or CRP), and possibly a serum uric acid level if gout is clinically suspected. Routine serologic testing for antinuclear antibodies (ANAs) or rheumatoid factor (RF) should be discouraged unless warranted by the clinical picture. Advanced serologic testing (e.g., ANCA, HLA-B27, ASO) is only indicated in selected clinical situations. Finally, arthrocentesis and synovial fluid analysis should be considered for patients with monarthritis, suspected infection, or crystal-induced arthritis or when the diagnosis is uncertain. Chapter 1.4 (p. 75) reviews the use, indications, and interpretation of commonly used diagnostic tests and imaging modalities.

REFERENCES

Cush JJ, Lipsky PE. Approach to articular and musculoskeletal disorders. In: Fauci AS, Braunwald E, Isselbacher KJ, et al., eds. Harrison's principles of internal medicine. 14th ed. New York: McGraw-Hill, 1998:1928–1935.

Fries JF, Mitchell DM. Joint pain or arthritis. JAMA 1976;253:199–204.

Lipsky PE, Alarcon GS, Bombardier C, et al. Algorithms for the diagnosis and management of musculoskeletal complaints. Am J Med 1997;103:49S–85S.

Pincus T. A pragmatic approach to cost-effective use of laboratory tests and imaging procedures in patients with musculoskeletal symptoms. Prim Care 1993;20:795–814.

Wernick R. Avoiding laboratory test misinterpretation. Geriatrics 1989;44:61.

COMMON REGIONAL AND SYSTEMIC RHEUMATIC PRESENTATIONS

NECK PAIN

Overview

Neck pain is a relatively common complaint, affecting approximately 1/3 of the population at some time in their lives.

Anatomic Considerations

Neck pain can derive from several structures within the neck, including bone, joints, ligaments, nerves, tendons, and muscles. Pain originating in the neck may be referred to other locations, including the suboccipital and interscapular regions or shoulder and arm. Whereas cervical rotation is primarily due to craniocervical and C1–C2 articulations, flexion and extension are largely accomplished at the C5–C6 and C6–C7 articulations.

Etiology

Inciting stimuli for pain in these structures include degenerative arthritis, inflammatory arthritis, bony hypertrophy, trauma, muscle spasm, and other causes, such as infection and tumor.

History

Acute onset of neck pain is often related to injury to muscle or other soft tissues. Such pain may be caused by direct trauma, indirect trauma (e.g., rapid deceleration or "whiplash"), or overuse (e.g., keeping the head in an unusual position for a period of time). It is sometimes referred to as a "sprain," and patients may refer to having a "crick" in the neck. In this condition, neurologic examination should be normal. Patients often try to resist motion and will keep their head/neck in a single position. They may report tenderness on palpation of the paraspinous muscles, and these muscles may feel "tight" on examination. As is true for other painful spinal conditions, most pain probably derives from continuous contraction ("spasm") of the paraspinous musculature. Acute neck pain may also result from infection, fracture, vertebral collapse, or meningitis.

Chronic conditions (e.g., cervical osteoarthritis) may also be associated with acute soft tissue strain or spasm, thereby contributing to the patient's overall perception of pain.

Chronic neck pain may result from fibromyalgia, osteoarthritis (OA), inflammatory arthritis (e.g., rheumatoid), or bony metastases.

Examination

A number of joints in the neck (e.g., uncovertebral, facet, or disc joints) may be a source of pain. These joints can be affected by inflammatory arthritis (e.g., juvenile arthritis) or OA. The exact diagnosis may be inferred from clinical findings elsewhere or review of radiographs. However, radiographic changes consistent with cervical OA are quite common, particularly among the elderly. Many patients with radiographic evidence of OA are asymptomatic, and even in patients with neck pain, finding bony spurs or sclerosis on x-ray does not establish OA as the source of pain.

Patients with neck pain should be evaluated by assessing for range of motion (flexion, extension, lateral bending, lateral rotation), muscle spasm, tender trigger points (indicating myofascial pain syndrome or fibromyalgia), focal vertebral tenderness, and neurologic deficit. A detailed neurologic examination is indicated for all patients with neck pain.

Most neck pain is benign. However, patients with neurologic deficits tend to have greater morbidity. Neurologic findings may result from cervical myelopathy, radiculopathy, or spinal cord trauma or transection following trauma (e.g., in ankylosing spondylitis patients). Cervical myelopathy may be seen in RA patients with C1–C2 subluxation due to destruction of the transverse ligament or erosion of the odontoid. Subaxial subluxation (usually at C4–5, C5–6) may result from apophyseal joint damage at these levels. Myelopathy should be suggested by either upper extremity weakness, paresthesias, hyperactive reflexes or *Lhermitte's sign* (the induction of paresthesias or electric sensations down the thoracic spine upon cervical flexion). Patients with OA of the neck may form bony spurs or ligamentous hypertrophy that may cause impingement of the spinal cord or nerve root. If such lesions are central, they may result in spinal stenosis. More commonly, bony spurs near the neural foramina impinge on the exiting nerve root, resulting in radiculopathy. Depending upon the severity, there may be demonstrable impairment of neurologic function.

Diagnostic Testing

Because most neck pain is due to a benign process, workup need not be extensive. In general, a history eliciting trauma and symptoms associated with systemic diseases in conjunction with a physical examination that includes a thorough neurologic examination will suffice. If necessary, laboratory testing should be guided by the diagnostic considerations.

Imaging

Roentgenograms are not routinely recommended because of their low yield (i.e., most patients with neck pain do not have visible diagnostic radiographic findings) and low specificity (as stated above, many older patients have radiographic changes of OA that may be of no consequence). Radiographs should be obtained if there is history of trauma, suspicion of malignant disease, infection, or vertebral collapse or if a neurologic deficit is found. If abnormalities are seen on plain films, tomograms or CT scans may give further delineation. If neurologic impairments are suspected (e.g., cervical spinal stenosis), magnetic resonance imaging (MRI) may be the imaging procedure of choice, as it provides greater definition of bone, nerve, and soft tissue.

Differential Diagnosis

See Table 1.

Table 1
Differential Diagnosis of Neck Pain

Soft tissue injury ("sprain")
    Traumatic (e.g., "whiplash")
    Secondary to strain or overuse
    Associated with other diseases (e.g., OA)
Arthritis
    Osteoarthritis (with or without osteophyte formation)
    Inflammatory arthritides
Ankylosing spondylitis
Other spondyloarthropathies
    Juvenile arthritis (juvenile rheumatoid arthritis)
    Rheumatoid arthritis
Neurologic
    Radicular (nerve root) entrapment (i.e., radiculopathy)
    Spinal stenosis
    Syringomyelia
Bone disease
    Fracture/dislocation
    Diffuse idiopathic skeletal hyperostosis (DISH)
    Osteoporosis (with compression fracture)
    Metastatic cancer
    Infections of bone (osteomyelitis)
Other
    Discitis
    Meningitis
    Thyroiditis
    Fibromyalgia/myofascial pain syndrome

Treatment

Several modalities may be used. Many patients respond to nonsteroidal antiinflammatory drugs (NSAIDs) or simple analgesics. Because muscle spasm may be an important contributor to the pain, muscle relaxants are sometimes useful adjuncts. Some patients with cervical soft tissue injury report good pain relief with short-term use of a soft cervical collar. Patients with arthritis, either inflammatory or degenerative, are treated for cervical involvement as they would be for arthritis elsewhere in the body. Surgical interventions are seldom indicated and usually not effective. Surgical stabilization may be indicated for patients with severe C1–C2 subluxation or with marked cephalad migration of the odontoid and a neurologic deficit.

SHOULDER PAIN

Overview

Pain referred to the shoulder is very common in the general population, particularly among the elderly. After back pain, it is the second most common acute musculoskeletal complaint in general practice. The prevalence of shoulder complaints among normal older persons is approximately 20%. With some forms of arthritis, such as rheumatoid arthritis (RA), the prevalence of shoulder complaints exceeds 80%.

Anatomic Considerations

Pain may originate from the shoulder joint or overlying structures or be referred from the neck, chest (e.g., Pancoast tumor), or even abdomen (e.g., gall bladder, hepatic, or diaphragmatic lesions). Understanding the anatomy of the shoulder joint is relevant to the evaluation of shoulder pain. The shoulder is an incomplete ball-and-socket type of joint, with the head of the humerus held against the glenoid labrum of the acromion by the surrounding muscles. This can be compared with the more completely formed and thus more stable ball and socket of the hip joint. In primates, this design allows abduction of the humerus, which in turn allows free movement of the hands in many planes. The downside to this design is that the shoulder is less stable than the hip. In addition, the complex range of arm movements is offset by the multiple surrounding structures that may be potential sources of shoulder pain. Finally, the shoulder area defines a relatively narrow space through which many muscular, neurologic, and vascular structures must pass. Impingement of the rotator cuff, between the humeral head and the acromioclavicular arch, may occur with modest pathologic changes.

Etiology

Shoulder pain can derive from numerous structures in the area of the shoulder, including tendons, bursae, joints, nerves, ligaments, and muscles (Table 1). In-

Table 1
Differential Diagnosis of Shoulder Pain

Bursitis/tendinitis
    Rotator cuff dysfunction (including tendinitis, tendon tears, impingement syndrome,
       frozen shoulder)
    Subacromial bursitis
    Bicipital tendinitis
Arthritis (degenerative or inflammatory; e.g., RA, gout, spondyloarthropathy)
    Glenohumeral arthritis
    Acromioclavicular (AC) joint arthritis
    Sternoclavicular (SC) joint arthritis
Bone disease
    Fracture
    Dislocation/separation
    Metastatic cancer
    Osteonecrosis (e.g., humeral head)
Neurologic/vascular
    Suprascapular nerve entrapment
    Thoracic outlet syndrome
    Brachial plexus injury (brachial plexopathy)
Other (including referred pain)
    Cervical spine disease
    Polymyalgia rheumatica
    Fibromyalgia
    Reflex sympathetic dystrophy (also known as shoulder-hand syndrome)
    Intrathoracic etiology (e.g., Pancoast tumor, myocardial infarction)
    Intraabdominal etiology (e.g., perihepatitis, cholecystitis)

citing stimuli for pain in these structures include inflammation, degeneration, trauma, and overuse.

The most common source of shoulder pain is the rotator cuff apparatus (see p. 334), which may be affected in up to 75% of patients with shoulder pain. Rotator cuff dysfunction represents a spectrum of conditions, from rotator cuff tendinitis, rotator cuff tear, to frozen shoulder. Many patients have an associated subacromial bursitis.

History

A focused history and physical examination often succeed in defining the cause of shoulder pain. Shoulder pain is often exacerbated by activity and is most prominent late in the day or at night. Many patients report an inability to sleep in a recumbent position, and many sleep upright or in a reclining chair. Any history of trauma should raise suspicion of fracture or rotator cuff damage. Acute shoulder pain may result from acute bursitis or tendinitis from overuse or rotator cuff damage. Less commonly, septic, inflammatory, or crystal-induced arthritis may cause acute shoulder pain. Causes of chronic shoulder pain include rotator cuff dysfunction, adhesive capsulitis, fibromyalgia, RA, and OA.

Examination

The cause of shoulder pain can often be determined from physical examination. Testing for pain and range of motion on abduction, internal rotation, and external rotation of the humerus may establish rotator cuff dysfunction as the cause of the pain. Tenderness of the subacromial bursa will be apparent on direct palpation laterally below the acromion. Patients with glenohumeral arthritis often have substantial pain and resist any movement of the shoulder joint. Arthritis of other joints about the shoulder (acromioclavicular (AC), sternoclavicular (SC)) can be elicited on palpation. In severe cases of inflammatory arthritis, other signs of inflammation (e.g., swelling) may be present. Neurovascular function should be tested to rule out those structures as the cause of shoulder pain. If no cause is found by these examinations, a more thorough evaluation for other causes should be undertaken.

Diagnostic Tests

Laboratory testing is seldom useful in the diagnosis of shoulder pain. If referred pain from a radiculopathy is being considered, then nerve conduction studies may be indicated.

Imaging

Plain radiography can be used to detect fracture or arthritis (degenerative or inflammatory). Standard views include an anteroposterior (AP) view and an AP view with external rotation. The glenohumeral joint may also be viewed in an axillary view. MRI has largely replaced other imaging procedures for evaluation of persistent rotator cuff dysfunction.

Differential Diagnosis

See Table 1.

Treatment

Treatment of shoulder pain depends on the cause and often involves several modalities. In many cases, temporary rest followed by physiotherapy to achieve optimal range of motion is indicated. For treatment of pain, many patients respond to NSAIDs or simple analgesics. Local injection with corticosteroids may be of value in bursitis or monarticular arthritis of the shoulder. Surgery is most often considered with severe rotator cuff dysfunction or impingement syndrome. Common procedures include excision of the distal clavicle, acromioplasty (e.g., impingement), glenohumeral synovectomy (e.g., RA), or total shoulder arthroplasty (replacement).

WRIST AND HAND PAIN

Overview

Disorders of the wrist and hand are a common cause of medical consultation. Pain, swelling, dysfunction, or structural abnormalities may incite such an evaluation.

Anatomic Considerations

Sources of pain and swelling may include diarthrodial joints, tendons, tenosynovium, bone, nerve, skin, or other soft tissue structures. A detailed physical examination is required to determine whether there is articular or nonarticular (periarticular) involvement.

History

It is important to note the chronology of involvement, so that acute, chronic, intermittent, additive, or migratory joint involvement may identified. Musculoskeletal disorders often manifest a distinctive pattern of joint involvement (Fig. 1). For example, RA commonly involves the PIP, MCP, and wrist joints, whereas OA tends to involve the DIP, PIP, or first CMC (base of the thumb) joints. A history of trauma should suggest the possibility of a fracture or a degenerative (OA) or overuse (carpal tunnel) condition. Patients should describe the functional limitations associated with their complaint. The past medical history may disclose disorders with prominent musculoskeletal manifestations. For example, diabetics may develop flexion contractures of the fingers—the so-called syndrome of limited joint mobility.

Examination

Articular abnormalities often demonstrate obvious clinical findings. Bony, nodular enlargement of the DIP (Heberden's nodes) or PIP (Bouchard nodes) joints may suggest OA. By contrast, soft tissue swelling and effusion of the MCP or PIP joints, with or without swan-neck or boutonnière deformities, should suggest RA. Degenerative changes at the MCP joint may be related to OA (a rare manifestation of a common disease) or hemochromatosis (a common manifestation of a rare disease). Soft tissue abnormalities may include nodular swellings due to ganglion cysts (see p. 215), rheumatoid nodules (see p. 331), nodules associated with methotrexate use, or gouty tophi. Nodular or fibrotic changes involving the flexor tendons may result in episodic "catch" or "trigger finger" when the finger is flexed and extended. Trigger fingers may be seen in both RA and OA. Thickening of the palmar fascia may result in a Dupuytren's contracture of the fourth or fifth flexor tendons with a fixed flexion deformity of the involved digits. Tendon rupture of the fingers results in an unopposed reducible malposition or deformity away from the involved side. Thus, rupture of the ex-

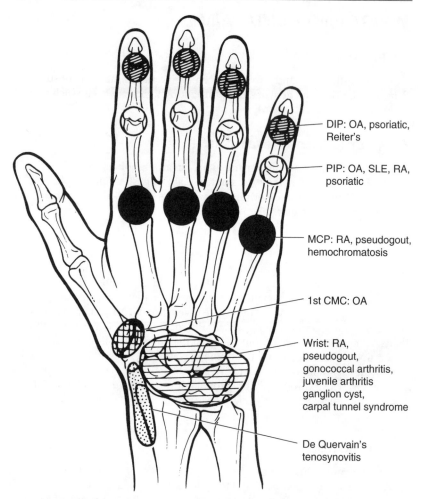

DIP: OA, psoriatic, Reiter's

PIP: OA, SLE, RA, psoriatic

MCP: RA, pseudogout, hemochromatosis

1st CMC: OA

Wrist: RA, pseudogout, gonococcal arthritis, juvenile arthritis ganglion cyst, carpal tunnel syndrome

De Quervain's tenosynovitis

Figure 1. Sites of hand/wrist involvement and their disease associations.

tensor tendons over the dorsum of the hand (as in RA) results in the fingers being held in a position of unopposed flexion. A common cause of periarticular wrist pain is De Quervain's tenosynovitis (Fig. 1) manifest as distal radial pain, with or without swelling, and a positive "Finkelstein's test" (Table 7, p. 13). Examination of the hand and wrist should also reveal the presence of cutaneous abnormalities. Common skin lesions indicating a systemic disorder may include Gottron's papules over the MCP joints (dermatomyositis), erythema or hyperpigmentation over inflamed joints (RA), periungual erythema (systemic lupus erythematosus (SLE), myositis, scleroderma, Reiter's syndrome, psoriatic arthritis), vasculitic lesions (digital infarcts, painful Osler's nodes, Janeway lesions), psoriatic lesions (scaly plaques, nail pitting, onycholysis), nail abnormalities (psoriasis, Reiter's syndrome), sclerodactyly and distal digital pulp scars (scleroderma), and Raynaud's phenomenon. Neurologic examination should seek muscle atrophy (from disuse or neuromuscular disease), signs of carpal tunnel syndrome (Tinel's sign, thenar muscle wasting), and brachioradialis reflex (C5–C6 innervation) and include careful sensory and motor examination of the hand and digits.

Diagnostic Testing

Testing should be guided by the results of the history and physical examination. Routine serologic testing and rheumatic "screens" or "panels" should be avoided. Nailfold capillaroscopy (see p. 129) should be done in all patients suspected of having Raynaud's phenomenon or scleroderma. Nerve conduction velocity testing may be useful in evaluating a potential neuropathy. Patients with acute or chronic monarthritis may benefit from synovial fluid aspiration

Table 1
Differential Diagnosis of Wrist/Hand Pain

Periarticular
   De Quervain's tenosynovitis
   Tenosynovitis (RA, gonococcal, gout)
   Trigger finger
   Dupuytren's contracture
   Syndrome of limited joint mobility (diabetes)
Articular
   Rheumatoid arthritis (PIP, MCP, wrist)
   Osteoarthritis (DIP, PIP, 1st CMC)
   Psoriatic arthritis (DIP, PIP, MCP)
   Hemochromatosis (2nd and 3rd MCP)
Bone
   Avascular necrosis (i.e., Kiembock's necrosis of the lunate)
   Fracture (e.g., Colles)
   Sarcoid (cystic lytic lesions)
   Periostitis (osteomyelitis, hypertrophic osteoarthropathy)
Neurologic/vascular
   Carpal tunnel syndrome
   Raynaud's phenomenon
   Subacute bacterial endocarditis with emboli
   Digital vasculitis (RA, SLE, cholesterol emboli)
   Reflex sympathetic dystrophy
Soft tissue
   Ganglion cysts
   Rheumatoid nodules
   Gouty tophi
   Clubbing (hypertrophic osteoarthropathy)

and analysis, and those with undiagnosed chronic monarthritis may benefit from arthrocentesis or synovial biopsy to exclude indolent infection.

Imaging

Radiographs of the hands are seldom revealing with acute presentations and may only show soft tissue swelling. Nonetheless, they should be considered if there is a history of trauma, if the condition is chronic, if there are vasomotor changes suggesting reflex sympathetic dystrophy, or if a baseline assessment is needed for a chronic osseous/articular disorder. MRI is largely an investigative tool and should be reserved for situations in which osteonecrosis or osteomyelitis is being considered.

Differential Diagnosis

See Table 1.

LOW BACK PAIN

Overview

Low back pain (LBP) is the most common acute musculoskeletal complaint in general practice. Overall, it is second only to upper respiratory ailments as the most common reason why patients seek medical attention. LBP is most prevalent in persons between 45 and 64 years of age. The annual incidence of LBP is approximately 5%. Moreover, between 60 and 85% of the population experience this symptom at some time in their lives. While symptoms resolve acutely in most, approximately 10% of patients may develop chronic pain. The societal ramifications of LBP in disability, psychosocial impact, and legal implications are enormous. It has been estimated that the total annual costs related to patients with LBP exceed $24 billion.

The primary objective in the assessment of a patient with LBP is to make a timely diagnosis, relieve pain, and return the patient to regular activity as soon as possible. Secondarily, it is important to identify the uncommon, but serious, causes of LBP, including the cauda equina syndrome, abdominal aortic aneurysm, fracture, infection, or tumor.

Anatomic Considerations

Back pain can derive from many structures in the area of the lower back, including joints, bursae, ligaments, nerves, tendons, and muscles (Table 1).

Etiology

Inciting stimuli for pain in these structures can include acute trauma, repetitive trauma, degeneration, inflammation, bony hypertrophy, infection, and tumor. In about 90% of patients with LBP, the etiology relates to a mechanical or degenerative cause; 10% have pain associated with a systemic illness.

Table 1
Differential Diagnosis of Back Pain

Soft tissue injury (affecting ligaments, muscles, and other nonosseous structures)
    Also known as myofascial pain (injury sometimes referred to as "sprain")
    Fibromyalgia
    Often secondary to trauma or overuse (mechanical pain)
Arthritis (e.g., affecting facet, uncovertebral, sacroiliac joints)
    Osteoarthritis (with or without osteophyte formation)
    Inflammatory arthritis
      Ankylosing spondylitis
      Other spondyloarthropathies
      Rheumatoid arthritis
      Infectious
Intervertebral disc disease
    Herniation (of the nucleus pulposus)
    Infection (discitis)
Neurologic/spinal cord injury
    Cauda equina compression syndrome
    Radicular (nerve root) entrapment ("sciatica")
    Spinal stenosis
    Tumors (intramedullary/extramedullary)
    Infection (meninges, epidural space)
    Syringomyelia
Bursitis
    Trochanteric
    Ischial
    Iliopsoas
Lumbosacral bone disease
    Spondylosis, spondylolysis, spondylolisthesis
    Fracture
    Diffuse idiopathic skeletal hyperostosis (DISH)
    Osteoporosis (with compression fracture)
    Metastatic cancer
    Infections (vertebral body)
Pelvic bone disease
    Insufficiency fractures (e.g., sacral) due to trauma or osteoporosis
    Metastatic cancer
    Infections (sacroiliac)
Other
    Abdominal/pelvic sources of pain
      Uterus
      Prostate
      Aorta
      Kidney
    Piriformis syndrome (pain from the piriformis muscle)

Evaluation

Because most patients with LBP have a benign process as the cause, workup need not be extensive. Generally, a history focusing on recent overuse, strain, or trauma will identify the inciting cause. In concert with a focused physical examination, this will also frequently identify the involved pathology. A thorough neurologic examination is indicated, as it will not only define the severity of the problem, but also provide some guidance for optimal therapy. In unusual cases or in patients without a clear inciting cause, a history and physical examination looking for systemic conditions associated with back pain (e.g., infection, tumor, autoimmune disease) are indicated.

History

The vast majority of patients with LBP have "myofascial pain"; that is, pain originating in muscles, ligaments, or other soft tissues as opposed to bones or joints. The pain may occur acutely, with stress or related to excess lifting or turning. In addition, many patients experience similar symptoms recurrently or chronically, sometimes with minimal exertion. Patients with myofascial pain uncomplicated by spine or nerve involvement should have a normal neurologic examination. They may report tenderness on palpation of the paraspinous muscles, and a good deal of the pain probably derives from continuous contraction ("spasm") of the paraspinous musculature. Several factors may predispose patients to development of myofascial injury, including occupational factors (work that requires repetitive lifting in the forward bent and twisted position), exposure to vibrations, deconditioning, obesity, and poor posture. Psychologic factors such as job dissatisfaction and depression are often associated with chronic LBP. Variations in spinal posture such as scoliosis do not appear to increase the risk of LBP.

Several joints in the lumbosacral spine and pelvis may be involved in LBP. These joints can be affected by inflammatory (e.g., rheumatoid arthritis or ankylosing spondylitis) or, more commonly, by degenerative arthritis (DJD) of the spine. However, radiographic changes consistent with OA are quite common, particularly among the elderly. Many patients with radiographic evidence of OA are asymptomatic, and even in patients with LBP, finding "DJD" on x-ray does not establish it as the source of pain in a given patient.

The intervertebral disc may be a source of LBP. Classically, patients with discogenic pain have increased pain with maneuvers that increase intraabdominal pressure (e.g., Valsalva, coughing, laughing). Also, in contrast to some other causes of back pain such as spinal stenosis, patients may find relief by walking around. Degeneration of the intervertebral disc is common with ageing. Tears of the circumferential annulus fibrosus may allow herniation of the central nucleus pulposus. Mild bulging or protrusion of the disc into the spinal canal is common and can be demonstrated in about half of asymptomatic normal persons by sensitive techniques such as MRI. Therefore, demonstration of such findings does not prove that the disc is the source of the pain.

Patients with arthritis (particularly with bony spur formation), disc disease, and other pathophysiologic changes may have impingement on the spinal cord or nerve roots and consequent neurologic symptoms. If such lesions are central, they may cause spinal stenosis. More commonly, bony spurs near the neural foramina impinge on the exiting nerve root, resulting in radiculopathy. Depending upon the severity, impairment of neurologic function may be demonstrable. Radicular pain originating in the lower lumbar nerve roots is commonly known as sciatica.

Sciatica, defined as pain that radiates from the gluteal region, down the posterolateral leg below the knee, is often associated with mechanical impingment of nerve. Sciatica may exacerbated by flexion or extension. Lumbar flexion- or sitting-induced pain may be caused by a herniated intervertebral disc (often involving L5 or S1 nerve roots). Extension- or standing-induced pain may be related to spinal stenosis. Both forms of sciatica should be treated with conservative measures, NSAIDs, and muscle relaxants. If these are ineffective, epidural injection with corticosteroids may be helpful.

LBP associated with anterior thigh (with or without groin) pain may be caused by hip disease, inguinal hernia, femoral neuropathy, tumor, aortic aneurysm, kidney disease, or retroperitoneal fibrosis. Anterior thigh pain may imply involvement of nerve roots L1–L3.

LBP associated with posterior thigh pain (above the knee) may be due to lumbosacral strain or a herniated lumbar disc (usually L3–L4).

The uncommon and serious causes of LBP may be suggested by findings of incontinence and saddle anesthesia (e.g., cauda equina syndrome), fever, weight loss (e.g., tumor), pain exacerbated by sleep or recumbency (e.g., tumor), prolonged morning stiffness (e.g., ankylosing spondylitis), focal bone pain worsened by manual pressure (i.e., fracture), or periodic pain related to menses or eating (e.g., gastrointestinal or genitourinary causes).

Diagnostic Testing

Laboratory testing seldom helps to determine the cause of LBP unless clinical evidence suggests a systemic disorder (i.e., infection, neoplasm, inflammatory arthritis). In such cases, the ESR or C-reactive protein (CRP) may provide nonspecific evidence of a systemic process. HLA-B27 should not be routinely obtained (see p. 118), as it is found in 8% of normal individuals and is poorly predictive of spondyloarthropathy. In those suspected of having a neurologic deficit (e.g., radiculopathy), nerve conduction velocity testing may provide supportive data.

Imaging

Roentgenograms are not routinely recommended because of their low yield (i.e., most patients with LBP do not have conditions visible on radiographs as the cause) and low specificity (as above, many older patients have findings of OA that may be of no consequence). Radiographs should be obtained if there is history of serious trauma, suspicion of malignant disease, suspicion of infection or fracture, or neurologic deficit. If abnormalities are seen on plain films, tomograms or CT scans may give further delineation. If neurologic impairments are suspected (e.g., spinal stenosis), MRI may be the imaging procedure of choice, as it allows definition of bone, nerve, and soft tissue.

Treatment

Historically, patients with LBP were put at strict bed rest for several weeks to "rest" the affected structures. However, more-recent studies have shown that most patients with acute back pain do as well with continuing ordinary activities, as well as bed rest or back-mobilizing exercises. No more than 2 days of bed rest is advised and should be followed by progressive mobilization and exercise. Treatment of back pain often involves several modalities. Local pain may respond well to cold or warm compresses and should be determined by patient preference. Many patients respond to NSAIDs or simple analgesics, such as acetaminophen. More-potent analgesics such as narcotics may be necessary in the acute setting. However, many patients have chronic symptoms, and such agents must be used with caution. Because muscle spasm may be an important contributor to the pain, muscle relaxants are sometimes useful adjuncts. Spinal manipulation is effective for some patients. Although there has been anecdotal support for the analgesic efficacy of electrical stimulation (TENS units), controlled trials have not shown it to be beneficial. Chronically, back-strengthening exercises may be of some value. Although they are widely used, lumbar belts have not been shown to be of proven benefit.

Surgery is rarely indicated and should be reserved for those proven to have tumor, infections, fractures, or dislocations.

REFERENCES

Borenstein DG. A clinician's approach to acute low back pain. Am J Med 1997;102(Suppl 1A):16S–22S.

HIP PAIN

Overview

Hip pain is one of the most often misdiagnosed joint complaints, primarily because of the public misconception that the "hip" is located in either the gluteal or trochanteric region. True hip pain is sensed anteriorly and may radiate medially into the groin or to the anteromedial thigh. This is to be distinguished from the more common complaint of "buttock pain" that is often referred from the lumbosacral impingement of nerve roots. Trochanteric pain is sensed over the upper lateral thigh with point tenderness and usually indicates trochanteric bursitis (Fig. 1).

Anatomic Considerations

Hip pain may originate in the femoral-acetabular joint or joint capsule, proximal femur or acetabulum, pelvic rami, surrounding bursae (e.g., trochanteric, ischiogluteal, iliopsoas), ligaments (e.g., inguinal, iliofemoral), and intraabdominal or vascular structures.

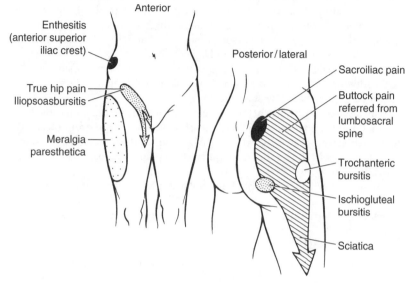

Figure 1. Origins of hip pain.

Etiology

Pain in the hip may result from traumatic, mechanical/degenerative, inflammatory, reactive, infectious, or neoplastic disorders affecting the joint or juxtaarticular structures.

History

In elderly individuals, hip pain is commonly due to OA of the hip, referred lumbosacral pain, trochanteric bursitis, or osteoporotic fractures. Young and middle-aged adults are often affected by trochanteric bursitis, adductor tendinitis, or inflammatory arthritis (e.g., RA, Reiter's). Hip pain in children is commonly caused by toxic synovitis of the hip, juvenile arthritis, or congenital anomalies of the joint. Toxic synovitis of the hip is common in children 1 to 13 years of age and typically follows an upper respiratory infection. It manifests as an acute inflammatory arthropathy that is self-limiting and lasts between 2 and 4 weeks. This condition responds well to rest and aspirin or NSAID therapy.

Referred pain accounts for many cases of hip pain. Whereas involvement of the T12–L1 nerve roots may result in buttock/trochanteric pain, L2–L4 nerve roots may produce inguinal or anterior thigh pain. Thus, it is important to detect lumbosacral spine, vascular, or intraabdominal disorders that may masquerade as hip pain. Buttock pain may result from the lumbosacral spine, sacroiliac joint, ischiogluteal bursa, or vascular insufficiency. Groin pain may be due to true hip disease, iliopsoas bursitis, hernia, adductor tendinitis, pelvic fracture, osteitis pubis, ureteral stones, or pain referred from L2–L4 nerve roots.

Trochanteric bursitis manifests as lateral thigh pain, often with radiation downward to the knee. It is worsened by general activity, sleeping on the affected side, or sitting with the affected leg crossed.

Ischiogluteal bursitis will manifest as lower buttock pain, possibly with radiation down the leg. Pain is worsened by prolonged sitting with legs uncrossed and may be exacerbated by standing on tiptoes.

The iliopsoas bursa lies between the psoas muscle and hip joint capsule. Inflammation of the psoas bursa may manifest as pain in the groin or anterior thigh that is exacerbated by extension of the hip or flexion against resistance. Patients may hold the joint in flexion to reduce pain. Iliopsoas bursitis is unaffected by rotation.

Acute monarticular presentations should lead the examiner to consider urgent noninflammatory (e.g., fracture) or inflammatory (e.g., septic arthritis) causes. Severe hip pain associated with weight bearing should suggest a fracture.

Examination

By virtue of its deep location, inspection and palpation is unlikely to yield diagnostic findings. Examination of periarticular bursae may disclose point tenderness over the greater trochanter laterally or ischial tuberosity posteriorly. Palpation and auscultation should identify abnormal bruits or pulsatile masses involving the abdominal aorta or iliac arteries. Palpable masses over the anterior groin may suggest a hernia or iliopsoas bursitis. Adductor tendinitis is common in young individuals who assume a "straddling" position (e.g., gymnasts, horseback riders) and manifests as pain in the groin or anterior thigh. Pain is elicited over the insertion of adductor musculature and is exacerbated by passive abduction or active adduction.

Range-of-motion testing (flexion, internal and external rotation, abduction) may disclose true hip joint involvement, as bursitis seldom causes true limitation of motion. True hip (and sacroiliac) disorders and range of motion are best assessed using the Patrick (or Fabere) test (see Table 7, p. 12). Notably, nondisplaced fractures may demonstrate a normal range of motion, until extremes in rotation are achieved. A pelvic tilt may indicate true hip disease, scoliosis, or a leg length discrepancy. Leg length discrepancies may be ascertained by comparative measurements from the anterior superior iliac crest to the lateral malleolus. Normally there is less than 1 cm variation between limbs. A flexion contracture of the hip may indicate antecedent trauma or undiagnosed articular inflammation and is best diagnosed by the Thomas test (flexion of the contralateral hip results in involuntary flexion of the involved hip).

Diagnostic Testing

Laboratory testing should be guided by the clinical findings. The examiner should avoid using routine laboratory screening tests. Inflammatory or infectious conditions may be associated with nonspecific elevation of acute-phase reactants (e.g., ESR, CRP). If acute infectious arthritis is suspected, synovial fluid aspiration (under fluoroscopic guidance), culture, and analysis should be strongly considered (see p. 61).

Imaging

For nontraumatic acute presentations, radiographs are not indicated, as they are seldom revealing. Those suffering trauma or who have undiagnosed chronic hip pain should undergo radiography of the hip and pelvis. Lumbosacral spine films should be obtained if there is a history of low back pain, if hip and pelvic radiographs are unrevealing, and if referred lumbosacral pain is suspected. MRI has largely replaced the bone scan in evaluation of hip disorders and may be useful in the diagnosis of osteonecrosis, osteomyelitis, or early fractures not yet apparent by routine radiography.

Differential Diagnosis

See Table 1.

Treatment

Depending on the condition, nonpharmacologic modalities of cold or warm compresses, immobilization, ambulatory-assist devices, physical therapy, and range-of-motion exercises may be indicated. Symptomatic control of pain may be achieved with NSAIDs or simple analgesics (e.g., acetaminophen). In selected instances, judicious use of local corticosteroid injections may be helpful in treating trochanteric or ischiogluteal bursitis. Surgery may be indicated for some pelvic, acetabular, or femoral fractures. Total hip replacement may be indicated in those with advanced joint damage and pain.

Table 1
Common Causes of Hip Pain

Arthritis
    Inflammatory: RA, spondyloarthropathy, septic arthritis, juvenile arthritis, toxic synovitis of the hip, sarcoidosis
    Noninflammatory: OA, osteonecrosis, fracture (femur, acetabulum, pelvic rami), hemochromatosis, osteoid osteoma, hemarthrosis
Periarticular
    Inflammatory: Septic bursitis, enthesitis, polymyalgia rheumatica, osteomyelitis
    Noninflammatory: Trochanteric bursitis, iliopsoas bursitis, ischiogluteal bursitis, adductor tendinitis
Abdominal/genitourinary: Aortic aneurysm, hernia, pelvic inflammatory disease, ureteral nephrolithiasis, retroperitoneal disorders, lymphadenopathy (inguinal, paraaortic)
Bone: Fracture (osteoporotic), Paget's, osteitis pubis, osteomyelitis, osteoid osteoma
Referred pain: Sciatica, degenerative disc disease, lumbar facet OA, spinal stenosis, vascular insufficiency, meralgia paresthetica, sacroiliitis

REFERENCES

Schon L, Zuckerman JD. Hip pain in the elderly: evaluation and diagnosis. Geriatrics
    1988;43:48–62.

KNEE PAIN

Overview

The knee joint is the largest and most frequently affected peripheral joint. This
primarily relates to its importance in ambulation and weight bearing and its numerous supportive periarticular structures.

Anatomic Considerations

The knee is often divided into the medial compartment, lateral (femorotibial)
compartment, and patellofemoral compartment. Articular structures within
these compartments include synovium, synovial effusion, articular cartilage,
meniscal cartilage, cruciate ligaments, and the joint capsule. The term *internal
derangement of the knee* implies mechanical damage to one of these structures.
Outside the joint, periarticular structures that are common sources of pain may
include a variety of bursae (e.g., anserine, prepatellar, and the superficial and
deep infrapatellar), ligaments (e.g., collateral), tendons (e.g., semimembra-
nosus, semitendinosus), bones (e.g., patella, femur, tibia), muscles (e.g., quadriceps), vessels (e.g., popliteal artery), and other soft tissue structures (e.g.,
popliteal cysts) (see Fig. 1, p. 68).

Etiology

Pain in the knee may result from traumatic, mechanical/degenerative, inflammatory, reactive, infectious, or neoplastic disorders affecting the joint or juxtaarticular structures.

History

Knee pain in middle-aged and elderly individuals is likely to be caused by periarticular bursitis, traumatic or degenerative meniscal cartilage tears, or degenerative arthritis of the knee. In children, disorders commonly involving the
knee may include Osgood-Schlatter's disease (osteochondritis at the insertion
of the patellar tendon on the tibial tubercle), benign "growing pains," or juvenile arthritis. Young adults are most likely to complain of pain from chondromalacia patellae or trauma-induced internal derangement, with possible damage to menisci and cruciate or collateral ligaments.

It is important to ask about the presence of low back or hip pain with
"referred pain" to, or below, the knee. A history of recent trauma may suggest
fracture, internal derangement, bursitis, tendinitis, or even septic bursitis or
arthritis. A history of remote, repetitive trauma and occupational or athletic

contributions to knee pain should be sought. Although many individuals complain of fine or coarse joint crepitus, this is rarely associated with pain and thus has little diagnostic significance. However, pain associated with a sudden "pop" or "snap" may indicate severe ligamentous or tendinous injury or rupture. Most chronic articular disorders are accompanied by stiffness. However, prolonged morning stiffness (>1 h) may indicate an inflammatory process.

Often patients complain of "locking," "buckling," or "giving way". Such complaints should primarily suggest a meniscal tear but may also result from loose bodies, cruciate tear, severe quadriceps weakness, or patellar dislocation.

Acute monarticular presentations should lead the examiner to consider urgent noninflammatory (e.g., fracture) or inflammatory (e.g., crystal-induced or septic arthritis) causes.

Examination

Pain involving articular structures is likely to be diffuse and deep, while periarticular disorders may manifest focal or "point" tenderness. A careful search of periarticular bursae may disclose point tenderness, with or without local signs of inflammation, possibly indicating a bursal or tendinous condition. Palpation should also include examination of the popliteal fossa to detect any fluctuant mass indicating a Baker's cyst. The examination should identify limb alignment or the presence of contracture. A contracture may indicate antecedent trauma or undiagnosed articular inflammation. Range of motion is best assessed with the patient supine. Hypermobility of the patella and hyperextension at the knee may indicate a hypermobility syndrome. Ligamentous laxity may lead to excessive medial, lateral, forward, or posterior "play" at the knee. A series of specific maneuvers (i.e., Drawer sign or McMurray test) may be used to detect damage to the meniscal cartilages or cruciate ligaments (see Table 7, p. 12). Synovial effusion or proliferation is best palpated on either side of the patella and, if large enough, causes a "bulge sign," or distention of the suprapatellar pouch.

Diagnostic Testing

Laboratory testing should be guided by clinical findings. The examiner should avoid using routine laboratory screening tests. Inflammatory or infectious conditions may be associated with nonspecific elevation of acute-phase reactants (e.g., ESR, CRP). If an acute or chronic monarthritis exists, synovial fluid aspiration and analysis should be strongly considered (see p. 67).

Imaging

For nontraumatic acute presentations, radiographs are not indicated, as they seldom reveal more than soft tissue swelling or effusion. An AP and lateral view of the knees should be obtained in those suffering trauma or who have undiagnosed chronic knee pain. If tolerable, weight-bearing films are preferred, because they yield information on articular alignment and the degree of cartilage damage

Table 1
Common Causes of Knee Pain

Articular disorders
    Inflammatory: RA, gout, pseudogout, SLE, Reiter's, juvenile arthritis, sarcoidosis, and
        psoriatic, viral, or septic arthritis
    Noninflammatory: OA, osteonecrosis, internal derangement, fracture, genu valgum
Periarticular disorders
    Inflammatory: Septic bursitis, enthesitis, osteomyelitis
    Noninflammatory: Fracture, prepatellar bursitis, infrapatellar bursitis, anserine bursitis,
        patellar tendinitis, patellar tendon rupture, quadriceps tendinitis, chondromalacia
        patella, fibromyalgia, Osgood-Schlatter's disease, hypermobility syndrome, referred
        pain

(resulting in uni- or bicompartmental joint space narrowing). Arthroscopy and MRI are powerful imaging tools best reserved for those with severe internal derangement of the knee. MRI may be indicated to diagnose osteonecrosis, osteomyelitis, pigmented villonodular synovitis, or early fractures not yet apparent by routine radiography.

Differential Diagnosis

See Table 1.

Treatment

Depending on the condition, nonpharmacologic modalities of cold or warm compresses, immobilization, and quadriceps-strengthening exercises may be indicated. Symptomatic control of pain may be achieved with NSAIDs or simple analgesics (e.g., acetaminophen). In selected instances, infrequent use of local corticosteroid injections may enhance therapeutic results. Surgery (arthroscopic, etc.) may be indicated with acute internal derangement or fractures or chronically with advanced joint and cartilage damage.

REFERENCES

McCune WJ, Matteson EL, MacGuire A. Evaluation of knee pain. Prim Care 1988;15:795–808.

CENTRAL NERVOUS SYSTEM AND ARTHRITIS

Overview

The association of arthritis and central nervous system (CNS) abnormalities is seldom encountered. However, this association often heralds the presence of disorders with significant morbidity.

Evaluation

The most common neurologic findings in patients with rheumatic diseases include the neuropathies (entrapment, drug induced, or autoimmune). A careful history and physical examination should disclose the nature of the neurologic complaint and associated articular and extraarticular features that define the diagnostic possibilities. Neurologic complaints should be promptly evaluated to determine the anatomic site of involvement and degree of neurologic compromise, so early corrective measures can be taken.

Diagnostic Testing

Diagnostic testing may include assessment of acute-phase reactants (i.e., ESR), serologic tests (ANA, RF, antineutrophil cytoplasmic antibodies [ANCA], HIV, hepatitis, Lyme, etc.), nerve conduction velocities, electromyogram, lumbar puncture (with CSF studies, see p. 98), nerve biopsy, or angiogram. Many of these investigations are expensive, if not invasive, and thus should be used only to answer a specific diagnostic question.

Imaging

Radiographs and MRI may be useful in assessing vertebral and spinal disorders and CNS parenchymal or vascular conditions.

Differential Diagnosis

See Table 1.

Table 1
Differential Diagnosis of CNS Disorders and Arthritis

Peripheral neuropathies
    Entrapment neuropathy: Carpal tunnel syndrome, tarsal tunnel syndrome
    Sensory neuropathy: RA, SLE, amyloidosis, neuropathic arthritis
    Mononeuritis multiplex: RA, polyarteritis nodosa, cryoglobulinemia, Sjögren's
    Infection: Lyme disease, HIV, hepatitis B, leprosy, herpes zoster
Cranial neuropathies: Bell's palsy (Lyme disease), trigeminal neuralgia (scleroderma)
Myelopathy: C1–C2 subluxation (RA), spinal stenosis (OA), syringomyelia,
    transverse myelitis (SLE, vasculitis)
Vascular/vasculitis: Polyarteritis nodosa, Churg-Strauss vasculitis, giant cell (temporal)
    arteritis, Takayasu's arteritis, Wegener's granulomatosis, primary CNS angiitis, reflex
    sympathetic dystrophy, antiphospholipid syndrome, Behçet's syndrome
Autoimmune CNS disease: Multiple sclerosis; Guillain-Barré syndrome; chronic
    inflammatory polyneuropathy; neuropsychiatric lupus (lupus cerebritis); Behçet's
    syndrome (neuro-Behçet's); Sjögren's syndrome
Drugs[a]: Colchicine, penicillamine, gold salts, cyclosporine, corticosteroids, dapsone

[a] Antirheumatic drugs with neuromuscular side effects.

"HURTS ALL OVER"

Overview

One of the most challenging of presentations is the evaluation of patients with widespread arthralgias and/or myalgias. This challenge is compounded when such complaints are not supported by physical findings. The examiner should search for revealing historical features or evidence of articular or periarticular pathology (i.e., swelling, erythema, warmth) before considering the disorders mentioned herein.

Etiology

The most common cause of widespread arthralgias and myalgias is fibromyalgia (see p. 207). Other possibilities to be considered are drug-induced, infectious, endocrine/metabolic, autoimmune, neoplastic, psychiatric, and other miscellaneous disorders (Table 1).

Evaluation

Patients should be evaluated in a routine manner, and the source of articular and periarticular pain should be identified (see "Evaluation of Musculoskeletal Complaints," pp. 3–15). When faced with prominent joint complaints but few physical findings, the examiner should initially use conservative, symptomatic measures and serial observation. Serious medical conditions ultimately develop obvious clinical symptoms or signs to aid in diagnosis. The clinician should avoid the temptation to undertake expensive laboratory investigations or imaging procedures early in the evaluation of widespread pain.

History

Many patients manifest moderate-to-severe fatigue and morning stiffness (lasting minutes to hours); thus these features have little discriminant value. The patient should be questioned about fever (i.e., >100°F) or weight loss, as these may suggest conditions with significant morbidity. Symptoms suggesting endocrinopathies should be sought (i.e., heat or cold intolerance). Symptomatic rashes, muscle weakness, myalgias, muscle cramping, depression, or sleep disturbance may also provide important clues. It is equally important to review the patient's medication history, past medical and surgical history, health maintenance, and social history when evaluating diffuse musculoskeletal complaints.

Examination

Efforts should be directed toward identifying the source and extent of joint or muscle pain—many patients in this group will have periarticular rather than articular pain. The clinician should carefully examine for the trigger point tender areas of fibromyalgia. Signs of ligamentous laxity may indicate the hy-

Table 1
Differential Diagnosis of Arthralgias and Myalgias ("Hurts All Over")

Drug induced
    Antiinfectives: Quinolones, amphotericin, acyclovir
    Biologic agents: Interferon, interleukin (IL)-2, IL-6, immunotoxins
    Supplements: Excessive vitamin A, fluoride
    Lipid-lowering agents: Clofibrate, lovastatin
    Cardiac: Quinidine, propranolol, nicardipine
Infectious
    Viral syndromes
    Dengue fever
    Vaccines
Endocrine/metabolic
    Hypothyroidism/myxedema
    Hyperparathyroidism
    Hypercortisolism
    Corticosteroid withdrawal
    Adrenal insufficiency
    Hypophosphatemia
Autoimmune
    Systemic lupus erythematosus
    Polymyalgia rheumatica
    Inflammatory myositis
Neoplastic/hematologic
    Leukemia
    Lymphoma
    Multiple myeloma
    Metastases to bone
    Sickle cell crisis
Psychiatric
    Depression
    Psychogenic rheumatism
    Malingering
    Somatization disorder
Other
    Fibromyalgia
    Chronic fatigue syndrome
    Hypermobility syndrome
    Silicone implant syndrome (most have fibromyalgia)

permobility syndrome. Lymphadenopathy, masses, organomegaly, and stigmata of thyroid, adrenal, or muscle disease should be sought.

Diagnostic Testing

Routine laboratory testing should include a complete blood count, chemistries, and an ESR. Serologic testing for ANA or RF is unlikely to yield useful information. Similarly, thyroid function studies should only be done if symptoms and signs (beyond arthralgias) warrant.

Imaging

Imaging will seldom reveal diagnostic information not gleaned from the physical examination. Rarely, bony metastases are found by plain radiographs or scintigraphy.

Differential Diagnosis

See Table 1.

Treatment

Patients should be treated symptomatically, and narcotic analgesics should be avoided until a confident diagnosis is made. Thereafter, therapeutic choices are defined by the diagnostic entity rather than the general complaint. If the complaint is drug induced, then drug withdrawal usually results in rapid improvement. Treatment of the underlying condition may also improve the musculoskeletal complaint.

FEVER, RASH, AND ARTHRITIS

Overview

A number of autoimmune, infectious, and neoplastic processes can result in the clinical presentation of fever, rash, and arthritis (Table 1). As many of these disorders are associated with significant morbidity, their timely and efficient diagnosis is highly desirable.

Evaluation

In many cases, the particular characteristics of the dermatologic lesion provide important clues to the etiology (Table 1). Likewise, the pattern or type of arthritis may help distinguish among the conditions. Although fever frequently accompanies these disorders, its magnitude or pattern is seldom specific enough to aid in the diagnosis.

Diagnostic Testing

The most important diagnostic maneuver is focused history and physical examination. Laboratory studies may be helpful in specific conditions (e.g., ANA testing in SLE) but should not be used to "screen" for specific diseases without supportive clinical features.

Imaging

Imaging studies are generally of little value in differentiating among these conditions.

Table 1
Causes of Fever, Rash, and Arthritis

Condition	Characteristic Rash(es)	Typical Pattern of Arthritis	Other Diagnostic Clues
Autoimmune/idiopathic			
Systemic lupus erythematosus (SLE)	Malar (acute) discoid and subacute forms of rash exist; painless oral ulcers; photosensitivity; leukocytoclastic vasculitis	Symmetric, polyarticular, small joint, nondeforming	Prominent involvement of other organ systems; serologic testing (ANA, etc.)
Progressive systemic sclerosis (PSS; scleroderma)	Sclerodactyly; truncal and acral scleroderma; digital infarcts; dilated nailfold capillary loops	Oligo- or symmetric polyarticular, small joints	Raynaud's; esophageal dysfunction; serologic testing
Vasculitis	Depends on size of vessel involved: capillaries (leukocytoclastic vasculitis, palpable purpura), arterioles (erythema nodosum, subcutaneous nodules)	Oligoarticular, large or small joints	Other organ systems involved (depending on type of vasculitis); serologic testing in some cases (e.g., ANCA)
Dermatomyositis	Heliotrope rash (violaceous rash on sun-exposed areas); Gottron's papules; "mechanic's hands"	Oligo- or polyarticular, small joints	Muscle weakness; ↑ CPK; serologic testing, confirm by EMG or muscle biopsy
Psoriatic arthritis	Psoriatic plaques; associated nail changes	5 distinct forms (see p. 307)	Rash improved by sun exposure
Sarcoidosis	Early, erythema nodosum; late, sarcoid plaques and papules	Mono- or oligoarticular, large joint (ankles and knees most common)	Pulmonary involvement characteristic
Cryoglobulinemia	Acral leukocytoclastic vasculitis	Arthralgias more common than frank arthritis	Laboratory testing for cryoglobulins
Behçet's syndrome	Painful oral and genital ulcers; pathergy	Oligoarticular	Arterial/venous thromboses, CNS symptoms may be seen

continued

Table 1 (continued)
Causes of Fever, Rash, and Arthritis

Condition	Characteristic Rash(es)	Typical Pattern of Arthritis	Other Diagnostic Clues
Inflammatory bowel disease	Pyoderma gangrenosum	May be axial (with spondylitis) or peripheral (oligoarticular, large joint)	Bowel symptoms (may precede or follow arthritis)
Adult-onset Still's disease	Faint, salmon-colored, evanescent rash on trunk, extremities; Köebner's phenomenon	Oligoarticular or polyarticular	Quotidian fever, hepatosplenomegaly, leukocytosis
Infectious/reactive			
Parvovirus B19	"Slapped cheek" rash	Acute, generally self-limited, symmetric polyarticular	Serologic testing
Lyme disease	Erythema chronicum migrans	Episodic monarticular or oligoarticular	Serologic testing; neurologic involvement
Acute rheumatic fever (post-streptococcal arthritis)	Erythema marginatum	Migratory, oligoarticular, or polyarticular	Other manifestations (see Jones criteria)
Reiter's syndrome	Circinate balanitis; keratoderma blenorrhagicum	Oligoarticular, large joints	Urethritis, conjunctivitis
Gonorrhea	Pustules (painful)	Oligoarticular; tenosynovitis also seen	Urethral or cervical discharge
Meningococcemia	Petechiae	Oligoarticular (usually)	CNS symptoms
Rubella ("German measles")	Pale maculopapular rash; often spreads from face to trunk	Symmetric polyarthritis	Arthritis self-limited
Bacterial endocarditis	Septic emboli (necrotic vasculitic lesions)	Oligoarticular (septic); diffuse arthralgias	Heart murmur
HIV	Severe psoriasiform or seborrheiform rashes	Reiter's syndrome, psoriatic arthritis patterns most common	Serologic testing; immunocompromised host

Mycobacterial	Variable	Spondylitis; large joint monarthritis	Exposure history; immunocompromised host; other organ involvement
Fungal	Erythema nodosum; disseminated lesions	Spondylitis; large joint monarthritis; polyarticular (varies with organism)	Exposure history; immunocompromised host
Brucellosis	Variable	May be septic or reactive; sacroiliitis, oligoarthritis	Exposure (raw dairy products)
Hepatitis B	Diffuse erythematous rash or urticaria	Oligoarticular; may be migratory; arthalgias common	Arthritis usually improves with onset of jaundice
Neoplastic			
Cutaneous lymphoma/ leukemia (e.g., ATLL)	Extensive proliferative skin lesions; isolated maculopapular lesions	Oligoarthritis	Involvement in other organ systems; biopsy
Associated with solid-organ cancer	Variable	Oligoarthritis; polyarthritis; hypertrophic osteoarthropathy	Involvement in other organ systems

Differential Diagnosis

See Table 1.

Treatment

Treatment of these varied conditions is specific for the individual disease (e.g., for infectious causes) or class of disease (many autoimmune conditions share a therapeutic approach).

LIVER DISEASE AND ARTHRITIS

Overview

A variety of primary hepatobiliary diseases may manifest musculoskeletal symptoms. Conversely, many rheumatic disorders may involve the hepatobiliary system. Moreover, serologic abnormalities commonly accompany hepatobiliary disorders and may be a source of diagnostic confusion.

History

The following historical data should be obtained in such clinical situations:

- Family history of liver disease: relevant in hemochromatosis
- Risk factors for viral hepatitis: household exposure, blood transfusions, parenteral drug use, tattoos, or hemodialysis
- Alcohol consumption: may be associated with hepatotoxicity
- Medications: a variety of drugs may cause liver damage
- Symptoms of chronic liver disease: pruritus, peripheral edema, ascites, encephalopathy, gastrointestinal bleeding, gynecomastia, testicular atrophy, jaundice, easy bruisability, and palmar erythema; palmar erythema is poorly specific and may also be seen in normal individuals and those with inflammatory disease
- Surgical history: prior jejunoileal bypass surgery
- Medical history: gallstones, pancreatitis

Evaluation of Primary Hepatobiliary Disease and Arthritis

In acute viral hepatitis, arthritis may occur as a transient phenomenon, either alone or as part of a serum sickness–like syndrome with urticaria or a maculopapular rash. Joint and cutaneous symptoms usually resolve with the onset of jaundice and icterus.

Arthritis may be the first manifestation of previously unsuspected *chronic hepatitis B or C infection* and, in the presence of risk factors for viral hepatitis or abnormalities in liver function, should prompt testing for the presence of hepatitis B surface antigen and anti-HCV antibody. Similar testing should be done in all cases of *cryoglobulinemia* and *polyarteritis nodosa*. Renal function should also be assessed, since glomerulonephritis may be present.

Chronic calcium pyrophosphate dihydrate (CPPD) crystal-deposition disease has been associated with *hemochromatosis*. All patients with CPPD crystal-deposition disease should be screened for hemochromatosis. Screening should be done initially with transferrin saturation (100 × serum iron/total iron-binding capacity); if below 50%, measure serum ferritin (in hemochromatosis, serum ferritin is >200 ng/mL in males, >100 ng/mL in females). The diagnosis can be confirmed by liver biopsy.

Primary biliary cirrhosis (PBC) has been associated with rheumatoid arthritis (5–10%), limited scleroderma (CREST) (20–30%), anticentromere antibodies, and occasionally other connective tissue diseases. Infrequently, the rheumatic syndrome is the presenting feature. In cases of RA, limited scleroderma, and other connective tissue diseases, cholestatic laboratory abnormalities should alert the clinician to the potential diagnosis of PBC. Antimitochondrial antibodies are positive in 90 to 95% of cases of PBC.

Autoimmune chronic active hepatitis (CAH), or "lupoid hepatitis," may be associated with a positive antinuclear antibody in up to 70% of cases and a symmetric polyarthritis resembling SLE. In CAH, anti–smooth muscle antibody is frequently positive.

Persons with a history of *jejunoileal bypass surgery* may develop chronic liver disease and an arthritis-dermatitis syndrome. Obtaining such a surgical history should suggest this diagnosis.

Degenerative arthritis of large joints and the spine frequently accompanies *Wilson's disease.* Serum ceruloplasmin is decreased in most cases.

Hepatic hypertrophic osteoarthropathy accompanies some chronic liver diseases; clubbing may be present.

Evaluation of a Primary Rheumatic Disorder with Hepatic Abnormalities

First consideration is often given to possible medication-related hepatotoxicity, especially when ASA, NSAIDs, acetaminophen, or methotrexate is part of the drug regimen (Table 1). Abnormalities in liver function that persist after withdrawal of suspected medications may imply a disease-associated liver abnormality.

RA usually does not involve the liver; however, hepatomegaly has been reported in 10% of patients. There is a 5 to 10% overlap with PBC (antimitochondrial antibody is positive in such instances). Rheumatoid vasculitis may involve the liver. Nodular regenerative hyperplasia occurs in 25% of cases of Felty's syndrome (most patients have abnormal liver function tests).

Juvenile chronic arthritis, especially Still's disease, frequently causes abnormalities in liver function tests.

Subclinical liver involvement is common in SLE. Antiribosomal P antibodies have been associated with chronic liver disease. Antiphospholipid antibodies may cause the Budd-Chiari syndrome (hepatic vein thrombosis).

Table 1
Differential Diagnosis of Liver Disease and Arthritis

Elevated serum transaminases and arthritis
  Drug-related hepatotoxicity: ASA, NSAIDs, acetaminophen, methotrexate,
    azathioprine, gold, D-penicillamine, cyclosporine, cyclophosphamide, and allopurinol
  Viral hepatitis: Hepatitis A, B, C; Epstein-Barr virus; cytomegalovirus.
  Subclinical liver disease: Autoimmune chronic active hepatitis, primary biliary
    cirrhosis, hemochromatosis, Wilson's disease
Chronic liver disease and arthritis
  Chronic hepatitis B, chronic hepatitis C
  Autoimmune chronic active hepatitis
  Primary biliary cirrhosis
  Hemochromatosis
  Wilson's disease
  Liver disease following jejunoileal bypass surgery
Primary rheumatic disorder and abnormal liver function
  Rheumatoid arthritis
  Felty's syndrome
  Systemic lupus erythematosus
  Juvenile arthritis
  Polyarteritis nodosa
  Cryoglobulinemia

Diagnostic Testing

Liver disease is evaluated by assessing the degree of cellular damage, reflected by serum transaminase levels. Elevated transaminases may also be seen with muscle damage (i.e., polymyositis). Conjugated serum bilirubin and serum alkaline phosphatase are markers of cholestasis. Serum albumin and prothrombin time reflect synthetic liver functions. γ-Glutamyltransferase (GGT) is a sensitive indicator of liver disease and often parallels the alkaline phosphatase. GGT is easily induced by drugs (i.e., phenytoin, acetaminophen, tricyclic antidepressants) or alcohol and may be elevated in primary biliary cirrhosis, obstructive jaundice, hepatic metastasis, hepatitis, and primary carcinoma of the liver. GGT is not increased in bone disease. Hepatitis serology is sensitive and specific for viral hepatitis. Useful autoantibody tests include antimitochondrial antibodies (PBC) and anti–smooth muscle antibody (CAH). Diagnostic tests include serum ceruloplasmin (Wilson's disease) and transferrin saturation and serum ferritin (hemochromatosis).

Imaging

Ultrasonography is useful in assessing cholestasis, detecting gallstones, and suggesting parenchymal abnormalities (focal or diffuse). Computerized axial tomography is useful in evaluating focal lesions. Doppler ultrasonography may detect hepatic vein thrombosis. Radionuclide liver scans can assess liver and spleen size and shape and evaluate the extent of cirrhosis and portal hypertension.

Differential Diagnosis

See Table 1.

Treatment

Arthritis associated with liver disease usually responds to NSAIDs. The minimum effective dose should be used, since most NSAIDs are extensively metabolized by the liver and may undergo enterohepatic circulation. In chronic liver disease, half-lives are frequently prolonged. If available and effective, therapy should also be directed at the underlying cause.

NEOPLASIA AND ARTHRITIS

Overview

Musculoskeletal manifestations account for almost one-quarter of all paraneoplastic syndromes. Table 1 lists both the direct and indirect associations between rheumatologic syndromes and cancer.

Differential Diagnosis

See Table 1.

REFERENCES

Canoso JJ. Tumors of joints and related structures. In Koopman WJ, ed. Arthritis and allied conditions: a textbook of rheumatology. Baltimore: Williams & Wilkins, 1996: 1867–1887.

Naschitz JE, Rosner I, Rozenbaum M, et al. Cancer-associated rheumatic disorders: clues to occult neoplasia. Semin Arthritis Rheum 1995;24:231–241.

PREGNANCY AND ARTHRITIS

Overview

The hormonal alterations accompanying pregnancy may affect disease activity in patients with several rheumatic conditions. In addition, anato-mic changes associated with pregnancy may produce musculoskeletal symptoms.

Disease Associations

Disease Improvement: Amelioration in the activity of RA has been noted anecdotally for more than half a decade. It has been reported that most RA patients experience improvement in their arthritis during pregnancy. In about half

Table 1
Associations between Neoplasia and Arthritis

Diagnostic Entity	History/Presentation	Diagnostic Testing	Treatment/Prognosis
Direct associations			
Synovial tumors			
Pigmented villonodular synovitis (PVNS) (benign)	May present (a) diffuse articular—has equal sex distribution; (b) localized articular; or (c) localized nodular tenosynovial—female predominance; most common location is a finger joint	Synovial fluid of diffuse PVNS has a bloody or rust-colored appearance; T2-weighted MRI shows a diminished signal	Tumor is locally aggressive only; surgical resection has a 50–70% cure; intra- and extraarticular radiation tried with varying success
Synovial sarcoma (malignant)	Most common malignant joint neoplasia; occurs as a slow-growing, occasionally painful, periarticular mass; most common location is a lower extremity (knee preferred) in a young adult	Speckled soft-tissue calcifications often seen by plain radiography	Combination surgical resection, radiation, and systemic chemotherapy results in 40% overall cure rate; metastasis to the lung is a frequent cause of death
Leukemia	Severe bone pain; occasional oligoarticular arthritis; osteoarticular disease more common in children	Radiographs show juxtaarticular osteopenia, periosteal reaction, lytic lesions; synovial fluid occasionally contains blasts	Leukemia treatment; NSAIDs as adjuvant analgesia
Lymphoma	Non-Hodgkin's lymphoma has skeletal involvement in up to 25% of cases; synovial reaction secondary to adjacent bone disease common; direct synovial involvement is rare	Bone or synovial biopsy	Local radiotherapy and/or systemic chemotherapy
Primary tumors of bone			
Osteoid osteoma (benign)	Affects male adolescent children more commonly; most common in lower extremities and vertebra, with severe nighttime pain; symptoms may persist undiagnosed for months to years	Radiographs show subperiosteal thickening with central radiolucency.	Aspirin provides symptomatic relief; definitive therapy is resection; outcome is good

Osteosarcoma (malignant)	Most common malignant primary bone tumor; predominantly male children and adolescents; Paget's disease progresses to osteosarcoma in <1% of cases	Mixed sclerotic and lytic lesions with occasional "sunburst" appearance due to new bone	Wide resection with pre- and postoperative chemotherapy; 40–80% have a 5-year disease-free survival; metastatic to lungs
Metastatic disease Synovial joint involvement	Majority secondary to bronchogenic cancer; usually asymmetric with metastases in paraarticular bone	Synovial fluid may rarely yield diagnosis if tumor has intraarticular extension, rheumatoid factor elevated in up to 20% of cases	Treat underlying malignancy
Cartilaginous joint involvement	Up to 40% of malignant neoplasms have vertebral metastases	Plain radiographic detection if at least 30% of bone is lost; bone scan and MRI more sensitive	Treat underlying malignancy; local irradiation
Indirect associations *Carcinoma polyarthritis*	Breast cancer accounts for about 80%; explosive, predominantly lower extremity arthritis with asymmetric involvement	Usually seronegative; ESR often markedly elevated; radiographs without distinctive features	Palliate underlying malignancy; control arthritis symptoms with NSAIDs or corticosteroids
Palmar fasciitis	Known association with ovarian cancer	May be confirmed by MRI or scintigraphy	Treatment of underlying malignancy; occupational therapy
Hypertrophic osteoarthropathy	Seen in 10% of all pulmonary malignancies; clubbing and long bone pain, especially in the lower extremities is most common.	Elevated ESR and alkaline phosphatase; bone scan shows pericortical linear concentration	Treatment of underlying malignancy; aspirin and NSAIDs, followed by corticosteroids for symptom control; surgical vagotomy uncommonly tried
Amyloidosis	Amyloid arthropathy results in symmetric soft tissue swelling with decreased range of motion. Carpal tunnel syndrome is common	Serum and or urine monoclonal proteins; if amyloid is secondary to myeloma, bone marrow has plasma cell dyscrasias and radiographs show lytic lesions; fat pad or rectal biopsy to detect amyloid fibrils	Systemic corticosteroids; treatment of underlying myeloma (if applicable); colchicine sometimes helpful

continued

Table 1 (continued)
Associations between Neoplasia and Arthritis

Diagnostic Entity	History/Presentation	Diagnostic Testing	Treatment/Prognosis
Secondary gout	Seen in myeloproliferative disorders and after chemotherapy of hematologic malignancies (tumor lysis syndrome); acute gouty arthritis with exquisitely painful oligoarthropathy	Negatively birefringent crystals seen in synovial fluid with polarizing microscopy	Prophylactic hydration, urine alkalinization, and allopurinol prior to chemotherapy for leukemia; acute gout treated with NSAIDs, colchicine, or corticosteroids
Dermatomyositis/ polymyositis	Associated with solid tissue malignancy: lung, ovarian, breast most common; presents as proximal muscle weakness and related connective tissue manifestations	Elevations in creatine kinase, abnormal electromyography, and characteristic muscle biopsy findings	Screening for malignancy in patient with newly diagnosed myositis should include routine history, examination, and testing appropriate for age and health maintenance
Vasculitis	Systemic necrotizing vasculitis associated with lympho/ myeloproliferative disorders; hairy cell leukemia and Hodgkin's disease have strongest associations; characteristic systemic manifestations of polyarteritis nodosa (PAN) with the potential for skin, nervous system, joint, renal, and visceral involvement	Elevated creatinine, anemia, increased acute-phase reactants; characteristic visceral angiogram in PAN; biopsy of affected organ showing vasculitis	High-dose systemic corticosteroids and alkylating agents; these agents may be part of the treatment of the underlying malignancy
Cryoglobulinemia	Monoclonal cryoglobulinemias seen in myelomas and lymphomas; may lead to acrocyanosis, digital infarcts, arthritis, renal impairment	Cryoglobulins isolated from serum	Corticosteroids for cryoglobulinemia associated complications; plasmapheresis occasionally considered in severe cases; management of primary malignancy

Sjögren's syndrome	May progress from a benign B-cell exocrinopathy to a pseudolymphoma to a frank B-cell lymphoma; symptoms include keratoconjunctivitis sicca with xerostomia; persistently enlarged exocrine glands, lymphadenopathy, splenomegaly may herald onset	Monoclonal gammopathy with cryoglobulinemia, reversion to negative of previous positive rheumatoid factor; positive ANA, SSA, and/or SSB antibodies	Ocular, oral, and vaginal moisturizing agents for Sjögren's syndrome; aggressive systemic combination chemotherapy if transformation to B-cell lymphoma
Scleroderma	Scleroderma patients at increased risk for adenocarcinoma of lung (50% alveolar cell carcinoma) and carcinoid; scleroderma skin changes and internal organ manifestations	Abnormalities in renal pulmonary function studies if involvement in these organs; positive Scl-70 antibody portends worse prognosis	No effective disease-modifying therapy for scleroderma; treatment aimed at complications
Eosinophilic fasciitis	Associated with myeloproliferative disorders; hide-bounding of midextremities with peau de orange appearance	Peripheral and tissue eosinophilia, hypergammaglobulinemia	May respond to high-dose corticosteroids, H2 blockers, and/or antimalarial agents

of cases, the improvement occurs in the first trimester, although some patients improve only in the third trimester. The improvement in symptoms is almost always transient; recurrence of arthritis following delivery is the rule. Other disorders reported to improve during pregnancy include psoriasis, psoriatic arthritis, and sarcoidosis.

Exacerbation: Patients with other rheumatic diseases may have increased activity during pregnancy. Although there is some controversy, a large body of literature suggests that many SLE patients experience a flare during pregnancy. Controversy comes from the fact that any group of SLE patients, not only pregnant ones, observed over a period of 9 months, is likely to include many with flares of disease over that time period. Nevertheless, it does appear that some SLE patients flare during their third trimester and in the immediate postpartum period. Moreover, patients with an increased level of disease activity before pregnancy appear to be susceptible to flare during pregnancy. Thus, many rheumatologists recommend that patients wait until their disease has been quiescent for at least 6 months before becoming pregnant. This is also relevant because many medications used to treat severe SLE are contraindicated during pregnancy. Lupus patients also have a higher incidence of spontaneous abortion, prematurity, and intrauterine death. Distinguishing between a lupus renal flare and preeclampsia may be difficult. Although the data are less clear, other diseases reported to worsen during pregnancy include polymyositis and dermatomyositis.

Back Pain: Changes in posture related to pregnancy are thought to play some role in the high prevalence of low back pain among pregnant women. Approximately 50% of pregnant women complain of low back pain during pregnancy, typically during the late second and third trimesters. Pain is usually sacral or lumbar. Excess lumbar lordosis, direct pressure on the spine, the weight of the fetus, and pelvic ligament laxity have all been suggested as potential contributing factors.

Therapy

Most pharmacologic agents are best avoided during pregnancy. However, if necessary, corticosteroids may be used throughout pregnancy. Acetaminophen and NSAIDs may also be used, but NSAIDs should be discontinued beyond the 30th week to avoid premature closure of the ductus arteriosus. Drugs contraindicated during pregnancy include methotrexate, hydroxychloroquine, penicillamine, gold, cyclophosphamide, and cyclosporine. Use of azathioprine during pregnancy is controversial. It appears that sulfasalazine may be used safely, if necessary, during pregnancy.

REFERENCES

Cecere FA, Persellin RH. The interaction of pregnancy and the rheumatic diseases. Clin Rheum Dis 1981;2:747–768.

PULMONARY-RENAL SYNDROMES

Overview

A number of distinct conditions are characterized by significant pulmonary and renal involvement (Table 1). Typically, they present with hemoptysis related to alveolar hemorrhage, and extensive alveolar infiltrates on chest roentgenogram. Renal involvement in these syndromes is usually a form of proliferative glomerulonephritis and may be asymptomatic at initial presentation. Nephritis often manifests with hematuria, proteinuria, and, in some cases, azotemia. Although the pathogenesis of the various conditions may be quite distinct, their presenting signs and symptoms tend to be similar and do not usually allow differentiation. Nevertheless, optimal treatment of these various diseases may differ; thus an early specific diagnosis may favorably influence the outcome.

Etiology

See Table 1.

Disease Associations

The presence of symptoms in other organ systems may provide clues to the correct diagnosis. For example, patients with Wegener's granulomatosis may have nasal airway involvement or sinusitis in addition to the pulmonary and renal signs. Patients with SLE who have severe renal and pulmonary disease often have additional manifestations of lupus in other organ systems. Patient demographics sometimes also provide diagnostic clues. Goodpasture's syndrome tends to occur in Caucasian men in their twenties. SLE affects women 10 times as commonly as men, primarily during their childbearing years. Wegener's granulomatosis and cryoglobulinemia tend to affect older persons more commonly

Table 1
Differential Diagnosis of Pulmonary/Renal Syndromes

Goodpasture's syndrome (anti-GBM antibody disease)
Systemic lupus erythematosus
Vasculitis
   Wegener's granulomatosis
   Churg-Strauss syndrome
   Microscopic polyarteritis
   Hypersensitivity vasculitis
Rapidly progressive glomerulonephritis
Cryoglobulinemia
Infection (e.g., subacute bacterial endocarditis)
Diffuse thromboembolic disease
Congestive heart failure

than SLE and Goodpasture's syndrome. However, males and females of all races and ages can be affected by each of these conditions.

Biopsy

That the pathophysiologic processes involved in these conditions are distinct is borne out by histopathology. Wegener's granulomatosis is characterized by granulomatous vasculitis in affected tissues. Goodpasture's syndrome is characterized by antibodies to the glomerular basement membrane (GBM). Immunofluorescent staining of biopsy specimens from the lungs and kidneys of patients with Goodpasture's syndrome reveals a characteristic linear pattern of antibody deposition at the basement membrane. In contrast, diseases such as SLE and cryoglobulinemia are characterized by immune complex formation. Biopsy of affected tissues may reveal a "lumpy-bumpy" pattern of immunofluorescence in these conditions, consistent with immune complex formation.

Histopathology, particularly of renal lesions, may provide important diagnostic clues. For example, cryoglobulinemia may be associated with pathognomonic findings on electron microscopic (EM) analysis of renal biopsy specimens. The renal pathologic findings of SLE are not seen commonly in other diseases and, in the correct clinical setting, can provide strong support for diagnosis of SLE.

There is an important caveat to the use of biopsy specimens to provide a diagnosis in patients with pulmonary/renal presentations. Obtaining biopsies, particularly pulmonary biopsies, may be difficult and also dangerous in some cases. For example, in both Wegener's granulomatosis and Goodpasture's syndrome, transbronchial biopsy has a low diagnostic yield and has been associated with uncontrolled bleeding and death. If necessary, open lung biopsy would be preferred.

Diagnostic Testing

Laboratory studies are often useful in evaluating patients with pulmonary/renal syndromes. "Routine" types of laboratory studies may not help to pinpoint the cause, but they can be quite important in defining the severity of end-organ involvement. For example, patients with most of these conditions have a hypoproliferative anemia, consistent with the anemia of chronic disease. In addition, those with significant blood loss from the lungs or kidneys may have a superimposed iron deficiency anemia. Urinalysis will reveal hematuria, pyuria, and proteinuria, and serum creatinine will reflect the extent of renal impairment. These indices are useful not only in establishing renal involvement, but also in following the course of the disease and the response to therapy. Arterial blood gases are important for establishing the severity of pulmonary compromise and the need for specific therapies such as supplemental oxygen. Serum complement protein (C3, C4) levels reflect activation of the complement cascade. They tend to be depressed in conditions characterized by immune complex formation, such as SLE and cryoglobulinemia, and normal or elevated in other conditions.

Specific immunologic laboratory testing can be of great help in defining the etiology underlying a pulmonary/renal syndrome. Anti-GBM antibodies are seen in more than 95% of patients with Goodpasture's syndrome and are rarely seen in other conditions. In the correct clinical setting, the presence of cryoglobulins in the serum offers strong support for this diagnosis. Routine use of an ANA without regard for clinical symptoms or signs may be of little help in establishing the diagnosis of SLE. However, when used in selected patients (e.g., a young woman with a pulmonary/renal syndrome and a malar rash), ANA results have greater predictive value. Other tests, such as anti-DNA and anti-Sm antibodies, are more specific for SLE. Finding antineutrophil cytoplasmic antibodies (ANCA) may help establish the diagnosis of a pulmonary renal syndrome. Finding a C-ANCA (cytoplasmic pattern) or anti-proteinase-3 antibody offers strong support for the diagnosis of Wegener's granulomatosis. P-ANCA (peripheral pattern) antibodies may suggest the presence of other vasculitic conditions associated with pulmonary and renal involvement, including Churg-Strauss syndrome, microscopic polyarteritis, and idiopathic crescentic glomerulonephritis.

Treatment

Treatment generally consists of nonspecific therapies in conjunction with specific immunomodulatory therapies. Interventions such as red cell transfusion, supplemental oxygen, tight control of blood pressure, appropriate therapy with antibiotics, and others may be critical to the patient's outcome. Immunomodulatory interventions generally include corticosteroids, plasmapheresis, and cytotoxic drugs such as cyclophosphamide and azathioprine. The choice of agents, dosage, and other variables may differ among the various pulmonary/renal syndromes.

REFERENCES

Gravelyn TR, Lynch JP. Alveolar hemorrhage syndromes. IM Intern Med Special 1987; 8:63–83.

RENAL DISEASE AND ARTHRITIS

Overview

Numerous systemic disorders manifest renal and musculoskeletal features (Table 1). This listing is further augmented by commonly used musculoskeletal medications that may adversely affect the kidneys. Moreover, approximately 60 to 80% of patients with chronic renal failure have musculoskeletal complaints. Although the most common symptom by far is arthralgia, patients with end-stage renal disease (ESRD) are susceptible to a variety of arthropathies discussed below (Table 2).

Table 1
Conditions Associated with Renal Disease and Arthritis

Autoimmune: SLE, scleroderma, Sjögren's syndrome, cryoglobulinemia, serum
    sickness, hepatitis, thrombotic thrombocytopenic purpura, Goodpasture's syndrome,
    antiphospholipid syndrome (with renal vein thrombosis)
Vasculitis: Polyarteritis nodosa, microscopic polyarteritis, Henoch-Schönlein purpura,
    Wegener's granulomatosis, Takayasu's arteritis
Metabolic/endocrine: Urate nephropathy (gout), renal osteodystrophy
Rhabdomyolysis: Drug induced (e.g., cocaine), traumatic, inflammatory (e.g., myositis)
Drugs: NSAIDs, cyclosporine, gold, penicillamine, analgesic nephropathy
    (acetaminophen)
Other: Amyloidosis, sarcoidosis, nail-patella syndrome

Table 2
Musculoskeletal Conditions Associated with End-Stage Renal Disease

Crystalline arthritis
    Calcium pyrophosphate deposition disease (CPPD; pseudogout)
    Monosodium urate arthritis (gout)
    Calcium oxalate arthritis
Arthropathy
    Hemodialysis associated arthropathy
    Secondary hyperparathyroidism (especially involving hand joints)
    Axial arthritis
Tendinitis/periarthritis
Amyloidosis (e.g., with carpal tunnel syndrome)
Calciphylaxis (calcium deposition in blood vessel walls may mimic vasculitis)

Etiology

See Tables 1 and 2.

Disease Associations

Several types of crystals tend to deposit in and about the joints of patients with
ESRD. Reduced renal clearance of urate leads to hyperuricemia and a predisposition to gout. The excess calcium and phosphorous seen in patients with
ESRD may be associated with deposition of crystals containing these compounds. CPPD is associated with hyperparathyroidism. Calcium oxalate crystal deposition, which is not a common cause of arthritis in normal persons, is associated with chronic hemodialysis and ascorbic acid supplementation.

Renal osteodystrophy due to secondary hyperparathyroidism associated
with ESRD may be associated with several musculoskeletal complaints. These
may include arthritis, particularly of the hand joints, as well as arthralgia and
bony lesions. Up to 20% of such patients develop an erosive arthropathy involving the finger, shoulder, wrist, and knee joints.

Amyloidosis occurs in ESRD patients receiving chronic hemodialysis or peritoneal dialysis and often manifests as carpal tunnel syndrome, large-joint synovitis (shoulders), erosive arthritis, or tenosynovitis.

Calciphylaxis is considered elsewhere (see p. 171).

WEAKNESS

Overview

The subjective complaint of weakness may be an important clue to an underlying musculoskeletal disorder or a relatively nonspecific component of a variety of chronic medical conditions. Differentiating between these possibilities requires careful attention to elements of the history and physical examination and, in some cases, may require selected laboratory testing. Initially, it must be resolved whether the symptoms expressed are from pain, fatigue, or muscle weakness.

Anatomic Considerations

Weakness may result from myopathic, neuropathic, articular (i.e., pain), constitutional (e.g., anemia), or psychiatric (e.g., malingering) disorders.

History

Directed questioning is usually required to elucidate the nature of the symptoms. Patients with fatigue, but without weakness, can generally complete their required activities of daily living at home and work. However, they often cannot pursue leisure time activities and often retire to bed at an unusually early hour. Patients with weakness, on the other hand, typically cannot perform many of their daily activities. The disability may be mild, as in the patient who cannot climb stairs but instead uses the elevator. It may be more severe, as in an individual who cannot dress without assistance or get in and out of a bath or car.

Once it is clear that weakness is the underlying problem, further questioning should establish whether these problems are associated with soft tissue or joint pain and identify the location or distribution of the weakness. Morning stiffness and pain in the joints rather than muscles, for example, should suggest a diagnosis of early RA rather than a primary muscle disorder. Weakness of proximal muscles with minimal pain is consistent with polymyositis or dermatomyositis, while weakness of distal muscles is more typical of neurologic disorders (e.g., muscular dystropy) or the relatively rare syndrome of inclusion body myositis. Metabolic myopathies, such as carnitine palmityltransferase deficiency, are associated with periodic weakness, often during exertion; between these episodes, strength is usually normal. Current and past medications should be recorded. Drugs may also cause muscle weakness (Table 1).

Table 1
Differential Diagnosis of Muscle Weakness

Inflammatory myopathies
    Dermatomyositis
    Polymyositis
    Inclusion body myositis
Metabolic myopathies
    McArdle's disease (myophosphorylase deficiency)
    Acid maltase deficiency
    Phosphofructokinase deficiency
    Carnitine palmityl transferase deficiency
    Familial periodic paralysis
Neurologic disorders
    Muscular dystrophies
    Myasthenia gravis
    Eaton-Lambert syndrome
    Guillain-Barré syndrome
Endocrine disorders
    Hypothyroidism
    Hyperthyroidism
    Cushing's syndrome
    Hypokalemia
Toxic myopathies
    Alcohol
    Corticosteroids
    Hydroxychloroquine, chloroquine
    Cocaine
    Colchicine
    Penicillamine
    Lovastatin
    Zidovudine (AZT)
Infectious myopathies
    Viruses (influenza, EBV, HIV)
    Bacteria (staphylococci, streptococci, clostridia)
    Parasites (*Toxoplasma, Trichinella,* cysticercosis)

Physical Examination

A simple test of proximal muscle strength in the lower extremities is to observe the patient's ability to rise from a sitting position in a chair to a full standing position without using the hands. Patients who are weak also slide their feet backward and rock forward to shift their center of gravity and allow them to rise from the seated position. The chair used for this test should be firm and of standard height. Proximal muscle weakness in the arms may not be as apparent as that in the lower extremities. Watching patients comb their hair or remove or replace articles of clothing or jewelry may be instructive. Commonly, patients are unaware of adaptations they have made to perform these simple activities. The ability to resist force applied to the extremities can be assessed at the bedside or in the clinic, and degrees of weakness can be graded on a 5-point scale (see Table 9, p. 14). More quantitative testing can be done using robotic dynamometers that measure forces applied by the patient as well as resistance to forces applied by the machine. Such testing is usually done in a physical therapy facility. Grip strength may be tested semiquantitatively by simply having the patient squeeze the examiner's fingers. Other portable/hand-held quantitative devices are also available.

Identification of muscle atrophy or fasciculations may provide important clues to chronicity or etiology. Inflammatory muscle disorders rarely cause muscle fasciculations and are more suggestive of a neurologic disorder. Quadriceps atrophy may occur with polymyositis or dermatomyositis, while atrophy of the intrinsic muscles of the hands suggests other possibilities such as inclusion body myositis or disuse atrophy.

Other systemic findings should be sought. A rash, for example, may be the primary clue to a diagnosis of dermatomyositis. Thyroid enlargement suggests an underlying abnormality of this gland, while moon facies or truncal obesity could indicate Cushing's syndrome.

Diagnostic Testing

Selected laboratory tests should be performed based on clues derived from the history and physical examination. Generalized symptoms of weakness and fatigue may indicate thyroid dysfunction, which is best assessed by the appropriate laboratory tests (free T4, TSH). Proximal muscle weakness should be evaluated by measuring serum levels of the muscle enzyme creatine kinase (CK) or may be incidentally suggested by elevated hepatic transaminases (AST, ALT). If the CK is normal and myositis is suspected, aldolase measurement may be useful. For patients with metabolic myopathies, muscle enzyme levels are often normal except during periods of exertion, when a rhabdomyolysis syndrome can occur. Urine myoglobin and renal function should be measured in these individuals. Further testing such as electromyography or muscle biopsy should be done in consultation with a rheumatologist or neurologist, as indicated.

Differential Diagnosis

See Table 1.

SYNOVIAL FLUID ANALYSIS, ARTHROCENTESIS, AND JOINT INJECTION TECHNIQUES

SYNOVIAL FLUID ANALYSIS

Description: Synovial fluid (SF) analysis is often used to aid differential diagnosis and therapy. SF, the transudative product of type B synoviocytes, serves as a local lubricant and medium for nutrient replenishment to cartilage and other intraarticular structures. The primary goal of SF analysis is to discern whether a synovial effusion is noninflammatory, inflammatory, septic, or hemorrhagic.

Method: SF is primarily obtained by needle aspiration. (See Table 1 for a description of the procedure.) Joint fluid may also be obtained during other diagnostic and therapeutic procedures (i.e., arthrogram, arthroscopy, arthroplasty). SF usually will not clot but may with high fibrinogen levels (inflammatory states). Aspirated SF should be promptly divided among plain (red top) tubes (for glucose, if necessary), sodium (not lithium) heparin tubes (for crystals), EDTA (for cell count, differential, complement), or sterile culture tubes. If gonococcal arthritis is suspected, immediate inoculation on Thayer-Martin media is recommended. Delay in SF analysis may lower WBC counts and increase the number of birefringent artifacts. Whereas calcium pyrophosphate dihydrate (CPPD) crystals may decrease over time (i.e., weeks), Monosodium urate (MSU) crystals will not. If the sample cannot be promptly analyzed, refrigerate at 4°C.

Crystal Analysis: A wet preparation requires only a few drops of SF. Glass slides and cover slips should be clean and free of dust and other potentially birefringent debris. Crystals can been seen under plain light microscopy but are best seen under the polarizing microscope.

—*Gout:* MSU crystals, seen in gouty effusions, are long, needle shaped, and negatively birefringent; they are usually intracellular during acute attacks.

—*Pseudogout:* CPPD crystals, found in pseudogout and chondrocalcinosis, are usually shorter, rhomboid or needle shaped, and positively birefringent.

—*Cholesterol crystals:* These appear as "stacked panes of glass."

—*Calcium oxalate crystals:* These are positively birefringent and bipyramidal in shape.

—*Hydroxyapatite crystals:* These are not routinely seen and may only be identified by electron microscopy or by staining with alizarin red.

Table 1
Procedure for Arthrocentesis and Joint Injection

- Inform patient of purpose, expected benefits, and side effects of the procedure
- Have patient sign informed consent form
- Check for allergies: iodine, lidocaine, or adhesives?
- Position patient; maximize patient comfort and joint exposure
- Identify bony landmarks with pen
- Identify puncture site with imprint from retracted end of ballpoint pen
- Wash hands before procedure and wear gloves (required by OSHA)
- Prepare and lay out syringes, needles, corticosteroid, and anesthetic to be used
- Cleanse injection site with povidone-iodine solution
- Begin with topical anesthetic (i.e., ethyl chloride) and spray until a light frost appears
- Swab site with alcohol preparation
- Keep the injection site sterile
- Speak to the patient and inform of each step; pain may be felt while lidocaine is instilled (described as "burning") or when needle penetrates an inflamed joint capsule or bursa (described as "sharp")
- Use 22-g, 23-g, or 25-g needle for local anesthesia and joint injection
- Slowly infiltrate anesthetic (lidocaine), pausing before each advance of the needle
- With each advance, draw back on the plunger before injecting
- Switch to an 18-g needle (or largest possible) if aspirating joint fluid
- Use hemostat to clamp and stabilize needle while changing syringes
- Use a 5- or 10-mL syringe to aspirate joint fluid; reposition needle if necessary
- Synovial fluid may not always be obtained once inside the joint; if large amount of fluid remains, leave needle in place, use 20- or 30-mL syringes to withdraw
- Once "tapped dry," a corticosteroid preparation, with or without a small amount of lidocaine, can be instilled by leaving the needle in place, stabilizing it with a hemostat, and changing syringes
- Remove needle and apply local pressure for 2–4 min (longer if patients are on NSAIDs or Coumadin)
- Process synovial fluid specimen promptly (i.e., laboratory workup, cultures, polarized microscopy)
- Advise home (bed/chair) rest and ice to injected site (20 min q. 2–3 h) for the next 24–36 h
- Immobilization for 24–72 h following injection may improve outcome
- Counsel patient to call or return if fever or local pain/erythema develops
- Record volume withdrawn, color, appearance, viscosity, microscopic findings, and tests ordered in the patient's chart

—*Negative birefringence (i.e., MSU crystals):* Present if the crystal appears yellow when parallel to the axis of the compensator and blue when perpendicular.

—*Positive birefringence (i.e., CPPD crystals):* Present if the crystal appears blue when parallel to the axis of the compensator and yellow when perpendicular.

Normal Values: Normal SF is transparent, clear, and colorless or pale straw colored. It is normally viscous, owing to high levels of hyaluronate. Expression of a drop of fluid from the syringe tip will produce a long, viscous, stringlike tail ("string sign"). Viscosity, hyaluronate, and string sign are lost with inflammatory states. Normal SF WBC counts are below 200 cells/mm^3, with a predominance of mononuclear cells. Normally, small amounts (<5 mL) of joint fluid are present in large (i.e., knee) joints and may also be obtained from small (i.e., finger) joints. When available, SF should be examined for appearance, viscosity, and WBC cell count and differential. The clinician should determine the need for polarized microscopy, bacteriologic cultures, fungal cultures, and cytology. Whenever infection is suspected, SF should be gram-stained and cultured appropriately.

Not Recommended: Synovial fluid protein, albumin, glucose, lactate dehydrogenase (LDH), complement, and serologic tests are of no diagnostic value in the analysis of SF. Nonetheless, protein, albumin, and complement levels are lower than serum values; the glucose concentration is normal and usually within 10 to 15 mg/dL of serum values.

Abnormal Synovial Fluid: SF is abnormal in a variety of conditions, including osteoarthritis, meniscal and cruciate tears, inflammatory arthritis (i.e., RA), crystal arthritis (i.e., gout), and hemorrhagic conditions. Table 2 details SF abnormalities and their disease associations. In noninflammatory conditions, SF WBC counts are between 200 and 2000 cells/mm^3. In inflammatory states, SF WBC counts range from 2,000 to 75,000 cells/mm^3 and show a predominance of neutrophils. Septic effusions often have WBC counts from 60,000 to 500,000 cells/mm^3, with an even greater percentage of neutrophils. In most bacterially induced septic arthritides, SF has more than 90% neutrophils. SF WBC counts between 20,000 and 60,000 cells/mm^3 may be seen in some infectious arthritides

Table 2
Synovial Fluid Analysis

	Noninflammatory Type I	Inflammatory Type II	Septic Type III	Hemorrhagic Type IV
Appearance	Yellow	Yellow	Purulent	Bloody
Clarity	Clear	Cloudy	Opaque	Opaque
Viscosity	High	Decreased	Decreased	Variable
Cell count	200–2000	2000–75K	>60K	RBC >>
(% PMNs)	(<25% PMNs)	(>50% PMNs)	(>80% PMNs)	WBC
Examples[a]	Osteoarthritis, trauma, osteonecrosis, SLE	RA, Reiter's, crystal arthritis, SLE, viral arthritis, fungal arthritis, Tb	Bacterial arthritis, crystal arthritis	Trauma, fracture, ligament tear, hemophilia, Charcot arthritis, PVNS

[a] Abbreviations: Tb, tuberculosis; PVNS, pigmented villonodular synovitis.

(i.e., gonococcal, fungal, tuberculous) or previously treated (i.e., antibiotics) septic arthritis. Gouty effusions occasionally yield SF WBC counts above 60,000 cells/mm^3.

Indications: SF should be analyzed when available. Indications for arthrocentesis are given below.

Comment: With only a few drops of SF, the examiner can do a visual inspection, assess viscosity, and perform SF culture, polarized microscopy, and a peripheral smear to gauge the number and type of cells present. Crystal arthritis may coexist with septic arthritis or other inflammatory arthritides; however, coexistence of gout and RA is very rare.

REFERENCES

Schmerling RH, Delbanco ML, Tosteson ANA, Trentham DE. Synovial fluid test: what should be ordered? JAMA 1990;264:1009–1014.

ARTHROCENTESIS AND JOINT INJECTION TECHNIQUES

Description: Techniques for needle aspiration and injection of joints.

Indications: Indications for needle aspiration and injection of joints include (a) acute or chronic monarthritis (with effusion), (b) suspected infection or crystal-induced arthritis, (c) unexplained exacerbation of preexisting polyarthritis, (d) joint effusion following trauma, (e) intraarticular treatment (e.g., corticosteroids), (f) injection of contrast media for diagnostic arthrography, and (g) uncertain diagnosis. Clinical situations in which joint aspiration and injection with corticosteroids may be beneficial include painful monarticular osteoarthritis, focal pain/swelling in RA, acute gout or pseudogout, acute bursitis or tendinitis, early adhesive capsulitis, and possibly reflex sympathetic dystrophy.

Contraindications: Relative contraindications for intraarticular injection include suspected septic arthritis or bursitis, overlying cellulitis, neuropathic (Charcot) joint, joint pain secondary to referred pain, known bacteremia, thrombocytopenia (platelets <50,000/mm^3), coagulopathy, anticoagulant therapy, uncontrolled diabetes, lack of response to previous injection, prosthetic joints, and inaccessible joints (i.e., hip, sacroiliac).

Method: Access to periarticular structures (i.e., bursae), joint cavity, or SF is best achieved by percutaneous needle aspiration. Table 1 details the steps involved in arthrocentesis. Preparation of commonly used materials into an "arthrocentesis tray" facilitates the process (Table 3). Many large (i.e., knee, shoulder) and small (i.e., MCP, sternoclavicular) joints are easily aspirated. Difficult or inaccessible joints should not be attempted by routine needle aspiration. Thus, fluoroscopically guided arthrocentesis is best for the hip, sacroiliac,

Table 3
Contents of Arthrocentesis Tray

Gloves (nonsterile)
Povidone-iodine solution
Alcohol preparations
Gauze
Ethyl chloride spray (topical anesthetic)
Hemostat
1.5″ sterile needles (18 g, 22 g, 23 g)
1″ sterile needles (21 g, 23 g, 25 g)
Syringes
   3 mL (to inject steroid or lidocaine)
   5 mL (to instill lidocaine)
   10 mL (for initial SF withdrawal)
   20 or 30 mL (withdraw large amount of SF)
Tubes
   EDTA/lavender—cell count
   Heparin/green—crystals, in vitro studies
Single-dose vials of 1% lidocaine (without epinephrine)
Single-dose vials of corticosteroid preparation
Sterile container, culture media
Glass slides/cover slips
Band-Aids
Ballpoint pen
Cup or basin (for waste)

apophyseal, toe interphalangeal, and temporomandibular joints. The operator should select an injection site after identifying anatomic landmarks and the point of maximal fluctuance or tenderness. Prepare all syringes before starting. Povidone-iodine solution and alcohol swabs should be used to maintain a sterile field. (See below for methods used in arthrocentesis of selected joints.)

Precautions: Occupational Safety and Health Administration (OSHA) guidelines state that gloves (sterile or nonsterile) should be worn by the clinician and assistant(s) throughout the procedure and that sterile technique should be observed when handling needles, syringes, and joint fluid. Gloves and all materials contaminated by blood or SF should be disposed of in appropriate "sharps" or biohazard containers. Patients with a history of valvular heart disease should receive appropriate antibiotic prophylaxis prior to the procedure. Hand washing before and after arthrocentesis is advised.

Record: When applicable, the volume withdrawn, color, appearance, viscosity, cell count and differential; crystal appearance by light or polarized microscopy; gram stain, culture, and sensitivity results; culture for acid-fast bacilli or fungi; and cytology should be recorded.

Avoid: SF protein or glucose; SF urate, LDH, autoantibodies (i.e., RF, ANA, LE cells); mucin clot test; pH; or complement should not be done. A low SF glucose level (<50% of serum value) may be seen in RA, tuberculosis, and other forms of septic arthritis but is infrequent and not specific.

Complications: Although infrequent, the most common complications include allergic reactions (to iodine, adhesive, lidocaine), vasovagal episodes, local ecchymoses, and exacerbation of hyperglycemia in diabetics. Uncommonly, postinjection flares, corticosteroid crystal–induced synovitis, depigmentation of overlying skin, and subcutaneous atrophy are seen. Skin or joint infection, hemarthrosis, and calcification or rupture of periarticular structures are rare events with proper technique.

Therapy: Corticosteroid injection may provide significant relief as sole therapy or adjunctive therapy in many conditions. Steroid preparations vary in equivalent potency and diluent. (See Table 4 for a comparison of common parenteral steroid preparations.) Ideally, single-dose vials or ampules of steroids and lidocaine should be used to avoid medication sharing between patients. Whereas water-soluble steroids tend to be absorbed rapidly and have shorter durations of action, the converse is true for the insoluble steroid preparations (Table 4). The needle size and volume of steroid to be instilled depend on the relative size of the joint (Table 5). Lidocaine (1% solution) without epinephrine may be used for local anesthesia during the procedure. Depending on the size of the joint, 0.5 to 3 mL of lidocaine may be used for soft tissue anesthesia. Soft tissue anesthesia is recommended if aspiration of SF or difficulty with joint access is anticipated. Intraarticular steroid may be mixed with 0.25 to 0.5 mL (depending on size of joint/bursa) of 1% lidocaine to provide immediate pain relief, improve range of motion, and confirm the adequacy of injection. Corticosteroids should not be instilled into joints that are potentially septic, unstable, or neuropathic. Bed/home rest for 24 to 36 hours is recommended, with immobilization and local application of ice every 2 to 3 hours. An extended period of immobilization may enhance

Table 4
Comparison of Commonly Used Intraarticular Corticosteroids Preparations

Trade Name	Generic Name	Concentration (mg/mL)	Equivalent Doses	Water Solubility	Range of Dosing (mg/mL)
Depo-Medrol	Methylprednisolone acetate	20, 40, 80	4	Insoluble	10–80
Aristospan	Triamcinolone hexacetonide	20	4	Insoluble	5–40
Kenalog, Aristocort	Triamcinolone acetonide	20	4	Soluble	5–40
Celestone	Betamethasone acetate	6	0.6	Insoluble	1.5–6
Hydeltra	Prednisolone tebutate	20	5	Soluble	5–50

Table 5
Materials and Doses for Joint Injections

Joint	Needle Length (gauge)[a]	Volume of Intraarticular Injection (mL)	Dose of Depo-Medrol (mg)
Knee	1.5″ (22/18)	1–3	40–80
Shoulder	1.5″ (22/18 or 19)	1–3	40–60
Wrist	1–1.5″ (22/19)	0.5–2	20–40
Ankle	1.5″ (22/19)	0.5–2	20–40
Elbow	1.5″ (22/18)	0.5–2	20–40
MCP	5/8–1″ (25/21)	0.25–0.5	5–10
PIP	5/8–1″ (25/23)	0.25–0.5	5–10
MTP	5/8–1″ (25/21)	0.25–0.5	5–10

[a] Sizes suggested apply to needle gauge during instillation only or aspiration/instillation, respectively.

the outcome of the procedure but should be combined with nontraumatic, non-weight-bearing range-of-motion exercises.

Comment: The maximum number of steroid injections per site is not known but should kept to a minimum. A safe recommendation is to limit intraarticular/periarticular steroid injections to three or less per year per site, not to be repeated in consecutive years. Repetitive injections may become less effective, may adversely effect cartilage, and may increase the risk of infection or tendon rupture.

REFERENCES

Gatter RA. Arthrocentesis technique and intrasynovial therapy. In: Koopman WJ, ed. Arthritis and allied conditions. Baltimore: Williams & Wilkins, 1996:751–760.

Pfenninger JL. Injections of joints and soft tissue: part I. General guidelines. Am Fam Physician 1991;44:1196–1202.

Pfenninger JL. Injections of joints and soft tissue: part II. Guidelines for specific joints. Am Fam Physician 1991;44:1690–1702.

KNEE (PATELLOFEMORAL) ARTHROCENTESIS

Patient Position: Patient should lie supine and be made comfortable with the head supported and slightly inclined. If a flexion contracture exists, use pillows to support and position the knee so that the quadriceps is relaxed during the procedure.

Limb Position: The leg should be parallel to the ground and the knee may be slightly flexed. The foot should be perpendicular to the ground so that the leg is neither externally nor internally rotated.

Bony Landmarks: Mark the medial, lateral, superior, and inferior borders of the patella (Fig. 1).

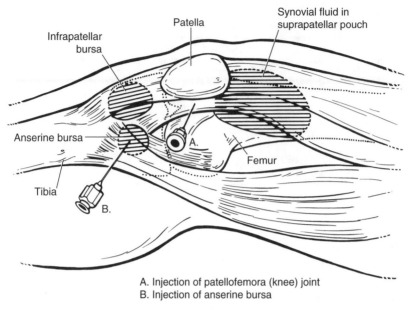

A. Injection of patellofemora (knee) joint
B. Injection of anserine bursa

Figure 1. Knee arthrocentesis.

Site/Angle of Entry: Use a medial or lateral approach. Site selection should be based on maximum fluctuance (for aspiration) or tenderness (for injection). The needle should be placed between the midpoint and superior pole, 1 cm below the edge of the patella. The axis of entry is perpendicular to the leg, with a 20 to 25° downward tilt to avoid the underside of the patella. The needle should be advanced more than 3 cm to enter the joint space. Aspirate before injecting.

Amount of Injection: Use 40 to 80 mg of Depo-Medrol^{TM} (or equivalent), with or without 0.5 mL of 1% lidocaine, in a total volume of 1 to 3 mL.

Other Injectable Sites: With anserine bursitis, the bursae may be injected with the patient seated or supine. The bursa may be entered from the medial side, tangentially, at a 30° angle, injecting 20 to 40 mg of Depo-Medrol (Fig. 1).

Comment: SF aspiration may be facilitated by manually compressing fluid downward ("milking") from the suprapatellar pouch into the joint space.

SHOULDER (GLENOHUMERAL) ARTHROCENTESIS

Patient Position: The patient should be seated upright with the shoulder joint fully exposed.

Limb Position: Place the patient's arms at the side, with hands on lap and palms facing upward so that the glenohumeral joint is partially externally rotated.

Bony Landmarks: Palpate the acromion (laterally), humeral head and coracoid process (anteriorly), bicipital tendon and groove (anterolaterally), and the acromioclavicular (AC) joint (superiorly). The humeral head is best palpated by placing the thumb over the joint anteriorly and having the patient internally and externally rotate the humerus.

Site/Angle of Entry: The entry site is anterior to where the humeral head can be felt to rotate inward (under the thumb) during rotation. This site is just inferior and lateral to the coracoid process (Fig. 2). The axis of entry is parallel to the ground, directly into the shoulder but angled (10–15°) toward the midscapula. The needle should be fully advanced (>3 cm) to enter the joint. Aspirate before injecting.

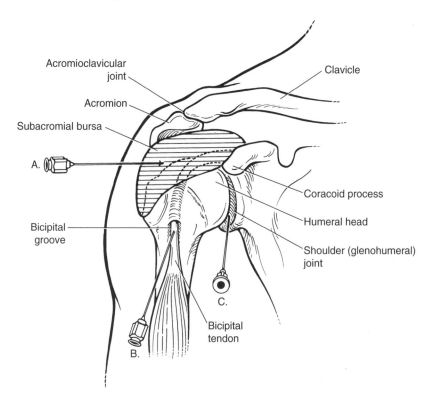

A. Injection of subacromial bursa
B. Injection of bicipital tendon
C. Injection of glenohumeral joint

Figure 2. Shoulder arthrocentesis.

Amount of Injection: Use 20 to 40 mg of Depo-Medrol (or equivalent), with or without 0.5 mL of 1% lidocaine, in a total volume of 1 to 3 mL.

Other Injectable Sites: The subacromial (subdeltoid) bursa may be injected using the same patient/limb position (Fig. 2). Use 20 to 40 mg of Depo-Medrol (or equivalent) with 0.5 mL of 1% lidocaine. After locating the point of maximal tenderness, enter laterally 1 cm beneath the acromion, with the needle axis parallel to the ground. The bicipital tendon may be injected tangentially after palpating the tendon, bicipital groove, and point of maximal tenderness. Do not inject into the tendon, but rather, inject close to the tendon sheath by advancing the needle until the tendon is felt, then withdrawing 1 to 2 mm.

Comment: Concomitant use of lidocaine allows the operator to gauge the adequacy of injection, as many patients can "suddenly" move the shoulder more freely and without pain at the completion of the procedure.

WRIST (RADIOCARPAL) ARTHROCENTESIS

Patient Position: The patient may be seated or lying supine.

Limb Position: The wrist, hand, and forearm should be comfortable and parallel to the ground. A small towel can be rolled into a 3- to 4-cm elevation and put under the wrist, leaving it slightly flexed (10°).

Bony Landmarks: Medially, palpate the tip of the ulnar styloid; laterally, the tip of the radial styloid; and dorsally, the extensor pollicis longus tendon. Draw a line (visually) from the tip of the ulnar to radial styloid (Fig. 3). Ask the patient to fully extend the thumb and note where the extensor pollicis longus tendon rises to bisect this line. The injection site is to the ulnar side of this intersection. Confirm this site by palpating along the radius, moving distally until the depression of the radiocarpal joint is felt.

Site/Entry Angle: Using a dorsal (extensor) approach, enter downward at a 90° angle to the ulnar side of the extensor pollicis longus tendon (away from the anatomic "snuff box"). The needle should be advanced more than 2 cm into the joint space. Aspirate before injecting.

Amount of Injection: Use 10 to 40 mg of Depo-Medrol (or equivalent), with or without 0.25 mL of 1% lidocaine, in a total volume of 0.5 to 2 mL.

Other Injectable Sites: De Quervain's tenosynovitis, affecting the extensor pollicis brevis and abductor pollicis longus tendons, may be injected with the same amount of steroid preparation. Rotate the hand 90° (thumb up) and place the wrist in slight ulnar deviation. Locate the point of maximal tenderness over the affected tendon. Enter tangentially at a 30° angle. Do not inject into the tendon but close to the tendon sheath.

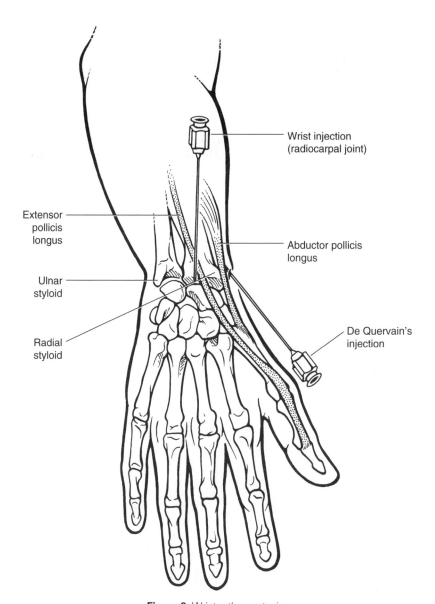

Figure 3. Wrist arthrocentesis.

ANKLE ARTHROCENTESIS

Patient Position: The patient should lie supine (or be seated) on the examination table.

Limb Position: In a lying position, the foot should be perpendicular to the floor and partially plantar flexed (75°).

Bony Landmarks: Medially, palpate the tip of the medial malleolus; laterally, the tip of the lateral malleolus; and anteriorly, the extensor hallucis longus tendon. Draw a line (visually) from medial to lateral malleoli. Ask the patient to dorsiflex the big toe and note where the extensor hallucis longus tendon rises to bisect this line (Figure 4). The injection site is medial to the tendon intersection.

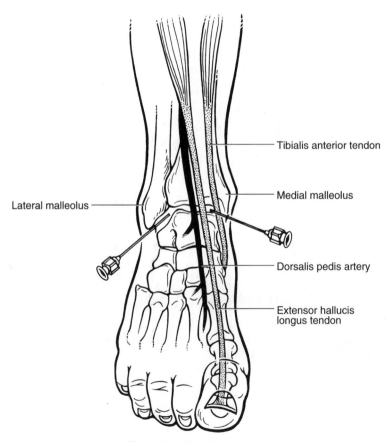

Figure 4. Ankle arthrocentesis.

Site/Angle of Entry: To inject the true ankle joint, use an anteromedial approach and place the needle at the injection site described above. Enter at a 90° angle (perpendicular to floor) and direct the needle slightly laterally (toward the Achilles tendon). The needle should be advanced more than 3 cm into the joint space. The ankle may also be approached laterally (adjacent to the subtalar joint) using the same positioning, but entering just anterior to and beneath the lateral malleolus, with a slight inward angle. Aspirate before injecting.

Amount of Injection: Use 20 to 40 mg of Depo-Medrol (or equivalent), with or without 0.25 mL of 1% lidocaine, in a total volume of 0.5 to 3 mL.

TROCHANTERIC BURSAL INJECTION

Patient Position: The patient should lie on his or her side, with the painful trochanter ("hip") facing up.

Limb Position: Legs should be comfortably extended, side by side.

Bony Landmarks: Usually the greater trochanter is the most elevated point over the hip curvature. Using one finger, identify the point of maximal tenderness over the bony greater trochanter.

Entry Angle: The needle should be directed downward at a 90° angle and slowly advanced until the tip pierces the painful bursa or touches the trochanter. Aspirate before injecting.

Amount of Injection: Use 40 to 60 mg of Depo-Medrol (or equivalent) and 0.5 mL of 1% lidocaine in a total volume of 0.5 to 1.5 mL.

Comment: When entering an inflamed bursa, the operator may feel a "pop" or the patient may note a sudden sharp pain. Rarely is there sufficient bursal fluid to aspirate.

DIAGNOSTIC TESTS GUIDE

ANGIOTENSIN CONVERTING ENZYME

Description: Angiotensin converting enzyme (ACE) catalyzes the conversion of angiotensin I to the potent vasopressor angiotensin II. ACE also inactivates the vasodilator bradykinin. Although it is produced primarily by endothelial and epithelial cells, ACE may also be synthesized in substantial quantities by activated macrophages in certain pathologic conditions such as sarcoidosis.

Method: ACE is measured by bioassay; for example, an inhibitor-binding assay. Normal values may vary, and results must be interpreted according to laboratory standards.

Increased In: Elevated serum ACE levels are often associated with sarcoidosis and may be found in approximately 80% of patients with sarcoid, primarily in those with lung involvement. However, increased serum ACE levels are not specific for sarcoidosis and may also be found in conditions such as interstitial lung disease of various etiologies (e.g., asbestosis, silicosis), hematologic malignancies (e.g., Hodgkin's disease), endocrine diseases (e.g., hyperthyroidism and diabetes mellitus), and infections (e.g., leprosy). Moreover, patients with sarcoidosis may have normal serum ACE levels, depending upon the organ involvement and extent and activity of disease. Also, although ACE levels have been reported to decrease following successful treatment of patients with sarcoidosis, this is not universally true. Thus, serum ACE levels must be interpreted carefully in sarcoidosis. Decreased serum levels of ACE have been suggested to indicate endothelial injury; for example, in patients with scleroderma.

ACE has also been measured in fluids other than serum, including cerebrospinal fluid (CSF) and bronchoalveolar lavage (BAL) fluid. Although suggested to be of diagnostic utility (e.g., increased ACE levels in the CSF suggesting neurosarcoidosis), interpretation of results of these tests is somewhat controversial. Until their utility is established, they are probably most appropriately considered research tools.

Confounding Factors: Factors that affect ACE levels include storage temperature, and samples kept frozen overnight or longer may have spuriously high values when tested.

Cost: $40–60.

REFERENCES

Lawrence EC. Serial changes in markers of disease activity with corticosteroid treatment in
    sarcoidosis. Am J Med 1983;74:747–756.

ACUTE-PHASE REACTANTS (ESR, CRP)

Description: Acute-phase reactants are a group of plasma proteins normally
produced by the liver. Synthesis of these diverse proteins increases greatly in
response to inflammatory stimuli in both acute and chronic settings. Examples
of acute phase reactants include (*a*) coagulation proteins: fibrinogen, prothrombin; (*b*) transport proteins: haptoglobin, transferrin, ceruloplasmin; (*c*) complement components: C3, C4; and (*d*) miscellaneous proteins: fibronectin, serum
amyloid-A, C-reactive protein (CRP), ferritin.

Acute-phase reactants are commonly used as an indirect measure of the extent of inflammation. For rheumatic diseases, the most commonly used acute-
phase reactants are the CRP and the erythrocyte sedimentation rate (ESR). The
ESR measures the rate of gravitational settling of erythrocytes, which is accelerated by a variety of factors, the most important of which is fibrinogen.

Method: In practice the two most often used clinical tests for the acute-phase
reactants are the ESR and CRP. The CRP is most often (and accurately) measured by rate nephelometry (an automated antigen/antibody-mediated reaction). The ESR is performed by the Westergren method (recommended by the
International Committee for Standardization in Hematology) and uses anticoagulated venous blood, diluted 4:1 with sodium citrate and placed in a 200-mm
glass tube with a 2.5-mm internal diameter. At the end of 1 hour, the distance
(in millimeters) from the meniscus (plasma and sodium citrate) to the top of
the column of erythrocytes is recorded as the ESR. The modified Westergren
method substitutes EDTA for sodium citrate and enables the same sample of
blood to be used for other tests. Both methods yield identical results.

Normal Values: CRP is normally less than 0.8 mg/dL and is unaffected by age
or sex. The ESR is affected by age and sex. In young men, the ESR ranges from 0
to 13 mm/h, and in women, 0 to 20 mm/h. Importantly, the ESR increases with
advancing age. Rough formulas for age-adjusted estimates of ESR follow:

    Men: ESR = age in years/2
    Women: ESR = (age in years + 10)/2

Increased In: The ESR and CRP are increased in a variety of disorders including:

—*Acute or chronic inflammatory disorders:* Gout, rheumatoid arthritis
    (RA), rheumatic fever, spondyloarthropathies, polymyalgia rheumatica, giant
    cell arteritis and other forms of vasculitis, inflammatory bowel disease, etc.

—*Tissue injury/necrosis:* Acute myocardial infarction, tissue ischemia or infarction, transplant rejection, malignant tumors, following surgery, burns, and trauma

—*Infections:* Bacterial (e.g., endocarditis, osteomyelitis, intraabdominal infections) and some viral infections (e.g., acute viral hepatitis)

—*Miscellaneous:* May also be elevated in late pregnancy and postpartum, hyper- and hypothyroidism, azotemia, nephrotic syndrome. *Note:* Over 10% of very high ESR (>75 mm/h) values lack an identifiable cause. This is particularly true in the elderly. The physician should wait and repeat the test in 3 to 6 months and not routinely embark on an exhaustive, expensive, or invasive search for an occult neoplastic, infectious, or inflammatory process.

Decreased In: The ESR may be low in CHF, cachexia, and those on high-dose corticosteroids. The ESR and CRP may be normal in patients with systemic lupus erythematosus (SLE), polymyositis, scleroderma, pregnancy, osteoarthritis, and most viral infections.

Confounding Factors: The ESR may be increased by macrocytosis, hypercholesterolemia, increased fibrinogen, and high ambient temperatures. The ESR may be decreased by disorders of RBC morphology (sickle cells, spherocytosis, microcytosis) polycythemia, high leukocyte counts, hyperviscosity states, or a delay (>2 h) in testing.

Indications: The acute-phase reactants may be used in distinguishing inflammatory and noninflammatory disorders. Although nonspecific, they may be diagnostically or therapeutically useful.

The American College of Physicians recommends that the ESR be used in the diagnosis and monitoring of polymyalgia rheumatica, temporal arteritis, and Hodgkin's disease. With inflammatory disorders such as RA, the ESR should primarily be used to resolve conflicting clinical data (e.g., the patient whose examination improves but subjective complaints do not). Nonetheless, there is a long history of experience with the ESR in diagnosis and monitoring of inflammatory disorders such as RA.

The CRP is useful in monitoring disease activity and response to therapy in chronic inflammatory disorders (e.g., RA). Some prefer the CRP to the ESR in monitoring inflammatory disease because changes are more acute. The CRP increases rapidly following an inflammatory stimulus and returns to normal within days; the ESR may take days to rise and may return to normal values over weeks. Also, the CRP is more dynamic (the difference between the levels seen in inflammatory and normal states is greater). Surgeons sometimes prefer to monitor the CRP and use very high elevations in CRP to indicate postoperative infection, as the ESR may be elevated due to the surgery itself. In inflammatory conditions associated with protein-losing nephropathy, such as SLE, the ESR may always be elevated, and the CRP may be a better indicator of superimposed infection.

Cost: ESR $18–36; CRP $25–48; Ferratin $45–55.

Table 1
Comparison of the CRP and ESR

Acute-Phase Reactant	Advantages	Disadvantages

CRP	Rises and falls early
	Age independent
	Few confounding factors
	Uninfluenced by
	  RBC shape
	Fewer technical errors
		Results may take longer
		Physicians less familiar
		Not well studied in
		  diseases other than RA
		  (e.g., SLE)
		Slightly more expensive
		  than ESR

ESR	Simple to perform
	Readily available
	Greater familiarity
	Cheap
		Rises and falls slowly
		Age and sex dependent
		Potential confounding
		  factors
		Influenced by RBC
		  morphology
		Technical errors can give
		  false results

Comments: While the CRP generally parallels the ESR, it rises earlier than the ESR (4–6 h) and returns to normal first. It is especially useful in situations in which the ESR results may be affected by confounding variables (anemia, polycythemia, abnormal RBC morphology, hypergammaglobulinemia, and CHF). The CRP is superior to the ESR in assessing disease activity and therapy in RA (Table 1).

The ESR is never diagnostic of a single disease, and trends may be more valuable than a single result. Extreme elevations (>100 mm/h) may suggest cancer, vasculitis (e.g., giant cell arteritis), adult-onset Still's disease, spondyloarthropathy, or serious infections. Normal values do not exclude disease. It is not useful as a screening test in asymptomatic individuals.

REFERENCES

Otterness IG. The value of C-reactive protein measurement in rheumatoid arthritis. Semin Arthritis Rheum 1994;24:91–104.

Sox HC, Liang MW. The erythrocyte sedimentation rate: guidelines for rational use. Ann Intern Med 1986;104:515–523.

Wallach J. Core blood analytes: alterations by diseases. In: Wallach J, ed. Interpretation of diagnostic tests. 6th ed. Boston: Little, Brown and Co, 1996:73–76.

ALDOLASE

Synonyms: ALD, fructose biphosphate aldolase

Description: Aldolase is an enzyme that is elevated in certain forms of muscle disease. Aldolase can be found in many tissues including skeletal muscle, liver, erythrocytes, and brain.

Method: Aldolase determinations are not routine in most laboratories. Several automated methods have been used including ultraviolet and coupled enzymatic determinations. Serum should be collected in a red-top tube.

Normal Values: Reference values are age related and may vary among laboratories. Newborns may have values up to four times the adult value. Adult values usually range from 1.7 to 4.9 U/L.

Increased In: Levels are increased in polymyositis, dermatomyositis, inclusion body myositis, eosinophil-myalgia syndrome, progressive Duchenne's muscular dystrophy, limb-girdle and facioscapulohumeral muscular dystrophy, and muscle damage induced by infection (e.g., trichinosis, toxoplasmosis) or drug toxicity (e.g., cocaine). Levels are elevated in hepatitis (hepatitis B and C) but not cirrhosis or biliary obstruction. Aldolase may also be elevated in pancreatitis, myocardial infarction, delirium tremens, gangrene, myelogenous leukemia, renal cell carcinoma, eosinophilic fasciitis, measles, malignant hyperthermia, muscle trauma, and strenuous exercise.

Confounding Factors: Erythrocytes contain aldolase, which thus may be falsely elevated with hemolysis. Aldolase values are proportional to muscle mass and may decline with muscle wasting.

Indications: Aldolase determinations are useful in evaluating patients with muscle disease, especially when wasting or weakness is present. Aldolase is less sensitive than creatinine phosphokinase (CPK) in evaluating muscle disease. With the inflammatory myopathies, it may be useful in gauging response to corticosteroid therapy.

Cost: $30–48.

ANGIOGRAM

Description: Angiography is a radiographic imaging technique that uses intravenous or intraarterial contrast media to visualize the vasculature.

Indications: Arteriography is most useful in supporting a diagnosis of vascular occlusion. It is particularly helpful in diagnosing the vasculitides, such as polyarteritis nodosa (mesenteric and renal vessels imaged), isolated CNS angiitis (brain), Takayasu's arteritis (aortic arch and subclavian vessels), and rarely giant cell arteritis (aortic arch and its proximal branches). Irregularities of the vascular lumen (taperings and dilatations), aneurysms, and non–atherogenic appearing occlusions may help establish a vasculitic diagnosis. Characteristic arteriographic findings in the distal extremities are also seen in thromboangiitis obliterans (Buerger's disease). Pulmonary angiography may help diagnose pulmonary embolisms and allow concurrent measurement of right-sided intracardiac pressure useful in establishing the diagnosis of pulmonary hypertension. Venography is occasionally needed as a follow-up procedure to noninvasive vascular studies when a deep venous thrombosis is suspected (such as in the antiphospholipid antibody syndrome).

Cost: Depending on the procedure, $500–1500.

Comment: Angiography is a moderately safe approach to vascular imaging that may provide considerable assistance in substantiating certain diagnoses. All patients should be questioned about hypersensitivity to intravenous contrast agents. Newer digital subtraction techniques minimize contrast load. Careful monitoring of renal function and volume status is needed after all intravascular radiographic contrast procedures.

ANTI–GLOMERULAR BASEMENT MEMBRANE (GBM) ANTIBODY

Synonyms: Anti-GBM

Description: Autoantibodies that react with components of the alveolar and glomerular basement membranes are known as GBM antibodies or anti-GBM antibodies. Recently, the specific antigenic epitopes recognized by GBM antibodies have been demonstrated on the $\alpha3$ chain of type IV collagen.

Method: GBM antibodies, as well as antibodies specifically to type IV collagen are measured by enzyme-linked immunosorbent assay (ELISA).

Increased In: Anti-GBM antibodies are found in Goodpasture's syndrome, which is characterized by pulmonary hemorrhage and rapidly progressive glomerulonephritis (RPGN) (see p. 216). In addition to being a marker for Goodpasture's syndrome, anti-GBM may also play a pathogenic role in causing the pulmonary and renal damage in this disease.

Indications: GBM antibodies are a sensitive test for Goodpasture's syndrome, as they occur in more than 95% of patients. Moreover, they are specific, and they are rarely seen in normal persons or patients with other pulmonary-renal syndromes (see p. 53).

Cost: The test is typically performed in a specialized reference laboratory and costs approximately $125 ($80–180).

ANTI-MITOCHONDRIAL ANTIBODIES (AMA)

Description: AMAs are antibodies to a variety of mitochondrial autoantigen complexes, designated M1–M9; M2 is the best characterized.

Method: Methods of detecting AMAs include indirect immunofluorescence (IIF) using rat kidney tissue substrate. Other methods include complement fixation, ELISA, and radioimmunoassays.

Normal Values: Negative (titers < 1:20)

Abnormal In: AMA is not specific and may be seen in a variety of disorders.

—*Primary biliary cirrhosis (PBC):* Antibodies to M2 are sensitive for PBC, as they are detected in over 90% of patients with this disorder and rarely seen in other diseases or normal persons. Titers in PBC typically exceed 1:160.

—*Autoimmune chronic active hepatitis:* AMAs are found in 5%.

—*Scleroderma:* Subsets of patients with scleroderma (diffuse and limited) may have an overlap with PBC. In such patients the AMA may be positive.

—*Mitochondrial myopathy:* A rare subset of patients demonstrate mild PBC and severe progressive myopathy and are positive for AMA.

—*Other diseases:* AMAs have been detected in some patients with SLE, Sjögren's syndrome, autoimmune thyroiditis, and myasthenia gravis.

Indications: AMA is most useful in the diagnosis of PBC and its differentiation from sclerosing cholangitis, a disease that can be clinically similar. It may be useful in distinguishing between PBC and extrahepatic biliary obstruction.

Cost: $30–100.

ANTI-NEUTROPHIL CYTOPLASMIC ANTIBODY (ANCA)

Synonyms: C-ANCA, P-ANCA, myeloperoxidase (MPO), proteinase-3 (PR3)

Description: ANCA comprises a group of antibodies that bind to enzymes present in the cytoplasm of neutrophils. ANCAs are found in patients with several types of vasculitis and other conditions. These ANCAs may be of diagnostic and prognostic value.

Method: ANCA are assayed using human neutrophils (or monocytes) fixed on a glass slide. Patient serum is added to the slide, and the presence of antibodies binding to the neutrophil. ANCAs are cytoplasm determined by IIF. Because of an artifact that occurs during fixation of slides with ethanol, distinct staining patterns are observed (Table 1). With C-ANCA, a granular, diffuse, cytoplasmic staining pattern is observed. By contrast, P-ANCA exhibits perinuclear staining. An atypical perinuclear pattern sometimes referred to as A-ANCA or X-ANCA may also be observed. The different staining patterns are associated with binding to different antigens.

Abnormal Results

—*C-ANCA:* The antigen associated with C-ANCA is proteinase-3 (PR3); antibody testing specifically for this enzyme can confirm C-ANCA. Positive C-ANCA is associated with Wegener's granulomatosis, particularly in patients with active disease. Depending upon the extent and activity of disease, C-

Table 1
Anti-Neutrophil Cytoplasmic Antibodies

	Staining Pattern	Target Antigen	Clinical Association
C-ANCA	Granular, diffuse cytoplasmic	Proteinase-3	Wegener's granulomatosis
P-ANCA	Perinuclear	MPO, lactoferrin, elastase, cathepsin, other antigens	Microscopic PAN, Churg-Strauss syndrome, idiopathic crescentic GN, inflammatory bowel disease, Felty's syndrome
A-ANCA or X-ANCA	Atypical perinuclear	Unknown	HIV, endocarditis, inflammatory bowel disease

ANCA has approximately a 50 to 90% sensitivity for Wegener's granulomatosis. Moreover, although C-ANCA may be seen rarely in some other vasculitides (e.g., Churg-Strauss syndrome, polyarteritis nodosa), it is relatively specific for Wegener's granulomatosis with a specificity above 90%. In some, but not all patients with Wegener's granulomatosis, the titer of C-ANCA may correlate with disease activity. In addition to being a diagnostic marker, C-ANCA may play an etiopathogenic role in Wegener's granulomatosis.

—*P-ANCA:* P-ANCA is associated with binding to various enzymes, including myeloperoxidase (MPO), lactoferrin, cathepsin, elastase, and others. P-ANCA and particularly MPO antibodies are seen in approximately 60% of patients with microscopic polyarteritis and Churg-Strauss syndrome. P-ANCA may also be observed in a variety of other conditions, including inflammatory bowel disease, polyarteritis, and idiopathic crescentic glomerulonephritis.

Indications: A serum ANCA, MPO, or PR3 assay may be useful in evaluating patients with suspected Wegener's granulomatosis (see p. 381), pulmonary-renal syndromes, or systemic vasculitis. A positive ANCA assay should not supplant use of biopsy or angiography in the diagnosis of Wegener's granulomatosis or vasculitis. In selected patients, serial ANCA testing may be useful in assessing disease activity or the success of therapy.

Cost: ANCA $110–220; PR3 $70–165; MPO $60–165; elastase $160.

ANTINUCLEAR ANTIBODIES (ANAC)

Synonyms: ANA, FANA, LE preparation

Description: Autoantibodies that react with various components of the cell nucleus are called antinuclear antibodies (ANAs). ANA is the characteristic laboratory finding of SLE. However, ANA may be found in patients with a variety of other autoimmune conditions as well as in normal persons. The ANA test defines a population of autoantibodies that react with specific intracellular constituents (Table 1). This is clinically relevant, as the presence of specific autoantibodies may correlate with particular organ involvement and prognosis. Some manifestations are more typical of patients possessing particular autoantibodies, such as the presence of renal disease in patients with anti-DNA antibodies.

Table 1
Autoantibodies[a]

Specificity	Antigen Recognized	Frequency in SLE	Frequency in Other Diseases	Clinical Associations
DNA	dsDNA	50–60%	Very uncommon	Associated with lupus nephritis, severe disease
Sm	U1, U2, U4–6 snRNP	30–40%	Very uncommon	Interstitial lung disease
RNP	U1 snRNP	30–40%	100% in patients with MCTD	Symptoms are an overlap of SLE, DM/PM, PSS
Ro (SS-A)	60-kDa RNA-binding protein	25–30%	70% Sjögren's	Subacute cutaneous lupus, neonatal lupus
La (SS-B)	50-kDa RNA-binding protein	10–15%	60% Sjögren's	
Histone	Histone proteins H1, H2A, H2B, H3, H4	50–70%	≥95% drug-induced lupus	Also common in idiopathic SLE
Scl-70	Topoisomerase I	<5%	40–70% PSS (diffuse)	
Centromere/ kinetochore (staining pattern)	70/13-kDa nuclear proteins	<5%	70–85% in limited scleroderma (CREST)	Raynaud's phenomenon
Jo-1	Histidyl tRNA synthetase	<5%	20% PM/DM	Myositis, interstitial lung disease, arthritis

[a]Abbreviations: snRNP small nuclear ribonuclear proteins; MCTD, mixed connective tissue disease (see p. 256).

Method: The ANA test was superseded by the discovery of the LE cell (a leuko-cyte that phagocytizes a nucleus) in 1948 as the first diagnostic test for SLE. When it was later realized that the LE cell phenomenon was mediated by high titers of antinuclear antibodies, the LE cell test was replaced by more sensitive immuno-fluorescent tests specific for antibodies capable of binding various nuclear con-stituents. Hence, the LE cell preparation is seldom performed any more, but LE cells may be coincidentally found in body fluids (e.g., pleural fluid).

Initially, ANA tests were performed on rodent tissue sections. Of note, some nuclear antigens (e.g., Ro) are absent in rodents, and some organelles (e.g., nucleoli, centromeres) are present in limited numbers in normal tissue. Thus, prior to the mid-1980s there were patients who had clinical manifestations char-acteristic of SLE and anti-Ro antibodies but a negative ANA test. With replace-ment of rodent tissues by the human HEp2 tumor cell as the standard substrate for ANAs, the concept of "ANA-negative lupus" has largely disappeared. The generic ANA test is now universally performed by IIF, using an HEp2 substrate.

Tests for the antigens to which specific ANAs react (e.g., Sm, RNP, Ro, La) can be performed by several methods, including ELISA.

Interpretation: In addition to being "positive" or "negative," the ANA test is quantitatively reported as a titer. The clinical significance of the ANA test often parallels the strength of the titer reported. Typically, positive ANA results are reported in terms of both titer and pattern. Higher titers are more consistent with, but not diagnostic of, SLE. Typically, titers of 1:160 and above are consid-ered positive, whereas titers of 1:80 or less are equivocal and often nonspecific.

The ANA test is also interpreted according to the pattern of nuclear staining observed. These patterns may correlate with different antigen reactivity (Table 1). A *speckled* pattern of immunofluorescence is most commonly seen with the Hep2 substrate but is perhaps least specific. A speckled ANA result is associated with various of the so-called extractable nuclear antigens (ENAs; so named because they can be "extracted" from the nucleus by saline). These include Ro (SS-A), La (SS-B), Sm (anti-Smith), RNP, Scl-70, Jo-1, and many others. Anti-Ro and anti-La antibodies are also observed in patients with Sjögren's syndrome (hence the des-ignations SS-A and SS-B). Anti-Ro may also be seen in neonatal lupus and suba-cute cutaneous lupus erythematosus (SCLE). Anti-Sm is relatively specific for the diagnosis of SLE, as it is infrequent in other diseases or in normal persons. Along with anti-RNP antibodies, SLE patients with anti-Sm may be more prone to de-velop interstitial lung disease. Anti-RNP antibodies were also previously associ-ated with mixed connective tissue disease, or MCTD (now better termed *undiffer-entiated connective tissue disease*). Anti-Scl-70 antibodies are associated with the diffuse form of systemic sclerosis. A *nucleolar* pattern of ANA test is also seen in systemic sclerosis, SLE, and inflammatory myositis. A *centromere* pattern is asso-ciated with the limited form of systemic sclerosis (previously referred to as the CREST syndrome). The *homogeneous* (or *diffuse*) ANA is also very nonspecific and is often associated with antibodies to histones. Such antibodies are seen in SLE, and reactivity to specific histone proteins is characteristic of drug-induced lupus. A *rim* (or *peripheral*) pattern of immunofluorescence is associated with antibodies to "native" or double-stranded DNA (dsDNA). Anti-dsDNA antibodies are useful for the diagnosis of SLE as they are uncommon in other diseases. In addition, patients with high titers of anti-dsDNA antibodies are more prone to develop proliferative lupus nephritis. The titer of anti-dsDNA antibodies may vary with the activity of disease, particularly lupus nephritis, and sequential anti-DNA determination is sometimes used to follow the activity of SLE. Anti-DNA antibodies may be specifically determined by several assays, including the *Crithidia lucilae* assay and the Farr test. Results from these various tests are reported in different units, and it is important to be familiar with the laboratory performing these tests.

Normal Values: Local laboratories should establish positive and negative titers such that less than 5% of normal individuals have a positive result. For most clinical laboratories, an ANA result is said to be negative when the titer is 1:160 or below.

Increased In: ANAs are found in patients with SLE and a variety of autoimmune diseases (e.g., Hashimoto's thyroiditis, inflammatory myositis). A positive ANA result may be seen in patients with chronic liver disease (e.g., chronic active hepatitis, primary biliary cirrhosis), chronic renal disease, chronic interstitial lung disease, and drug-induced lupus, and among intravenous drug abusers. The incidence of positive ANA results is 3-fold higher (15%) in the elderly. In addition, first-degree relatives of patients with autoimmune disease and normal persons (particularly women and older persons) may have a positive ANA result with no associated autoimmune disease.

ANA titers do not generally correlate with disease activity, and there is little value in repeating an ANA test in a patient known to be positive.

Indications: The ANA test is most commonly used in the diagnosis of SLE. It is almost 100% sensitive, as virtually all SLE patients have a positive ANA result. However, ANA are not specific at all, since they may be seen in other connective tissue diseases such as drug-induced lupus (>95% of patients are ANA positive), scleroderma (70–90%), inflammatory myositis (40–60%), and Sjögren's syndrome (75–90%). Moreover, even some healthy persons have positive ANA results, particularly at low titer. The ANA test should not be used to screen patients with joint pain or presumed systemic illness.

Cost: Performed by immunofluorescence on an HEp2 substrate, ANA tests are widely available and typically cost $35–75.

ANTIPHOSPHOLIPID (APL) ANTIBODIES/LUPUS ANTICOAGULANT (LAC)

Synonyms: APL or anticardiolipin (ACL) antibodies, LAC, biologic false-positive test for syphilis (BFP-STS).

Description: APLs are antibodies that bind to negatively charged phospholipids, including cardiolipin. LAC is a functional description of abnormalities in several hematologic tests often found in patients with APL antibodies. Patients may possess all or only one of these laboratory abnormalities in clinical association with the antiphospholipid syndrome.

Method: APL antibodies are detected by ELISA. Such tests may be used to detect antibodies not only to cardiolipin, but also to phosphatidylcholine and other negatively charged phospholipids. Although several antibody isotypes (e.g., IgG, IgA, IgM) can have ACL activity, high-titer IgG ACL most strongly correlates with the clinical antiphospholipid syndrome (APS). Recently, it has been demonstrated that most pathogenic ACL antibodies have binding activity only in the presence of another serum protein, β_2-glycoprotein-I (β_2GP-I). Antibodies that react with β_2GP-I may be important to the thrombotic tendency in APS patients, as they are not seen among patients with nonpathogenic ACL (i.e., ACLs not associated with clinical APS). Moreover, some patients with clinical APS may have antibodies that bind β_2GP-I (which are also detected by ELISA) and do not bind cardiolipin at all.

"Lupus anticoagulant" refers to abnormalities in several hematologic laboratory clotting tests. The name is derived from observations that blood from some patients with SLE clotted more slowly than normal in vitro, suggesting an anticoagulant factor. This was a misnomer, as not only did many of the patients not have lupus, but this laboratory finding was associated clinically with thrombosis rather than a bleeding tendency. To understand this phenomenon, recall that several in vitro clotting assays require addition of negatively charged phospholipids to potentiate clot formation. Antiphospholipid antibodies bind to these phospholipids, interfering with their ability to promote clotting in the test tube. Thus, despite their association with thrombosis in patients, these antibodies demonstrate anticoagulant properties in the laboratory. Currently, several laboratory tests are widely performed that define the presence of a "lupus anticoagulant." A prolonged partial thromboplastin time (PTT) with a normal prothrombin time (PT) is often the first suggestion of such an abnormality. If the PTT does not correct with a 1:1 dilution with normal serum (as expected with a deficiency of clotting factors), the presence of an inhibitor such as the lupus anticoagulant is suggested.

A variety of other dynamic clotting tests are available that are more phospholipid dependent than the PTT. Such tests are also used to confirm the presence of the lupus anticoagulant and include the dilute Russell viper venom time (DRVVT) and the kaolin clot time. Finally, correction of a prolonged PTT by addition of excess phospholipid, as is done in the platelet neutralization test and the hexagonal phospholipid test, suggests the lupus anticoagulant.

Tests for RPR (rapid plasma reagin) and VDRL (venereal disease research laboratory) also identify ACL.

Increased Values: APL antibodies are uncommon in normal persons. Normal values on the ELISA for APL antibodies are defined with abnormal values being more than 5 standard deviations above the mean. This value is designated 10 PL units (these units are known as GPL for IgG antibodies, MPL for IgM, and

APL for IgA). Antiphospholipid antibodies are elevated in most patients with APS. High-titer IgG APL antibodies are most strongly correlated with clinical syndromes. Uncommonly, patients with clinical APS may have abnormalities only on lupus anticoagulant testing or antibodies only to β_2GP-I.

Elevated levels of APL antibodies are seen in patients with SLE. The reported prevalence of IgG or IgM APL antibodies varies from 17 to 60%, with most studies reporting more than 30%. The prevalence of APL is also elevated in patients with RA, being found in approximately 17% of patients (with a range of 4–49%). In other autoimmune diseases, the prevalence of APL antibodies is not substantially above normal. APL antibodies may also be found in a variety of infectious diseases, including syphilis, tuberculosis, and HIV and other viral infections. They may also be found in patients with cancers. In these nonautoimmune conditions, APL antibodies are rarely associated with APS (thrombotic events, etc.).

Abnormal LAC test results are not common in autoimmune diseases. They may be abnormal in patients with dysfibrinogenemia or in patients with other types of clotting inhibitors.

Indications: APL antibodies may be sought in patients with symptoms suggesting APS syndrome, such as recurrent arterial or venous thromboses, fetal wastage, and thrombocytopenia. Testing for LAC and a false-positive RPR may also help secure such a diagnosis.

Cost: Lupus anticoagulant panel $100–190; cardiolipin Abs $100–190.

REFERENCES

Buchanan RR, Wardlaw JR, Riglar AG, et al. Antiphospholipid antibodies in the connective tissue diseases. J Rheumatol 1989;16:757–761.

Merkel PA, Chang Y, Pierangeli SS, et al. The prevalence and clinical associations of anticardiolipin antibodies in a large inception cohort of patients with connective tissue diseases. Am J Med 1996;101:576–583.

Petri M. Diagnosis of antiphospholipid antibodies. Rheum Dis Clin North Am 1994;20:443–469.

ANTI–SMOOTH MUSCLE ANTIBODY (ASMA)

Description: ASMA is autoantibody to cytoskeletal components of smooth muscle (principally actin). The etiology and function of these antibodies is unknown.

Method: ASMA is detected by IIF using smooth muscle tissue as substrate.

Normal Values: A negative result has a titer less than 1:20.

Abnormal In

—*Autoimmune chronic active hepatitis:* Titers are greater than 1:160 in >95% of cases.

—*Primary biliary cirrhosis (PBC):* ASMA may be seen in up to 30% of patients.

—*Other conditions:* Acute viral infections (e.g., mononucleosis), chronic viral hepatitis (especially hepatitis C), other autoimmune diseases.

Indications: ASMA assay may be useful in diagnosing autoimmune chronic active hepatitis and distinguishing it from PBC. The lack of specificity lowers its clinical usefulness.

Cost: $30–100.

Comment: Identification of specific cytoskeletal antigens and their antibodies may improve the usefulness of ASMA tests.

ANTI–STREPTOLYSIN O (ASO)

Description: ASO is antibody to an extracellular streptococcal product, hemolysin O.

Method: A rapid latex-agglutination slide test is currently used most commonly. Older methods used tube dilutions with red blood cell hemolysis. Todd units are expressed as the reciprocal of the last tube showing hemolysis. International units (IU) using newer rapid latex are equivalent to Todd units.

Normal Values: Normal values are below 200 to 240 IU (varies by laboratory) using the latex method. With the older methodology, normal values are below 240 Todd units in adults and 320 Todd units in children.

Increased In: With streptococcal infection, titers peak 4 to 5 weeks after infection (this is usually second or third week after the onset of acute rheumatic fever). Titers are elevated in 80% of patients with acute rheumatic fever and are usually *not* increased after streptococcal skin infection. ASO may be nonspecifically elevated in patients with hypergammaglobulinemia or those with heightened immunologic activity.

Confounding Factors: Titers of ASO vary with age, season, and geography. Higher values are seen in children and in those living in crowded living conditions and in temperate climates. Serum contamination and cross reactivity with muscle sarcolemma can rarely yield false-positive results.

Indications: ASO is useful along with other antistreptococcal antibodies such as anti-DNase B, anti-NADase, anti-streptokinase, and antihyaluronidase to demonstrate evidence of recent streptococcal infection.

Cost: ASO $30–75; DNase B $40–65.

Comments: There is a 90 to 95% likelihood that at least one out of three antistreptococcal antibodies will be elevated in the setting of acute rheumatic fever.

ARTHROGRAM

Description: Arthrography is an imaging technique used to define local anatomy and structures within, or disruption of, the synovial cavity. The arthrogram has been used to evaluate shoulder, knee, ankle, and prosthetic joints. However, it has been replaced in most clinical conditions by MRI or arthroscopy.

Method: Radiopaque (Hypaque or Renografin-M) and/or radiolucent (air) contrast may be used. The double-contrast method is common for examining shoulder, knee, and small joints. Joints should be aspirated prior to injection, and a small amount of 1:1000 epinephrine may be instilled to improve contrast retention and image resolution. The procedure is done with fluoroscopic guidance, and the joint is imaged by radiography, CT scanning, or digital radiography.

Abnormal In: Rotator cuff tears, tendon rupture, meniscal tears, loose bodies, inflammatory synovitis, adhesive capsulitis, and loosening of prosthetic joints can be visualized by arthrography.

Indications: Arthrography is useful for suspected rotator cuff tear, internal derangement of joint (i.e., cartilage or ligamentous tears), evaluation of painful prosthetic joints, identification of soft tissue masses or intraarticular loose bodies. MRI has replaced arthrography as the diagnostic procedure of choice for rotator cuff tears and meniscal tears. It is contraindicated in patients with bleeding disorders.

Complications: Local pain, swelling, subcutaneous emphysema, flare of synovitis, or allergic reaction to contrast agent may occur. Rarely, infection or air embolism is seen.

Cost: $180–300.

REFERENCES

Resnick D. Arthrography, tenography, and bursography. In: Resnick D, Niwayama G, eds. Diagnosis of bone and joint disorders. 2nd ed. Philadelphia: WB Saunders, 1988:303–440.

BASIC CALCIUM PHOSPHATE CRYSTALS

Description: Basic calcium phosphate (BCP) crystals have three main chemical formulae:

Hydroxyapatite	$Ca_5(PO_4)_3OH2H_2O$
Octacalcium phosphate	$Ca_8H_2(PO_4)_65H_2O$
Tricalcium phosphate	$Ca_3(PO_4)_2$

These are normally involved in formation of bone and enamel. Tissue deposition of these crystals is associated with a variety of disorders.

Method: Plain radiography is useful in visualizing calcification associated with larger deposits but is neither sensitive nor specific. Polarized light microscopy is not useful because BCP crystals are too small to differentiate from urate and CPPD crystals. Scanning electron microscopy or transmission electron microscopy, the best means of visualizing BCP crystals, show typical microspheroidal crystal aggregates.

Observed In: These crystals are found in different anatomic sites and clinical disorders.

—*Periarticular BCP crystal deposition:* Calcific periarthritis, calcific tendinitis, and bursitis

—*Intraarticular BCP crystal deposition:* Milwaukee shoulder/knee syndrome, acute BCP arthritis, osteoarthritis

—*Secondary BCP crystal arthropathies/periarthropathies:*

Metastatic: Hyperphosphatemic states (e.g., renal failure, hypoparathyroidism), hypercalcemic states (e.g., hyperparathyroidism)

Dystrophic states: Connective tissue diseases (scleroderma, dermatomyositis), metabolic diseases (e.g., diabetes mellitus, hypothyroidism, ochronosis, acromegaly, myositis ossificans progressiva)

Indications: BCP crystal detection is still investigational.

Comments: It is still unclear whether BCP crystals play a primary role in articular disorders or simply represent epiphenomena.

Cost: Testing for BCP crystals is not routinely available.

REFERENCES

Halverson PB, McCarty DJ. Basic calcium phosphate (apatite, octacalcium phosphate, tricalcium phosphate) crystal deposition diseases. In: Koopman WJ, ed. Arthritis and allied conditions: a textbook of rheumatology. 13th ed. Baltimore: William & Wilkins, 1997: 2127–2146.

BIOPSY

Overview: Tissue biopsy is often a useful means of establishing the diagnosis or degree of disease activity in selected rheumatic disorders (Table 1). Tissue samples may reveal histologic evidence of inflammation, vasculitis, fibrosis, atrophy, necrosis, or infection. For all sites, one must determine how the tissue must be processed before obtaining the sample. This can be accomplished by contacting the pathologist beforehand. Specimens for culture, for example, cannot be put in fixative, and samples that are to undergo immunofluorescent analysis may require freezing rather than fixation. The most useful biopsy sites are skin, muscle, blood vessels, synovium, and nerves, as described below.

Table 1
Indications for Tissue Biopsy in the Rheumatic Diseases

Biopsy Site	Suspected Diagnosis
Skin	Systemic lupus erythematosus
	Dermatomyositis
	Cutaneous vasculitis
	Panniculitis
Muscle	Inflammatory myopathies
	Metabolic myopathies
	Muscular dystrophy
Blood vessel	Temporal arteritis
Synovium	Rheumatoid arthritis
	Mycobacterial or fungal arthritis
	Neoplasms
	Pigmented villonodular synovitis
Nerve	Systemic vasculitis
Kidney	Systemic lupus erythematosus
	Acute renal failure
	Progressive nephrotic syndrome
	Acute nephritic syndrome
	Renal allograft rejection

Skin: Histologic examination of skin using light or immunofluorescent microscopy may be helpful in the diagnosis of SLE, discoid lupus, dermatomyositis, scleroderma, cutaneous vasculitis, or panniculitis. The lupus band test uses skin biopsy to detect deposition of immunoglobulins at the dermal-epidermal junction of uninvolved skin. Although useful in the diagnosis of SLE, the lupus band test is seldom necessary. Inflammation in walls of small cutaneous blood vessels can be used to diagnose cutaneous vasculitis, which is usually of the leukocytoclastic type. While many issues can be successfully addressed using a 4-mm punch biopsy specimen, a deeper, incision wedge biopsy specimen may be required to evaluate some problems such as eosinophilic fasciitis panniculitis. Tissue samples should be taken from fresh new lesions, with an edge of normal skin included. Both punch and wedge biopsies are usually performed by dermatologists.

Muscle: Biopsy of involved muscle is often required to diagnose inflammatory myositis, metabolic myopathies, muscular dystrophies, or vasculitis. The biopsy site should be the most symptomatic area. End-stage or atrophic areas should be avoided. Also, muscles previously used for injection or electromyography should be avoided as they may yield false-positive results. Needle aspiration of muscle is useful for histologic evaluation, and the diagnostic yield may be improved by taking up to four samples from the same cutaneous puncture site. Open surgical biopsies are usually required to obtain sufficient tissue to measure functional enzyme levels for evaluation of metabolic disorders. Contraction of the biopsied muscle should be avoided (as this causes artifact) by using a surgical muscle clamp. The biopsy specimen should delivered to the pathologist immediately (within 30 min) after collection, for proper specimen handling for histology by light microscopy, electron microscopy, and enzyme analysis.

Blood Vessels: Histologic analysis of the vasculature is routinely done whenever tissue biopsies are obtained. Blind tissue biopsies (i.e., muscle, skin, testes) are uncommonly useful in identifying significant vascular pathology. Hypersensitivity (also known as leukocytoclastic) vasculitis (inflammation of venules) is one of the most common vascular abnormalities seen on skin biopsy. Temporal artery biopsy is useful in establishing a diagnosis of giant cell arteritis. The diagnostic yield of the procedure is maximized by taking a large section of vessel (at least 3 cm in length) and examining at least 20 to 25 cross sections. Multiple section analysis is required as "skip" vascular lesions may be missed. This procedure is usually done in the operating room under local anesthesia.

Synovium: As the synovial fluid often reflects processes active within the synovium, synovial fluid analysis is often attempted prior to considering synovial biopsy. Although synovial histology was once used as a diagnostic criterion for RA, this diagnosis is now easily made on clinical grounds without synovial biopsy. However, synovial tissue biopsy is essential for the diagnosis of synovial neoplasias or chronic joint infections such as those caused by mycobacteria, or evaluation of chronic undiagnosed monarthritis. Synovial biopsy may be necessary when synovial fluid is unrevealing or not accessible. Synovial tissue culture is more often positive for mycobacterial or fungal infection than synovial fluid culture. Blind needle or arthroscopically guided biopsies usually yield sufficient tissue for histologic analyses and cultures; open surgical biopsies are only rarely required. Tissue samples are usually fixed in formalin, or in alcohol if gout is suspected.

Nerve: Biopsy of the sural nerve is useful for evaluating suspected vasculitis. The yield of such a procedure is likely to be enhanced in the setting of a foot drop or lower extremity neuropathy. Thus, an abnormal nerve conduction study is likely to improve the diagnostic yield of a sural nerve biopsy. Usually, the biopsy is performed under local anesthesia, at the bedside or in the clinic. There may be residual local hypesthesia present after the procedure.

Kidney: Renal biopsies are occasionally necessary to determine the underlying pathology in acute renal failure, progressive nephrotic syndrome, SLE, acute nephritic syndrome (hematuria, red cell casts, proteinuria, hypertension), and undiagnosed hematuria and to assess renal allograft and possible rejection. Kidney biopsy is not necessarily indicated in all SLE patients with renal or urine abnormalities. It is most helpful in determining whether current renal abnormalities are due to coexistent conditions (e.g., diabetes, hypertension, NSAID therapy) or if lupus renal lesions are reversible (high activity score) or irreversible (high chronicity score). Prior to the procedure, the patient's CBC, PT, PTT, and bleeding time should be checked. Relative contraindications for biopsy may include active infection, uncontrolled hypertension, thrombocytopenia, bleeding diathesis, and pregnancy. Biopsy is usually percutaneous, with ultrasound guidance. The most common complication, gross hematuria, occurs in 5 to 10% of patients and usually resolves in 2 to 3 days.

Cost: Depending upon whether done as an outpatient or inpatient/operating room procedure; skin $150; muscle $250–350; kidney $325–625.

REFERENCES

Velthuis PJ, Kater L, van der Tweel I, et al. Immunofluorescence microscopy of healthy skin from patients with systemic lupus erythematosus: more than just the lupus band. Ann Rheum Dis 1992;51:720–725.

BONE SCAN

Synonyms: Bone scintigraphy, radionuclide scintigraphy

Description: Bone scanning is an imaging method used to detect metabolic, inflammatory, or osseous skeletal abnormalities.

Method: Scintigraphy requires intravenous administration of technetium-99m diphosphate. ^{99m}Tc diphosphate is a bone-seeking radionuclide whose uptake is enhanced by blood flow and bone turnover/remodeling or proliferative bone formation. Patients are assessed immediately postradionuclide (measures blood flow) and 2 to 3 hours later (bone uptake). The procedure takes 3 to 4 hours to complete, and patients need not fast or be NPO.

Normal Results: Normally there is a low level of homogeneous, symmetric tracer uptake in bone. Tracer normally concentrates in the bladder. Normal bone scan is seen in multiple myeloma.

Increased Uptake: Paget's disease, reflex sympathetic dystrophy, osteomyelitis, septic arthritis, infected prosthetic joints, inflammatory arthritis, sacroiliitis, enthesitis, osteoarthritis, metastasis to bone, osteoid osteoma, and osteonecrosis show increased uptake. Whereas early (infarctive stage) osteonecrosis shows no uptake, later (repairative) stages may demonstrate increased uptake. Increased uptake is seen with inflammatory, degenerative, infectious, and neoplastic spinal disease. Occult fractures (including compression or stress fractures) may be found with delayed imaging (72 h).

Complications: Allergic reaction to radionuclide is uncommon.

Indications: Bone scans may be used in the diagnosis of the above-noted conditions. It may provide useful information regarding the metabolic status of bone or detecting infectious or neoplastic involvement of bone and periarticular structures. It may be indicated in total-body skeletal assessments of musculoskeletal disease. Scintigraphy may be useful in the serial evaluation of Paget's disease or neoplastic disease or response to treatment in osteomyelitis. Infrequently, a bone scan may be used to assess patients with persistent polyarthralgia and repeatedly normal joint examinations or radiographs.

Cost: $400–800.

COMPLETE BLOOD COUNT (CBC)

Synonyms: Hemogram, blood count, hematology profile

Description: CBC is a profile of tests providing quantitative measures of red blood cell (RBC), white blood cell (WBC), and platelet indices. The CBC is useful for diagnosis of anemia, bleeding disorders, infection, connective tissue disorders, and neoplasia and to monitor clinical status or response to medication.

Method: Most clinical laboratories use an automated electronic multichannel analyzer with aperture-impedance or laser beam to estimate cell counts, size, and complexity. Venous blood should be collected in a lavender-top tube (containing the anticoagulant EDTA) and gently inverted several times to prevent coagulation. A peripheral smear of anticoagulated blood may be examined with Wright stain to evaluate RBC, WBC, and platelet morphology and relative cell number.

Normal Values: Consult local reference laboratory values.

RBC Abnormalities: See Table 1. RBC indices and abnormalities are defined below:

—*MCV (mean corpuscular volume):* Useful in diagnosis of microcytic or macrocytic anemias, drug effects (i.e., MTX, SSZ, and dapsone increase MCV), or occult alcohol abuse

—*RDW (RBC distribution width):* Measures anisocytosis (variation in RBC size); increased in iron deficiency and macrocytic anemias

—*Heinz bodies (due to precipitated hemoglobin):* Seen in thalassemia, glucose-6-phosphate (G6PD) or pyruvate kinase deficiency, postsplenectomy, drug-induced RBC injury (antimalarials, sulfonamides, etc.)

—*Schistocytes (fragmented RBCs):* caused by microangiopathic hemolytic anemia, DIC, TTP, prosthetic heart valves, hemolysis, severe burn, and snake bite

—*Acanthocytes (spiculated RBCs from abnormal membrane lipids):* Seen with hyposplenism, abetalipoproteinemia, severe liver or renal disease, and hereditary acanthocytosis

—*Target cells (increase in cell membrane in relation to cell volume):* May be artifactual or due to Hgb C, Hgb S, thalassemia minor, iron deficiency, or liver disease, or postsplenectomy

—*Howell-Jolly bodies (precipitated DNA in mature RBC):* Seen postsplenectomy and in hyposplenism, megaloblastic anemia (pernicious anemia), sickle cell, hemolytic anemia, and hereditary spherocytosis

—*Burr cells (regularly scalloped, crenated RBCs):* May be artifactual or due to uremia, GI bleeding, or gastric carcinoma

—*Elliptocytes (ovalocytes, oval-shaped RBCs):* May be hereditary or seen with iron deficiency anemia

—*Sickle cells (due to polymerization of Hgb S):* Seen in sickle cell syndromes (not in S trait)

—*Teardrop RBCs:* Consider polycythemia, myelofibrosis, thalassemia

—*Basophilic stippling:* May be seen in heavy metal poisoning (e.g., lead), severe hemorrhage, or hemolysis

Anemia: Anemia in patients with rheumatic disease may be due to rheumatic disease, coexistent disorders, or the adverse effects of medication.

—*Anemia of chronic disease (ACD):* With ACD, the hematocrit (Hct) seldom drops below 27%. RBC morphology is normal or hypochromic. ACD results from ineffective erythropoiesis due to inability to mobilize and use bone marrow iron (BM) stores. BM iron content is normal. ACD may be present in patients with chronic infection, neoplasia, or active inflammatory disorders such as RA or SLE. ACD does not accompany noninflammatory disorders such as osteoarthritis or fibromyalgia. Therapy should be primarily directed at the underlying disorder. Supplemental iron is of little value.

—*Iron deficiency anemia (IDA):* Commonly caused by GI blood loss (especially with NSAID use) or menstrual blood loss. Morphology reveals hypochromic and microcytic RBCs and low serum ferritin levels. However, normal ferritin levels are seen with inflammatory states, as ferritin behaves as an acute-phase reactant. There is usually an elevated TIBC.

—*Hemolytic anemia:* May be due to hemoglobinopathies (i.e., sickle cell, thalassemia, Hgb C), hereditary spherocytosis or elliptocytosis, paroxysmal nocturnal hemoglobinuria, transfusion reaction, autoimmune hemolytic anemia (i.e., Coombs positive, SLE, viral infection, lymphoma, drugs, idiopathic), prosthetic heart valves, DIC, TTP, scleroderma renal crisis, hemolytic-uremic syndrome, malaria, snakebite, G6PD or pyruvate kinase deficiency.

—*Aplastic anemia:* May be seen with NSAIDs (phenylbutazone, diclofenac, etc.), gold, penicillamine, azathioprine, cyclophosphamide, chlorambucil, methotrexate, viral infections, hepatitis

WBC Abnormalities

—*LE cells:* phagocytic cells that have ingested an opsonized nucleus. Although rarely done or available, they may be incidentally found in joint, pleural, or pericardial fluid. They are found in 75% of SLE patients but also seen in MCTD, RA, Sjögren's syndrome, chronic active hepatitis, primary biliary cirrhosis, and drug-induced lupus or with ANA-inducing drugs.

—*Hypersegmented neutrophils:* With macrocytic anemia

—*Toxic granulation:* Seen with severe bacterial or viral infections and sepsis

—*Atypical lymphocytes:* Seen in viral infections (mononucleosis, mumps, CMV, hepatitis), drug reactions, serum sickness, pertussis, and brucellosis

Table 1
Diagnostic Clues from Hemogram Components

Test	Increased In	Decreased In	Comment
Hgb/Hct	Polycythemia, hemoconcentration	Iron deficiency anemia, anemia of chronic disease, hemolysis	Hgb may be falsely elevated with lipemic plasma or with WBC > 50K
MCV	Drugs (MTX, SSZ, dapsone, Dilantin, estrogen), megaloblastic anemia, liver disease, alcoholism, myxedema, cold agglutinin disease	Microcytic anemia, iron deficiency, thalassemia, sideroblastic anemia, lead poisoning	May be increased (with marked leukocytosis, reticulocytosis, or hyperglycemia) or decreased (with hemolysis or fragmented RBCs)
RDW	IDA, sideroblastic, B₁₂/folate deficiency, alcoholism, liver disease	Thalassemia or ACD (normal or low RDW)	Usually normal or low in ACD; more sensitive in microcytic anemias
Reticulocyte count	Acute blood loss, hemolysis, sickle cell, RBC sequestration; Rx of IDA	SLE, BM aplasia, pancytopenia, megaloblastic anemia, alcoholism, liver disease, chronic renal failure, myxedema	Reticulocytes indicate effective erythropoiesis; useful in gauging response to iron, B₁₂, folate therapy or blood loss
WBC neutrophils	Corticosteroids, epinephrine, lithium, acute infection, seizures, stress, myeloproliferative disorders, leukemia, vasculitis (PAN), Reiter's syndrome, acute gout, septic arthritis, rheumatic fever, adult Still's disease, Sweet's syndrome, Kawasaki disease, familial Mediterranean fever	MTX, azathioprine, chlorambucil, cyclophosphamide, gold salts, NSAIDs (rare), SLE, drug-induced lupus, MCTD, overlap syndrome, RA, Sjögren's syndrome, Felty's syndrome, cyclic neutropenia, bacterial sepsis, viral infection, hypersplenism, aplastic anemia, radiation, CLL, hemodialysis, nutritional deficiency (folate, copper, etc.)	Falsely elevated WBC may be due to clumping associated with monoclonal gammopathy, cryoglobulins, cold agglutinins, or nucleated RBCs; African Americans may manifest lower WBC counts than Caucasians
Lymphocytes	Mononucleosis, viral (EBV, CMV, mumps), pertussis, Crohn's disease, ulcerative	Chemotherapy (azathioprine, cyclophosphamide,	Absolute lymphocyte counts may be helpful in diagnosing

Test	Increased	Decreased	Comments
	colitis, hypersensitivity drug reactions, serum sickness vasculitis	chlorambucil), corticosteroids, radiation, SLE, MCTD, renal failure, myasthenia gravis	certain disorders (e.g., SLE) or gauging response to chemotherapy
Monocytes	RA, SLE, sarcoidosis, inflammatory bowel disease, myeloproliferative disorders, postsplenectomy, SBE, Rocky Mountain spotted fever, tuberculosis, brucellosis	Corticosteroids, acute stress, acute infection, aplastic anemia, myelotoxic therapies	
Eosinophils	SLE, polyarteritis nodosa, Churg-Strauss angiitis, RA, Sjögren's syndrome, eosinophilic fasciitis, Wegener's granulomatosis, eosinophil myalgia syndrome, pemphigus, allergic disorders, asthma, Hodgkin's disease, polycythemia vera, hypereosinophilic syndrome, parasitic infection, inflammatory bowel disease	Corticosteroids, acute stress, bacterial infection	
Basophils	CML, polycythemia, myelodysplasia, Hodgkin's disease	Hyperthyroidism, pregnancy, acute infection, chemotherapy, radiation	
Platelets	Inflammation (i.e., RA), infection, malignancy, sarcoidosis, essential thrombocytosis, polycythemia vera, CML, postsplenectomy, iron deficiency anemia, oral contraceptives	Drugs (gold salts, penicillamine, chloroquine, sulfasalazine, penicillin, heparin, quinidine, estrogen, cyclophosphamide, chlorambucil), infection (EBV, herpes), SLE, hypersplenism, aplastic anemia, ITP, TTP, DIC, radiation, toxemia of pregnancy	May be falsely elevated with cryoglobulins, malaria, or fragmented RBCs; platelet clumping may decrease counts and be caused by EDTA collection tubes, cold agglutinins
MPV	ITP, recovery from thrombocytopenia, myeloproliferative disorders, hyperthyroidism, massive hemorrhage, splenectomy, preeclampsia, smokers, vasculitis	Wiskott-Aldrich syndrome, autoimmune thrombocytopenia, leukemia, hypersplenism	Increased with effective thrombopoiesis.

Platelet Abnormalities

—*Platelet clumping:* May falsely lower platelets but increase leukocyte counts; may be induced by EDTA and large platelets associated with thrombocytopenia

—*Giant/large platelets:* Recovery of thrombocytopenic states, myeloproliferative syndromes, hyperthyroidism, Bernard-Soulier syndrome

—*MPV (mean platelet volume):* MPV is increased with large (young/immature) platelets and with increased platelet turnover. MPV is inversely proportional to platelet count.

Confounding Factors: CBC is rendered inaccurate by hemolysis, hemodilution with intravenous fluids, and hypercalcemia (causes coagulation). Accuracy is lowered when numbers approach critical values (i.e., platelets $< 10,000/mm^3$).

Indications: CBC is useful in evaluation or diagnosis of anemia, infection, connective tissue disorders, or neoplasia, and monitoring the effects of medication.

Cost: $20–30.

Comment: A peripheral smear should be requested and examined when evaluating anemia, suspected hemolysis, leukemia, or thrombocytopenia.

REFERENCES

ARA Glossary Committee. Miscellaneous tests in the rheumatic diseases: A. Blood studies. In: ARA Glossary Committee, JL Decker, chairman. Dictionary of the rheumatic diseases, vol II: Diagnostic testing. American Rheumatism Association. Atlanta: Contact Associates International Ltd. 1985:2–6.
Wallach J. Interpretation of diagnostic tests. 6th ed. Boston: Little, Brown and Co, 1996.

CEREBROSPINAL FLUID (CSF) STUDIES

Description: CSF tests may be used in diagnosing or distinguishing between benign, infectious, autoimmune, inflammatory, hemorrhagic, obstructive, and neoplastic disorders.

—*Method.* The clinician should look for signs of increased intracranial pressure (i.e., papilledema) or perform cranial imaging (CT or MRI) before doing lumbar puncture. CSF should be aseptically obtained, with the opening pressure and appearance of fluid recorded. Routine CSF studies include cell and differential counts; glucose and protein determinations, and serologic tests for syphilis. When infection is considered, microbiologic assays may include gram staining; culture for bacteria, fungi, or mycobacteria; or detection of microbial antigens (e.g.,, cryptococcal, pneumococcal, meningococcal, or *Haemophilus influenzae*) by latex agglutination. With suspected inflammatory or autoimmune causes, oligoclonal bands or quantitation of IgG and albumin may be useful.

Table 1
CSF Findings in Selected Neurologic Conditions

Disorder	Opening Pressure (mm Hg)	WBC (cells/mm^3)	Predominant Cell Type	Glucose	Protein (mg/dL)	IgG Index	Q albumin	Oligoclonal Bands (% +)
Normal results[a]	60–180	0–5	Lymphocytes, monocytes	> 60% of serum value	15–45	< 0.7	< 9.0	Negative
Bacterial meningitis	High	100–10,000	PMNs	Low or normal	100–500	< 0.7	>15.0	Negative
Cryptococcal or tuberculous meningitis	High	50–500	Lymphocytes	Low or normal	100–500	Normal or high	15–100	Negative
Lupus cerebritis	Normal or high	0–50	Lymphocytes	Normal or low	Normal	65% > 0.7	67% < 9.0 33% 9–15	0–40%
Multiple sclerosis	Normal	0–20	Lymphs	Normal	Normal	80% > 0.7	75% < 9.0	> 90%
Neuro-Behçet's syndrome	Normal	> 100	Lymphocytes, monocytes	Normal	Increased	20–50% > 0.7	40% > 9.0	< 10%
Neurosarcoid	Normal or high	100–500	Lymphocytes, monocytes	Normal or low	40–100	25–80% > 0.7	12–80% > 9.0	0–50%
Neurosyphilis	Normal or high	< 100	Lymphocytes, monocytes	Normal or low	40–200	> 80%	>80%	50%

[a] Normal reference values may vary according to laboratory.

—*Q albumin:* Estimates the state of the blood-brain barrier (or the rate of albumin transfer between compartments); requires a paired sample of serum and CSF for analysis

$$Q \text{ albumin} = \frac{(CSF \text{ albumin} \times 1000)}{\text{serum albumin}}$$

—*IgG index:* Calculates the amount of in situ IgG production within the CSF; requires a paired sample of serum and CSF for analysis; tends to be increased in a variety of conditions including multiple sclerosis, neuropsychiatric lupus, and neurosyphilis

$$IgG \text{ Index} = \frac{[CSF \text{ IgG}/\text{serum IgG}]}{CSF \text{ albumin}/\text{serum albumin}}$$

Another measure of in situ IgG production is the IgG synthetic rate. Many advocate this calculation as the more reliable indicator of IgG synthesis.

$$IgG \text{ synthetic rate} = \left[\left(IgG_{CSF} - \frac{IgG_{serum}}{369} \right) - \left(albumin_{CSF} - \frac{albumin_{serum}}{230} \right) \times \right.$$

$$\left. \left(\frac{IgG_{serum}}{albumin_{serum}} \right) \times 0.43 \right] \times 5$$

—*Oligoclonal bands:* Indicate the presence of clonally restricted immunoglobulins identified by high-resolution electrophoresis or isoelectric focusing. Test requires a paired sample of serum and CSF for analysis. Oligoclonal bands are seen in nearly 90% of patients with multiple sclerosis. They are also found in a minority of patients with SLE, neuro-Behçet's syndrome, neurosyphilis, cerebral vasculitis, Guillain-Barré syndrome, and encephalitis.

Normal Values: See Table 1. CSF is normally clear, colorless, and without cells. Blood or RBCs may indicate a traumatic tap or subarachnoid or intracerebral hemorrhage. Xanthochromia indicates hemorrhage.

Abnormal In: See Table 1. Tests should be used selectively to establish/confirm clinical suspicions. Ordering *all* CSF tests is likely to be expensive and provide misleading, rather than diagnostic, information.

Confounding Factors: A traumatic tap alters the reliability of cell counts, glucose and protein determinations, IgG index, and Q albumin.

Indications: In patients with suspected meningitis, encephalitis, subarachnoid or intracerebral hemorrhage, neurosyphilis, multiple sclerosis, neuropsychiatric lupus, primary CNS vasculitis, or inflammatory conditions with suspected CNS involvement (i.e., Behçet's syndrome, sarcoidosis).

Cost: Cell count $20–30; CSF protein $55; IgG index $60–110; antineuronal Ab $140.

REFERENCES

Andersson M, Alvarez-Cermeno J, Bernardi G, et al. Cerebrospinal fluid in the diagnosis of multiple sclerosis: a consensus report. J Neurol Neurosurg Psychiatry 1994;57:897–902.

CHLAMYDIA *TESTS*

Description: A variety of tests are useful in diagnosing infection or past exposure to chlamydial species (*C. trachomatis, C. psittaci,* and *C. pneumoniae*).

Method: Chlamydial infection is best detected by analysis of specimens taken from urethral, cervical, conjunctival, nasopharyngeal, or rectal swabs. Genitourinary (GU) specimens are most reliable when not contaminated with urine. In males, urethral swabs should be inserted more than 2 cm into the urethra. In females, swabs of the cervix/endocervix should be sufficient to collect infected epithelial cells. Serum antibody assays are also available but are less reliable. Available tests include:

—*Enzyme immunoassay (EIA) or direct fluorescent antibody (DFA) testing of urethral or cervical swabs:* Useful and >80% sensitive in diagnosing active infection

—*PCR (using DNA probe for chlamydial RNA):* Very sensitive and reliable; recommended if available. Specimens are collected in special medium provided by laboratory.

—*Culture:* Definitive, difficult, unreliable, 2- to 7-day turnaround time

—*Serologic tests for IgG or IgA anti-Chlamydia* antibodies: Most useful in the diagnosis of systemic infection (i.e., infantile pneumonia, lymphogranuloma venereum, or psittacosis)

—*Infrequently used:* Microimmunofluorescence or complement fixation assays

Positive In: More than 50% of reactive arthritis (Reiter's syndrome) patients have positive results, as do those with nongonococcal urethritis, ocular infections, psittacosis, or lymphogranuloma venereum. Acute and convalescent serum titers may be necessary to prove infection. Titers of 1:640 or above suggest active infection.

Confounding Factors: Recent antibiotic therapy may alter culture but not serologic or PCR results.

Indications: Tests may be useful in patients with suspected reactive arthritis, ocular and urogenital infections, or psittacosis. Serologic or culture evidence of infection may be an indication for antibiotic therapy.

Cost: EIA $70–110; DNA probe $50–80; culture $100–120.

CHOLESTEROL CRYSTALS

Description: Crystals of cholesterol are occasionally found in joints, bursae, tendons, pericardial and pleural fluid, and skin. Two morphologic forms occur: highly birefringent, large, flat, rectangular plates, with notched corners (80–100 μm) and needle-shaped, strongly birefringent crystals (2–20 μm). The former are more common and appear as "stacked pains of glass."

Method: Crystals are best identified by polarized light microscopy but may be seen with ordinary light microscopy.

Found In: Cholesterol crystals are often found in:

—*Synovial fluid, joints, bursae, tendons:* Patients with RA, SLE, OA, hyperlipidemia, chronic tophaceous gout

—*Skin:* Found in xanthomas, cholesterol tophi, calcinosis cutis (scleroderma, dermatomyositis), rheumatoid nodules

—*Pleural and pericardial effusions:* RA, malignant effusions, tuberculosis

Indications: Crystals are usually an incidental finding, and testing is rarely requested.

Comments: The importance lies in not confusing the less common needle-shaped cholesterol crystals with CPPD or monosodium urate (MSU) crystals. They are most often seen in chronic rheumatoid effusions. Their contribution to inflammation and their significance is unclear.

REFERENCES

Reginato AJ. Calcium oxalate and other crystals or particles associated with arthritis: cholesterol crystals. In: Koopman WJ, ed. Arthritis and allied conditions: a textbook of rheumatology. 13th ed. Baltimore: Williams & Wilkins, 1997:2154–2155.

COMPLEMENT

Synonyms: C3, C4, total hemolytic complement activity (CH_{50})

Description: Complement is an organized system of more than 20 serum proteins (mostly made in the liver) that helps protect the host from invading organisms. Historically, the name "complement" is derived from the notion that factors present in the serum "complemented" the ability of immunoglobulin to destroy bacteria. Activation of complement depends on sequential cleavage of individual components. This amplifies the ultimate response and generates many "complement split products," a number of which serve important biologic functions. The complement system is organized into classical and alternate pathways, both of which merge and activate C3 and lead to formation of the membrane attack complex. The cascade is regulated by a variety of inhibitory factors and cell surface receptors.

In the classical pathway, complement is normally inactive in the serum until it becomes activated by immune complexes or antibody-coated surfaces. C1 recognizes either of these and activates the classical pathway components—C4, C2, and C3. C1 esterase inhibitor (C1-inh) regulates the classic pathway and is dysfunctional in hereditary angioedema.

The alternate pathway is activated by endotoxin, bacterial cell wall polysaccharides, and proteolytic enzymes.

Complement is an important part of the antigen-nonspecific part of the immune response and helps control infections by several mechanisms: (a) complement components and complement split products bound to the surface of bacteria function as opsonins, enhancing phagocytosis of bacteria; (b) complement split products C3a and C5a (anaphylotoxins) activate mast cells, leading to recruitment and activation of neutrophils and other cells; (c) the membrane attack complex (C5b-9) can punch a hole in the membrane of pathogens; and (d) immune complexes with complement fragments attached are more easily cleared by the reticuloendothelial system.

Method: Individual complement components (C3, C4) may be directly quantified by such specific immunologic methods as rate nephelometry or radial immunodiffusion. Complement consumption, which is probably the most common clinical indication for complement testing, is best assessed by measuring serum C3 and C4.

The overall complement cascade can be functionally assessed by the CH_{50}, which measures the ability of a patient's serum to lyse foreign blood cells. While this test has the advantage of assessing the function all of the components, it is labor intensive and performed infrequently in many laboratories. Thus, it is best used to indicate deficiency of one of the terminal complement proteins (e.g., in a patient with recurrent neisserial infections and a C5–9 deficiency, C3 and C4 determinations will be normal, but CH_{50} will be very low). In the future, complement consumption will likely be assessed by direct measurements of complement split products (e.g., C3a), which are more specific and sensitive for this purpose.

Normal In: Complement is normal in Henoch-Schönlein purpura, Goodpasture's syndrome, polyarteritis nodosa, and Wegener's granulomatosis.

Abnormal In: While complement is important in host defense, activation of the complement system is detrimental to the host in a variety of diseases. Conditions associated with specific serum complement profiles are shown in Table 1.

—*SLE:* Serial determinations of C3 and C4 are often performed in SLE patients. Depressed C3 and C4 levels may indicate disease activity and tissue damage (e.g., glomerulonephritis). Patients with SLE whose complement proteins are within the normal range may fare better than those with persistent complement

Table 1
Complement Profiles in Various Disease States

Condition	C3	C4	C1	C1-inh (antigenic)	C1-inh (functional)
Immunologic activation of the classical pathway (e.g., by immune complexes in SLE)	↓	↓	↓	N	N
Alternate pathway activation (e.g., by bacterial cell walls)	↓	N	N	N	N
Tissue injury (proteolytic cleavage of C3, e.g., in DIC)	↓	N	N	N	N
Hereditary angioedema type I (85% of cases)	N	↓	N	↓	↓
Hereditary angioedema type II (15% of cases)	N	↓	N	N	↓
Acquired angioedema type I (paraprotein related)	N or ↓	↓	↓	↓	↓
Angioedema type II (anti-C1 inhibitor antibody related)	N or ↓	↓	↓	N or ↓	↓

consumption. Among SLE patients, however, there is a higher than normal prevalence of null alleles for C4; therefore C3 may be a better measure. Immune complex formation further activates the complement cascade and contributes to tissue damage.

—*Other diseases:* Associated with immune complex formation, complement consumption and low serum complement levels are serum sickness, active viral hepatitis, mixed cryoglobulinemia, rapidly progressive and poststreptococcal glomerulonephritis, and infective endocarditis. Low levels may be seen with advanced liver disease. In addition, direct enzymatic activation of the alternate pathway and low serum complement levels may be seen in conditions such as DIC or myocardial infarction. Low complement levels may be seen in IgA nephropathy and hypersensitivity vasculitis.

—*Complement deficiencies:* Deficiencies of the early components of the classical pathway (C1, C4, C2) interfere with the ability to handle immune complexes, which results clinically in an SLE-like condition. Deficiencies of the terminal components (C5, C6, C7, C8) lead to increased susceptibility to infection, particularly with neisserial organisms. Deficiencies or abnormal function of the inhibitor of C1 (C1inh) lead to unrestrained activation of the classical pathway and the clinical syndrome of angioedema.

—*Inflammation:* Many complement components function as acute-phase reactants (e.g., ESR or CRP) and may be elevated in inflammatory conditions (e.g., RA, ulcerative colitis, rheumatic fever, thyroiditis).

Indications: Tests of individual complement proteins such as C3 and C4 are used to assess the activity of diseases characterized by immune complex formation and consumption of these components. Complement assays are useful in diagnosing and monitoring SLE and diagnosing hereditary angioedema.

Cost: C3 $25–70; C4 $25–80; CH_{50} $80–140; C1-inh $60–115.

REFERENCES

Frank MM. Complement in the pathophysiology of human disease. N Engl J Med 1987;316:1625–1630.
Glovsky MM. Applications of complement determinations in human disease. Ann Allergy 1994;72:477–486.

CREATINE PHOSPHOKINASE

Synonyms: CPK, CK, creatine kinase

Description: Creatine phosphokinase (CK) is an intracellular enzyme found in high concentrations in skeletal muscle, myocardium, and brain. Damage to these tissues results in elevated serum levels of CK. Three isoforms are used to determine the tissue origin of serum CK: skeletal muscle, MM; myocardium, MB; and brain, BB.

Method: Analysis may be part of a selected automated chemistry profile or may be ordered separately. Serum should be collected in a plain red-top tube. Avoid hemolysis. All determinations of CK levels should be done prior to invasive diagnostic procedures such as electromyography or muscle biopsy.

Method: Ultraviolet spectrophotometry is most common.

Normal Values: Values depend on the method used but generally range from 50 to 200 U/L for males; values for females are 25% lower. Black individuals (males more so than females) may have CK levels above normal values. Such values do not correlate with muscle mass and are not associated with an occult myopathic process. Normal values are seen in renal or pulmonary infarction, pericarditis, thyrotoxicosis, and steroid myopathy.

Increased In: Most patients with dermatomyositis (DM) or polymyositis (PM) have elevated serum levels of CK. Unless the clinical picture is unclear (e.g., in a patient with chest pain as well as limb weakness), determination of the isoenzyme pattern is not necessary. Although skeletal muscle (MM) is the usual isoenzyme pattern in patients with myositis, elevated MB fractions may occur because of inflammatory damage to, or regeneration of, skeletal muscle, which can express the MB isoform. If CK levels are elevated at the outset of myositis, serial measurements may provide a useful index of therapeutic response.

A significant minority (≤35%) of patients with active DM or PM do not show CK elevations, and in these cases, measurement of other muscle enzymes such as aldolase may be useful. Low levels of CK, sometimes below the normal range, may predict a poor prognosis, especially in patients with malignancy-associated DM. Reasons for the lack of CK elevation in some PM/DM patients are not clear but may include the loss of muscle mass or the presence of circulating inhibitors of this enzyme.

Other causes of CK elevation include alcoholic myopathy, myxedema (hypothyroidism), malignant hyperthermia syndrome, Duchenne's muscular dystrophy, postseizure, eosinophil-myalgia syndrome, late pregnancy (parturition), moderate to severe hemolysis, cocaine use, rhabdomyolysis, CVA, myocardial injury, cardioversion, or muscle trauma. Intramuscular injections and vigorous exercise can also cause CK elevations and should be avoided prior to phlebotomy.

Decreased In: Those with low muscle mass, severe DM or PM, alcoholic liver disease, early pregnancy (<20 weeks), and RA may show low CK values.

Indication: CK may be useful in the diagnosis and treatment of inflammatory myositis, muscular dystrophy, myocardial disease, and rhabdomyolysis.

Cost: $20–65.

REFERENCES

Wei N, Pavlidis N, Tsokos G, et al. Clinical significance of low creatine phosphokinase values in patients with connective tissue diseases. JAMA 1981;246:1921–1923.

Worrall JG, Phongsathorn V, Hoope RJL, Paice EW. Racial variation in serum creatine kinase unrelated to lean body mass. Br J Rheumatol 1990;29:371–373.

CRYOGLOBULINS

Definition: Cryoglobulins are immunoglobulins that reversibly precipitate in the cold (4°C). The reversibility of precipitation by warming the sample to body temperature (37°C) distinguishes cryoglobulins from other cold-precipitable proteins such as cryofibrinogen.

Classification: Cryoglobulins are usually classified into one of three categories, depending on the characteristics of their component immunoglobulins (Table 1).

Type I includes monoclonal antibodies, which can be of any of the major immunoglobulin classes (IgA, IgG, IgM). Such monoclonal proteins may be produced by malignant clonal expansion of B lymphocytes. Monoclonal cryoglobulins are commonly seen in multiple myeloma and Waldenström's macroglobulinemia.

Type II cryoglobulins are referred to as mixed, indicating that both monoclonal and polyclonal antibodies are present. The most common mixed cryoglobulin consists of a monoclonal IgM with rheumatoid factor activity that binds polyclonal IgG. Such complexes are associated with idiopathic mixed cryoglobulinemia, hepatitis C, Sjögren's syndrome, and lymphoproliferative disorders.

Type III cryoglobulins do not contain any monoclonal components and are most commonly associated with connective tissue diseases such as RA and SLE. Type III cryoglobulins are usually present in low concentrations, often with cryocrits below 1%.

Table 1
Classification of Cryoglobulins

Type	Immunoglobulin Components	Other Features
I	Monoclonal only	High levels may be seen
II	Mixed (monoclonal-polyclonal)	IgM-RF often present
III	Mixed polyclonal	Levels usually below 1%

Method (Collection of Sample): Serum samples to be processed for detection of cryoglobulins must be collected carefully to ensure accurate quantitation. Samples cannot be collected during routine scheduled phlebotomy. The laboratory that is to receive the sample must be notified in advance to prepare for processing. Since some cryoprecipitation may occur even at room temperature (22°C), collection must be in a Vacutainer tube prewarmed to 37°C in a portable water bath. The bath can be fashioned from a small covered Styrofoam box or jug with an indwelling thermometer. Blood is drawn into the prewarmed tube, which is then placed in the warm water bath for immediate transport to the laboratory. Samples may be rejected if the specimen has cooled to less than 36°C. Once received, the blood is allowed to clot completely at 37°C. This procedure is designed to keep all cryoprecipitable proteins in the serum rather than in the blood clot. The clotted sample is spun in a warm centrifuge, and serum is removed and placed at 4°C. Samples are usually kept in the cold for 72 hours to allow precise quantitation, although cryoprecipitate accumulation can often be detected visually after 24 hours. The volume of cryoprecipitate is quantitated in a tube similar to a hematocrit tube, and results are expressed as a percentage of the serum volume. High levels may reach values of 10% or more; levels below 1% are difficult to quantitate accurately. Alternatively, the precipitate can be centrifuged out of the cold serum, washed, and resuspended in warm buffer. The amount of protein is then determined spectrophotometrically, and values are expressed as milligrams per total volume of serum.

Typing: After quantitation, cryoprecipitate components may be characterized by counterimmunoelectrophoresis. Specific antibodies are used to detect heavy chains identifying the major immunoglobulin classes as well as the accompanying light chains. Expression of exclusively λ or κ light chains by an immunoglobulin in the precipitate indicates monoclonality. Detection of rheumatoid factor positivity within the cryoprecipitate (tested under warmed conditions) is often useful in characterization.

Normal Values: Values are usually negative (cryocrit < 1%; serum < 80 μg/mL.

Clinical Associations: Cryoglobulins are found in a wide variety of disorders, including infection (e.g., infective endocarditis, hepatitis, EBV, syphilis), autoimmune disorders (e.g., SLE, RA, polyarteritis nodosa, Sjögren's syndrome, scleroderma, Kawasaki's disease), lymphoproliferative disorders (e.g., multiple myeloma, lymphoma, Waldenström's macroglobulinemia), and hyperviscosity syndrome, or it may be idiopathic (essential mixed cryoglobulinemia).

The most clinically important syndromes associated with cryoglobulins are nephritis and cutaneous vasculitis (see p. 185). Essential mixed cryoglobulinemia may demonstrate an acute glomerulonephritis, and patients with this syndrome should be screened for the presence of cryoglobulins in serum. Cryoproteins present a unique appearance in renal biopsies and are usually recognized without special staining. Cutaneous vasculitis with palpable purpura, especially in the lower extremities, should suggest cryoglobulinemia. Biopsy of the rash commonly demonstrates leukocytoclastic vasculitis. Recently, associations of hepatitis C virus infection with type II mixed cryoglobulins have been reported, and this viral infection may represent a significant number of cases previously considered to be idiopathic or essential.

Indications: Cryoglobulin testing should be considered in patients suspected of cryoglobulinemia (i.e., palpable purpura and systemic illness) or those with no known cause for acute glomerulonephritis, severe Raynaud's phenomenon, cutaneous vasculitis, or hyperviscosity syndrome.

Cost: $25-65.

CYTOKINES

Synonyms: Other names such as interleukins, reflect the importance of cytokines in intercellular interactions between WBCs. Other names reflect the predominant cell type from which they derive (e.g., monokines, lymphokines), or the functions with which they were first associated (e.g., B cell growth factor, endogenous pyrogen, or chemokine).

Definition: To perform their functions optimally, cells of the immune system must communicate with each other. Such communication can be accomplished in two ways. Cells may physically touch each other, relaying information via specific cell-surface receptors (e.g., adhesion molecules). Alternatively, cells may secrete molecules (cytokines) that interact with receptors on other cells. Many cytokines are small glycoproteins with varying cellular origins (Table 1) that bind with high affinity to specific receptors.

Role: Cytokines serve critical roles in (*a*) immune reactions (they modulate antigen presentation, activation of immunocompetent cells, and the determination of whether immune reactions are predominantly humoral or cellular); (*b*) inflammatory reactions (cytokines cause recruitment and activation of cells and also initiate the acute-phase response); and (*c*) hematopoiesis (several cytokines promote the growth and maturation of various cell lineages).

More than 50 cytokines and their receptors have been identified, and the range of functions of these molecules expands continuously. Cytokines may exert their varied effects in an *autocrine* (acting on the cell from which they were secreted), *paracrine* (acting on cells in the same area), or *endocrine* (acting on dis-

Table 1
Major Cytokines, Cellular Sources, and Biologic Functions

Cytokine[a]	Major Sources	Functions
IL-1	Macrophages, many other cell lines	Activates lymphocytes, stimulates acute-phase response, CNS effects (fever, increased sleep, anorexia), bone and cartilage destruction, stimulates various inflammatory mediators (leukotrienes, prostaglandins), increases IL-6, activates endothelium
IL-2	T cells, NK cells	Critical autocrine growth factor for T cells; increases killing of tumors by NK cells (creating LAK cells)
IL-3	T cells	Stimulates growth of multiple cell lineages
IL-4	T cells, mast cells	Increases antibody synthesis (e.g., IgE), may inhibit cell-mediated T-cell responses
IL-5	T cells, mast cells	Promotes maturation, activation, and survival of eosinophils
Il-6	Macrophages, lymphocytes	Promotes terminal B-cell maturation, synthesis of acute-phase reactants
IL-8	Macrophages, endothelial cells	A "chemokine," promotes chemotaxis of neutrophils to inflammatory sites
IL-10	Macrophages, T cells	Inhibits synthesis of other cytokines (e.g., IL-2, IFN-γ)
TNF	Macrophages, lymphocytes, endothelial cells	Stimulates acute-phase response, CNS effects (fever, increased sleep, cachexia), bone and cartilage destruction, increases IL-1, IL-6, IL-8, activates endothelium
IFN-γ	T cells	Critical cytokine for macrophage activation, activates endothelium, inhibits humoral response
GM-CSF	T cells, endothelial cells	Stimulates growth of macrophage, granulocyte precursors

[a]Abbreviations: IL, Interleukin; TNF, tumor necrosis factor; IFN, interferon; GM-CSF, granulocyte-macrophage colony-stimulating factor.

tal cells) manner. Cytokines are typically pleiotropic; that is, a single cytokine typically has numerous functions and acts on various cell types. In addition, there is significant redundancy; several cytokines may have overlapping functions. Rather than acting in isolation, cytokines act in an organized network. Some cytokines have antagonistic functions; others are synergistic.

Disease Associations: The role of cytokines in various diseases has been illustrated by demonstrating increased concentrations of certain cytokines in specific conditions. For example, the synovial fluid of patients with inflammatory arthritides such as RA contains elevated amounts of the proinflammatory cytokines interleukin-1 (IL-1) and tumor necrosis factor–alpha (TNF-α). In addition, the efficacy of various immunosuppressive therapies depends in large part upon their ability to inhibit cytokines (e.g., corticosteroids inhibit IL-1, IL-6, and other cytokines; cyclosporine inhibits IL-2). Moreover, specific therapies directed against cytokines, such as anticytokine monoclonal antibodies or receptors, will probably be used for various inflammatory diseases in the near future.

Method: Several of the cytokines listed in Table 1 are available from special clinical laboratories. Most assays for secreted circulating cytokines are enzyme immunoassays performed on serum or plasma.

Indications: Cytokine levels are not clinically indicated in diagnosis or monitoring of patients with rheumatic or autoimmune disease. They are primarily used in certain research situations to evaluate a patient's immunologic status or response to biologically specific therapies.

Cost: These tests are expensive. IL-1 $150; IL-6 $155; IL-8 $255; IL-2 $100; IL-2R $100; IFN-γ $155.

DENSITOMETRY

Synonyms: Single-photon absorptiometry (SPA), dual-energy x-ray absorptiometry (DEXA)

Description: Densitometry is a noninvasive procedure that uses a radiation source to quantitate bone mineral density. This imaging technique is widely used in evaluation of osteoporosis and other metabolic bone disorders. Densitometry is far superior to radiography in estimating bone mass. Newer techniques for measuring bone density that do not use radiation (ultrasound, MRI) are under development.

Method: Bone is exposed to a radiation source (photons or gamma rays), and as the rays pass through the bone, the amount of attenuation is quantitated. Observed results are compared with sex- and age-specific normal values. The differences between observed and expected values may be used to assess the risk of fracture. The most common method currently in use is DEXA, which allows shorter scanning time and is more precise than SPA. SPA produces a radiation dose of 15 mrem and DEXA produces less than 5 mrem. Unlike some other methods, DEXA can be used to assess both trabecular and cortical bone.

Commonly, two sites (lumbar spine and hip) are evaluated. These are common sites of fracture, and each represents a different bone type—trabecular bone in the spine and cortical bone in the hip. The patient is positioned with the hips flexed to reduce the normal lumbar lordotic curvature and a posterior-anterior view is obtained. Vertebral bodies with compression fractures should be avoided. The procedure usually takes 10 to 20 min. Intravenous contrast is not used.

Normal Values: Most equipment reports standards for normal individuals of both sexes in age-specific categories. Results are expressed relative to both the age-matched, sex-matched group and to normal young controls of the same sex. Deviation from these norms is calculated as a *Z-score,* corresponding to the number of standard deviations from the mean. Current FDA recommendations suggest initiation of treatment in women with a Z-score that is more than 2 units below that of normal premenopausal women (not age-matched controls).

Increased In: Z-scores may be increased in rare bone disorders such as osteopetrosis.

Decreased In: Z-scores may be low in postmenopausal women, hypogonadal men, patients with excess endogenous or exogenous glucocorticoids, immobilized patients (or limbs), hyperthyroidism, and primary hyperparathyroidism.

Confounding Factors: Fractures, even in very thin bones, can cause false elevations in calculated bone density. Heavy calcification in the abdominal aorta can confound readings for the lumbar spine. Residual barium may produce significant artifact.

Indications: With the advent of numerous therapies to treat osteoporosis, diagnosis of this condition has become more important, but there is no universal agreement on when to perform densitometry. New guidelines for testing have been developed by the National Osteoporosis Foundation and will be available on their internet site. An initial 2-site DEXA is reasonable for high-risk patients or individuals who have already sustained a fracture. Following initiation of treatment, it is also reasonable to repeat the examination at yearly intervals to determine whether the chosen therapy has been effective.

Cost: The usual cost is $150 to $200 per site. Medicare allots $124 for the entire examination, regardless of the number of sites.

REFERENCES

American College of Rheumatology Task Force on Osteoporosis Guidelines. Recommendations for the prevention and treatment of glucocorticoid-induced osteoporosis. Arthritis Rheum 1996;39:1791–1801.
Lane NE, Jergas M, Genant HK. Osteoporosis and bone mineral assessment. In: Koopman WJ, ed. Arthritis and allied conditions: a textbook of rheumatology. Baltimore: Williams & Wilkins, 1996:153–171.

DNA ANTIBODIES

Synonyms: anti-DNA, dsDNA, native DNA, nDNA Farr assay, Crithidia assay, DNA-binding assay

Description: Autoantibodies that react with dsDNA (anti-DNA or anti-dsDNA) are important in both the diagnosis and the pathogenesis of SLE. Diagnostically, anti-dsDNA antibodies are relatively specific for SLE and are part of the

American College of Rheumatology classification criteria for SLE (see p. 363). The presence of anti-dsDNA antibodies defines a subset of SLE patients expected to have more severe disease. In particular, these antibodies are associated with development of lupus nephritis. The concentration (or titer) of DNA antibodies may give some indication of disease activity when followed serially. Some lupus patients demonstrate higher titers of dsDNA antibodies and lower serum complement levels during disease flares, and conversely, these indices normalize with appropriate medication and clinical improvement. Pathogenically, immune complexes containing anti-dsDNA antibodies can be found in the circulation and deposited in the tissues of patients with SLE. Specific characteristics of anti-DNA antibodies (e.g., their isotype and overall electrical charge) predispose to renal disease. Single stranded DNA (ssDNA) antibodies are commonly found in SLE, but are distinctly different from dsDNA antibodies and are not specific for SLE or associated with nephritis.

Method: Several methods can assess the presence of anti-dsDNA antibodies. The *Crithidia lucilae* assay uses immunofluorescence to detect antibodies binding to a structure called the kinetoplast (that is rich in dsDNA) near the tail of this organism. It has been used for many years and is relatively specific for anti-dsDNA antibodies (antibodies to denatured or single-stranded DNA do not give positive results in this assay). Results are reported as titers (i.e., the highest dilution of serum that still gives positive staining). Other tests for DNA antibodies include radioimmunoassay (the Farr assay) and ELISA. Results from these various tests are reported in different units, and one must be familiar with the laboratory performing these tests.

Increased In: Anti-DNA antibodies are relatively specific for SLE. On rare occasion, low titers are found in healthy older persons or in patients with Sjögren's syndrome autoimmune or infectious hepatic disease.

Indications: Anti-DNA antibodies may be of value in establishing the diagnosis of SLE in difficult cases, determining the prognosis of patients known to have SLE, and indicating disease activity in SLE. These are not absolutes; SLE patients without anti-DNA antibodies may have severe lupus nephritis and vice versa. Also, anti-DNA titers do not correspond to disease activity in every SLE patient.

Relative Cost: The *Crithidia lucilae* assay, Farr assay, and ELISA all cost approximately $50.

ELECTROMYOGRAPHY

Synonyms: EMG, electrodiagnostic studies

Description: Electromyography (EMG) is a diagnostic test used to evaluate patients with suspected muscle disease. SMG is often performed in conjunction with nerve conduction testing (see p. 131).

Method: This test assesses the electrical activity and physiologic function of muscle by placing needle electrodes into selected muscle groups. The procedure does not use external electrical stimulation. Muscle action potentials are produced as waveforms (recorded on an oscilloscope), with specific patterns corresponding to various types of pathologic processes in muscle tissues. EMG is generally performed by specially trained individuals (i.e., neurologist or physiatrist). Since the test is relatively nonspecific, it is important that the clinician provide as much clinical information as possible along with the EMG request to aide in interpretation of the findings.

Normal In: EMG is not useful in fibromyalgia, polymyalgia rheumatica, restless legs, muscle cramps.

Abnormal In: For patients with inflammatory muscle disorders such as polymyositis or dermatomyositis, characteristic EMG findings include (a) generally increased insertional activity and spontaneous discharges (indicating muscle irritability); (b) decreased amplitude and duration of motor unit action potentials; and (c) an increased number of polyphasic potentials. Although none of these findings is necessarily specific for a given myopathic diagnosis, other potential causes of muscle weakness, such as neuropathies, can often be excluded from further consideration.

Indications: EMG is primarily used to distinguish between weakness caused by disorders of muscle (e.g., muscular dystrophy, inflammatory myositis), peripheral motor neuron (e.g., peripheral neuropathy, radiculopathy), or neuromuscular junction (e.g., myasthenia gravis, Eaton-Lambert syndrome).

Contraindications: EMG is contraindicated with thrombocytopenia, severe coagulopathy, and anticoagulant use.

Confounding Factors: If muscle biopsy is contemplated, the EMG needles should be placed on the side opposite the biopsy site, as low-grade inflammatory infiltrates may result from needle insertion. EMG itself may also result in *minor* elevations of the CPK.

Relative Cost: $$$

Comments: While EMG testing is generally considered noninvasive, patients should be told that mild-to-moderate discomfort may be noted. If possible, aspirin and NSAIDs should be stopped (5 half-lives) prior to the procedure.

FUNCTIONAL ASSESSMENT

Synonyms: ACR functional classification, AIMS, HAQ, MHAQ, SF36

Description: A variety of validated scales have been developed to assess the functional status of patients with arthritis. These are of three main types: (a) assessment of functional capacity by either patient self-report or physician; (b) quantitative joint examinations; (c) measurement of performance. Although these assessment tools have been applied primarily in clinical trials of new drugs and evaluation of disability status, they are now being used in clinical practice where functional and clinical outcomes may be easily measured, recorded, and studied longitudinally.

Assessment of Capacity: The American College of Rheumatology (ACR) has devised a 4-class scale to determine the global functional status, primarily in patients with RA. This physician-determined scale is based on the patient's ability to perform activities of daily living including self-care and vocational and avocational activities (Table 1).

Global scales measuring pain or overall functional status may be determined using a 10 cm visual analog scale ranging from no problems (score = 0 cm) to very severe limitations (score = 10 cm). These are often used in clinical trials but can be applied to numerous diseases and situations and can be independently completed by the patient or physician or both.

The most established self-report scale is the Health Assessment Questionnaire (HAQ). A total of 20 items regarding activities of daily living are scored by the patient on a scale of 0 (no problem), 1 (some difficulty), 2 (much difficulty), or 3 (extreme difficulty or unable to do). A shorter modified version of

Table 1
ACR Functional Classification in RA

Class	Description
I	Able to perform all activities of daily living
II	Able to perform activities of daily living and vocational activities; limited in avocational activities
III	Able to perform activities of daily living but not vocational or avocational activities
IV	Limited in all activities, including self-care

Table 2
Modified Health Assessment Questionnaire

Please check the column which is the best answer for your abilities at this time:

AT THIS MOMENT, are you able to:	Without ANY difficulty (1)	With SOME difficulty (2)	With MUCH difficulty (3)	UNABLE to do (4)
Dress yourself, including tying shoelaces and doing buttons?	_____	_____	_____	_____
Get in and out of bed?	_____	_____	_____	_____
Lift a full cup or glass to your mouth?	_____	_____	_____	_____
Walk outdoors on flat ground?	_____	_____	_____	_____
Wash and dry your entire body?	_____	_____	_____	_____
Bend down to pick up clothing from the floor?	_____	_____	_____	_____
Get in and out of a car?	_____	_____	_____	_____
Turn regular faucets on and off?	_____	_____	_____	_____

the HAQ, the MHAQ (Table 2), with 8 questions scored from 1 through 4, has been advocated as easier to perform in usual clinical situations. The MHAQ score is the mean value of these 8 questions. This scale has been very useful in following patients with RA in both clinical trials and practice settings.

The Arthritis Impact Measurement Scales (AIMS) involves a longer questionnaire and has been validated in both RA and psoriatic arthritis. Patients with relatively low educational levels may have difficulty completing this scale without assistance.

A more generalized assessment of overall health is the Short-Form 36 (SF-36) Health Status Questionnaire, which can be administered in person or by telephone and covers general aspects of function in life activities, including social interactions. It has been used in large studies assessing health care delivery as well as in evaluating responses to new treatments in clinical trials.

Various disease-specific questionnaires have been developed. For instance in lupus, the SLE Disease Activity Index (SLEDAI) and SLAM are two indices of activity and severity that have also been used in clinical trials. A questionnaire for patients with fibromyalgia, the Fibromyalgia Impact Questionnaire (FIQ), has been validated and tested in small studies. In those with osteoarthritis of the knee, the Western Ontario and McMaster Universities (WOMAC) Osteoarthritis index is a commonly used, validated functional assessment tool.

Quantitative Joint Examination: Counts of tender and swollen joints are a standard means for measuring disease activity and response to therapy in patients with RA. These indices can also be applied to other forms of arthritis, including osteoarthritis and lupus arthritis. Generally, 66 and 68 joints are scored for swelling and tenderness, respectively. A joint is assigned a value of 1 if abnormal (tender or swollen) and 0 if normal. The sum of these is called the (tender or swollen) "joint count." A tender or swollen "joint score" is the sum of the individual joints scored on a scale of 1 to 3. Joint pain is scored as 0 (no pain), 1 (tenderness), 2 (tenderness with wincing), or 3 (wince and withdrawal). Joint swelling is scored as 0 (none), 1 (swelling, just appreciable), 2 (swelling within normal joint contours), or 3 (swelling outside of normal joint contours). Recent studies suggest that evaluation of fewer accessible joints (e.g., the 28 joint count that examines only the upper extremities and knees) provides as much information as examining all joints.

Assessment of Performance: In RA, the walking time (for 25 or 50 feet) and grip strength (measured using a modified sphygmomanometer) are commonly used functional measures that show correlations with other measures of disease status and are reliable and reproducible.

Confounding Factors: Most validation studies of questionnaires have been done in Caucasian, English-speaking populations. Their applicability to those who are non–English speaking or of low educational levels cannot be assumed. However, some forms have been validated in Spanish and French.

Indications: These assessments have been used in trials of new therapeutic agents, especially in patients with RA. Applications in other diseases such as SLE or fibromyalgia are less well established. Insurance companies, other third-party payers, and disability assessment organizations have begun to use these outcome measures. Thus, their use in evaluating patient outcomes in clinical practice is likely to become more common.

Cost: Time is the major cost involved, but even the longer questionnaires such as the AIMS or HAQ can be completed in less than 20 minutes. Some questionnaires can be completed by telephone or through the mail. A computerized data entry system may facilitate longitudinal and comparative analyses.

REFERENCES

Bellamy N, Buchanan WW. Clinical evaluation in the rheumatic disease. In: Koopman WJ, ed. Arthritis and allied conditions: a textbook of rheumatology. Baltimore: Williams & Wilkins, 1996:47–79.

Hochberg MC, Chane RW, Dwosh I, et al. The American College of Rheumatology 1991 revised criteria for the classification of global functional status in rheumatoid arthritis. Arthritis Rheum 1992;25:498–502.

Pincus T, Brooks RH, Callahan LF. Prediction of long-term mortality in patients with rheumatoid arthritis according to simple questionnaire and joint count measures. Ann Intern Med 1994;120:26–34.

HEPATITIS: SEROLOGIC TESTS

Description: Serologic tests are used in the diagnosis and management of viral hepatitis A, B, and C. Serologic tests are also available for viral hepatitis D, E, and G, but they have limited clinical application in rheumatology.

Method: Methods include immunodiffusion, ELISA, recombinant immunoblot assays (RIBA), polymerase chain reactions (PCRs), and branched DNA assays (bDNA).

Normal Value. Tests are normally negative in healthy persons.

Abnormal In: Serologic pattern varies with hepatitis type and duration.

—Hepatitis A virus (HAV)
- Anti-HAV IgM is detected in acute hepatitis A. It appears with onset of symptoms, is detectable up to 24 weeks, and confirms the diagnosis.
- Anti-HAV IgG is detected after the acute period and persists for life. It indicates previous exposure, recovery, and immunity to hepatitis A.

—Hepatitis B virus (HBV)
- Hepatitis B surface antigen (HBsAg) is the earliest indicator of HBV infection; it appears in 27–41 days, persists during acute illness, and disappears within 6 months with recovery. Persistence after 6 months implies chronic carrier state.
- Antibody to HBsAg (anti-HBs) indicates clinical recovery and immunity to HBV; it appears after immunization against HBV.
- Hepatitis B "e" antigen (HBeAg) is associated with infectivity. It appears shortly after HBsAg and disappears before HBsAg disappears, being present for 3–6 weeks. Persistence beyond 10 weeks suggests progression

Table 1
Diagnostic Approach in Suspected Acute Viral Hepatitis

Screening	Result	Secondary Test	Diagnosis[a]
Anti-HAV IgM HBsAg Anti-HBc IgM	Positive Negative Negative		Acute HAV infection
Anti-HAV IgM HBsAg Anti-HBc IgM	Negative Positive Positive		Acute HBV
Anti-HAV IgM HBsAg Anti-HBc IgM	Negative Positive Negative	Anti-HBc IgG Positive Anti-HBc IgG Negative	Chronic carrier Acute HBV
Anti-HAV IgM HBsAg Anti-HBc IgM	Negative Negative Positive	Anti-HBs Positive Anti-HBs Negative	Convalescence "Window" period
Anti-HAV IgM HBsAg	Negative Negative	Anti-HBs Positive	Convalescence, immune, passive transfer
Anti-HBc IgM	Negative	Anti-HBs Negative	Possible HCV infection

[a]Diagnosis based on screening and secondary test results.

to chronic carrier state, chronic hepatitis. Presence correlates with neonatal transmission of HBV.

- Antibody to HBeAg (anti-HBe) correlates with decreasing infectivity and good prognosis.
- Antibody to core antigen includes anti-HBc total, anti-HBc IgM, and anti-HBc IgG. Anti-HBc total appears early in infection and persists lifelong. The IgM component is found for a short time during acute viral infection and persists during the "window" period (after disappearance of HBsAg and before appearance of anti-HBs) and is thus a marker of recent infection. The IgG component persists lifelong and indicates prior exposure to HBV.

—*Hepatitis C virus (HCV):* Four assays are available for the diagnosis of HCV: ELISA, RIBA, PCR, and a bDNA assay:

- Antibody to HCV (ELISA) reflects actual viral replication and infectivity rather than immunity. Its sensitivity is about 80% in chronic carriers and only about 15% in the first 6 months following acute infection. It is present in several high-risk groups: post-transfusion hepatitis (70–85%), intravenous drug users (70%), hemodialysis patients (20%), homosexual men positive for HIV-1 (8%). Its prevalence in normal blood donors is between 0.5 and 2%.
- RIBA is used as a supplemental test if the ELISA is borderline positive (differentiates false-positive from true-positive results).
- PCR and bDNA assays both measure the amount of HCV. PCR efficiently detects very low levels of the virus.

Confounding Factors: False positives are common with anti-HCV and are seen in many autoimmune diseases, with passive antibody transfer, and with prolonged blood storage. False negatives may occur in early infection and in immunosuppression.

Indications: Serologic tests are used for diagnosis of acute hepatitis (Table 1), screening potential blood donors, gauging the response to therapy in chronic hepatitis, monitoring for immunization, investigation of polyarteritis nodosa (25% of cases, usually intravenous substance abusers, are HBsAg, anti-HBs, or HCV positive), suspected cryoglobulinemia (anti-HCV or HCV-RNA occurs in more than 80% of patients with essential mixed cryoglobulinemia).

Cost: HAVAb $30–73; HB$_s$Ag $25–68; HCVAb $36–60; HCV RIBA $140–190.

Comments: HCV testing continues to improve with newer generations of ELISA and RIBA, with decreasing numbers of false positives. A logical stepwise approach is preferred to indiscriminate testing.

REFERENCES

Wallach J. Hepatobiliary diseases and diseases of the pancreas. In: Interpretation of diagnostic tests. 6th ed. Boston: Little, Brown, and Co, 1996:187–205.

HLA-B27

Description: HLA-B27, one of the HLA-B alleles, is expressed on all human cells and is involved in presentation of antigen to CD8+ T cells. HLA-B27 is often associated with spondyloarthropathies such as ankylosing spondylitis, Reiter's syndrome, psoriatic arthritis, and enteropathic arthritis.

Method: Collect 15 mL of blood into tubes containing acid-citrate-dextrose solution B and mix to avoid coagulation. Do not refrigerate or freeze. HLA-B27 may be detected by a microcytotoxicity assay in which mononuclear cells are exposed to test antiserum and complement. B27 also can be detected by flow cytometry using HLA-B27-specific antibodies.

Normal Values: HLA-27 is a normal gene found in up to 8% of normal individuals (6–8% of Caucasians, 3–4% of African Americans, and 1% of Orientals).

Increased In: HLA-B27 is associated with a variety of spondyloarthropathies. The frequency of this allele is shown in Table 1. HLA-B27 positivity is associated with a propensity for axial disease (spondylitis) and uveitis. The actual risk of an HLA-B27(+) person developing ankylosing spondylitis is estimated to be 1 to 2%. Only 20% of HLA-B27(+) individuals infected with arthritogenic bacteria (salmonella, shigella) develop a reactive arthropathy. Also, only 20% of HLA-B27(+) first-degree relatives of HLA-B27(+) spondylitis patients develop ankylosing spondylitis. B27 positivity may be associated with more aggressive disease in Reiter's syndrome but not in ankylosing spondylitis.

Confounding Factors: There are none.

Table 1
Population Frequency of HLA-B27

Population	Frequency of HLA-B27 (%)
Ankylosing spondylitis (AS)	90
AS with uveitis/aortitis	>95
Reiter's syndrome	75–80
Juvenile spondylitis	80
Psoriatic arthritis	
Peripheral arthritis	<10
Spondylitis	50
Enteropathic arthritis	
Peripheral arthritis	<10
Spondylitis	50
General population	
Caucasians	6–8
African Americans	3–4
Orientals	1

Indications: HLA-B27 assay is used infrequently as a diagnostic test in suspected cases of spondyloarthropathy. It should not be routinely ordered for evaluation or screening of patients with low back pain, because the prevalence of HLA-B27 may be as high as 8%, yet the prevalence of spondyloarthropathy is perhaps 1 per 1000 individuals. Ordering this test is more likely to yield more false-positive than true-positive results. It is diagnostically valuable when the incomplete syndrome is present or when the pretest probability lies between 30 and 70%. It has no value for screening (low pretest probability) or in patients with classic disease presentations (high pretest probability).

Cost: $50–130.

REFERENCES

Shmerling RH, Liang MH. Laboratory evaluation of rheumatic disease. In: Schumacher HR Jr, ed. Primer on the rheumatic diseases. 10th ed. Atlanta: Arthritis Foundation, 1993:64–66.
Taurog JD. Seronegative spondyloarthropathies: epidemiology, pathology and pathogenesis. In: Schumacher HR Jr, ed. Primer on the rheumatic diseases. 10th ed. Atlanta: Arthritis Foundation, 1993:151–154.

HLA-DR4

Definition: The major histocompatibility complex (MHC) locus designated HLA-DR4 was first associated with RA in studies reported by Stastny in 1978. Using the technique of mixed lymphocyte culture, patients with RA were found to be more alike than were normal individuals, suggesting the presence of a shared cell-associated antigen. This shared antigen was later identified on chromosome 6 as a member of the MHC "D" locus, designated HLA-DR4. The DR molecule consists of two transmembrane chains, designated α and β. The β chain shows extensive polymorphisms and is used to identify subtypes of DR4.

Normal Values: The prevalence of HLA-DR4 is highest in northern European Caucasians and lowest in those of Mediterranean ancestry.

Increased In: Studies in diverse ethnic groups show that the incidence of HLA-DR4 is significantly higher in patients with RA than in the matched normal control population. In Caucasian populations of North America, most published series indicate that 60 to 65% of RA patients are positive for HLA-DR4, which is more than twice the incidence of this allele in the normal population. Moreover, the presence of this allele seems to define a more aggressive variant of RA, with a greater incidence of articular erosions, rheumatoid nodules, secondary Sjögren's syndrome, and other extraarticular features of RA. Molecular techniques have been used to identify subtypes of the serologically identified HLA-DR4 molecule that are associated with a significantly elevated risk of RA. These include the HLA-DR4 alleles designated DRB1*0401 and DRB1*0404 as well as the closely related alleles of HLA-DR1 designated DRB1*0101.

- Sequence analyses have further demonstrated that the above alleles known to be associated with increased susceptibility and severity of RA also share a common amino acid sequence at positions 67, 70, 71, and 74 in the β chain of the DR4 molecule. This common sequence has been called the "shared epitope." Identification of the antigen recognized by the shared motif carries the potential to reveal the causative antigen in RA. Furthermore, interference with the pathogenetic binding site through production of blocking antibodies or peptides may offer therapeutic benefit. Studies examining the feasibility of this approach are currently in progress.
- The association of HLA-DR with other arthropathies is weaker but, when present, seems to define individuals with a greater risk of chronic, severe polyarthritis (e.g., Lyme disease, psoriatic arthritis).

Clinical Applications: At the present time, HLA typing is not useful in the clinical management of RA patients. It appears that patients with DR4, especially those with two copies of the disease-related shared epitope, have more severe disease than RA patients without any shared epitope alleles. Nonetheless, patients show significant variability in clinical course, and no predictive or prognostic value has been demonstrated. Therefore therapeutic decisions should be made on the basis of clinical disease features, not the HLA type.

Cost: HLA-DR4 (DRβ1) $110–230; full HLA typing $350–690.

REFERENCES

Olsen NJ, Callahan LF, Brooks RH, et al. Associations of HLA-DR4 with rheumatoid factor and radiographic severity in rheumatoid arthritis. Am J Med 1988;84:257–264.

Weyand CM, Hicok KC, Conn DL, Goronzy JJ. The influence of HLA-DRB1 genes on disease severity in rheumatoid arthritis. Ann Intern Med 1992;117:801–806.

Winchester R. Genetic determination of susceptibility and severity in rheumatoid arthritis. Ann Intern Med 1992;117:869–871.

IMMUNE COMPLEXES

Description: Immune complexes composed of antibody and antigen are responsible for pathophysiologic findings in various autoimmune and infectious diseases. The ability of immune complexes to cause injury depends upon their deposition in certain tissues and subsequent activation of the complement system, phagocytic leukocytes, and other inflammatory mediators.

Deposition of immune complexes in specific tissues depends on a number of factors related to the immune complex itself as well as local factors. For example, the size of immune complexes is critical. Very small immune complexes (typically seen early in an immune response, in states of antigen excess) are readily eliminated and seldom cause tissue injury. Very large immune complexes (usually seen late in the immune response, in states of antibody excess) are efficiently removed by phagocytic cells of the reticuloendothelial system and seldom cause tissue injury. Immune complexes that are prone to deposit and cause injury are often those formed when circulating antigen and antibody are present in roughly equal amounts. Thus, in a immune reaction to a foreign protein, the clinical picture of immune complex deposition may be seen transiently as the immune response switches from a state of antigen excess to one of antibody excess. Other factors that affect tissue deposition of immune complexes include the electric charge of the complex, local blood pressure, and flow patterns (e.g., turbulence).

Methods: Circulating immune complexes may be detected by several methods. Physical methods, such as precipitation with high-molecular-weight polymers such as polyethylene glycol, take advantage of the large size of immune complexes and allow direct quantification of the protein concentration in the complex. Other physical methods include gel filtration, cryoprecipitation, and nephelometry. Immune complexes activate the complement cascade via interaction with the C1q component of complement. Thus, C1q can be used in various assays such as a solid-phase radioassay to estimate the concentration of immune complexes in samples. As they activate the complement cascade, complement fragments such as C3d become bound to immune complexes. Assays such as the Raji cell assay take advantage of this by quantifying the amount of immune complex that binds to cell surface complement receptors. Samples should be sent to the laboratory immediately or refrigerated, as complement and immune complexes deteriorate at room temperature.

Normal Value: Immune complexes are normally not present or not detected.

Clinical Associations: Clinical expression of immune complex disease varies with the tissues involved. For example, deposition of immune complexes in the kidney (e.g., in bacterial endocarditis) causes glomerulonephritis. Serum sickness, a constellation of symptoms that includes arthralgias, arthritis, lymphadenopathy, fever, and urticarial, petechial, or macular skin lesions results from widespread deposition of immune complexes in various organs.

Immune complex formation and deposition play a part in a number of diseases. The relevant antigens include exogenous antigens (e.g., drugs, foreign proteins, vaccines); infectious agents (e.g., bacteria such as staphylococci, streptococci, mycoplasma, treponemes; parasites such as plasmodia, toxoplasma, schistosoma; viruses such as hepatitis B, Epstein-Barr, cytomegalovirus); endogenous or self antigens (as in SLE, RA, cryoglobulinemia, tumor antigens). In some cases, specific antigens may be typically associated with certain end-organ manifestations, such as arthritis associated with hepatitis B or the glomerulonephritis associated with staphylococcal endocarditis. In other cases, many antigens may produce a similar constellation of symptoms, such as serum sickness related to various endogenous or infectious agents.

Confounding Factors: Some rheumatoid factors, cryoglobulins, cold agglutinins, and paraproteins may cause false-positive results.

Cost: Panel $140–250; Raji $80–165; C1q $60–140.

Comment: Immune complex assays are seldom used in clinical practice because they are expensive, etiologically nonspecific, poorly correlated with each other, and slow, as many are performed primarily in reference laboratories. Some investigators and researchers still use these assays as sequential indicators of disease activity in diseases characterized by immune complex formation (e.g., SLE) or to aid in the diagnosis of patients with multisystem disease. Because circulating immune complexes are very efficient at activating the complement system, some investigators use direct measurements of complement proteins or their split products (see Complement, p. 102) to provide indirect evidence of immune complex involvement in disease processes.

IMMUNOGLOBULINS (IgG, IgA, IgM, IgE)

Description: Immunoglobulins are serum antibodies produced by plasma cells and are the major component of the humoral immune response. Measurement of serum immunoglobulins of different isotypes (i.e., IgG, IgA, IgM, and IgE) may be useful in a variety of immunodeficiency, infectious, allergic, and lymphoproliferative diseases.

Method: Serum immunoglobulins are currently measured by specific immunologic methods, such as ELISA.

Normal Values: Concentrations may vary slightly depending upon the laboratory and the particular methods used, but in general, normal values for serum immunoglobulins in healthy adults are as follows: IgG, 550 to 1900 mg/dL; IgM, 50 to 150 mg/dL; and IgA, 60 to 350 mg/dL. IgE is usually present in far smaller amounts.

Serum immunoglobulin concentrations depend on a number of developmental, genetic, and environmental factors, among which the most important is age. IgG synthesized by the mother crosses the placenta in increasing amounts beginning at about 3 months of fetal development. At birth, this maternal contribution to the newborn's IgG stops, and total IgG levels slowly decrease until the contribution from the newborn increases at about 4 to 6 months of age. Levels of immunoglobulins increase throughout childhood, generally reaching adult concentrations by age 12.

Abnormal Values: Values vary according to clinical situation, therapy, and isotype.

—*IgE:* Most methods currently used do not ascribe any significance to very low concentrations of IgE (i.e., normal persons may have undetectable serum concentrations of IgE). Elevated serum IgE concentrations correlate with a proclivity to allergic conditions such as allergic rhinitis, asthma, atopic skin disease, anaphylactic shock, and certain parasitic infections. However, determination of IgE specific for particular antigens is of greater significance in evaluating patients with allergic diseases than measurements of total IgE. Antigen-specific IgE may be determined by in vivo tests such as the cutaneous scratch tests using particular allergens or by in vitro methods such as the radioallergo-sorbent test (RAST).

—*IgM:* IgM usually circulates in a large-molecular-weight pentamer and remains almost entirely within the vasculature and does not cross the placenta. It is the earliest immunoglobulin synthesized in response to antigenic challenge. Decreased IgM levels may be seen in humoral immunodeficiencies such as common variable immunodeficiency (CVID) or in conditions of excess protein loss, such as the nephrotic syndrome. Polyclonal increases in IgM may be seen during the course of various infections or autoimmune disorders in which there is polyclonal stimulation of the immune response. Monoclonal elevations in IgM are seen in neoplastic proliferations of B cells, for example, Waldenström's macroglobulinemia. Because of their large size, IgM aggregates are more likely to affect plasma viscosity and cause clinical symptoms than are other immunoglobulin isotypes. Clinically important IgM antibodies are directed against rheumatoid factor and the ABO blood groups.

—*IgA:* Serum concentrations of IgA reflect the amounts of two isotypes, IgA1 and IgA2. While these are present in roughly equal amounts in serum, IgA1 is the predominant IgA isotype secreted onto mucosal surfaces. This secreted form is an important part of the immune response to pathogens present on mucosal surfaces. Serum IgA levels, therefore, may not reflect the functional status of IgA-mediated responses. Indeed, serum concentrations of IgA below the lower limits of normal, the most commonly observed humoral immunodeficiency, are found in 1/700 persons. While the vast majority of these patients are asymptomatic, decreased serum levels of IgA may also be seen in immunodeficient patients; for example, those with CVID.

—*IgG:* IgG is present in approximately equal amounts in the intravascular and extravascular compartments and comprises nearly 80% of the circulating immunoglobulin. It is the most important immunoglobulin isotype in secondary (anamnestic) immune responses. Total serum IgG represents the sum of the four IgG subclasses (IgG1, IgG2, IgG3, and IgG4), which are numbered in descending order of their concentration in normal serum. Thus, isolated deficiencies of IgG1 typically are evidenced as a decrease in total IgG (as well as decreased gamma fraction of the SPEP). By contrast, deficiencies of IgG3 or IgG4 may be masked within a normal total IgG concentration.

Confounding Factors: Leaving samples at room temperature for hours may result in lower immunoglobulin levels. Radiation therapy, chemotherapy, and high-dose corticosteroids may also lower serum immunoglobulin levels.

Indications: Quantitative serum immunoglobulin (IgG, IgA, IgM) determinations are appropriate for initial evaluation of a patient with suspected humoral (antibody) immunodeficiency (see p. 238). If these are normal but there is a very high clinical suspicion of humoral immunodeficiency, it may be appropriate to obtain IgG subclasses or antigen-specific antibody titers (e.g., serum titers of antipneumococcal antibody in patients who have been appropriately vaccinated). Testing is also indicated in the diagnosis of some paraproteinemias such as multiple myeloma and Waldenström's macroglobulinemia.

Cost: $50–90.

LABIAL SALIVARY GLAND BIOPSY

Synonyms: Labial or lip biopsy, minor salivary gland biopsy

Description: Incisional biopsy of minor salivary glands in the lower lip is useful in the evaluation of xerostomia and the diagnosis of Sjögren's syndrome.

Method: Patients should suspend aspirin or NSAIDs 3 to 7 days before the procedure. This outpatient procedure is usually done by a surgeon, using local anesthesia. The lower lip is everted, and normal mucosa is incised with a 2-cm horizontal incision. At least five minor salivary glands are removed and sent for histopathologic examination.

Complications: Complications include numbness in the lower lip (<1%), local bleeding, infection, and pain.

Abnormal Pathology: A diagnosis of Sjögren's syndrome can be entertained if there is more than one focus of lymphocyte clusters ($\geq$50 round cells in $\geq$4 mm^2 of glandular tissue), with acinar atrophy and hypertrophy of ductal epithelial and myoepithelial cells. The reliability of the biopsy is improved if normal-appearing acini are also seen adjacent to foci of inflammation. Myoepithelial islands may not be seen with minor salivary gland biopsies. Focal lymphocytic sialoadenitis is graded as a "focus score," indicating the number of inflammatory foci seen. A focus score above 1 has a 95% specificity and 63% sensitivity for Sjögren's syndrome. A focus score of 10 or more implies near confluent inflammation.

Confounding: False positive results may be seen with lichen planus or mucosal trauma.

Indications: The procedure is indicated when Sjögren's syndrome is suspected, especially when the clinical presentation is incomplete or other tests are inconclusive or negative.

Contraindications: Coagulopathy, anticoagulant therapy, local infection, mouth ulcers, and sensitivity to lidocaine or epinephrine are contraindications.

Alternative Procedures: Noninvasive procedures include salivary flow rate, sialography, or salivary scintigraphy.

Cost: $80–200 (does not include hospital charges or consultation).

Comment: Positive labial salivary gland biopsy does not imply coexistent ocular inflammation. In patients with parotid swelling, biopsy of the parotid may be considered, especially if other diagnoses (e.g., parotid tumors) are suspected.

REFERENCES

Daniels TE. Labial salivary gland biopsy in Sjögren's syndrome. Arthritis Rheum 1984;27:147–156.

LYME DISEASE ANTIBODY

Description: A serologic test that may be used to confirm the diagnosis of Lyme disease (LD).

Method: Screening for serum antibodies against *Borrelia burgdorferi* is done using ELISA or, less commonly, an indirect immunofluorescent assay (IFA). Additional specificity is provided by western immunoblot confirmation (more than three bands is considered confirmatory). PCR has been used to confirm *B. burgdorferi* DNA in ticks but is not yet standardized for routine clinical use in humans.

Normal Values: This test is normally negative.

Increased In: Specific IgM antibody peaks within 3 to 6 weeks after LD onset. IgG titers rise more slowly and are often present when arthritis begins. CSF antibody levels help confirm neuroborreliosis.

Confounding Factors: Serology may be normal in early disease or with an attenuated immune response to a partially treated infection. Cross reactivity with other spirochetes such as *Treponema pallidum* can lead to false-positive results. False positives also occur in less than 20% of patients with high-titer rheumatoid factor. High serum lipid levels and hemolysis may interfere with results.

Indications: LD serologic testing should only be done when individuals are strongly suspected of having Lyme disease because of (*a*) the low prevalence of

LD in nonendemic areas; (*b*) significant false-positive and false-negative rates; and (*c*) considerable intra- and interlaboratory variation in results.

Cost: EIA $55–100; Western blot $60–120; PCR $130–180.

Comments: LD remains a clinical diagnosis with laboratory studies helpful for confirmation. Half of patients with early LD (ECM, constitutional features) and nearly all of those with late LD (carditis, neuritis, arthritis) or in remission have positive serologic test results.

MAGNETIC RESONANCE IMAGING (MRI)

Synonyms: Nuclear magnetic resonance (NMR)

Description: MRI is an imaging method that uses a magnetic field to detect changes in the spin orientation of hydrogen nuclei, or protons, located in living tissues. Patients are placed within a magnetic coil and then exposed to pulsed radiofrequency waves that cause the protons in tissues to change spin orientation. After the pulse, the magnet measures the time required for protons to return to baseline, which is translated into a signal used to characterize tissue composition.

Methods: Most studies involve acquisition of two or more types of images, the most common of which are designated T1- and T2-weighted. These images use different repetition times (TRs) and sample after different echo times (TEs). The T1-weighted image usually provides greater anatomic detail, but the T2-weighted image is more likely to show common tissue pathology such as inflammation, which is associated with increased free water content.

Confounding Factors: Patients with indwelling magnetic metal cannot be evaluated; this includes those with pacemakers, insulin pumps, sutures or artificial components in the eye, wire sutures in brain tissues, and rods or screws in bones. Most joint replacement components in current use are made of nonmagnetic materials, so these patients can be safely scanned. Wire sutures in areas such as the abdomen also do not present problems.

Adverse Effects: No radiation exposure is involved, and at present, there are no known health risks associated with exposure to the magnetic field. A minority of patients may experience claustrophobia or other discomfort. At times, these reactions require stopping the examination; in other cases, use of sedative agents is required to complete the scan.

Indications: Unlike standard radiographs, MRI can define soft tissues in great detail, so joint structures such as ligaments, tendons, synovium, and articular cartilage can be evaluated. Examples of joint abnormalities that can be delineated with MRI include meniscal tears, ligamentous damage, tendon rupture, Baker's cysts, pigmented villonodular synovitis, and simple effusions. MRI has largely replaced invasive radiologic procedures (e.g., arthrography) in evaluation of rotator cuff and shoulder disorders. Inflammation in muscles can be detected in patients with myositis and related syndromes. MRI may be useful in evaluating the integrity of bone and nerve tissues in the spine.

Cost: $1000–2000. Expense is significantly greater than with other techniques. MRI should therefore be used selectively.

Comment: MR spectroscopy, a related application, is currently a research tool but may be adapted for clinical use. Spectroscopy is useful in evaluation of the biochemical and functional properties of muscle tissues (Park et al. 1994).

REFERENCES

An HS, Haughton VM. Nondiscogenic lumbar radiculopathy: imaging considerations (review). Semin Ultrasound CT MR 1993;14:414–424.

Park JH, Vital T, Ryder N, et al. Magnetic resonance imaging and P-31 magnetic resonance spectroscopy provide unique quantitative data useful in the longitudinal management of patients with dermatomyositis. Arthritis Rheum 1994;37:736–746.

Peterfy CG, Genant HK. Magnetic resonance imaging in arthritis. In: Koopman WJ, ed. Arthritis and allied conditions: a textbook of rheumatology. Baltimore: Williams & Wilkins, 1996:115–151.

MYOGLOBIN

Description: Myoglobin is an oxygen-binding intracellular muscle protein that stores and delivers oxygen to mitochondria. It is found in skeletal and cardiac muscle and may be released into the circulation following damage to muscle cells.

Method: Myoglobin is measured by radioimmunoassay in serum and by dipstick in urine. Myoglobin is chemically similar to hemoglobin and is detected by the usual dipsticks used for urinalysis. A strongly positive hemoglobin indicator on the dipstick in the absence of erythrocytes may signal myoglobinuria and should prompt measurement of urine myoglobin.

Normal Values: Concentration in serum is normally 90 ng/mL or less; in urine, 0 to 2 mg/mL.

Increased In: Myoglobin is released into the circulation following muscle damage, most commonly caused by injuries such as blunt trauma, heat stroke, ischemia, or inflammation. Release may occur during the course of inflammatory muscle disorders such as polymyositis. In some but not all cases, muscle swelling or tenderness occurs.

Elevated serum levels are also seen in patients with overlap disease with myositis, alcoholic myopathy, hypothermia, shock, severe renal failure, myocardial infarction, or recent cardioversion.

Myoglobinuria may be detected in any instance of excessive serum myoglobin and may also be found in those with familial myoglobinuria, transient "march" myoglobinuria, diabetic ketoacidosis, marked hypokalemia, and severe infections.

Indications: Myoglobin is determined to assess the magnitude of muscle damage or the risks to renal function following muscle damage.

Comment: Myoglobin is cleared by the kidney and excreted in the urine. For reasons that are not well understood, myoglobin is toxic to renal tubular cells, and excess myoglobin (myoglobinuria) may cause acute tubular necrosis and renal failure.

Cost: Urine dipstick is inexpensive; Serum RIA $50-100; Urine RIA $90-130.

MYOSITIS-SPECIFIC AUTOANTIBODIES

Synonym: Anti-synthetase antibodies

Description: Approximately 60 to 80% of patients with inflammatory myopathies have autoantibodies. Some of these, such as antinuclear antibodies (ANAs) are seen in other syndromes and are not specifically associated with muscle disorders. However, about half of patients with autoantibodies show antibody specificities that are exclusively seen in association with inflammatory muscle disease. Most myositis-specific autoantibodies (MSAs) are directed against intracellular (usually cytoplasmic) ribonucleoproteins that are involved in protein translation. The most common are a family of antibodies directed against aminoacyl-tRNA synthetases. Antibodies to histidyl-tRNA, also called Jo-1 antibodies, are the most common and most clinically assayed of these "anti-synthetase antibodies." Other MSAs include anti-Mi-2 and anti-SRP (signal-recognition particle) antibodies.

Method: MSAs are detected by indirect fluorescent antibody (IFA) assay.

Normal Values: MSAs are normally not present.

Clinical Associations: Some researchers suggest that MSAs may be more useful in defining clinical subsets of inflammatory muscle disorders than currently used clinical categories, such as polymyositis and dermatomyositis. This proposal is based on observations indicating that the clinical disease course, including mortality rates, is correlated with the pattern of autoantibody expression. Some of these clinical associations are summarized in Table 1.

—*Jo-1:* Jo-1 is seen in patients with polymyositis, interstitial lung disease, and arthritis; 20% of all inflammatory myositis patients are Jo-1(+). Patients with antibodies to synthetases have a higher incidence of interstitial lung disease than patients in the other groups; responses to treatment interventions are intermediate. The antisynthetase syndrome is characterized by the occurrence of inflammatory myositis, arthritis, interstitial lung disease, Raynaud's phenomenon, photosensitive facial rashes, "mechanics (or machinists) hands" (cracked, fissured, hypertrophic changes over the distal fingers), and fever.

—*Mi-2:* Antibodies to Mi-2 are seen almost exclusively in patients with the clinical syndrome of dermatomyositis. These patients tend to respond best to treatment.

Table 1
Syndromes Associated with Myositis-Specific Autoantibodies

Autoantibody	Characteristic Clinical Features	Response to Treatment
Anti-Jo-1 and other antisynthetases	Relatively acute onset; frequent interstitial lung disease, fever, arthritis, Raynaud's phenomenon	Moderate response to therapy, but persistent disease
Anti–signal recognition particle (SRP)	Very acute onset, severe weakness, palpitations (no rash)	Poor response to therapy
Anti-Mi-2	Relatively acute onset, classic dermatomyositis rash, cuticular overgrowth	Good response to therapy

—*SRP:* Patients with antibodies to SRP tend to have the clinical syndrome of acute onset polymyositis without a rash, have variable cardiac involvement, and generally respond poorly to treatment. Limited studies in children suggest a similar clinical pattern in juvenile myositis syndromes.

Indications: MSA assays are primarily used in research to characterize subsets of inflammatory myositis. The utility of anti-synthetase antibodies has largely been investigated at tertiary academic sites, and it is unknown if the same associations will be seen in a primary care practice setting. Since MSAs are relatively expensive, not readily available, and of uncertain prognostic value, their routine in patients with myositis is not recommended.

Cost: Jo-1 $48–120; Mi-2 $150–190.

REFERENCES

Love LA, Leff RL, Fraser DD, et al. A new approach to the classification of idiopathic inflammatory myopathy: myositis-specific autoantibodies define useful homogeneous patient groups. Medicine 1991;70:360–374.

Plotz PH, Rider LG, Targoff IN, et al. Myositis: immunologic contributions to understanding cause, pathogenesis and therapy. Ann Intern Med 1995;122:715–724.

Rider LG, Miller FW, Targoff IN, et al. A broadened spectrum of juvenile myositis: myositis-specific autoantibodies in children. Arthritis Rheum 1994;37:1534–1538.

NAILFOLD CAPILLAROSCOPY

Synonym: Wide-field nailfold capillaroscopy

Description: Easily performed, this test examines nailfold capillary architecture by microscopy. While not truly specific, the test is useful in distinguishing primary and secondary Raynaud's phenomenon. Secondary Raynaud's disease refers to Raynaud's phenomenon in the setting of another connective tissue disorder (e.g., systemic sclerosis, CREST, RA, or SLE).

Method: A clean nailbed from the 3rd and 4th (preferred) fingers should be examined at room temperature using low-power magnification from either an ophthalmoscope (+40 diopters), hand-held illuminating microscope (10–40×— available from Radio Shack), or a wide-field stereomicroscope (12–14×) using a low-voltage lamp that does not heat the skin. Videomicroscopy has also been used. Place a drop of grade B immersion oil, mineral oil, or lubricant gel (e.g., K-Y Jelly) proximal to the cuticle. Look for evenly arranged capillary loops arising from the nail bed with a "hairpin" appearance. There may be finger to finger variation.

Normal: Normal vessels are thin, uniform, evenly spaced, and symmetric in distribution (Fig. 1). Normal capillary loops have a hairpin appearance. Normal vessels are seen in most rheumatic disorders, including fibromyalgia, osteoarthritis, gout, primary Raynaud's phenomenon, and eosinophilic fasciitis. Minor vessel abnormalities and a few avascular areas are uncommonly seen in normal individuals. However, extensive hemorrhage and avascular dropout and bizarre or giant vessels are rarely seen in normal controls.

Abnormal: Commonly seen abnormalities may include absent ("dropout" areas) or dilated capillary loops. Vessel architecture may be described as irregular, tortuous, elongated, bizarre, bushy, engorged, or corkscrew in appearance. Spacing between loops may be uneven or irregular (Fig. 1).

—*Primary Raynaud's Phenomenon:* Normal capillaries are most common and suggest a good prognosis and low risk for future development of scleroderma and related disorders.

—*Scleroderma:* The scleroderma pattern (also seen with CREST and MCTD) is one of enlarged or dilated capillary loops with areas of intervening vessel dropout. Dropout is specific for scleroderma. Tortuous vessels, distortion, or "budding" of capillaries may be seen. Capillary hemorrhages and bizarre vessel architecture are common. The extent of capillary lesions may correlate with the severity of end-organ damage and survival rates.

—*Dermatomyositis (DM):* DM patients are frequently abnormal, with vessel changes similar to scleroderma. Giant, engorged vessels with hemorrhage may be seen macroscopically. SLE patients may be abnormal with corkscrew-appearing capillaries.

—*Others:* Nailfold capillary abnormalities have also been described in patients with diabetes mellitus, RA, psoriasis, and Behçet's syndrome.

Indications: Nailfold capillaroscopy is useful as a bedside aid to the differential diagnosis of Raynaud's phenomenon or an undifferentiated connective tissue disease. Many undifferentiated patients with abnormal capillary findings progress to a fully manifest syndrome. Capillaroscopy may be of some value in documenting the extent of microvascular disease in patients with scleroderma, CREST, MCTD, and dermatomyositis.

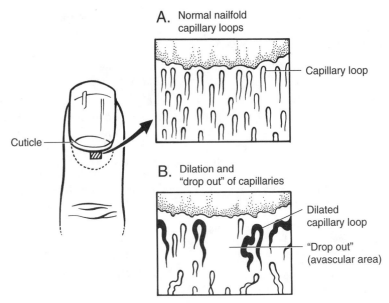

Figure 1. Nailfold capillaroscopy.

Cost: This is a cheap procedure using an ophthalmoscope or hand-held microscope (≤$10); more expensive and sophisticated stereomicroscopic equipment ($2000–3000) is available for office use.

REFERENCES

Kabasakal Y, Elvins DM, Ring EFJ, McHugh NJ. Quantitative nailfold capillaroscopy findings in a population with connective tissue disease and in normal healthy controls. Ann Rheum Dis 1996;55:507–512.
Maricq HR. Widefield capillary microscopy: technique and rating scale for abnormalities seen in scleroderma and related disorders. Arthritis Rheum 1981;24:1159–1165.

NERVE CONDUCTION TESTING

Synonyms: Nerve conduction velocity (NCV), latency studies

Definition: Evaluation of peripheral nerves by nerve conduction testing involves measurement of the velocity of an electrical stimulus in a target nerve.

Method: The test is done by percutaneous stimulation of a nerve at two separate points along its course and recording the electrical response (evoked action potentials) on the skin (for sensory nerves) or an associated muscle (for motor nerves). This test helps to evaluate both generalized and localized neuropathies that might affect peripheral nerves or muscle function. Nerve conduction testing is usually performed by a specially trained physiatrist or neurologist, often at the same time as electromyography (see p. 112). Referrals should include a clinical history and reason for the procedure.

Normal In: Nerve conduction is normal in primary muscle disorders, myastheniagravis radiculopathies, and amytrophic lateral sclerosis.

Abnormal In: Detection of abnormalities in all extremities suggests generalized disorders such as polyneuropathy, mononeuritis multiplex, or Guillain-Barré syndrome. If only localized abnormalities are found, then mechanical problems with nerve entrapment (e.g., carpal tunnel syndrome) or localized inflammatory problems such as mononeuritis multiplex should be considered. Measurements to confirm a diagnosis of carpal or tarsal tunnel syndrome can be limited to the involved extremity, whereas a more generalized problem requires evaluation of all limbs.

Confounding Factors: A cardiac pacemaker (or implanted defibrillator) may influence evoked potentials. Results are unreliable or unobtainable in agitated or uncooperative patients. Results are not affected by medications.

Indications: NCV testing is a noninvasive procedure appropriate for evaluating peripheral neuropathies. Specifically, NCV is useful in determining the extent of nerve involvement (i.e., polyneuropathy vs. mononeuritis multiplex), whether demyelinating or axonal process is present. It is often useful in distinguishing neuropathic from myopathic causes of muscle weakness. Diagnostic findings may occur in patients with entrapment syndromes (e.g., carpal tunnel syndrome), Guillain-Barré syndrome, Eaton-Lambert syndrome, and myasthenia gravis.

Cost: $200–500 per limb. (Cost includes evaluation by the neurologist or physiatrist.)

PROTEIN: URINE

Description: Quantitative tests for proteinuria are commonly performed. Normal persons may secrete approximately 150 mg of protein into the urine in a 24-h period. Albumin constitutes only a fraction of this (15–40 mg); the remainder is composed of many different proteins derived predominantly from the renal cells. The most prevalent of these is the Tamm-Horsfall mucoprotein derived from the loop of Henle, which is made in amounts up to 50 mg/day. Increased amounts of protein in the urine result most commonly from glomerular damage that allows plasma proteins to enter the urine.

Method: Proteinuria is initially screened for by dipstick testing. This colorimetric chemical reaction depends on urine protein concentration rather than absolute amount. Thus results may vary considerably depending on how concentrated the urine is. The test is semiquantitative, with results typically reported as 0, trace, + (or 30 mg/dL), ++ (or 100 mg/dL), and +++ (or >300 mg/dL). Proteinuria can be better quantified with a 24-h urine collection. A close estimate of 24-h protein excretion may also be obtained from a single ("spot") urine sample if the amount

Table 1
Causes of Proteinuria

Glomerular disease
  Minimal change disease
  Mesangial proliferative glomerulonephritis (e.g., IgA nephropathy)
  Focal segmental glomerulonephritis/glomerulosclerosis
  Membranous glomerulonephritis
  Crescentic glomerulonephritis
Glomerular disease associated with systemic conditions
  Autoimmune
    SLE (lupus nephritis)
    Wegener's granulomatosis
    Henoch-Schönlein purpura
    Goodpasture's syndrome
    Amyloidosis
    Sjögren's syndrome
    Microscopic polyarteritis
    Rheumatoid arthritis
  Infectious/postinfectious
    Poststreptococcal
    Subacute bacterial endocarditis
    HIV
  Neoplastic
    Leukemia/lymphoma
    Wilms' tumor
Hereditary proteinuria
Proteinuria associated with drugs
  Intramuscular gold salts
  D-Penicillamine
  Impure heroin
  Amphotericin B
  Aminoglycosides
Benign proteinuria (typically < 2.0 g/day)
  Orthostatic

of protein is correlated with the concentration of creatinine in the same sample. This gives an estimate of the amount that would be excreted in 24 hours.

Individual proteins in a urine sample may be determined by protein electrophoresis (similar to serum protein electrophoresis, see "Serum Protein Electrophoresis," p. 140). This distinguishes proteinuria reflecting glomerular injury (largely albumin) from tubular proteinuria (diverse proteins that migrate in the α, β, and γ regions) from proteinuria related to myeloma (proteins that typically migrate in the γ region). The specific type of immunoglobulin in the urine may be identified by immunoelectrophoresis. Patients with diabetes mellitus often secrete increasing amounts of albumin in their urine as the disease progresses. Albumin present in the urine in the early stages of diabetes is often missed by dipstick. "Microalbuminuria" can be detected by several test reagents now available that allow detection of concentrations as low as 5 mg/dL.

Normal Values: Normally, approximately 150 mg of protein is excreted into the urine in a 24-h period. Amounts greater than 500 mg/day are often considered clinically significant. Excretion of more than 3.5 g of protein is considered massive proteinuria. Massive proteinuria associated with hypoalbuminemia, edema, and hyperlipidemia is known as the nephrotic syndrome.

Increased In: Proteinuria may be seen in a variety of conditions (see Table 1).

Confounding Factors: Dipstick analysis of urine for protein is most sensitive to albumin, so substantial amounts of other proteins may be missed. Because dipstick urinalysis is so dependent on protein concentration, significant amounts of excreted protein may be missed in a dilute urine sample. Analysis of a concentrated early morning urine specimen is one way to address this problem. The common assumption that microhematuria itself causes proteinuria is usually false; 1 mL of blood contains 5 million red blood cells but only 70 mg of protein. When diluted in urine, this usually falls below the level of detection for proteinuria. Thus, proteinuria in the setting of microhematuria (as opposed to massive hematuria) almost always reflects glomerular damage. Lastly, certain drugs may cause false-positive dipstick results (e.g., tolbutamide, chlorpromazine, high-dose penicillin, sulfonamide, cephalosporin, and iodine contrast).

Indications: Determination of proteinuria is useful in a number of diseases. In rheumatology, it is most commonly used to determine the extent of glomerular injury from diseases such as SLE or drugs such as gold (Table 1).

Cost: Urinalysis $13–28; 24 hr. urine protein quantification $25–40.

RADIOGRAPHY

Synonyms: X-ray, conventional radiography, roentgenograms

Description: Radiography is an imaging method used in assessment of osseous and soft tissue structures. Conventional radiography is useful in the diagnosis and staging of articular and osseous disorders.

Method: Symptomatic structures should be imaged from several views to allow a circumferential view of articular structures. Both the imaging equipment and film used in conventional radiography vary, as does the clarity and resolution of films obtained. The quality of radiographs can be enhanced by using faster machines and single-emulsion film cassettes without an intensifying screen. Ensuring patient comfort during the imaging procedure results in more reliable images. Those in pain or with severe deformities that limit proper positioning may have difficulty complying with the imaging process.

Recommended Views: The use of proper technique, patient positioning, and selected views may eliminate the need for further diagnostic studies. The following is a list of commonly requested views during routine radiography. These may be modified in accord with the clinical picture or after consultation with an experienced musculoskeletal radiologist.

—*Hand/wrist:* Posteroanterior (PA) and oblique ("pincer" or "ball-catchers") views

—*Elbows:* Anteroposterior (AP) and lateral views

—*Shoulders:* AP (with internal and external rotation) views; consider axillary view

—*Cervical spine:* AP, obliques, lateral (extension and flexion), and open-mouthed views

—*Lumbar spine:* AP, obliques, lateral, and L5-S1 views

—*Hips:* AP of the pelvis and "frog leg" (external rotation) views

—*Sacroiliac joints:* AP pelvis and AP with 30° cephalad angle

—*Knees:* Standing AP and lateral views; axial ("sunrise") view is best for the patella

—*Ankles:* AP and lateral views

—*Feet:* AP, oblique, and lateral views

Abnormal Findings: A limited number of abnormalities can be identified by standard radiography. Such reports often comment on soft tissue alterations (e.g., effusions, calcification), articular malalignment (e.g., swan neck deformity), bone stock (e.g., osteopenia, osteoporosis), joint space (implying cartilage thickness), changes in cortical bone (e.g., fracture, erosions, osteophytes, periosteal reaction), or subcortical bone (e.g., cysts). A poor correlation exists between clinical symptoms and radiographic changes in many disorders, but this is especially true in osteoarthritis. Findings of osteopenia are nonspecific as it is seen in a variety of inflammatory and metabolic disorders.

Indications: Plain x-rays are most appropriate when there is a history of prior trauma, suspected chronic infection, progressive disability, or monarticular involvement, when therapeutic alterations are considered, or as a baseline assessment for what appears to be a chronic process. Diagnostic patterns of radiographic change may be seen in conditions such as gout, pseudogout, RA, psoriatic arthritis, spondyloarthropathy, reflex sympathetic dystrophy, osteonecrosis, OA, and diffuse idiopathic skeletal hyperostosis. Generalized bone surveys are not routinely recommended, unless evidence of skeletal metastases or Paget's disease of bone is sought. In most inflammatory disorders, early radiographs rarely help to establish a diagnosis and may only reveal soft tissue swelling or juxtaarticular demineralization.

Alternatives: Bone scans (see p. 93), computerized tomography, and MRI (see p. 126) are other modalities often used in evaluation of rheumatic complaints. Such modalities are far more costly and also have limited indications.

Cost: $100–300 (depends on locale and extent).

RAPID PLASMA REAGIN (RPR)

Synonyms: VDRL (venereal disease research laboratory), Wassermann test, reaginic antibody test

Description: The RPR test detects antibodies that bind cardiolipin (so named because they were initially derived from cow heart). Historically, this test was of substantial importance, as results were positive in patients with syphilis. Subsequently, a variety of tests and techniques were developed to check for reactivity to this antigen.

Method: The RPR test is a flocculation test (results may be determined macroscopically or microscopically).

Normal Values: RPR is not normally detected. (Negative results may be seen in early primary and late syphilis.)

Abnormal In: The RPR is sensitive but nonspecific.

—*Syphilis:* The sensitivity of RPR depends on the stage: 75% in primary syphilis, more than 99% in secondary syphilis, and 70% in late latent or tertiary syphilis. The diagnosis of syphilis is suggested by high or rising titers in the correct clinical setting. Alternatively, patients suspected of having syphilis may be assessed using a more specific test for treponemal infection, such as the FTA-ABS and MHA-TP. Patients positive for the RPR but negative for these treponema-specific tests are said to have a "biologic false-positive" RPR. Although not specific for syphilis, the RPR may be a prognostic aid in following the response to therapy, as successful treatment of syphilis should be accompanied by reversion of the RPR to negative after a period of time (e.g., 1 year for primary syphilis).

—*Other:* Positive RPR results may be found in patients with a variety of other diseases, including mononucleosis, leprosy, hepatitis, SLE, and the antiphospholipid syndrome.

Confounding Factors: False-positive results are seen in 2% or less of pregnant women.

Indications: The RPR test may be used to screen for primary or secondary syphilis in asymptomatic individuals with multiple sexual partners, to confirm the diagnosis of secondary syphilis in the presence of syphilitic lesions, to gauge efficacy of therapy, or to identify a biologic false-positive RPR.

Cost: $20–32.

RHEUMATOID FACTOR

Description: Rheumatoid factors (RF) are autoantibodies that react with the Fc portion of IgG. The major immunoglobulin classes are capable of demonstrating RF activity, but the usual routine laboratory assays detect primarily IgM-RF.

Methods: Classically, IgM-RF in serum is detected by agglutination of IgG-coated particles. The source of IgG may be human or rabbit, as human IgM-RF reacts with IgG molecules from various species. The particles may be latex beads or tanned erythrocytes. Addition of test serum in graded amounts (dilutions) may lead to agglutination of the coated particles and a positive result. The most dilute serum concentration that causes agglutination is the titer reported. The Rose-Waler test or sensitized sheep cell agglutination test (SCAT) was used previously. Although less sensitive, it was more specific than current assays. It has been replaced by cheaper and methodologically simpler tests.

Other, more quantitative techniques include measurement of complexes that form between IgM-RF and IgG by rate nephelometry or by capture of IgM-RF on IgG-coated plastic wells, detected using enzyme-linked reagents (e.g., EIA, ELISA). Results from these assays may be reported in international units (IU) using standardized reagents. Normal ranges should be supplied for each assay.

Normal Values: RF is normally not detected.

Clinical Associations: RF is found in a variety of conditions (Table 1).

—*RA:* Approximately 80% of RA patients are seropositive for RF. The remaining 20% of RA patients are said to be "seronegative." Distinction between seropositive and seronegative RA has been considered of some importance, as patients without RF are thought to have milder disease and a less severe disease course. Nonetheless, some of the more severe extraarticular manifestations of RA, such as vasculitis and nodules, occur almost exclusively in high-titer seropositive patients. Treatment with some second-line drugs, notably gold salts and penicillamine, can lower or abolish RF positivity, while others (e.g., cyclosporine) do not affect RF titers.

—*Other conditions:* RF can be detected in patients with diseases other than RA (Table 1). These disorders can be grouped into four major categories: immune system disorders, infections, malignancies, and other miscellaneous conditions. These processes suggest that long-term stimulation of the immune system may lead to production of RF.

—*Normals:* RF positivity is seen in 5% of healthy, young individuals and up to 15% of elderly individuals. These "normal" individuals are not more likely to develop RA or arthritis. More-sensitive techniques (RIA, ELISA) can demonstrate RF production by mitogen-stimulated blood mononuclear cells from normal individuals, indicating that this autoantibody is part of the normal immune repertoire. Furthermore, sequences encoding immunoglobulins with RF activity exist in the normal human genome. These findings suggest that RF has an important role in the normal immune response, perhaps enhancing clearance of infectious agents or senescent cells from the circulation.

Confounding Factors: Prevalence of RF positivity increases with age. Some patients with cryoglobulinemia or very high lipid levels may demonstrate RF activity.

Table 1
Conditions Associated with Rheumatoid Factor Positivity

Immune system disorders
   Rheumatoid arthritis
   Sjögren's syndrome
   Systemic lupus erythematosus
   Sarcoidosis
   Waldenström's macroglobulinemia
Infectious diseases
   Subacute bacterial endocarditis
   Tuberculosis
   Leprosy
   Syphilis
   Lyme disease
   Viral infections
   Parasitic diseases (e.g., leishmaniasis)
Malignancies
   Leukemias
   Lymphomas
Miscellaneous conditions
   Elderly individuals
   Interstitial pulmonary fibrosis
   Chronic liver disease
   Chronic renal disease

Indications: RF is not specific for RA but can be seen in a wide variety of other conditions. Therefore, RF measurement should be ordered intelligently and reserved for individuals with possible RA based on the history and physical examination. Even in these situations, RF positivity should not be overinterpreted. RF should only be used as a confirmatory, rather than screening, test. For example, in patients with arthralgia only and a low pretest probability (i.e., 1%) of having RA, a positive RF result has a positive predictive value of 7% (only 7 patients in 100 with a positive result are likely to have RA). Conversely, in patients with new-onset symmetric polyarthritis of the knees and wrists and a moderate likelihood (pretest probability = 50%) of having RA, a positive test result has a positive predictive value of 89% (89 in 100 patients are likely to have RA).

Cost: $30–55.

Comment: High levels of RF somewhat increase the specificity of the RA test but do not correlate with more severe disease or with fluctuations of disease activity in an individual patient. Therefore, measurement of serial RF levels is rarely, if ever, indicated. Exceptions are during the first year of disease, when conversion from seronegativity to seropositivity may occur or with long-term use of some second-line drugs (as noted above), when conversion to seronegativity may correlate with a good therapeutic response. Some of the very highest RF titers are seen not in patients with RA but in those with other disorders such as Sjögren's syndrome, macroglobulinemias, or leishmaniasis. In these patients, titers may exceed 1:10,000 using the latex agglutination test.

REFERENCES

Carson DA, Chen PP, Kipps TJ. New roles for rheumatoid factor. J Clin Invest 1991;87:379–383.
Koopman WJ, Schrohenloher RE. In vitro synthesis of IgM rheumatoid factor by lymphocytes from healthy adults. Arthritis Rheum 1980;33:1340–1346.

ROSE-BENGAL STAIN

Description: Rose bengal, a vital stain that detects dead or dying cells, is used to evaluate corneal abnormalities in patients with symptomatic or suspected keratoconjunctivitis sicca.

Method: This test is performed by an ophthalmologist. After instillation of a topical anesthetic, the dye is introduced using sterile paper strips, and corneal staining is observed with a slit lamp.

Normal Results: A normal cornea does not take up the stain.

Abnormal Results: A punctate pattern of staining in the interpalpebral area is characteristic of the sicca syndrome.

Indications: Patients appropriate for referral include those with symptomatic dry eyes, usually manifested by a foreign body sensation, redness or pain; the patient may also note decreased tear formation. However, it is also likely that symptoms do not correlate with the ocular findings in some patients. Loss of the normal tear film can result in ocular problems such as infections, and thus, establishing a diagnosis allows institution of appropriate treatment and preventative measures. Keratoconjunctivitis sicca has multiple causes including inflammatory conditions such as Sjögren's syndrome (primary or secondary). Diminished tear secretion also occurs with normal aging.

Cost: $200–350. (Cost includes procedure and ophthalmology consultation.)

SCHIRMER'S TEST

Description: Schirmer's test is a simple, crude measure of ocular tear formation and is useful in evaluating patients with dry eye symptoms.

Method: Standardized, commercially available strips of filter paper are folded 5 mm from the end (usually indicated by a notch), and the short end of the fold is placed inside the lower palpebral-conjunctival sac. Normal tear formation spontaneously wets this strip, which will extend downward (at least 15 mm from the eyelid) over a period of 5 minutes. For most normal individuals, this amount of wetting actually occurs in far less than the suggested time. Less than 15 mm of wetting suggests deficient tear formation. This test is most commonly carried out by an ophthalmologist, although other physicians may perform it at bedside or in the clinic if the calibrated Schirmer's strips are available.

Abnormal In: Moistening less than 5 mm of filter paper is consistent with Sjögren's syndrome and keratoconjunctivitis sicca (KCS). A positive Schirmer's test result suggests, but is not diagnostic of, KCS and should be confirmed with a rose bengal dye test. Moistening of 5–10 mm is equivocal and may require further testing.

Indications: Schirmer's test is used for evaluation of suspected Sjögren's syndrome or dry eye syndrome (due to medications, blepharitis, allergies, autoimmune disorders, etc.)

Cost: Schirmer's strips can be purchased for less than $20.

Comment: Patients should discontinue artificial tear use prior to the procedure. Although topical anesthetic is not required for this test, some patients may find the strip uncomfortable in the eye unless an anesthetic is used. More-sensitive measures of tear formation include fluorescein dye staining and rose bengal staining.

SERUM PROTEIN ELECTROPHORESIS (SPEP)

Definition: SPEP measures the major blood proteins, albumin and globulins.

Method: Because proteins are heterogeneous in surface charge and size, they can be separated electrochemically. In zone electrophoresis, serum is placed on an inert surface such as cellulose acetate and exposed to an electrical current. Different proteins in the serum will move at different rates, thus migrating to different locations where they can be quantified. When proteins are present in normal concentrations, this yields the familiar pattern of SPEP that includes albumin and the globulins (α_1, α_2, β, and γ). α-Globulins include the acute-phase proteins. Immunoglobulins, (IgG, IgA, and IgM) migrate predominantly in the γ-globulin fraction and to a lesser extent in the β fraction (particularly IgM).

Normal Values: Variation may occur between laboratories. Total protein ranges from 6.6 to 7.9 g/dL; albumin, 3.3 to 4.5 g/dL; α_1, 0.1 to 0.4 g/dL; α_2, 0.5 to 1.0 g/dL; β, 0.7 to 1.2 g/dL; and γ, 0.5 to 1.6 g/dL.

Abnormal Findings: Analysis of the individual subfractions on the SPEP may yield important information about several disease states.

Total protein. A decrease in all protein fractions (which would also be seen as a decrease in total protein on chemistry profile) occurs during massive protein loss, typically from the kidney or gastrointestinal tract. An increase in total protein may result from increases in individual fractions, especially the γ-globulins. Increased protein levels are seen in chronic inflammatory diseases, infections, liver disease, and dehydration.

—*Albumin.* Decreases in albumin may be seen with renal diseases, particularly those associated with membranous glomerular lesions and resultant proteinuria. In such cases, there may be a compensatory increase in proteins in other fractions. Hypoalbuminemia may also be seen in severe liver disease, reflecting impaired synthetic capacity, and as a result of major dermatologic burns. α_1-Antitrypsin constitutes a substantial portion of the α_1-globulin fraction of the SPEP; thus decreases in this fraction may signal α_1-antitrypsin deficiency.

—*α-Globulins.* Various proteins synthesized during the acute-phase response migrate in the α_1-globulin fraction; therefore, this fraction increases in patients with inflammatory diseases, infections, or malignancies. Increases in the α_2-globulin fraction, which encompasses proteins such as haptoglobin, are commonly seen in patients with hypoalbuminemia; for example, secondary to the nephrotic syndrome.

—*γ-Globulins.* Decreases in γ-globulins reflect decreases in IgG, the immunoglobulin present in largest quantity. Decreases in IgG, or hypogammaglobulinemia, may indicate immunodeficiency of the antibody-mediated component of the immune response. Likewise, increases in the γ-globulin fraction largely reflect increases in serum IgG. When this increase is polyclonal (indicated by a diffuse "hump" on the SPEP), it often reflects a response to infection or an autoimmune disease. When a single clone of B cells produces excess amounts of IgG, as in multiple myeloma, the IgG molecules are identical and thus yield a sharp "spike" on SPEP. The immunoglobulin molecules can be specifically identified by immunoelectrophoresis (IEP).

—*Other Uses:* Urine protein electrophoresis (UPEP) is particularly useful in detecting light chains (Bence Jones proteins) secreted by some myelomas. Electrophoretic analysis of CSF for oligoclonal protein bands is used to support the diagnosis of multiple sclerosis.

Indications: SPEP is frequently used in the evaluation of weight loss, fever of unknown origin, hypoalbuminemia, elevated serum protein, or suspected multiple myeloma malignancy, autoimmune disease, or malnutrition.

Cost: $35–45.

URIC ACID

Synonyms: Urate, monosodium urate (MSU)

Description: Uric acid is the end product of purine metabolism and is excreted in the urine. It is primarily used in the diagnosis of gout. Uric acid is not soluble at a pH below 7.4.

Method: Uric acid may be measured singly or as part of an automated chemistry panel. These automated enzymatic methods depend on generation of peroxide during oxidation of urate by uricase.

Normal Values: In men, serum uric acid levels rise during childhood and reach adult levels following puberty. In women, urate levels remain constant until after menopause, when they rise (as does the incidence of gout). Gender differences are due to estrogen, which exerts a uricosuric effect. Although normal values vary between laboratories, serum values in men range from 4.0 to 8.6 mg/dL and in women from 3.0 to 5.9 mg/dL. Urinary uric acid levels are normally below 750 mg/24 h. Urinary levels above 750 mg/24 h in gout (or >1100 mg/24 h in asymptomatic hyperuricemia) indicates the patient is a urate overproducer and may need allopurinol therapy.

Abnormal In: Serum uric acid values may be abnormally high or low (Table 1). Although hyperuricemia may indicate gout, levels do not correlate with the severity of disease. Hyperuricemia levels above 9 mg/dL are associated with increased risk of gout and nephrolithiasis. Nonetheless, treatment of asymptomatic hyperuricemia may not be necessary until values are above 13 mg/dL in men or 10 mg/dL in women. Although nearly all patients with gout demonstrate hyperuricemia at some time during their illness, up to 40% of patients having an acute gouty attack have normal serum uric acid levels.

Indications: Serum uric acid assays are most useful in monitoring the response to treatment in gout, renal failure, neoplasia or during chemotherapy; 24-h urinary uric acid determinations may be valuable in assessing the risk of nephrolithiasis or in making therapeutic decisions in gout (e.g., whether to treat with probenecid or allopurinol).

Table 1
Abnormalities of Serum Uric Acid

Increased Values	Decreased Values
Renal failure	Drugs
Gout	Adrenocorticotropic hormone
Asymptomatic hyperuricemia	Uricosuric drugs (sulfinpyrazone,
Increased purine turnover	probenecid, high-dose salicylates)
Lymphoproliferative disorders	Allopurinol
Myeloproliferative disorders	Wilson's disease
Chemotherapy or radiotherapy	Fanconi's syndrome
Hemolytic anemia	
Toxemia of pregnancy	
Psoriasis	
Drugs	
Diuretics (except p spironolactone)	
Low-dose salicylates	
Ethanol	
Diet: Purine-rich foods (meat, legumes)	
Metabolic acidosis	
Lead poisoning	
Hypoparathyroidism	
Primary hyperparathyroidism	
Hypothyroidism	
Sarcoidosis	

Cost: $15–30.

Comments: Urinary uric acid determinations are most reliable when the patient is on a low-purine diet and not taking uricosuric drugs. Serum uric acid levels are labile and vary from day to day.

REFERENCES

Wallach J. Core blood analytes: alterations by diseases. In: Interpretation of diagnostic tests. 6th ed. Boston: Little, Brown, and Co, 1996:37–38.

VIRAL ARTHRITIS: SEROLOGIC TESTING

Description: Arthritis is an often observed consequence of viral infection. Viral pathogens most apt to demonstrate musculoskeletal manifestations include parvovirus B19, hepatitis B and C, rubella, HIV, and Epstein-Barr virus (EBV). Each entity demonstrates a distinctive clinical picture, and the diagnosis may require serologic confirmation as outlined below (Table 1).

Method: Most are detected by EIA, PCR, or RIA (see below)

Indications: Viral serologic testing is neither diagnostic nor conclusive in all instances. The strength of such evidence is strongly influenced by the clinical picture. Serologic testing should only be performed if such evidence will influence therapy or prognosis or help determine the infectivity of an individual patient.

Cost: EBV panel $100–175; Rubella $60–100; Parvovirus $70–100.

REFERENCES

Field BN, Knipe DM, Chanock RM, et al., eds. Virology. 2nd ed. New York: Raven, 1990.
Wiedbrauk DL, Johnston SLG. Manual of clinical virology. New York: Raven, 1993.

Table 1
Serologic Testing for Virus-Associated Musculoskeletal Disease

Virus	Primary Method/ Confirmatory Test[a]	Antibody Specificities	First Detected[b]	Persistence[b]	Interpretation	Confounding Factors
Parvovirus	EIA/DNA probe or PCR	IgG IgM Viral DNA	7 days 3 days	Life 2–3 months	Prior exposure Acute infection	IgG positivity found in 60% of U.S. adults
Hepatitis B	EIA or RIA	Surface antigen (HBsAg) Surface antibody (anti-HBs) Core antibody (anti-HBc) IgM Core antibody (anti-HBc) IgG E antigen (HBeAg) E antibody	3 weeks 6 months 2 months 6 months 6 weeks 4 months (anti-HBe)	6 months Life 6 months Life 4 months 6 months (<50%)	Active/persistent disease Prior exposure or immunization Active viral replication Present first in the "window" period Indicative of high infectivity Infectivity is low (used in chronic hepatitis)	A small number of hepatitis B vaccine recipients may acquire hepatitis B despite evidence of neutralizing anti-HBs
Hepatitis C	EIA/immunoblot or PCR (quantitative)	Antibody (anti-HepC) Viral RNA	Within 4 weeks	Life	EIA at least 94% sensitive	False negatives due to testing before seroconversion or immunosuppression blunting the antibody response; considerable interlaboratory variability for confirmatory PCR
Rubella	HAI or EIA	IgM IgG	1–5 days 1–3 days	6–12 weeks Life	Fourfold rise from acute to	Rheumatoid factors can give rise to false-positive

Organism	Test	Antigen/Antibody	Time	Duration	Comments
HIV	EIA	gp 120	3–12 weeks		convalescent sera or presence of IgM Abs indicating acute infection; IgM assay results; IgM may be detected for as long as 1 year using sensitive assays
	Western blot	p23, p24, gp41, gp 120/160			Western blot positive if at least 2 of 3 keys bands to p23, gp41, or gp 120/160 (CDC definition); Indeterminate western blot if single band; may indicate impending seroconversion in high-risk patient; but negative result in low-risk person (although follow-up testing is necessary)
	p 24 antigen	p24 antigen	Acute infection		
Epstein-Barr	Card agglutination	Heterophile antibody			Heterophile is a sensitive and specific test for infectious mononucleosis; False positive heterophile seen in other lymphoproliferative diseases and some lymphoid malignancies
	EIA	Viral capsid antigen (VCA IgM)	2–4 weeks	3 months	
		Viral capsid antigen (VCA IgG)	1–2 weeks	Life	
		Early antigen (EBV-EA)	4 weeks	3–6 months	
		Nuclear antigen (EBNA)	8 weeks	Years	

[a] EIA, enzyme immunoassay; HAI, hemagglutination inhibition; PCR, polymerase chain reaction; RIA, radioimmunoassay.

[b] With the exception of HIV, refers to time frame for acute uncomplicated infection in initially nonimmunocompromised host.

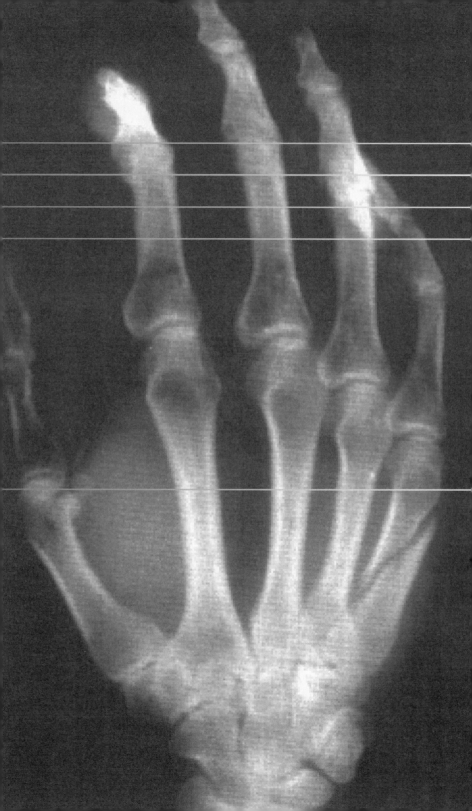

SECTION 2.

RHEUMATIC DISEASES

This section is devoted to specific musculoskeletal disorders. Each disease or topic is listed alphabetically for easy retrieval of the most commonly used or accepted diagnostic label. Disorders may also be found by searching the index for alternative terms or synonyms. The depth of information presented is roughly proportional to the prevalence and complexity of the disorder. Where appropriate, abbreviations are used and reflect the most commonly used abbreviations or acronyms in clinical practice. Abbreviations used throughout this text are listed on p. xi–xv.

Key clinical, diagnostic, and therapeutic information is presented under template headings that may include "Synonyms," "ICD9 Codes," "Definition," "Etiology," "Genetics," "Pathology," "Demographics," "Risk Factors," "Clinical Associations," "Disease Subsets," "Cardinal Findings," "Uncommon Findings," "Complications," "Diagnostic Tests," "Imaging," "Biopsy Findings," "Keys to Diagnosis," "Diagnostic Criteria," "Differential Diagnosis," "Therapy," "Surgery," "Prognosis," "Monitoring," or "Comments." When necessary, the reader is referred to other sections or appendices for supplemental information on related topics, diagnostic tests, or medications. Guidance on the dosing and use of pharmacologic agents is available in Section 3 of this text.

Selected references are provided at the end of each topic. For more complete information on these topics, the reader is referred to more expansive reference texts in rheumatology, such as:

Klippel JH, Weyand CM, Wortmann RL, eds. Primer on the rheumatic diseases. 11th ed. Atlanta: Arthritis Foundation, 1997.

Koopman WJ, ed. Arthritis and allied conditions: a textbook of rheumatology 13th ed. Baltimore: Williams & Wilkins, 1997.

CHAPTER 2

RHEUMATIC DISEASES

ACROMEGALY

Synonyms: Gigantism, acromegalia

ICD9 Code: 253.0

Definition: Overproduction of growth hormone by a pituitary tumor causes acromegaly. This syndrome is accompanied by distinct findings in the musculoskeletal system that may contribute to early detection and diagnosis.

Cardinal Findings: If the onset is during childhood, affected individuals manifest gigantism. This is usually not seen in pituitary tumors arising during adulthood. Clinically, patients develop distinctive coarse facial features, thickening of the skin, enlarged hands and feet, hirsutism, and excessive sweating. Nearly 50% of patients develop a mild proximal myopathy. The musculoskeletal complaints of patients with acromegaly usually result from premature osteoarthritis, kyphosis, pseudogout, or entrapment neuropathies (e.g., carpal tunnel syndrome). Many patients complain of nonspecific arthralgias affecting the shoulder, knees, and hips and back pain.

Diagnostic Tests: Serum somatomedin C (IGF-1) is more sensitive and cost-effective than serum growth hormone levels. Patients should be tested for increased prolactin levels (seen in 40% of patients); 80% of patients have evidence of insulin resistance, but only 20% develop clinical diabetes mellitus.

Imaging: Radiographic findings may be diagnostic and include generalized widening of the joint spaces because of overgrowth of cartilage. These changes in joint composition trigger secondary bone remodeling and spur formation. In later stages of the disease, osteoarthritis is obvious. In some cases, deposition of calcium pyrophosphate within joint tissues can lead to the clinical syndrome of pseudogout. Radiography or MRI may disclose an abnormal sella turcica and pituitary tumor.

Differential Diagnosis: Other causes of tall stature may include Marfan's syndrome and Klinefelter's syndrome.

Therapy: Treatment is primarily directed at the pituitary tumor and the need for radiation therapy or surgical intervention (transsphenoidal resection). Bromocriptine and long-acting somatostatin has also been used in selected instances. Musculoskeletal manifestations should be treated symptomatically.

Prognosis: In most cases, the joint findings of acromegaly are not reversed with correction of the growth hormone overproduction. One exception is the commonly observed carpal tunnel syndrome, which may show prompt improvement following surgical or medical ablation of the pituitary tumor.

REFERENCES

Melmed S. Acromegaly. N Engl J Med 1990;322:966.

ACUTE RHEUMATIC FEVER (ARF)

Definition: ARF, a febrile illness occurring as a delayed sequela to infection with group A streptococci, is characterized by inflammatory lesions of connective tissue.

ICD9 Codes: With arthritis, 390.0; with carditis, 391.9

Etiology: ARF occurs 2 to 3 weeks after untreated severe group A β-hemolytic streptococcal pharyngitis (in up to 3% of cases). It may be more common with certain streptococcal M serotypes.

Pathology: Exact mechanisms are unclear. Humoral response leads to immune-complex deposition. Cell-mediated immune damage to the heart is potentially due to molecular mimicry secondary to cross-reactive antigens. Streptococcal extracellular toxins, which can act as superantigens, may also be pathogenic. B cell alloantigen type 833 is present in a very high percentage of patients (but is nonspecific). Certain class II major histocompatibility complex antigens may also predispose to ARF.

Demographics: Peak age of incidence is 5 to 15 years. ARF remains endemic and is the major cause of valvular heart disease in the developing world. Incidence is very low in countries with good housing and economic conditions that lead to less crowding and better management of streptococcal pharyngitis. However, a recent resurgence of ARF has appeared in certain regions and populations in the United States.

Cardinal Findings: A migratory or additive polyarthritis is usually the earliest finding. Fevers and abdominal pain also occur early. Arthritis increases in frequency with age and has a predilection for large lower extremity joints as well as wrists and elbows. Joint pain may be out of proportion to physical findings. Jones' criteria serve as a guideline for diagnosis. Carditis is less common among adults, occurring in less than 15%. Only two-thirds of patients recall an antecedent pharyngitis. Poststreptococcal reactive arthritis (see p. 359) may be a form fruste of ARF, without carditis and with different extraarticular manifestations (i.e., tenosynovitis).

Uncommon Findings: Erythema marginatum (an evanescent, erythematous eruption of the torso with a serpiginous border and central clearing) and nodules are rare in adults. Most cases of (Sydenham's) chorea occur in women. Arthritis of the small joints of the hands or feet alone occurs in less than 1% of cases. Jaccoud's arthropathy, a nonerosive, reducible, deforming arthritis of the hands, occurs rarely when there are repeated episodes. Epistaxis and pneumonia are other uncommon findings.

Diagnostic Testing: Elevated levels of antistreptolysin "O" (ASO), anti-DNase B, anti-NADase, antistreptokinase, and antihyaluronidase all provide presumptive evidence of recent streptococcal infection. Although none of these tests is specific for ARF, at least one titer is elevated in 90% of streptococcal infections. Elevated levels of acute-phase reactants (ESR and/or CRP) and anemia of chronic inflammation are often present. Throat culture for streptococcal infection is usually negative at the time of ARF; if positive, it may only indicate noninfectious carriage. An ECG is necessary to evaluate for first-degree A-V block. A chest radiograph or ECHO cardiogram may also be necessary to diagnose carditis.

Diagnostic Criteria: Jones' criteria define classic features of ARF. Major manifestations include polyarthritis, carditis, chorea, subcutaneous skin nodules, and erythema marginatum. Minor manifestations include previous ARF or rheumatic heart disease, arthralgias, fever, elevated acute-phase reactants, and a prolonged PR interval on ECG. The presence of two major, or one major and two minor criteria indicates a high probability of ARF if supported by evidence of recent streptococcal infection (see testing above).

Keys to Diagnosis: A young patient with fever and painful migratory polyarthritis following pharyngitis may be suggestive of ARF.

Therapy: The underlying streptococcal infection should be treated with penicillin or an alternative antistreptococcal antibiotic. Although the arthritis is sensitive to high-dose salicylates (4–8 g/day in divided doses or a serum salicylate level of 20–30 mg/dL), other NSAIDs may be used. A prompt and prominent response to salicylates/NSAIDs supports the diagnosis. Refractory arthritis and severe carditis may require corticosteroids. Prevention and prompt management of recurrent pharyngitis is essential. Long-term prophylactic penicillin (or erythromycin if penicillin allergic) is often recommended. The cumulative duration of prophylaxis is controversial. Poststreptococcal reactive arthritis is less responsive to NSAIDs than ARF.

Prognosis: Acute mortality secondary to carditis is very uncommon. The most serious chronic sequela is rheumatic heart disease (RHD), which most commonly involves the mitral valve. RHD develops within 10 to 20 years of the initial attack. Joint disease in ARF is generally self-limiting, lasting less than 6 weeks on average, and chronic arthropathy is rare. Poststreptococcal reactive arthritis has a generally benign prognosis.

REFERENCES

Amigo MC, Martinex-Lavin M, Reyes P. Acute rheumatic fever. Rheum Dis Clin North Am 1993;19;333–350.

Gibofsky A, Zabriskie JB. Rheumatic fever: etiology, diagnosis and treatment. In: Koopman

WJ, ed. Arthritis and allied conditions: a textbook of rheumatology. 13th ed. Baltimore: Williams & Wilkins, 1997:1581–1594.

Veasy LG, Wiedmeier SE, Orsmond GS, et al. Resurgence of acute rheumatic fever in the intermountain area of the United States. N Engl J Med 1987;316:421–427.

ADULT-ONSET STILL'S DISEASE (AOSD)

Synonyms: Still's disease, systemic juvenile rheumatoid arthritis, Wissler-Fanconi syndrome, subsepsis hyperallergica

ICD9 Code: 714.3

Definition: AOSD is a systemic inflammatory disease that typically afflicts young adults. It is characterized by quotidian fevers, evanescent rashes, and chronic polyarthritis.

Etiology: Unknown. Many cases follow a prodromal sore throat without evidence of infection. AOSD infrequently has been associated with a variety of viral infections, including rubella, Epstein-Barr virus (EBV), Coxsackie B4 and mumps, although no single agent has been proven to be the cause.

Incidence: AOSD is uncommon. Between 5 and 9% of patients with "fever of unknown origin" are caused by AOSD. Most major medical centers may see one to two cases per year.

Demographics: Ninety percent of patients have their onset between 16 and 50 years of age. Males and females are equally affected. AOSD has been reported worldwide, affecting all races, including blacks, Orientals, and Latinos.

Cardinal Findings: Nearly 90% of patients have the triad of quotidian fevers, evanescent rash and, arthritis. Quotidian (spiking, daily) fevers may be as high as 102 to 105°F and usually occur at the same time each day—either late afternoon (3–6 PM) or late night (11 PM–2 AM). The evanescent rash is faintly erythematous or salmon pink, maculopapular, and maximal with febrile episodes. It commonly appears on the trunk, neck, or extremities and may be associated with dermatographism or Koebner's phenomenon (lesions arising at sites of trauma/pressure). Pruritus, urticaria, and fixed dermal plaques have been described. Arthritis tends to predominate with time and behaves like rheumatoid arthritis, involving the wrist, knee, ankle, and small joints of the fingers. Other prominent manifestations (seen in ≥50% of patients) include prodromal sore throat, myalgias, carpal ankylosis, weight loss, lymphadenopathy, hepatomegaly, splenomegaly, pleuritis, or pericarditis.

Diagnostic Tests: No test is "diagnostic." AOSD patients should be seronegative for RF and ANA. Neutrophilic leukocytosis, thrombocytosis, markedly elevated ESR or serum ferritin (acute-phase reactants), hypoalbuminemia, and elevated hepatic enzymes are common during active inflammatory disease. Ferritin levels above 1000 ng/mL are seen in 50% of patients, and very high levels (up to 30,000 ng/mL) are occasionally seen. Radiographs are nondiagnostic. Nearly half of patients develop carpal ankylosis with chronic arthritis.

Diagnostic Keys: This is a clinical diagnosis of exclusion. The evanescent rash may be the most distinctive feature of AOSD. Fever follows a circadian rhythm and occurs at the same time each day.

Differential Diagnosis: Acute viral infection (EBV, rubella, etc.), dermatomyositis, Reiter's syndrome, inflammatory bowel disease, and hematologic malignancies (i.e., acute leukemias) are most commonly confused with AOSD. Less common possibilities include bacterial endocarditis, sarcoidosis, Sweet's syndrome, tuberculosis, and granulomatous hepatitis.

Therapy: Initially, NSAID therapy at antiinflammatory doses can be used. Sustained-release indomethacin (75–150 mg/day) is effective in 40 to 60% of patients. Aspirin is seldom effective. Corticosteroids should be reserved for patients with markedly elevated hepatic enzymes, pericardial tamponade, severe serositis or pneumonitis, and those resistant to NSAIDs. High-dose prednisone (40–80 mg/day) may be necessary to control the systemic manifestations. Weekly oral methotrexate (7.5–20 mg/week) has been used successfully to limit steroid exposure. Active systemic manifestations may also be treated with hydroxychloroquine, azathioprine, or cyclosporine. Chronic, progressive polyarthritis can be managed in the same manner as that used for rheumatoid arthritis.

Prognosis: Flares of systemic disease may last from 6 to 24 months. In most, the clinical course displays either intermittent bouts of systemic disease or chronic arthritis. Death is uncommon (<9% of cases) and results from complications of therapy, pericardial tamponade, hepatic failure, or disseminated intravascular coagulation.

REFERENCES

Cush JJ, Medsger TA, Christy WA, et al. Adult-onset Still's disease: clinical course and outcome. Arthritis Rheum 1987;30:186–194.
Yamaguchi M, Ohta A, Tsunematsu T, et al. Preliminary criteria for classification of adult Still's disease. J Rheumatol 1992;19:424–430.

ALKAPTONURIA

Synonyms: Ochronosis

ICD9 Code: 270.2

Definition: This rare metabolic disorder is caused by accumulation of homogentisic acid in cells and body fluids because of a deficiency of the enzyme homogentisic acid oxidase. Homogentisic acid binds to collagen, resulting in deposition of a darkened pigment in joint cartilage, intervertebral discs, and soft tissues (e.g., skin).

Demographics: The disorder is transmitted as an autosomal recessive gene; heterozygotes do not have ochronosis. The incidence of homozygotes is estimated to be 1 in 200,000.

Cardinal Findings: Skin changes are usually first noted after age 20 years. The delayed onset of skin and cartilaginous changes leaves many undiagnosed until they are elderly, when the clinical findings are striking. The dark pigmentation may be seen in the pinna and external canal of the ear or in skin overlying the nasal and malar areas of the face. Pigmentation is often described as slate blue, gray, or coal colored. This pigment may even appear in axillary sweat and stain clothing. Articular manifestations usually begin in the spine. Peripheral joint pains and subsequent osteoarthritis may affect the knees, shoulders, and hips. Hands, feet, elbows, and ankles are usually spared.

Diagnostic Tests: The diagnosis is confirmed by demonstrating homogentisic aciduria. Urine samples may be dark colored or become dark if left to stand. Nearly 50% of patients develop a noninflammatory, yellow- or amber-colored synovial effusion.

Imaging: Radiographs of the spine show a characteristic pattern of densely calcified intervertebral discs with intervening osteoporotic vertebral bodies, giving the appearance of a "rugger jersy" spine. Late degenerative changes or chondrocalcinosis of involved peripheral joints may occur.

Therapy: Definitive medical therapies are not available; treatment of the arthritis is symptomatic.

REFERENCES

Schumacher HR, Holdsworth DE. Ochronotic arthropathy. I. Clinicopathologic studies. Semin Arthritis Rheum 1977;6:207–246.

AMYLOIDOSIS

ICD9 Code: 277.3

Definition: Amyloidosis is a multisystem disorder caused by deposition of fibrillar protein aggregates that interfere with structural integrity and function of targeted organs or tissues. Four major forms are distinguished by the deposited protein and the clinical associations (Table 1).

Etiology: Primary amyloidosis (AL) is commonly associated with plasma cell dyscrasias such as multiple myeloma or may be seen with other malignancies, such as medullary carcinoma of the thyroid. Secondary amyloidosis (AA) occurs most commonly in association with inflammatory syndromes such as familial Mediterranean fever or rheumatoid arthritis. β_2-Microglobulin amyloidosis occurs in association with hemodialysis.

Pathology: The various proteins associated with amyloidosis all show a characteristic fibrillary array, most clearly seen by electron microscopy. Under the

Table 1
Syndromes of Systemic Amyloidosis

Type	Clinical Syndromes	Protein
Immunoglobulin (AL)	Primary, myeloma-associated amyloidosis	Ig light chains
Reactive (AA)	Secondary to inflammatory disease	Amyloid A (also called serum amyloid A (SAA))
Hereditary	Familial	Various non-Ig proteins
β_2-Microglobulin	Hemodialysis associated	β_2-Microglobulin

light microscope, amyloid deposits are visualized by staining with Congo red. When viewed under polarized light, the stained fibers show a characteristic apple-green birefringence.

Demographics: Patients can be of almost any age, from childhood to elderly, depending on the underlying cause. Primary AL shows a male predominance.

Cardinal Findings: In primary AL, the most commonly involved organs are kidney, heart, and liver; skin, skeletal muscle, and tongue may also be affected. Peripheral neuropathies are seen, but the CNS is generally not involved. Secondary AA most commonly presents with nephrotic syndrome or gastrointestinal bleeding. Macroglossia is not seen with secondary AA. The initial finding in hemodialysis-associated amyloid is often carpal tunnel syndrome.

Uncommon Manifestations: In primary AL, amyloid deposits may be seen in the synovium and occasionally in the synovial fluid.

Diagnostic Tests: Biopsies of affected tissues are usually required. The tissues are stained with Congo red and viewed under polarized light. Kidney and peripheral nerve biopsy specimens can be useful, if there are known abnormalities in these tissues, otherwise a blind abdominal fat pad aspirate should be attempted. Tissues available from previous biopsies or surgical procedures may be recut and stained with Congo red to visualize amyloid that may have been missed on routine histologic examination.

Keys to Diagnosis: Suspect amyloid in a patient with multisystem disease, especially those with cardiomyopathy, peripheral neuropathy, and nephrotic syndrome. Biopsy demonstration of amyloid deposits is diagnostic.

Differential Diagnosis: Malignancies, idiopathic cardiomyopathies, and systemic vasculitis syndromes may present with some of the findings of amyloidosis.

Therapy: In primary AL, chemotherapy with melphalan and prednisone is usually recommended, although it is not clear that this treatment prolongs survival. Cardiomyopathy is especially resistant to medical therapy. In secondary AA, treatment should be directed at control of the underlying inflammatory process. Colchicine has some utility in patients with amyloid secondary to familial Mediterranean fever.

Surgery: Surgery is not generally indicated. During surgical procedures diagnostic biopsy specimens may be obtained. Organ transplantation (heart, kidney) may be attempted in some cases.

Prognosis: In primary AL, only 20% of patients are alive 5 years after diagnosis. Disease progression is generally slower in secondary forms, with some patients surviving 10 years after diagnosis.

REFERENCES

Benson MD. Amyloidosis. In: Koopman WJ, ed. Arthritis and allied conditions: a textbook of rheumatology. 13th ed. Baltimore: Williams & Wilkins, 1997:1511–1512.
Westmark P. Diagnosing amyloidosis. Scand J Rheumatol 1995;24:327–329.

ANKYLOSING SPONDYLITIS

Synonyms: AS; Marie-Strumpell disease; Bechterew's syndrome

Definition: Ankylosing spondylitis (AS) is a common inflammatory arthropathy that preferentially affects the axial skeleton, often beginning in the sacroiliac joints and ascending to involve the remaining spine.

Etiology: AS has a strong genetic component, as over 90% of Caucasian patients are HLA-B27 positive and a significant minority have a positive family history for AS also. AS develops in 1 to 2% of HLA-B27–positive individuals. There is a 20% risk of AS in HLA-B27–positive first-degree relatives of AS patients. Others have postulated that AS may result from exposure to certain arthritogenic bacteria that resemble HLA-B27, resulting in molecular mimicry.

Pathology: The spondyloarthropathies typically demonstrate erosive changes early and fibrous ankylosis with chronicity. Synovial changes are similar to that seen in RA, with synoviocyte proliferation, inflammatory cell infiltration into the sublining layer, and juxtaarticular erosive changes. AS and the other spondyloarthropathies share a propensity for new bone formation in response to injury. This is most evident at the entheses (sites of tendon attachment to bone), where local inflammatory changes may result in new bone formation (osteophytes).

Demographics: Epidemiologic studies suggest that the prevalence of AS in a Caucasian population is between 0.5 and 5 cases per 1000 persons. The age- and sex-adjusted incidence rate in Rochester, Minnesota, is 7.3 per 100,000 person-years. AS and HLA-B27 are lower in African Americans (see HLA-B27, p. 118). AS commonly affects young men more frequently than women, with an estimated male:female ratio ranging from 2.5:1 to 5:1. AS in women is often underdiagnosed, primarily because of milder axial disease and occult extraarticular manifestations. Although there is some debate whether AS differs between the sexes, several studies suggest that women with AS may have a delayed disease onset, less hip involvement, less-aggressive axial disease, more peripheral arthritis, severe osteitis pubis, and a higher incidence of isolated cervical spine disease. Peak age of onset is between 15 and 30 years. It is rare after age 50. Juvenile spondylitis, a minor subset of juvenile arthritis, includes those with onset of AS between the ages of 9 and 16 years.

Cardinal Findings: Symptoms often begin in young adulthood. The insidious onset of low back pain or stiffness is often the initial symptom of AS. Bilateral symmetric sacroiliitis is highly suggestive of AS. Although sacroiliitis begins at an early age, it may take up to 10 years to become evident by conventional radiography. Sacroiliac pain is localized over the sacroiliac joints and less commonly down the posterior thigh. Patients usually complain of prolonged morning stiffness that is only relieved by increased activity or antiinflammatory medications. Often these young patients actively pursue sports and physical activity as a means of lessening their symptoms. Constitutional complaints of fever, anorexia, and weight loss may also be seen. With progressive axial involvement, pain and stiffness result in difficulty with ambulation and activities of daily living. Fusion of the axial spine occurs in an ascending fashion, with early lumbar and late cervical spine involvement.

An asymmetric oligoarticular, inflammatory, peripheral arthritis is seen in 30% of AS patients. Synovitis of the hip can be destructive and may lead to concentric loss of joint space, especially in men. Involved joints also typically include the ankles, wrists, shoulders, elbows, and small joints of the hands or feet. Radiographically, peripheral articular changes may be erosive and similar to RA.

Extraarticular disease in AS primarily affects the eye. Ocular involvement is seen in up to 40% of patients and is more frequently observed in HLA-B27–positive individuals. Uveitis presents as acute, unilateral, orbital pain, accompanied by photophobia and progressive loss of vision if untreated.

Examination reveals restricted spinal movement from axial stiffness, fusion, and paraspinal muscular spasm. Often the earliest finding is a loss of normal lumbar lordosis and resultant "flattening" of the lumbar spine. Left untreated, progressive axial inflammation may lead to a fixed forward flexion posture, most evident in the hip and neck. Chest expansion, as measured by the inspiratory minus expiratory chest circumference, normally exceeds 5 cm. AS patients demonstrate diminished expansion (<4 cm).

Schober's test examines lumbar spine mobility. While the patient stands upright with heels together, a 10-cm span is marked from the 5th lumbar vertebra cephalad. Upon maximal forward flexion, the distance between marks is remeasured. Normal spinal flexion expands the surface area over the flexed spine to more than 15 cm. Flexion in patients with spondylitis and limitation of spinal motion measures 14 cm or less.

Uncommon Findings: Thoracocervical kyphoscoliosis, aortitis, aortic insufficiency, aortic root dilation, and conduction defects are uncommon. Other uncommon manifestations include mitral valve disease, myocardial dysfunction, pericarditis, pulmonary fibrosis, and amyloidosis.

Complications: Minor or incidental trauma may result in serious spinal fractures in those with advanced disease and ankylosis of the spine. Such fractures may result in spinal cord damage and carry a high mortality rate. Such fractures may be identified on plain radiographs, bone scans, or MRI. Other rare complications of AS include cauda equina syndrome, osteoporotic compression fractures, spondylodiscitis, restrictive lung disease, apical fibrosis, cardiac conduction defects, aortic insufficiency, and uveitis.

Diagnostic Tests: Laboratory tests support the inflammatory nature of the disease with an elevated ESR or C-reactive protein (CRP), anemia of chronic disease, or mild elevations of alkaline phosphatase. IgA levels may be elevated, but other autoantibodies are noticeably absent. HLA-B27 determination is seldom necessary to establish the diagnosis. However, in questionable cases without distinctive radiographic changes, the presence of HLA-B27 may be of diagnostic value.

Imaging: Radiographs are often normal early in the disease and demonstrate normal mineralization before the onset of ankylosis. Once present, ankylosis results in marked immobility and subsequent generalized osteoporosis. Sacroiliitis is indicated by early erosions (leading to "pseudowidening") and later by ileal sclerosis or fusion of the inferior, synovial lined portion of the sacroiliac joint. These findings are easily observed on plain radiographs of the pelvis and seldom require computerized tomography or MRI for diagnosis. Axial radiographic findings also include marginal bridging syndesmophytes, fusion of the posterior facet joints, and "squaring" of lumbar and thoracic vertebrae. Collectively, these findings may produce the classical appearance of a "bamboo spine." Articular damage or fibrosis tends to have a bilateral symmetric distribution.

Diagnostic Criteria: Two different sets of diagnostic criteria have been developed (Table 1)

Keys to Diagnosis: AS must be distinguished from other causes of mechanical or degenerative low back pain. As is suggested by *(a)* young age of onset; *(b)* strong family history of low back pain; *(c)* low back pain lasting more than 3 months; *(d)* prolonged morning stiffness; *(e)* symptomatic improvement with activity or exercise; *(f)* limited spinal mobility on examination; and *(g)* elevated ESR or CRP.

Differential Diagnosis: The differential diagnosis includes other spondyloarthropathies (enteropathic arthritis, Reiter's syndrome, psoriatic spondylitis), osteitis condensans ilii, diffuse idiopathic skeletal hyperostosis (DISH), and other causes of hyperostosis (e.g., fluorosis, hypervitaminosis A).

Therapy: The goal of treatment is to reduce pain and stiffness and maintain posture and mobility. Both nonpharmacologic and pharmacologic measures should be used in all.

Table 1
Diagnostic Criteria for Ankylosing Spondylitis

Rome Criteria, 1961
  Clinical criteria
  1. Low back pain and stiffness for more than 3 months, not relieved by rest
  2. Pain and stiffness of the thoracic region
  3. Limited motion in the lumbar spine
  4. Limited chest expansion
  5. History or evidence of iritis or its sequelae
  Radiologic criterion
  6. Radiographs showing characteristic bilateral sacroiliac changes
  Definite AS = grade 3–4 bilateral sacroiliitis and one clinical criterion; or at least 4
    clinical criteria
Modified New York, 1984
  1. Low back pain for at least 3 months; duration improved by exercise and not
    relieved by rest
  2. Limitation of the lumbar spine in sagittal and frontal planes
  3. Chest expansion decreased relative to normal values for age and sex
  4. Bilateral sacroiliitis grade 2–4
  5. Unilateral sacroiliitis grade 3–4
  Definite AS = unilateral grade 3–4 sacroiliitis; or bilateral sacroiliitis grade 2–4
    and one clinical criterion

—*Nonpharmacologic:* Each patient should be instructed on the importance of patient education, joint protection, appropriate exercise, intermittent rest, physical therapy, and dietary and vocational counseling. Patients with axial disease should engage in lifelong physical therapy to maintain posture and prevent slow deformity.

—*NSAIDs:* NSAIDs are effective in controlling inflammatory back pain/stiffness, peripheral arthritis, and enthesitis. These agents modify symptoms but do not suppress disease progression. NSAIDs are the mainstay of therapy for most patients. A few NSAIDs are FDA approved for use in AS and/or Reiter's syndrome. These include indomethacin, diclofenac, naproxen, sulindac, aspirin, and phenylbutazone. Of these, indomethacin, especially the sustained-release formula (1–2 mg/kg/day), is recommended because of its prolonged duration of effect and antiinflammatory potency. Other NSAIDs are used according to individual tolerability and efficacy. Phenylbutazone is very effective, but it is rarely used and is reserved for patients who do not respond to other NSAIDs, primarily because of the unacceptable risk of aplastic anemia. Unfortunately, phenylbutazone is no longer commercially available and may only be acquired through a few select compounding pharmacies.

—*Corticosteroids:* Systemic corticosteroids are seldom used in the spondyloarthropathies. They are most effective in controlling localized disease. They are used primarily as local therapy by intraarticular injection (i.e., mono- or oligoarthritis), topical management of ocular complications (conjunctivitis or uveitis), and on occasion, intralesionally to control enthesitis. Uncontrolled reports suggest beneficial effects of intraarticular corticosteroids administered into the sacroiliac joints.

—*Disease-modifying antirheumatic drugs (DMARDs):* When the condition is chronic, progressive, NSAID unresponsive, or associated with uncontrolled peripheral inflammatory arthritis, addition of a DMARD (i.e., sulfasalazine, methotrexate) should be considered. These agents have a delayed onset of action (2–6 months), and their efficacy in the spondyloarthropathies is based on limited numbers of controlled trials and numerous anecdotal reports. Randomized placebo-controlled trials of sulfasalazine indicate that efficacy is greatest in patients with peripheral arthropathy and enthesopathy. Equivocal results have been observed in patients with longstanding axial disease and evidence of severe radiographic destruction or ankylosis. Despite these results, sulfasalazine should be considered in patients with poorly controlled axial disease. The usual dose is 2 g/day initially, although after 2 to 3 months this may be gradually increased up to 3 or 4 g/day, according to GI tolerance. Methotrexate (7.5–20 mg/week) may also be effective in the treatment of AS patients with axial or peripheral arthritis. Other DMARDs (azathioprine, gold salts, antimalarials, cyclosporine) have not been well studied in AS.

Surgery: Surgical intervention in AS is primarily reserved for those with advanced peripheral arthritis, usually affecting the hip or knee. Total joint replacement may be indicated when pain and immobility markedly interfere with the patient's lifestyle. The success of arthroplasty may be limited by postsurgical heterotopic bone formation. Surgical stabilization of spinal fractures should be undertaken with extreme caution. Correction of spinal deformities due to advanced, aggressive ankylosis is not advised.

Prognosis: The clinical course and disease severity is highly variable. Inflammatory back pain and stiffness are prominent early in the disease, whereas chronic, aggressive disease may produce pain and marked axial immobility or deformity. Early age of onset and diagnosis portend a more severe outcome. Moreover, AS patients are at risk for complications, some of which may be life threatening.

REFERENCES

Clegg DO, Reda DJ, Weisman MH, et al. Comparison of sulfasalazine and placebo in the treatment of ankylosing spondylitis. A Department of Veterans Affairs cooperative study. Arthritis Rheum 1996;39(12):2004–2012.

Hammer RE, Malka SD, Richardson JA, et al. Spontaneous inflammatory disease in transgenic rats expressing HLA-B27 and human β2m: an animal model of HLA-B27-associated human disorders. Cell 1990;63:1099–1112.

Khan MA. Pathogenesis of ankylosing spondylitis: recent advances. J Rheumatol 1993;20:1273–1277.

Resnick D, Dwosh IL, Goergen TG, et al. Clinical and radiographic abnormalities in ankylosing spondylitis: a comparison of men and women. Radiology 1976;119:293–297.

ANTIPHOSPHOLIPID SYNDROME

Synonyms: Anticardiolipin syndrome, Hughes syndrome

ICD9 Code: 279.8

Definition: The antiphospholipid syndrome (APS) refers to a constellation of clinical findings, including vascular thrombosis, fetal wastage, and thrombocytopenia, that are seen in association with the lupus anticoagulant and anticardiolipin (aCL) or antiphospholipid antibodies.

Etiology: The etiology of APS is unknown. Patients with a variety of infections, cancers, and other conditions may develop aCL antibodies, but fewer develop clinical APS. aCL antibodies may be found in up to half of patients with systemic lupus erythematosus (SLE). Clinical APS occurs only in a minority of those with the antibody. The precise pathogenesis of the APS is unknown. It is hypothesized that antibodies to negatively charged phospholipids, such as cardiolipin, alter the normal anticoagulant function of the vascular endothelium. Alternatively, aCL and other antiphospholipid antibodies may potentiate platelet activation, resulting in thrombosis.

Demographics: The APS occurs most commonly among young women, but all ages and both sexes may become involved. The prevalence of antiphospholipid antibodies (without clinical symptoms) is far more common than APS (with an abnormal test).

Cardinal Findings: Clinical characteristics of the APS are shown in Table 1. Recurrent venous or arterial thromboses are the most prominent feature. A history of thrombosis in a patient thought to be otherwise at low risk of such an event often prompts the search for the APS. Other common presentations include recurrent spontaneous abortions and refractory thrombocytopenia.

Table 1
Characteristics of the Antiphospholipid Antibody Syndrome

Common
    Venous thrombosis (e.g., pulmonary embolus, deep venous thrombosis, retinal vein thrombosis, Budd-Chiari syndrome)
    Arterial thrombosis (e.g., cerebrovascular accident, myocardial infarction)
    Thrombocytopenia
    Recurrent fetal loss
Less common
    Livedo reticularis
    Cutaneous ulceration
    Hemolytic anemia
    Endocardial/cardiac valvular vegetations (Libman-Sacks endocarditis)
    Chorea, myelopathy

Diagnostic Tests: Diagnosis of the APS depends upon two distinct types of laboratory tests: functional hematologic tests (the lupus anticoagulant test) or assays for specific antibodies (e.g., aCL antibody test (see p. 85)). While many APS patients may have abnormal results in both types of test, others may manifest only one abnormal test result. Although they are not exactly the same, the terms *antiphospholipid* and *anticardiolipin* are often used interchangeably.

There are several laboratory tests that define the presence of a "lupus anticoagulant." A prolonged partial thromboplastin time (PTT) with a normal prothrombin time (PT) is suggestive. If the PTT does not correct with a 1:1 dilution with normal serum, as would be expected if the prolonged PTT were due to a deficiency of clotting factors, the presence of an inhibitor such as the lupus anticoagulant is suggested. The dilute Russell viper venom time (DRVVT) and the kaolin clot time are clotting tests that depend upon phospholipids and are thus interfered with when antiphospholipid antibodies are present. Finally, correction of a prolonged PTT by addition of excess phopholipids, as is done in the platelet neutralization test and the hexagonal phospholipid test, suggests that a lupus anticoagulant is present.

ELISA is used to identify antibodies that bind to negatively charged phospholipids, including cardiolipin, phosphatidylcholine, and others. Although several antibody isotypes (e.g., IgG, IgA, IgM) may have aCL activity, high-titer IgG aCL correlates most strongly with the clinical syndrome of APS. Recently, it has been demonstrated that most pathogenic aCL antibodies have binding activity only in the presence of another serum protein, β_2-glycoprotein-I (β_2GP-I) (see p. 85).

Differential Diagnosis: Other considerations for those experiencing recurrent thrombotic events might include protein C, protein S, or antithrombin III factor V leiden deficiency, dysfibrinogenemias, hyperhomocysteinemia nephrotic syndrome, malignancies, Behçet's syndrome, paroxysmal nocturnal hemoglobinuria, thrombotic thrombocytopenic purpura, Buerger's disease, sickle cell anemia, hyperlipidemia, severe diabetes, or hypertension. Recurrent fetal loss may also be associated with anti-Ro antibodies, coexistent infection or inflammatory diseases, or anatomic abnormalities of the female reproductive tract.

Therapy: Treatment of the APS depends to some extent on the occurrence and severity of the clinical manifestations. Acutely, patients with severe thromboembolic events (e.g., pulmonary embolism) are treated with anticoagulation in the same manner as those without APS. Because APS patients are prone to recurrent thromboses, many physicians recommend that patients suffering a single serious clotting event be treated with long-term oral anticoagulation, typically with Coumadin. Patients with recurrent events should receive anticoagulation unless there are compelling reasons not to do so. Treatment that achieves an INR greater than 2 appears to be more efficacious than less intense anticoagulation. When anticoagulation is not feasible, low doses of aspirin are commonly used as adjunctive therapy, although data supporting the efficacy of this approach are lacking. In some circumstances, for example pregnancy,

Coumadin is contraindicated because it crosses the placenta. Daily treatment with heparin is an alternative. Low-molecular-weight heparin therapy has also been successfully used in APS patients. Because the APS relates to antibody production, corticosteroids and other immunomodulatory agents have been tried for some patients. However, good data supporting this approach are lacking.

REFERENCES

Alarcon-Segovia D, Deleze M, Oria CV, et al. Antiphospholipid antibodies and the antiphospholipid syndrome in SLE: a prospective analysis of 500 consecutive patients. Medicine 1989;68:353–365.

Lockshin MD. Antiphospholipid antibody syndrome. Rheum Dis North Am 1994;20:45–59.

Mackworth-Young CG, Loizou S, Walport MJ. Primary antiphospholipid syndrome. Ann Rheum Dis 1989;48:362–367.

Sammaritano LR, Gharavi AF, Lockshin MD. Antiphospholipid antibody syndrome: immunologic and clinical aspects. Semin Arthritis Rheum 1990;20:81–96.

ATRIAL MYXOMA

Synonyms: Cardiac myxoma

ICD9 Code: 212.7

Definition: Atrial myxoma is a benign cardiac tumor that may lead to valvular obstruction or emboli. Embolic manifestations may be confused with a systemic necrotizing vasculitis.

Pathology: Tumors are typically found in left atrium (75%), right atrium (20%), or ventricles (5%), usually as single pedunculated tumor attached to the septum, valve, or chordae tendineae. Large myxomas may produce valve obstruction. They may also fragment, causing emboli. Microscopically, a collection of myxomatous cells (polygonal and stellate) are found in a vascular mucopolysaccharide matrix. Increased amounts of interleukin-6 (IL-6), produced by myxoma cells, are responsible for many of the systemic and constitutional manifestations. Tumors may be asymptomatic and only discovered at autopsy.

Demographics: Atrial myxomas usually affect adults between 30 and 60 years of age. They are uncommon in blacks and rarely familial (autosomal dominant). No sex preference exists.

Cardinal Findings: Atrial myxomas produce systemic, obstructive, and embolic symptoms. Fever, weight loss, arthralgia, myalgia, Raynaud's phenomenon, rash, and clubbing may occur. Cardiac findings include new-onset congestive heart failure, chest pain, and dyspnea that improves when supine. Arterial emboli may cause central neurologic deficits, mononeuritis multiplex, or skin lesions.

Complications: Complications include CHF, pulmonary emboli, and pulmonary hypertension.

Diagnostic Tests: Anemia, leukocytosis, increased ESR, thrombocytosis or thrombocytopenia, hypergammaglobulinemia, and hypocomplementemia are common.

Imaging: Diagnosis is usually made by echocardiography but CT scan or MRI can also be used. Occasionally, vasculitic findings may be seen on angiogram or in biopsy specimens.

Therapy: Tumors are surgically excised.

Comment: Tumors may recur.

REFERENCES

Burke AP, Virmani R. Cardiac myxoma. A clinicopathologic study. Am J Clin Pathol 1993;100:671–680.
Sack KE. Mimickers of vasculitis: cardiac myxoma. In: Koopman WJ, ed. Arthritis and allied conditions. 13th ed. Baltimore: Williams & Wilkins, 1997:1529–1530.

BACTERIAL ARTHRITIS

Synonyms: Septic arthritis, infectious arthritis, gonococcal arthritis

ICD9 Codes: Pyogenic arthritis, 711.0; gonococcal arthritis, 098.5; bacterial arthritis unspecified, 711.4

Definition: Bacterial arthritis is bacterial infection of the joint space, which may affect any type of joint.

Etiology: Most cases of bacterial arthritis are hematogenously disseminated. Others may occur by direct invasion (e.g., trauma) or contiguous spread (e.g., osteomyelitis). Reasons for invasion of the joint space by bacteria are not known, but preexisting articular abnormalities (e.g., RA, OA) or previous surgery may contribute to entry of the infectious agent. Comorbid conditions such as diabetes mellitus or drugs that impair immune function may be contributing factors.

At-Risk Populations: Those at risk include the very young, elderly, or immunosuppressed (e.g., by cytotoxics or corticosteroids); those with chronic arthropathies (e.g., RA, OA), prosthetic joints, repeated joint aspiration or injection, or systemic illness (e.g., chronic liver disease, neoplasia, sickle cell); intravenous substance abusers; and those engaged in high-risk sexual activity or who have had recent trauma or surgery.

Pathology: Joint cultures are usually positive for the causative agent unless prior antibiotics have been given. An important exception is gonococcal arthritis, wherein synovial fluid cultures are often negative, even with appropriate culture techniques. Common pathogens in septic arthritis include staphylococci (*S. aureus, S. epidermidis*), streptococci (*S. pyogenes, S. pneumoniae*), neisseria (*N. gonorrhoeae, N. meningitidis*), *Haemophilus influenzae*, salmonella, *Proteus mirabilis, and Bacteroides fragilis.*

Demographics: All age groups are susceptible. An increasing percentage of patients have a chronic underlying disease (e.g., RA, diabetes), but healthy individuals can also be affected. Septic arthritis in children is usually caused by *S. aureus,* group B streptococci, or *H. influenzae.* Young adults are likely to have gonococcal or staphylococcal infection. The elderly are commonly affected by bacterial arthritis due to staphylococcal, streptococcal, gram-negative, and polymicrobic infections.

Cardinal Findings: The classic presentation is an acute monoarticular arthritis with effusion, warmth, and erythema, often accompanied by fever. Polyarticular onset occurs in a minority of cases and carries a poorer prognosis.

—*Gonococcal (GC) Arthritis:* Typically seen in young, sexually active (often menstruating) females, GC arthritis often affects the knees, ankles, wrists, or elbows as a monarthritis or oligoarthritis. Tenosynovitis and migratory arthralgias are common, and there may be an associated characteristic pustular (often painful) rash. Fever may be absent, and a minority will have genitourinary, pharyngeal, or rectal symptoms on presentation. If suspected, every orifice should be swabbed and cultured for gonococcus on Thayer-Martin culture media. In most cases, a positive culture can be found from one of these orifices. Only a small minority of patients have a positive synovial fluid culture.

—*Staphylococcal Arthritis:* Usually monarticular (seldom polyarticular), staphylococcal arthritis affects the knee, hip, shoulder, elbow, wrist, or ankle, and more than 90% of patients exhibit high fevers. Involvement of the sternoclavicular joint, shoulder, or sacroiliac joint should raise suspicion of a staphylococcal infection and, possibly, intravenous substance abuse. Patients with preexisting arthritis (e.g., RA) are prone to infection with *S. aureus.*

—*Prosthetic Joints:* Less than 2% of those with joint replacements develop septic joint. Those at greatest risk are patients with RA, distant infections, or corticosteroid use or those undergoing revision arthroplasty. When septic arthritis immediately follows the procedure, *S. epidermidis, S. aureus,* or skin anaerobes are the most common pathogens. Prosthetic infection occurring more than 1 year postoperatively is most likely to be caused by *S. aureus,* non–group A streptococci, and gram-negative organisms.

—*Intravenous Substance Abuse:* Common sites of infection include the shoulder, sternoclavicular, and sacroiliac joints. Infections in the sacroiliac joint may present as low back or buttock pain with only subtle suggestions of infection. These patients are commonly infected by *S. aureus* and gram-negative organisms (e.g., *Pseudomonas aeruginosa*).

Uncommon Manifestations: Patients with RA and infected joints may not show classic signs of inflammation, possibly because of concomitant treatment with medications (e.g., corticosteroids) that blunt the inflammatory response.

Diagnostic Tests: Joint aspiration and culture of synovial fluid is usually diagnostic in those with nongonococcal septic arthritis (Table 1). Blood should also be cultured and is frequently positive in nongonococcal arthritis. Other

Table 1
Suspected Bacterial Arthritis: Important Tasks in the First 48 Hours

1. Aspirate fluid from the joint *unless*
   a. Overlying skin/soft tissues appear infected
   b. The joint has been surgically replaced
2. Send the fluid to the laboratory for
   a. Leukocyte count and differential
   b. Culture and sensitivity
   c. Crystal identification
3. Initiate presumptive antibiotic treatment
   a. Intravenous therapy
   b. Include coverage for *S. aureus*
4. Repeat joint aspiration in 24 hours and then daily for
   a. SF leukocyte count; repeat until declining
   b. Culture; repeat until sterile
5. Obtain orthopaedic consultation for
   a. Suspected septic hips (adults or children)
   b. Suspected infections of prosthetic joints
   c. Consideration of open drainage if WBC not declining

measures, such as the synovial fluid WBC count and ESR or C-reactive protein (CRP) elevations, are only suggestive. Joint aspiration and the interpretation of synovial fluid results is discussed on pp. 61–73. Aspiration should utilize a large-bore needle to remove as much purulent material as possible. Synovial fluid WBC counts should be above 30,000 cells/mm^3 with gonococcal arthritis and above 50,000 cells/mm^3 with nongonococcal arthritis. The percentage of neutrophils usually exceeds 85% in such cases. The presence of crystals in synovial fluid does not exclude a coexistent infection. Gram stains are useful in making initial antibiotic choices, but culture confirmation is required. Needle aspiration should not be performed through skin or soft tissues that show signs of infection. If the joint in question has been surgically replaced, orthopaedic consultation should be considered prior to any joint aspiration or injection.

Imaging: Radiographs are seldom revealing and may only show soft tissue swelling with acute septic arthritis. Radiographic changes may take 2 to 3 weeks to become apparent. Thus, an early diagnosis *must* be established on clinical grounds and synovial fluid culture. The presence of gas formation should suggest infection with *Escherichia coli* or anaerobes. Radiographs and other modalities may be necessary to diagnose an infected prosthetic joint. Radiographs may show bone resorption and radiolucency at the implant/bone interface, with or without evidence of overlying periosteal reaction. Technetium bone scanning may suggest an infected prosthesis prior to changes on plain radiography. MRI and gallium- and indium-labeled WBC scanning have not been shown to be of value in such patients.

Keys to Diagnosis: Acute monoarticular arthritis with fever is the most common presentation, but polyarticular and subacute afebrile presentations also occur. In patients with inflammatory types of arthritis (e.g., RA), activity in one joint that seems out of proportion to that in others should raise consideration of septic arthritis. An acute inflammatory monarthritis in the setting of positive blood cultures should strongly suggest septic arthritis.

Differential Diagnosis: Bacterial arthritis may often be confused with other forms of infectious arthritis (viral, fungal, mycobacterial). The infectious arthropathies are compared in Appendix F. Bacterial arthritis should also be distinguished from acute crystal-induced arthritis (e.g., gout, pseudogout), Reiter's syndrome, Lyme disease, septic bursitis, overlying cellulitis, osteomyelitis, foreign body reaction, fracture, or mechanical joint derangement.

Therapy: Parenteral antibiotics must be given as soon as possible after the initial joint aspiration. While culture results are pending (usually 24–48 h), the initial antibiotic should include coverage for *S. aureus* (Table 1). The initial choice of therapy is shown in Appendix E. Parenteral therapy is recommended for at least 3 weeks for *S. aureus* and gram-negative organisms, 7 days for gonococcal infection, and 2 weeks for most other organisms (e.g., *S. pyogenes, H. influenzae*). Follow-up therapy with oral antibiotics is of unproven benefit. With the availability of long-lasting intravenous access lines and home care teams, prolonged hospitalization is not required. Prior to hospital discharge, serial joint taps must show (*a*) a steady and marked decrease in synovial fluid WBCs and (*b*) sterile synovial fluid culture. There is no role for intraarticular antibiotics.

Surgery: The role of surgical drainage is controversial except in inaccessible sites such as the hip, where a surgical approach (open drainage or fluoroscopically guided needle aspiration) is often required. In children, all septic hips require arthrotomy to reduce intraarticular pressure and allow adequate drainage. Most other joints can be treated by serial needle aspirations and do not require surgical drainage unless the leukocyte count does not drop as expected or cultures do not rapidly become sterile.

Prognosis: In general, mortality rates are below 5%. Prognosis is poorest in the elderly and those with gram-negative infections, polyarticular involvement, prosthetic joints, or delayed diagnosis. If less than 1 week elapses prior to initiation of therapy, the prospect for maintaining normal joint function is very good; if the time prior to treatment is 1 month or more, outcome is usually poor. Infections of prosthetic joints present major surgical problems, usually requiring removal of the components, prolonged antibiotic treatment, and then revised reconstruction. Such cases should be referred to an orthopaedist at the outset.

REFERENCES

Ike RW. Bacterial arthritis. In: Koopman WJ, ed. Arthritis and allied conditions: a textbook of rheumatology. 13th ed. Baltimore: Williams & Wilkins, 1997:2267–2295.

Javors JM, Weisman MH. Principles of diagnosis and treatment of joint infections. In: Koopman WJ, ed. Arthritis and allied conditions: a textbook of rheumatology. 13th ed. Baltimore: Williams & Wilkins, 1997:2253–2266.

Rotrosen D. Infectious arthritis. In: Isselbacher KJ, Braunwald E, Wilson JD, et al., eds. Harrison's principles of internal medicine. 13th ed. New York: McGraw-Hill 1994:554–557.

BEHÇET'S DISEASE

Definition: Behçet's disease is a syndrome of recurrent, painful oral and genital lesions associated with uveitis and other forms of systemic inflammation.

ICD9 Codes: 136.1; with arthropathy, 711.2

Etiology: Behçet's disease is a relapsing small vessel vasculitis of uncertain etiology. There is evidence suggesting immune-complex deposition, hyperfunctioning neutrophils, increased levels of circulating IL-6, and a decreased CD4:CD8 T cell ratio. HLA-B5 and subtype HLA-B51 may be risk factors in afflicted Japanese.

Pathology: Histology of skin lesions may show perivascular inflammation or vasculitis, with both neutrophilic and monocytic infiltrates.

Demographics: Behçet's disease is most common in the eastern Mediterranean (Turkey) and Japanese (prevalence about 1/1000) populations. In the United States, the prevalence is 0.3 to 6.6 cases per 100,000. Male:female ratio is 2:1 to 5:1. Mean age of onset is about 40 years. Behçet's disease is one of the leading causes of acquired blindness in Japan.

Cardinal Findings: *Aphthous stomatitis* (100% prevalence) is usually the first manifestation. Very painful lesions occur in crops and resemble "canker" sores. Lesions last 1 to 2 weeks and often heal with scarring. Oral ulcers are most commonly found on the buccal or gingival mucosa or tongue. Painful *genital ulcers* (70–100%) occur on the vulva or vagina in women (often during menses) and penis or scrotum in men. Genital ulcers resemble oral aphthae but tend to recur less frequently. *Ocular* findings (50–90%) are usually bilateral and occur 2 to 3 years after initial symptoms. Anterior uveitis, with hypopyon, and posterior uveitis may result in visual loss and be caused by retinal, macular, or choroidal vessel vasculitis. *Arthritis* (40–50%) is usually episodic, monoarticular or oligoarticular. Large joints are more commonly affected than small joints. Arthralgias are more common than frank arthritis. *Cutaneous lesions* (30–65%) include pustules, erythema nodosum, papules/pseudofolliculitis, and severe acneform lesions. Nodules are also seen secondary to superficial phlebitis. *Pathergy,* nearly unique to Behçet's disease, occurs when pricking the skin with a needle leads to development of a sterile pustule. *Central nervous system* (5–30%) manifestations of headaches, meningoencephalitis, ocular and other cranial nerve palsies, seizures, cerebrovascular insufficiency, brainstem syndrome leading to cerebellar ataxia, and pseudobulbar palsy have all been reported. *Phlebitis/arteritis* (25%) as thrombosis of large veins/arteries and aneurysms (of the aorta and pulmonary arterial tree) may occur. Budd-Chiari syndrome, dural sinus thrombosis, limb ischemia, stroke, and renovascular hypertension have been reported.

Uncommon Findings: Colitis and epididymitis are seen in a minority of patients. Nephritis and amyloidosis have rarely been noted. The rarely seen MAGIC syndrome (*M*outh *A*nd *G*enital ulceration with *I*nflamed *C*artilage) has overlapping features of Behçet's disease and relapsing polychondritis.

Complications: The most feared common complication is blindness from eye manifestations. Neurologic and vascular complications (thrombotic events) are responsible for most of the severe morbidity and potential mortality.

Diagnostic Testing: Nonspecific measures of systemic inflammation include elevated acute-phase reactants (ESR and CRP), leukocytosis, anemia of chronic inflammation, and thrombocytosis. With significant CNS involvement, the cerebrospinal fluid typically shows a mononuclear cell pleocytosis and elevated protein levels. Patients with thromboses may have antiphospholipid antibodies (see p. 85).

Differential Diagnosis: Other forms of systemic vasculitis and connective tissue diseases (polyarteritis nodosa, SLE) should be considered. Oral and genital lesions may be confused with inflammatory bowel disease or Reiter's syndrome. The oral ulcers of SLE or Reiter's syndrome are usually painless and palatal. Uveitis should raise the possibility of other inflammatory disease (i.e., the spondyloarthropathies) as well as infectious causes. Skin manifestations resemble those of Sweet's syndrome or Stevens-Johnson syndrome. Large-vessel vasculitis may mimic Takayasu's arteritis.

Keys to Diagnosis: Look for the triad of oral ulcers, genital lesions, and uveitis. Although pathergy is nearly pathognomonic, it is infrequently seen among North American Caucasians.

Diagnostic Criteria: Criteria of the International Study Group are
A. Recurrent oral ulceration (at least three times in 1 year), plus
B. Two of the following four criteria:

1. Recurrent genital ulcerations
2. Eye lesions—uveitis or retinal vasculitis
3. Skin lesions—erythema nodosum, pseudofolliculitis, papulopustular lesions, or unexplained acne
4. Pathergy

Therapy: Active uveitis or CNS disease merits aggressive therapy with high-dose corticosteroids, cytotoxic agents (e.g., azathioprine, chlorambucil, or cyclophosphamide), or cyclosporine. Intermittent prednisone (10–40 mg/day) is effective in the control of recurrent ulcerations, but chronic use should be discouraged because of the resk of steroid toxicity. Colchicine, dapsone, and levamisole may also be used to treat skin/mucocutaneous manifestations. Thalidomide has been used successfully for refractory oral and genital ulcers. Colchicine, NSAIDs, or sulfasalazine may be effective for Behçet's disease–associated arthritis. Chronic anticoagulation may be required for thrombotic complications.

Prognosis: Oral and genital lesions frequently predate vascular and neurologic manifestations by months or years. Relapses are common over a 5 to 7-year period before a reduction in disease activity may occur.

REFERENCES

International Study Group for Behçet's Disease. Criteria for diagnosis of Behçet's disease. Lancet 1990;335:1078–1080.

Kastner DL. Intermittent and periodic arthritic syndromes. In: Koopman WJ, ed. Arthritis and allied conditions: a textbook of rheumatology. 13th ed. Baltimore: Williams & Wilkins, 1997:1291–1297.

Rigby AS, Chamberlin MA, Bhakta B. Behçet's disease. Ballieres Clin Rheumatol 1995;9: 375–395.

BRUCELLOSIS

Synonyms: Undulant fever, Malta fever, Mediterranean fever

ICD9 Code: 023.9

Definition: Systemic infection with *Brucella* is uncommon and may cause fever, peripheral arthritis, sacroiliitis, or spondylitis.

Etiopathogenesis: Humans may acquire Brucella from ingesting infected unpasteurized dairy products (e.g., cheese), aerosolized bacteria, or contact with broken skin or conjunctiva. *Brucella* is a gram-negative coccobacillus. Brucella arthritis is usually caused by direct seeding of the synovium. Some cases appear to be "reactive" (i.e., not due to direct infection). *Brucella* septic arthritis is usually monarticular or axial, is persistent, and requires antibiotic therapy. The reactive arthritis is usually intermittent, self-limited, sterile, nondestructive, and polyarticular.

Demographics: *Brucella* has a worldwide distribution. Most cases are reported from South America. *Brucella* spp. include *B. abortus* (zoonotic source, cow), *B. melitensis* (goat), and *B. suis* (pig). Although *B. abortus* is most common in the United States, *B. melitensis* is most common worldwide. Infection occurs in all ages and sexes. Those at risk include veterinarians, farm and slaughterhouse workers, and persons ingesting unpasteurized milk or cheese.

Cardinal Findings: Acute infection is associated with bacteremia and may show fever (101–104°F), arthralgias, headache, or malaise. Fever, diaphoresis, and weight loss may be undulant. Hepatosplenomegaly and uveitis are common. In the subacute form, fever is less common. Acute peripheral arthritis of the lower extremities (e.g., hip or knee) is common. Arthralgias and myalgias are seen in more than half of patients. Sacroiliitis is usually unilateral and nondestructive. Spondylitis commonly affects the lumbar spine.

Uncommon Findings: Lymphadenopathy, pulmonary symptoms, orchitis, tendinitis, bursitis, and epicondylitis.

Complications: Local microabscesses (i.e., paraspinal abscess often manifesting as antibiotic resistance), endocarditis, thrombophlebitis, hepatitis, and CNS infection may occur.

Diagnostic Tests: Routine laboratory test may show leukopenia, relative lymphocytosis, thrombocytopenia, or abnormal hepatic enzymes. Culture of organism from joint fluid is slow (3–4 weeks) and is positive in less than 50% of samples. Bone marrow culture may improve culture yield or show granulomas. Serologic tests (ELISA or agglutination reaction) for IgM or IgG (chronic) anti-*Brucella* antibody are usually positive.

Imaging: Sacroiliitis appears as blurring of articular margins of the sacroiliac (SI) joints, seldom with erosions. Spondylitis appears as intervertebral erosions, disc narrowing, and reactive osteophytes with a "parrot-beak" appearance. Scintigraphy may be useful in identifying spondylitis or sacroiliitis.

Keys to Diagnosis: Bacteriologic or serologic evidence of infection signals the diagnosis, which requires a high index of suspicion, especially in the at-risk population.

Differential Diagnosis: Spondyloarthropathies, septic arthritis, psittacosis, tuberculosis, HIV, and rickettsial infections must be considered.

Therapy: At least 4 to 6 weeks of combination antibiotic therapy with tetracycline (doxycycline) plus a second agent (rifampin, streptomycin, or trimethoprim) is effective in most.

Monitoring: Clinical response and serum antibody levels should be monitored for a year after treatment.

Prognosis: Most do very well. The relapse rate is 5%. Mortality is rare and usually due to endocarditis.

REFERENCES

Colmenero J, Reguera JM, Fernandez-Nebro A, et al. Osteoarticular complications of brucellosis. Ann Rheum Dis 1991;50:23–26.
Zaks N, Sukenik S, Alkan M, et al. Musculoskeletal manifestations of brucellosis: a study of 90 cases in Israel. Semin Arthritis Rheum 1995;25:97–102.

CALCIPHYLAXIS

ICD9: 440.20

Definition: Calciphylaxis is a rare disorder that affects patients with long-standing end-stage renal disease (ESRD), many of whom have secondary hyperparathyroidism. This condition primarily manifests painful nodular lesions.

Etiology: Acute calcium deposition in tissues is responsible.

Pathology: Soft tissue and medial vascular calcification occurs, with subsequent tissue necrosis.

Demographics: This is a rare disorder that occurs only in ESRD patients.

Cardinal Findings: Plaquelike, nodular, or bullous lesions progress to necrotic, ulcerative, painful, nodular lesions on the digits, extremities, and trunk. Patients may develop gangrene of the digits, extremities, buttocks, or abdomen. Uncommonly it manifests as painful myopathy or severe livedo reticularis that progresses to cutaneous gangrene.

Complications: Complications include cutaneous gangrene and sepsis. Unfortunately, there is a very high mortality rate due to secondary sepsis. Calcification of the lungs or ischemic infarction of major organs is rare. It may be associated with functional protein C or S deficiency.

Diagnostic Tests: Elevated parathyroid hormone levels occur in 90%. Look for hypercalcemia and hyperphosphatemia. The calcium-phosphate product $(Ca^{2+} \times PO_4)$ exceeds 70 in 80% of patients. Radiographs may demonstrate vascular and soft tissue calcifications. Deep incisional biopsies are preferred over punch biopsies.

Diagnostic Keys: Look for vascular calcifications or painful nodules in ESRD patients.

Differential Diagnosis: Vasculitis, panniculitis, type 1 primary hyperoxaluria must be distinguished from calciphylaxis.

Therapy: Proper wound care is indicated, and appropriate antibiotics used if secondarily infected. Steroids are not indicated and are not helpful!

Surgery: Subtotal parathyroidectomy is of questionable benefit.

REFERENCES

Hafner J, Keusch G, Wahl C, et al. Uremic small-artery disease with medial calcification and intimal hyperplasia (so-called calciphylaxis): a complication of chronic renal failure and benefit from parathyroidectomy. J Am Acad Dermatol 1995;33:954–962.

CALCIUM PYROPHOSPHATE CRYSTAL DEPOSITION DISEASE (CPPD)

Synonyms: Pseudogout, chondrocalcinosis, pyrophosphate arthropathy

ICD9 Codes: Pseudogout, 712.2; CPPD, 712.2; chondrocalcinosis, 712.3

Definition: CPPD includes arthritic syndromes associated with calcium pyrophosphate dihydrate crystal deposition in articular tissues. Nomenclature in this disease has been inconsistent. The following definitions are used here:

Chondrocalcinosis: Calcification of articular cartilage

Chronic CPPD: Structural bone and cartilage abnormalities associated with intraarticular deposition of CPPD crystals

Pseudogout: clinical syndrome of acute synovitis caused by intraarticular CPPD crystal deposition; the most common form of CPPD

Etiology: The cause of CPPD crystal deposition is unknown. Formation of CPPD crystals in cartilage may be related to matrix changes or result from elevated levels of calcium or inorganic pyrophosphate. Some cases appear to be hereditary, while others are idiopathic.

Pathology: CPPD crystals are found in joint capsules and fibrocartilaginous structures. The earliest deposition is seen at the lacunar margin of chondrocytes. Neutrophils can be seen invading matrix structures, with erosion of cartilage and degradation of collagen fibrils. Synovial proliferation can resemble rheumatoid pannus.

Demographics: Data on CPPD crystal deposition disease are largely derived from radiologic surveys of chondrocalcinosis of the knee. Predominantly a condition of the elderly, it has a peak age of 65 to 75 years and female predominance (F:M, 2–7:1). Prevalence of chondrocalcinosis in the general population is 5 to 8% and rises to over 15% by the 9th decade. It is ubiquitous in geographic distribution. Familial predisposition has been reported in several groups, some of whom have early-onset, severe, polyarticular disease (3rd–4th decades).

Disease Associations: Several conditions are associated with CPPD crystal deposition: hyperparathyroidism, hypocalciuria, hypercalcemia, hemochromatosis, hemosiderosis, hypophosphatasia, hypomagnesemia, hypothyroidism, gout, neuropathic joints, amyloidosis, trauma, OA, and aging.

Cardinal Findings: Findings vary according to the type of disease.

—*Pseudogout:* Pseudogout often begins as self-limited acute arthritic attacks lasting from 1 day to 4 weeks and may be as severe as, and resemble, acute gout. Attacks are often provoked by concurrent medical illnesses or surgery. The knee joint is involved in 50% of cases, followed by the wrist, shoulder, ankle, and elbow. Podagra (first MTP arthritis) has been reported. Patients are asymptomatic between attacks. Men are predominately affected. Up to 20% show concurrent hyperuricemia, and 5% have monosodium urate crystals in synovial fluid as well. The diagnosis is suggested by the clinical presentation and confirmed by synovial fluid analysis (CPPD crystals) or radiography (chondrocalcinosis).

—*Chronic CPPD:* Chronic CPPD predominately affects women, as a chronic, progressive, often symmetric polyarthritis affecting the knees (most common), but also the wrists, MCP (especially 2nd and 3rd) joints, hips, spine, shoulder, elbows, and ankles. Some patients have episodic pseudogout. Patients typically have chronic pain, morning and inactivity stiffness, limitation of movement, and functional impairment. Symptoms may be restricted to a few joints. Affected joints reveal signs of osteoarthritis with varying degrees of synovitis. Variations in compartmental knee involvement may cause valgus or varus deformities. Chronic CPPD differs from pseudogout in its chronicity, tendency to affect MCPs and spine, and the pattern of progressive osteoarthritis with intermittent inflammation/synovitis.

—*Chondrocalcinosis:* Generally an incidental radiographic finding, chondro-calcinosis is usually seen in asymptomatic individuals, typically in the elderly.

Uncommon Findings: Severe synovitis in chronic CPPD disease may produce a pseudorheumatoid pattern. Charcot-like arthropathy of the knee has been ascribed to CPPD in some patients. Rarely, a predominantly axial pattern is seen, simulating ankylosing spondylitis. Other uncommon patterns are tendinitis, tenosynovitis, bursitis, and tophaceous CPPD crystal deposition.

Diagnostic Tests: Synovial fluid usually shows a mean leukocyte count of $20,000/mm^3$ with more than 90% neutrophils, and "blood-tinged" effusions may be seen. Compensated polarized light microscopy reveals rhomboidal or rodlike intracellular crystals with weakly positive birefringence. A careful microscopic search is required, as these crystals are often missed. In pseudogout, joint fluid should always be gram stained and cultured to exclude a septic process.

An increase in acute-phase reactants (ESR or CRP) can be seen along with an elevated leukocyte count, but these are not diagnostic. In chronic arthropathy, an elevated serum ferritin level and a mild anemia are not uncommon. Routine screening for metabolic causes of CPPD crystal deposition disease should be reserved for those with early-onset arthritis (age <55 years), florid polyarticular disease, or recurrent acute attacks out of proportion to the degree of chronic arthropathy. In such patients, the following screening tests are suggested: serum calcium, serum alkaline phosphatase, serum magnesium, and serum ferritin levels and tests of liver function.

Imaging: Calcification of articular fibrocartilage may be visible as punctate and linear densities, most frequently seen in the fibrocartilaginous menisci of the knee. Other sites of calcification include the articular discs of the distal radioulnar joint (triangular fibrocartilage), the symphysis pubis, the glenoid and acetabular labra, and the annulus fibrosus of the intervertebral discs. Calcification of hyaline cartilage occurs in the midzonal layer, appearing as a radiopaque line that runs parallel to the cortex of the underlying bone. Typically the larger joints are involved. Degenerative arthropathy is similar to that observed in osteoarthritis, with visible subchondral cysts, sclerosis, osteophytes, and joint space narrowing, all of which are often pronounced.

Keys to Diagnosis

—*Pseudogout:* The presence of an acute synovitis in one or more joints, with radiologic chondrocalcinosis and/or synovial CPPD crystals strongly suggests pseudogout. Synovial fluid may be purulent, mandating exclusion of sepsis (which may coexist).

—*Chronic CPPD:* In most cases, a characteristic joint pattern, radiologic findings, and CPPD crystals in joint fluid easily establish a diagnosis. Polyarticular involvement with modestly elevated sedimentation rate and rheumatoid factor may cause confusion with RA. The infrequency of systemic features, lack of radiologic erosions, and periarticular osteopenia often permit differentiation from RA. Differentiation from osteoarthritis is possible by involvement of MCP joints, radiologic findings, and presence of superimposed acute attacks.

Diagnostic Criteria: See Table 1

Differential Diagnosis: Pseudogout and CPPD may be misdiagnosed as gout, pseudogout, OA, septic arthritis, inflammatory OA, neuropathic arthritis, or hypertrophic osteoarthropathy.

Therapy

—*Pseudogout:* General principles of management include relief of symptoms, identification and treatment of triggering illnesses, and rapid mobilization. Although, aspiration alone can relieve symptoms, intraarticular steroid injection is appropriate, either concurrently with the first aspiration or after gram staining and culture results are negative. Acetaminophen or NSAIDs can be of additional benefit. Colchicine may be used as acute therapy for pseudogout but is rarely necessary. Colchicine may also be useful as prophylaxis in those with recurrent attacks of pseudogout. Systemic corticosteroids can be used if other treatments are contraindicated, although their efficacy remains untested in controlled trials.

—*Chronic CPPD:* No specific therapy exists for chronic CPPD, and treatment of any underlying metabolic abnormalities usually does not reverse joint damage. The aims of management are to relieve symptoms and improve function. Chronic NSAID or colchicine therapy may be effective. Troublesome individ-

Table 1
Diagnostic Criteria for CPPD

I. Demonstration of CPPD crystals by definitive means (x-ray diffraction, chemical analysis)
II. A. Identification of CPPD crystals by compensated polarized light microscopy
   B. Presence of typical calcifications on roentgenograms
III. A. Acute arthritis, especially of the knees
    B. Chronic arthritis, especially of the knee, hip, wrist, carpus, MCPs, elbow, or shoulder; differentiated from OA by demonstrating the following features
       1. Uncommon site for primary OA (MCPs, wrist, elbow, shoulder)
       2. Radiographic appearance (isolated compartment narrowing in wrist, knee)
       3. Subchondral cyst formation
       4. Severe progressive degeneration (subchondral bony collapse, intraarticular radiodense bodies)
       5. Variable and inconstant osteophyte formation
       6. Tendon calcifications
       7. Involvement of the axial skeleton
Diagnosis:
   Definite CPPD: criteria I or II.A and II.B
   Probable CPPD: criterion II.A or II.B
   Possible CPPD: criterion III.A or III.B

ual joints can be managed with injection of intraarticular steroids. Joint arthroplasty may eventually be needed.

Prognosis: Although pseudogout usually responds well to therapy, chronic CPPD is often progressive and in some may lead to significant disability and deformity.

REFERENCES

Doherty M. Crystal arthropathies: calcium pyrophosphate dihydrate. In: Klippel JH, Dieppe PA, eds. Rheumatology. London: Mosby-Year Book Europe Limited, 1994:7.13.1–7.13.12.
Ryan LM, McCarty DJ. Calcium pyrophosphate crystal deposition disease, pseudogout, and articular chondrocalcinosis. In: Koopman WJ, ed. Arthritis and allied conditions: a textbook of rheumatology. 13th ed. Baltimore: Williams & Wilkins, 1997:2103–2125.

CARCINOMA POLYARTHRITIS

Synonyms: Cancer polyarthritis

ICD9 Code: 714.9

Definition: A polyarthritis resembling rheumatoid arthritis (RA) that occurs in the setting of underlying malignancy.

Etiology: Carcinoma polyarthritis may be secondary to antigenic cross-reactivity between synovium and tumor or be due to altered cellular and humoral immune mechanisms.

Demographics: Carcinoma polyarthritis occurs most commonly with solid tumors; breast cancer accounts for about 80% of cases.

Cardinal Findings: Characteristic features include (*a*) close temporal relationship of explosive-onset arthritis with malignancy diagnosis (joint symptoms seldom precede malignancy by more than 10 months); (*b*) late age of onset for inflammatory arthritis; (*c*) asymmetric joint involvement, often affecting lower extremity joints, with relative sparing of wrists and small joint of hands; (*d*) absence of rheumatoid nodules and absent or low titer of serum rheumatoid factor. Carcinoma polyarthritis is occasionally mistaken for hypertrophic osteoarthropathy or adult-onset Still's disease (when associated with high fever).

Diagnostic Testing: ESR is often nonspecifically elevated, reflecting the tumor burden. Up to 20% of patients may have low-titer RF or ANA. Synovial biopsy specimens show only nonspecific synovitis. As in RA, bone erosions may develop.

Therapy: Therapy is aimed at alleviating the underlying cancer (tumor resection may improve arthritis). NSAIDs or corticosteroids may be necessary to control arthritis inflammation.

REFERENCES

Bennet RM, Ginsberg MH, Thomsen S. Carcinoma polyarthritis. The presenting symptom of an ovarian tumor and association with a platelet activating factor. Arthritis Rheum 1976;19:953–958.

CARPAL TUNNEL SYNDROME (CTS)

Synonyms: CTS, Median nerve entrapment syndrome

ICD9 Code: 354.0

Definition: Entering the hand, the median nerve and the flexor tendons pass through the carpal tunnel within the wrist. The carpal tunnel is formed on the bottom by the volar surface of the carpal bones of the wrist and on top by the transverse carpal ligament (flexor retinaculum), which encloses the tunnel (Fig. 1). Carpal tunnel syndrome (CTS) is a constellation of symptoms that result from the compression of structures within this restricted space. In most cases, symptoms result from compression of the median nerve, which innervates the thenar muscles, the lumbricales on the radial side of the hand, and the skin overlying the radial side of the palm and the first, second, third, and radial side of the fourth digits.

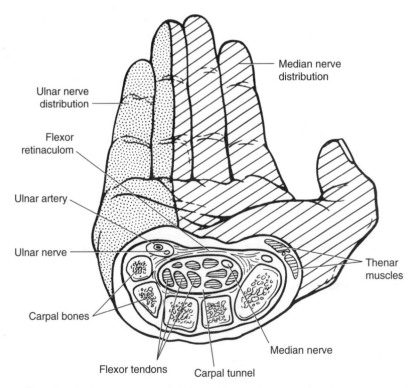

Figure 1. Anatomic cross section of the carpal tunnel. Median nerve (*hatched area*) and ulnar nerve (*stippled area*) innervation is shown.

Risk Factors: A number of conditions may be associated with development of this condition (Table 1). Among the most important may be overuse or repetitive stress injury, although this is somewhat controversial. Nevertheless, in some series, more than half of the patients evaluated were considered to have CTS of occupational origin. With the growing use of computer terminals in the workplace, it has been estimated that 1 in 10 office workers may develop CTS.

Demographics: CTS is the most common entrapment neuropathy, with a prevalence of approximately 250 to 500 cases per 100,000 population. It may affect as many as 2 million Americans every year.

Cardinal Findings: Early in CTS, patients may complain only of paresthesia or numbness of the fingers or hand, rather than frank pain. These symptoms may be accentuated at night and may be relieved by "shaking" the hand. Symptoms are more common in the dominant hand but may be bilateral. As the condition progresses, patients may report more-severe pain in the distribution of the median nerve that may be exacerbated by certain movements. Some patients may relate sensations of pain or numbness in areas that anatomically should not be affected (e.g., proximal to the wrist). As CTS becomes more chronic, frank muscle weakness, muscle atrophy (e.g., thenar muscle atrophy), and hypesthesia may develop. Tinel's sign or Phalen's sign is sometimes used to aid in the diagnosis of CTS. Tinel's sign is positive if repetitive tapping over the flexor retinaculum and medial nerve at the wrist (with the hand in slight dorsiflexion) elicits numbness, dysesthesia, or electric-like sensations in the first 3½ fingers. Phalen's test is positive if symptoms are elicited when the patient holds the dorsal surfaces (or backs) of the hands against each other with the wrists in forced flexion. Unfortunately, in several large research series, the sensitivity and specificity of these tests for diagnosing CTS were nearly 50%. Thus, a positive or negative result must be interpreted within the context of the clinical suspicion.

Table 1
Causes of Carpal Tunnel Syndrome

Repetitive motion injury[a]
Pregnancy[b]
Rheumatoid arthritis[b]
Hypothyroidism[b]
Diabetes mellitus[b]
Amyloidosis (e.g., with multiple myeloma)
Acromegaly
Infectious diseases (e.g., mycobacteria, fungi)
Ganglion cysts
Carpal bone osteophytes
Trauma
Idiopathic

[a]Accounts for >50% of cases.
[b]These conditions, in combination, account for nearly 25% of cases.

Diagnostic Tests: Because the pathophysiology relates to entrapment and impaired function of the median nerve, electrodiagnostic tests may be considered the gold standard for diagnosis of this disorder. Thus, nerve conduction velocity (NCV) testing would be expected to reveal findings such as prolonged distal nerve latency conduction times. In experienced hands, these tests may have a sensitivity of 90% and a specificity of 60%. The findings present on NCV vary with the extent of involvement and may progress over time. Laboratory studies may aid in the diagnosis of associated conditions (Table 1) and should be chosen on the basis of clinical presentation. Imaging studies are of little value in evaluating CTS.

Keys to Diagnosis: CTS should be strongly considered in any individual who presents with numbness or pain in the hand. Because it is so prevalent, many patients may be expected to have atypical presentations. A clinical history of pain or numbness affecting the hand in the distribution of the median nerve and pain or weakness of the thenar muscles (e.g., in flexing or opposing the thumb) should arouse clinical suspicion of CTS. Patients demonstrating classic symptoms and signs need not undergo further electrodiagnostic testing.

Differential Diagnosis: A variety of less common conditions may present with wrist or hand pain and be confused with CTS. Early, mild synovitis of the wrist, for example, with rheumatoid arthritis or crystalline arthritis, may mimic CTS. Likewise, ganglion cysts of the volar aspect of the wrist or bony osteophytes of the carpal bones may cause wrist pain. As noted above, all of these conditions may also be associated with true CTS, which may make determination of the exact cause of pain more difficult. Entrapment of the median nerve at another location or cervical radiculopathy may mimic CTS, but these are uncommon. Patients with ulnar or radial nerve entrapment may also report similar complaints. Ulnar nerve entrapment may produce pain, numbness, or clumsiness of the 4th and 5th fingers, hypothenar atrophy, or "clawing" of 4th and 5th digits. Radial nerve palsy may result in wrist drop, with flexion of the MCP joints and numbness of the thumb, index, and middle fingers.

Therapy: Treatment of CTS begins with avoiding overuse and splinting the wrist and hand in a neutral position (in slight extension). Nighttime splinting of the affected wrist(s) may suffice. Most physicians add an NSAID if there are no contraindications and wrist inflammation or arthritis exists. For those unresponsive to conservative maneuvers, local injection with a corticosteroid may be used. While steroid injections are often successful in the short term, many patients have recurrent symptoms.

A large number of cases arise from repetitive overuse at the workplace. Thus, correct ergonomics may be important in preventing CTS. For example, it is recommended that those who type at computer terminals for long periods of time sit with backs straight, feet flat on the floor, forearms parallel to the floor, and wrists "floating" (i.e., not resting continually on anything). In addition, it is important to take breaks every so often to stretch and rest the arms and hands.

Surgery: Surgical decompression of the carpal tunnel may be indicated when conservative measures fail or when there is evidence of persistent sensory loss or thenar atrophy. Surgical release of the transverse carpal ligament may relieve the compression on the nerve. Symptoms may recur after surgery. Although carpal tunnel release is usually an outpatient, open surgical procedure, newer techniques are being evaluated (e.g., arthroscopic decompression, balloon dilatation of the carpal tunnel, and laser stimulation of the affected nerve). The comparative efficacy and risks of these newer techniques remain to be determined.

REFERENCES

Dawson DM. Entrapment neuropathies of the upper extremities. N Engl J Med 1993;329: 2013–2018.
Golding RN, Rose DM, Selvarajah L. Clinical tests for carpal tunnel syndrome—an evaluation. Br J Rheumatol 1986;25:388–390.
Slater RR, Bynum DK. Diagnosis and treatment of carpal tunnel syndrome. Orthopaedic Rev 1993;(October):1095–1105.

CENTRAL NERVOUS SYSTEM (CNS) ANGIITIS

Synonyms: Primary CNS angiitis, isolated CNS angiitis, granulomatous angiitis of CNS

ICD9 Code: 437.4 (vasculitis)

Definition: The term *CNS angiitis* encompasses a variety of inflammatory conditions that result in decreased blood flow in cerebral vessels (Table 1). Neurologic defects may be focal or diffuse, depending upon the location and extent of the lesions. Primary CNS angiitis is an idiopathic inflammatory disorder with characteristic clinical, angiographic, or histologic findings of vasculitis limited to the CNS.

Pathology: Primary CNS angiitis may demonstrate granulomatous or nongranulomatous vasculitis affecting the leptomeningeal and cortical small and medium-sized vessels.

Demographics: This rare disorder is commonly seen in adults aged 20 to 60 years.

Cardinal Findings: Symptoms of primary CNS angiitis may include headache, confusion, neurocognitive dysfunction, cranial neuropathy, seizures, and focal motor or sensory defects. Physical examination may reveal fever, hypertension, focal neurologic deficits, papilledema, and fundoscopic abnormalities. Other systemic features, such as arthralgias or myalgias, are uncommon. Nearly 10% of patients exhibit a myelopathy.

Diagnostic Testing: In patients suspected of having CNS angiitis, routine laboratory test results are frequently normal. Nonspecific findings may include an elevated ESR or leukocytosis. Serology (ANA, RF, C-ANCA) should be normal. Cerebrospinal fluid analysis may reveal several abnormalities, including increased CSF protein, lymphocytic pleocytosis, and increased CSF immunoglobulins (see CSF studies, p. 98). The CSF results may also be normal and be of greatest value in excluding other causes.

The role of leptomeningeal biopsy is controversial. Although pathogno-

Table 1
Conditions Associated with or Resembling CNS Angiitis

Primary CNS angiitis
  Biopsy proven
  Angiographically proven
Secondary CNS angiitis
  Systemic vasculitides: Giant cell arteritis; Takayasu's arteritis; Wegener's
    granulomatosis; polyarteritis nodosa; Churg-Strauss angiitis; Behçet's syndrome
  Inflammatory disorders: RA; SLE; Sjögren's syndrome; sarcoidosis
  Infections: Tuberculosis; fungi (coccidioidomycoses, actinomycoses, cryptococcus);
    spirochetal disease (syphilis, Lyme disease); viruses (HIV, CMV, herpes)
  Drugs-induced: Cocaine; amphetamines; sympathomimetics (ephedrine,
    phenylpropanolamine); thiazides
Vasculopathic conditions
  Antiphospholipid syndrome
  Atherosclerotic disease
  Hypertension
  Thrombotic thrombocytopenia purpura
  Persistent or recurrent vasospasm
  CNS lymphoma
  Moyamoya disease

---

monic, granulomatous or nongranulomatous vasculitis with mononuclear infiltrates is found in less than 50% of patients. Sensitivity is increased by using biopsy specimens from both brain tissue and leptomeninges or by taking tissue samples from areas abnormal on MRI. However, the procedure may yield false-negative results in more than 25% of cases. Biopsy is particularly helpful in establishing or excluding other diagnoses such as lymphoma and sarcoidosis.

Imaging: CNS imaging results are often abnormal. However, they may not allow precise determination of the cause. CT scans may show infarcts or be entirely normal. It may be most useful in helping to rule out other conditions, such as subarachnoid hemorrhage or tumor. Up to 15% of patients have mass lesions on CT scans or MRI. MRI frequently reveals abnormal signals in the areas of affected vessels. MRI is most effective in identifying myelopathy due to vasculitis.

Angiography characteristically shows diffuse vascular "beading" with areas of alternating stenosis and dilatation. While these changes are consistent with vasculitis, they are not diagnostic; they may also be seen in noninflammatory vasculopathies.

Keys to Diagnosis: Primary CNS angiitis should be suspected in young to middle-aged individuals presenting with headache, focal neurologic findings, normal or slightly abnormal CSF results, and angiographic evidence of intracerebral vasculitis. Medications, infections, or associated inflammatory and noninflammatory vascular disorders must be considered and excluded.

Differential Diagnosis: See Table 1.

Therapy: Aggressive immunomodulatory therapy is indicated for proven primary CNS angiitis. Usual recommendations include high-dose prednisone in conjunction with cytotoxic drugs such as cyclophosphamide for a period of 6 to 12 months.

Prognosis: The prognosis of CNS angiitis can be variable. Primary CNS angiitis may be fatal if untreated. However, early diagnosis and aggressive treatment has led to more favorable outcomes, although some may be left with fixed neurologic deficits.

REFERENCES

Calabrese LH, Duna GF, Lie JT. Vasculitis in the central nervous system. Arthritis Rheum 1997;40:1189–1201.
Cohen SB, Hurd ER. Neurological complications of connective tissue and other "collagen-vascular" diseases. Semin Arthritis Rheum 1981;11:190–212.
Sigal LH. The neurologic presentation of vasculitic and rheumatologic syndromes. Medicine 1987;66:157–175.

CHOLESTEROL EMBOLI SYNDROME

Synonyms: Multiple cholesterol emboli syndrome, pseudovasculitis

ICD9 Code: 444.9

Definition: Cholesterol emboli syndrome is an uncommon complication of atherosclerosis with obstruction of small arteries and arterioles by cholesterol crystals. Symptoms are due to embolization from ulcerated or denuded large-vessel plaques and may mimic systemic necrotizing vasculitis.

Demographics: Cholesterol emboli syndrome occurs in adults (>50 years of age) with advanced atherosclerotic vascular disease, frequently following angiographic or other invasive vascular procedures. It may also follow anticoagulation or thrombolytic therapy. The lower aorta is the most common source of emboli.

Cardinal Findings: Skin and renal manifestations predominate. Skin manifestations include livedo reticularis, "blue toes," splinter hemorrhages, ulcerations, purpura/petechiae of the lower extremities, or gangrene. Renal impairment may initially be subacute but can progress over weeks to months to severe renal insufficiency. Up to 40% of patients may require dialysis. Less common clinical features include ischemia of the gut leading to perforation or hemorrhage and central nervous system involvement manifest as amaurosis fugax or stroke. Constitutional symptoms such as fever, weight loss, myalgias, and fatigue are occasionally seen and add to the difficulty in differentiating this entity from systemic necrotizing vasculitis.

Diagnostic Testing: Laboratory findings are nonspecific and include elevated acute-phase reactants (ESR and CRP) and eosinophilia. Urine may reveal granular or hyaline casts, proteinuria, and eosinophiluria. Skin, muscle, or less commonly renal biopsy shows pathognomonic findings of cholesterol clefts in the lumina of small vessels. Arteritis varies from a mild inflammatory response to obliterative endarteritis. Diagnosis is made premortem in only 30 to 40% of cases.

Therapy: Anticoagulation is contraindicated and, if already initiated, should likely be discontinued. It may be helpful to locate and resect the source of emboli. A role of steroid therapy has not been established. Treatment is largely supportive. Mortality may be as high as 60 to 90% because of renal involvement and frequent comorbidities.

REFERENCES

Cappiello RA, Espinoza LR, Adelman H, et al. Cholesterol embolism: a pseudovasculitic syndrome. Semin Arthritis Rheum 1989;18:240–246.
Sack KE. Mimickers of vasculitis. In: Koopman WJ, ed. Arthritis and allied conditions: a textbook of rheumatology. 13th ed. Baltimore: Williams & Wilkins, 1997:1525–1529.

CREST SYNDROME

Synonyms: Limited scleroderma (diffuse scleroderma is discussed on p. 343).

ICD9 Code: 710.1

Definition: "CREST syndrome" is more appropriately referred to as "limited scleroderma." In this variant of systemic sclerosis, skin thickening (sclerodactyly) is found distal to the elbow or knee and rarely affects the face or neck. The CREST constellation of findings includes calcinosis, Raynaud's phenomenon, esophageal dysmotility, sclerodactyly, and telangiectasias. Calcinosis is the least common of these findings. Table 1 compares features of limited and diffuse scleroderma.

Etiology: Unknown. (see etiology of scleroderma p. 343)

Demographics: Both diffuse and limited forms of scleroderma affect females more than males, with a female:male ratio of 3:1. The limited variant of scleroderma is more prevalent than the diffuse form, which is quite rare. Although Raynaud's phenomenon is quite common and affects up to 10% of female nonsmokers, only a small minority of Raynaud's patients develop limited or diffuse scleroderma.

Cardinal Findings: Virtually all patients manifest sclerodactyly and Raynaud's phenomenon (see p. 311). This should prompt a search for esophageal dysmotility and cutaneous telangiectasias, often found over the lips, tongue, hands, and face. Tight skin is usually most prominent in the fingers and toes and is less common over the hand or wrist. If severe, skin thickening may lead to problematic ischemic/traumatic ulcerations over the distal fingertips or DIP or PIP joints. Tendon friction rubs are rarely seen in limited scleroderma. Esophageal dysmotility manifests as food "sticking" substernally at the lower esophageal sphincter. Subcutaneous calcinosis is found in 30 to 40% of patients. Calcific deposits are usually "hard"; are located over the fingers, forearms, or lower extremities; and may be painful, intermittently inflamed, or ulcerate.

Table 1
Comparison of Limited and Diffuse Systemic Sclerosis

Feature	Limited[a]	Diffuse[a]
Sclerodactyly	+++++	+++++
Raynaud's phenomenon	+++++	+++++
Telangiectasias	++++	+++
Dysphagia	++++	++++
Calcinosis	++	+
Arthralgia/arthritis	++	++++
Pulmonary fibrosis	+	++
Pulmonary hypertension	+	0
Tendon friction rubs	0	+++
Renal crisis	0	+
Anticentromere Ab[b]	+++	+/0
Anti-Scl-70 Ab	+	++

[a]Relative percentages: +++++ 81–100%; ++++ 61–80%; +++ 41–60%; ++ 21–40%; + 1–20%.
[b]Ab, antibody.

Uncommon Findings: Small bowel disease is infrequently encountered in those with longstanding CREST syndrome and may manifest as bloating, cramping, diarrhea, or malabsorption. Interstitial lung fibrosis is much more common in diffuse scleroderma but has been described in the limited form. Those with longstanding CREST syndrome are at greatest risk for developing progressive pulmonary hypertension, usually late in the disease.

Diagnostic Testing: No abnormalities on hemogram, chemistry panel, or urinalysis are expected in a patient with limited disease. The vast majority of patients are ANA positive. In some, ANA subsets are correlated with the extent of scleroderma. Anticentromere antibodies are found in more than 50% of patients with limited scleroderma but only 10% of those with diffuse disease. Anticentromere antibodies may also be found in patients with primary biliary cirrhosis. A minority of CREST patients have anti-RNP antibodies. Pulmonary function test (PFT) results are abnormal in two-thirds of patients, with a reduced forced vital capacity or DLCO. Most patients have abnormal findings on nailfold capillaroscopy (see p. 129).

Imaging: Chest radiography (CXR) is indicated in those with pulmonary symptoms. Up to one-third of patients may show evidence of pulmonary fibrosis. High-resolution computerized tomography may be more sensitive than radiography in diagnosing pulmonary fibrosis but should only be used to resolve discrepancies between symptoms and PFTs or CXR.

Differential Diagnosis: CREST should be distinguished from diffuse scleroderma, eosinophilic fasciitis, overlap syndrome, drug-induced sclerodactyly, PBC, and other causes of pseudosclerodactyly (e.g., diabetes, hypothyroidism).

Therapy: Treatment of limited scleroderma is primarily directed at symptomatic relief of joint pain, Raynaud's phenomenon, and esophageal reflux and dysmotility (see "Scleroderma, Therapy," p. 346). Smoking cessation, hand warming (mittens, hand warmers, etc.), and care of the distal extremities should be emphasized. There is no proven role for penicillamine or other disease-modifying therapies in limited scleroderma. Cutaneous ulcerations may pose a therapeutic challenge. Treatment should hinge on warm soaks, vasodilator and antiplatelet agents, and treatment of superinfection.

REFERENCES

Furst DE, Clements PJ, Saab M, et al. Clinical and serological comparison of 17 chronic progressive systemic sclerosis (PSS) and 17 CREST syndrome patients matched for sex, age, and disease duration. Ann Rheum Dis 1984;43:794–801.

CRYOGLOBULINEMIA

ICD9 Code: 273.2

Definition: These clinical syndromes are associated with the presence of cryoprecipitable immunoglobulins (i.e., cryoglobulins).

Etiology: Cryoglobulins are produced by activated B cells, which may be oligoclonal or monoclonal. Some cases are associated with lymphoid malignancies, chronic immune-system disorders (e.g., RA or Sjögren's syndrome), or infection (e.g., hepatitis, infective endocarditis). Cryoglobulins are classified as type I (monoclonal), type II (mixed monoclonal and polyclonal), or type III (mixed polyclonal). Disease association with each type is discussed under "Cryoglobulins" (p. 106).

Pathology: Skin lesions often show leukocytoclastic vasculitis. Renal involvement is usually associated with a proliferative glomerulonephritis. Characteristic protein deposits in subendothelial regions are seen on electron microscopy. Serum samples contain reversibly precipitable immunoglobulins which may be monoclonal, polyclonal, or mixed. Hepatitis C or B antigenemia may be present.

Demographics: Most patients are in the fifth decade or older. Associations with an underlying disease, such as RA, follow the gender distribution characteristic of that disorder.

Cardinal Findings: Palpable purpura may be present on the lower extremities and rarely extends above the waist. Proteinuria may be present and in some cases can be accompanied by significant edema. Peripheral neuropathy with symptoms of pain, dysesthesia, or motor abnormalities may be the predominant finding in some patients. Cryoglobulinemia may present as a multisystem disorder with fever, cutaneous vasculitis, arthralgia, hepatosplenomegaly, lymphadenopathy, and glomerulonephritis.

Uncommon Manifestations: Raynaud's phenomenon and hyperviscosity syndrome are uncommon manifestations of cryoglobulinemia.

Diagnostic Tests: Serum collection, processing, and characterization of cryoglobulins must be carried out using proper procedure (see p. 106). Complement levels should be measured. Some cryoglobulins may demonstrate rheumatoid factor activity and should be tested for it. Hepatic enzyme elevations may be related to liver involvement or underlying hepatitis C or B infection, which should be assayed. Peripheral neuropathy or mononeuritis can be confirmed by nerve conduction tests. In some cases, biopsy of a nerve that is abnormal on EMG testing is useful. Skin biopsy evidence of leukocytoclastic vasculitis supports the diagnosis of cryoglobulinemia.

Keys to Diagnosis: Palpable purpura in a dependent distribution is most suggestive of cryoglobulinemia. A systemic disorder with involvement of the skin, kidney, peripheral nerves, and liver should suggest the possibility of cryoglobulinemia.

Differential Diagnosis: Conditions that may mimic cryoglobulinemia include vasculitis (e.g., polyarteritis nodosa, Henoch-Schönlein purpura), SLE, and lymphoma. Henoch-Schönlein purpura is more likely to be seen in young adults or children. Isolated renal involvement may occur with cryoglobulinemia and often requires renal biopsy for definitive diagnosis and exclusion of other forms of glomerulonephritis.

Therapy: If an underlying disorder is identified, therapy should be aimed at that process. Hepatitis C may be treated with IFN-α. Acute complications of the cryoglobulins themselves, such as rapidly progressive renal failure or symptoms associated with hyperviscosity, should be treated with a course of intensive plasmapheresis. Cyclophosphamide and steroids are used to treat patients with renal or nervous system involvement.

Surgery: Surgery is only used for diagnostic biopsy such as kidney or nerve.

Prognosis: In the absence of renal or neurologic involvement, many patients remain stable for years. Rapidly progressive glomerulonephritis is associated with a poorer prognosis. All patients should be monitored for transformation to neoplastic disease.

REFERENCES

Abel G, Zhang QX, Agnello V. Hepatitis C virus infection in type II mixed cryoglobulinemia. Arthritis Rheum 1993;36:1341–1349.

Anaya JM, Talal N. Sjogren's syndrome and connective tissue diseases associated with other immunologic disorders. In: Koopman WJ, ed. Arthritis and allied conditions: a textbook of rheumatology. 13th ed. Baltimore: Williams & Wilkins, 1997:1561–1580.

Brouet JC, Clauvel JP, Danon F, et al. Biologic and clinical significance of cryoglobulins: a report of 86 cases. Am J Med 1974;57:775–788.

CHURG-STRAUSS ANGIITIS

Synonyms: Allergic angiitis and granulomatosis

ICD9 Code: 287.0

Definition: Churg-Strauss angiitis is granulomatous vasculitis of small and medium-sized vessels associated with pulmonary disease and hypereosinophilia.

Etiology: This systemic vasculitis is of uncertain etiology.

Pathology: Churg-Strauss angiitis is necrotizing vasculitis with prominent eosinophilic tissue infiltrates and granulomas involving both medium and small arteries, capillaries, and venules.

Demographics: This very rare disorder is more prevalent in middle-aged men with antecedent asthma and rhinitis.

Cardinal Findings: Asthmatic manifestations with fluctuating pulmonary infiltrates (resembling Loeffler's syndrome), chronic eosinophilic pneumonia, and eosinophilic gastroenteritis may antedate frank vasculitis. Vasculitis may present with worsening respiratory status accompanied by systemic manifestations similar to those of polyarteritis nodosa (PAN). These include severe constitutional symptoms, arthralgias, mononeuritis multiplex, and occasional cardiac or gastrointestinal symptoms. Lung and skin findings are more common in Churg-Strauss angiitis than in PAN.

Uncommon Findings: In contrast to PAN, glomerulonephritis is *not* usually seen, and renal disease is present in only 40% of patients. In contrast to Wegener's granulomatosis, in Churg-Strauss angiitis the pulmonary lesions seldom cavitate, and the upper airway disease is less destructive.

Diagnostic Testing: Nonspecific measures of systemic inflammation include elevated acute-phase reactants (ESR and/or CRP), leukocytosis, anemia of chronic inflammation, and thrombocytosis. Peripheral blood eosinophilia and elevated IgE levels are often present. Circulating immune complexes, hypocomplementemia, and hyperglobulinemia have been observed but do not aid in the differential diagnosis. P-ANCA is occasionally present. A diagnosis is strongly supported by histopathologic evidence of small and medium vessel angiitis with eosinophils.

Keys to Diagnosis: The presentation is similar to that of PAN but with concomitant pulmonary involvement and a strong allergic component.

Diagnostic Criteria: 1990 ACR criteria include (*a*) asthma; (*b*) eosinophilia (>10% on WBC differential); (*c*) mononeuropathy or polyneuropathy; (*d*) migratory or transient pulmonary infiltrates; (*e*) paranasal sinus abnormalities; and (*f*) extravascular eosinophils on biopsy of a blood vessel. The presence of 4 or more of these 6 criteria constitutes a diagnosis for the purposes of classification (85% sensitivity; 99.7% specificity). A history of allergy is a criterion in other classification systems.

Therapy: High-dose corticosteroids are used ($\geq$1 mg/kg prednisone, occasionally started using a 1-g bolus of methylprednisolone). Cytotoxic therapy with cyclophosphamide or less commonly azathioprine is often used initially or added later as a steroid-sparing agent.

Prognosis: Survival is slightly better than in polyarteritis nodosa, with up to 90% of patients alive 1 year after the diagnosis.

REFERENCES

Gay RM, Ball GV. Vasculitis. In: Koopman WJ, ed. Arthritis and allied conditions: a textbook of rheumatology. 13th ed. Baltimore: Williams & Wilkins, 1997:1500–1501.

Lhote F, Guillevin L. Polyarteritis nodosa, microscopic polyangiitis and Churg Strauss syndrome: clinical aspects and treatment. Rheum Dis Clin North Am 1995;21:911–948.

Masi AT, Hunder GG, Lie JT, et al. The American College of Rheumatology 1990 criteria for the classification of Churg-Strauss syndrome (allergic granulomatosis and angiitis). Arthritis Rheum 1990;33:1094–1100.

DE QUERVAIN'S TENOSYNOVITIS

Synonyms: de Quervain's disease, stenosing tenosynovitis

ICD9 Codes: 727.04

Definition: de Quervain's tenosynovitis represents inflammation of the tendon sheath surrounding the abductor pollicis longus and extensor pollicis brevis muscles (see p. 24). It generally develops after overuse of the involved muscles (e.g., repetitive grasping with the thumb against resistance).

Demographics: Commonly affects women more than men. It is one of the most common forms of occupational overuse syndrome. It is also common during pregnancy, postpartum, and in other instances where no history of overuse can be elicited.

Cardinal Findings: Patients typically present with pain and tenderness in the area about the radial styloid that is worsened with movement. Uncommonly, local swelling of the involved tendons is seen. The diagnosis may be confirmed with the *Finkelstein test,* in which pain is elicited by stretching the involved tendons. To perform this test, the patient places the thumb inside a clenched fist and then moves or deviates the fist downward toward the ulnar side. Pain elicited with this maneuver suggests de Quervain's tenosynovitis.

Therapy: Treatment is guided by severity and may include splinting (to protect against further overuse), administration of topical analgesia (e.g., ice), NSAIDs, or local injection of corticosteroids (see p. 70). Surgery is rarely indicated.

REFERENCES

Moore JS. De Quervain's tenosynovitis. Stenosing tenosynovitis of the first dorsal compartment. J Occup Environ Med 1997;39:990–1002.

Schumacher HR Jr, Dorwart BB, Korzeniavski OM. Occurrence of de Quervain's tendinitis during pregnancy. Arch Intern Med 1985;145:2083–2084.

DIABETES MELLITUS: MUSCULOSKELETAL MANIFESTATIONS

Synonyms: Cheiroarthropathy, neuropathic joint, Charcot joints, diabetic amyotrophy, syndrome of limited joint mobility

ICD9 Codes: Neuropathic arthropathy, 250.6; diabetic complication NEC, 250.9; diabetic amyotrophy, 250.6 (358.1); arthropathy associated with endocrine disorder, 713.0

Definition: These are symptomatic abnormalities of skin, bones, joints and tendons that may associate with, or result from, type I or type II diabetes mellitus.

Etiology: Some abnormalities result from diabetes-induced nerve and blood vessel damage; others are due to excess collagen accumulation in periarticular structures and skin, which occurs with aging but is accelerated in diabetics. Others have hypothesized that nonenzymatic glycosylation of proteins leads to accumulation of advanced glycosylation end products that may contribute to the pathology.

Pathology: Skin and tendons show excessive fibrosis due to collagen accumulation. Muscle biopsy specimens may show type II fiber atrophy without significant inflammatory infiltrate.

Demographics: Musculoskeletal manifestations are most common in patients with longstanding type I diabetes but may also occur in some patients with type II diabetes.

Disease Associations: Associations between diabetes mellitus and gout, carpal tunnel syndrome, osteoporosis, or hyperostosis (DISH) have been suggested but are not well established.

Clinical Findings: The most common musculoskeletal conditions seen in diabetics include

Pseudosclerodactyly: Thickened, waxy skin changes are most apparent in the fingers. Motion of finger joints may be restricted because of thickened skin and tendons.

Syndrome of limited joint mobility (cheiroarthropathy or diabetic contractures): The small joints of the hand are commonly affected, with stiffness and an inability to completely extend or flex the fingers. Flexion contractures of the PIP and DIP joints results in the "prayer sign," an inability to close the gap between opposed palms and fingers. It is associated with advanced disease duration and diabetic microvascular disease elsewhere.

Periarthritis: Adhesive capsulitis of the shoulder is commonly seen in type I diabetics over 40 years of age. Patients complain of shoulder pain (especially at night) and difficulty raising their arms. Joint examination reveals limited range of motion (especially abduction).

Dupuytren's contractures (see p. 197) *and trigger fingers* are relatively common.

Neuropathic (Charcot) arthropathy (see p. 264) commonly affects the tarsal and metatarsal joints and manifests as bony swelling without pain. The diagnosis is made by radiography.

Diabetic neuropathy may cause pain and dysfunction in the extremities and may also lead to symptomatic muscle weakness.

Diabetic amyotrophy is an asymmetric ischemic myopathy that results in weakness and pain. Diabetic amyotrophy is typically seen in adults over 50 years of age and should be considered with pain, limb girdle muscle atrophy, and fasciculation. Prominent involvement of the iliopsoas, quadriceps, and adductor thigh muscles causes difficulty standing, rising from a seated position, or climbing stairs. The diagnosis may be made by MRI or muscle biopsy.

Uncommon Findings: There are reports of acanthosis nigricans and severe insulin resistance due to circulating antireceptor antibodies in patients with SLE and scleroderma.

Diagnostic Tests: Muscle biopsy or EMG may be required to confirm tissue involvement. Diagnosis of these manifestations does not depend upon the presence of hyperglycemia or an elevated hemoglobin-A1c.

Keys to Diagnosis: The onset of musculoskeletal symptoms in patients with established type I or II diabetes mellitus should lead to consideration of one of the above entities.

Differential Diagnosis: Skin changes (pseudosclerodactyly) in diabetics resemble those seen in scleroderma, but abnormalities on nailfold capillaroscopy are absent. Muscle weakness may suggest inflammatory myopathy, but the diabetic form is more likely to be asymmetric. The presence of neuropathic joints and neurologic changes in the extremities may resemble changes seen with syphilis.

Therapy: Some musculoskeletal manifestations may be slowed by improved glycemic control. Physical therapy may be helpful in managing or improving the range of motion in affected shoulders or fingers. Tendinitis is managed symptomatically with NSAIDs and physical therapy, but local application of heat is relatively contraindicated because of safety concerns. Neuropathic joints are treated primarily with rest and local measures to prevent infections.

Prognosis: Some manifestations show improvement or stabilization with improved glycemic control, and radiculopathy or weakness may spontaneously remit. Other problems, notably skin or tendon thickening and neuropathic joint abnormalities, are not likely to improve with glycemic control and may cause permanent dysfunction.

REFERENCES

Cronin ME. Rheumatic aspects of endocrinopathies. In: Koopman WJ, ed. Arthritis and allied conditions: a textbook of rheumatology. 13th ed. Baltimore: Williams & Wilkins, 1997:2233–2249.

Pastan RS, Cohen AS. The rheumatologic manifestations of diabetes mellitus. Med Clin N Am 1978;62:829–839.

Tsokos GC, Gordon P, Antonovych T, et al. Lupus nephritis and other autoimmune features in patients with diabetes mellitus due to autoantibody to insulin receptors. Ann Intern Med 1985;102:176–181.

DIALYSIS: MUSCULOSKELETAL MANIFESTATIONS

Synonym: Hemodialysis-related arthropathy

Definition: These are syndromes related to muscles and joint structures seen in patients undergoing renal dialysis.

Etiology: The cause of most hemodialysis-associated syndromes is unknown. Secondary hyperparathyroidism can lead to development of bone abnormalities. β_2-Microglobulin amyloidosis and crystal deposition arthritis result from abnormalities of renal clearance.

Pathology: Arthritic syndromes associated with dialysis show erosive bone changes in less than 25%. Most synovial fluids are noninflammatory, except those associated with crystals. β_2-Microglobulin deposits are observed in bone cysts and soft tissues such as those within the carpal tunnel.

Demographics: Affected patients are usually on long-term hemodialysis.

Cardinal Findings: Arthralgias are common. A minority of patients show erosive changes in small joints of the hands. Amyloid deposition most commonly presents as carpal tunnel syndrome or characteristic bone cysts seen on radiographs.

Uncommon Manifestations: Myelopathy with paresis due to amyloid deposition has been reported.

Diagnostic Tests: Biopsies of affected tissues are required to establish a diagnosis of amyloidosis. Radiographs of affected joints show bone cysts, erosions, or subperiosteal resorption of bone. Synovial fluid analyses are required to evaluate crystal deposition diseases.

Keys to Diagnosis: Persistent symptoms referable to joints or periarticular tissues in the setting of hemodialysis should prompt further investigation.

Differential Diagnosis: Hyperparathyroidism, idiopathic carpal tunnel syndrome (not related to amyloid deposition), and other metabolic disorders should be considered.

Therapy: Amyloid deposition in some patients may be slowed by changing the membrane used for dialysis. Symptomatic carpal tunnel syndrome may require surgical intervention. Nonspecific arthralgias and other joint complaints may be treated symptomatically, with use of analgesics dictated by the underlying medical condition. Treatment of crystal arthritis may also be limited by the underlying condition.

Prognosis: Patients with amyloid are difficult to treat and have a more limited prognosis than those with other dialysis-related syndromes, which probably do not significantly alter the patient's course.

REFERENCES

Menerey K, Braunstein E, Brown M, et al. Musculoskeletal symptoms related to arthropathy in patients receiving dialysis. J Rheumatol 1988;15:1848–1854.

DIFFUSE IDIOPATHIC SKELETAL HYPEROSTOSIS (DISH)

Synonyms: Forestier's disease, ankylosing hyperostosis

ICD9 Code: 721.8

Definition: DISH is not an arthropathy, but rather a bone-forming diathesis primarily affecting the spine, with ossification of tendons and ligaments. Diagnosis is often made incidentally during standard chest radiography.

Etiology: The etiology of DISH is unknown.

Demographics: This common disorder occurs in 12% of those over age 65 years. Men are more commonly affected than women by a ratio of 2:1.

Associated Disorders: DISH is associated with calcium pyrophosphate dihydrate deposit disease, gout, rheumatoid arthritis, and osteoarthritis but not ankylosing spondylitis (extremely rare). DISH may be associated with diabetes mellitus, obesity, hyperlipidemia, and hyperuricemia.

Cardinal Findings: Patients are usually asymptomatic but may complain of thoracolumbar or neck stiffness. Large osteophytes of the cervical spine may cause dysphagia in up to 25% of patients. Enthesopathy is common. Large osteophytes elsewhere may cause recurrent Achilles tendinitis or tennis elbow.

Complications: Excessive heterotopic bone formation may complicate hip surgery. Relatively minor trauma may result in fractures through ankylosed segments with subsequent neurologic impairment. Rarely, ossification of the posterior longitudinal ligament may result in myelopathy.

Diagnostic Tests: Test results are normal for age (e.g., ESR). No association with HLA-B27 is seen in most studies.

Diagnostic Criteria: Resnick has proposed the following. All three criteria are required.

1. Flowing spinal calcification involving at least four vertebrae
2. Preservation of disc height and lack of degenerative disc disease
3. Absence of apophyseal and sacroiliac joint ankylosis or erosions

Imaging: Radiographic findings are diagnostic in DISH and include spinal and extraspinal findings.

—*Spinal findings:* There is normal bone mineralization. Anterolateral ossification of the anterior longitudinal ligament (and surrounding soft tissues) of the spine results in flowing, bridging, often bulky osteophytes that involve at least four contiguous vertebrae. Disc spaces are preserved. Involvement of the thoracic (nearly 100%), lumbar (>90%) and cervical spine (75%) is common.

—*Extraspinal findings:* Pelvic films are frequently abnormal with "whiskering" of the iliac crests, ossification of the symphysis pubis, or large bony osteophytes at the acetabular margin of the hip. The lower third (synovial lined portion) of the sacroiliac joint should not be involved in DISH. Other sites of extensive ossification (or spurring) may include the calcaneus, patella, tibial tuberosity, and olecranon. Calcification of the sacrotuberous and iliolumbar ligaments may be seen.

Differential Diagnosis: Ankylosing spondylitis, other spondyloarthropathies, osteoarthritis, intervertebral osteochondrosis, hypoparathyroidism, retinoid therapy, fluorosis, and hypervitaminosis A must be distinguished.

Therapy: No specific therapy retards development of new bone. Analgesic agents and NSAIDs may be used for pain or stiffness. Rarely is surgical removal of calcific masses indicated. Although some have advocated low-dose radiation following hip surgery to minimize heterotopic bone formation, this has not been thoroughly tested.

REFERENCES

Paley D, Schwartz M, Cooper P, et al. Fractures of the spine in diffuse idiopathic skeletal hyperostosis. Clin Orthop 1991;267:22–32.

Resnick D, Niwayama G. Radiographic and pathologic features of spinal involvement in diffuse skeletal hyperostosis (DISH). Radiology 1976;119:559.

DRUG-INDUCED LUPUS

ICD9 Code: 695.4

Definition: Drug-induced lupus (DIL) is an uncommon complication of several commonly used medications. It is characterized by development of lupus-like symptoms, ANA positivity, and symptom resolution upon withdrawal of the offending drug. DIL differs from SLE by affecting an older population with milder symptoms and having a different autoantibody profile and a more favorable outcome.

Etiology: Numerous drugs have been implicated in causing DIL (Table 1). Mechanisms underlying this disorder remain unclear but may involve either (*a*) similarities between drug and self antigens, resulting in immunologic cross-reactivity; (*b*) drug-induced alteration in immunogenicity of autoantigens (i.e., drugs may react with histones or deoxyribonucleoprotein); or (*c*) altered immunoregulation by drug or its metabolites.

Risk Factors: Other factors may contribute to the onset of DIL. The slow acetylator phenotype clearly increases the risk of hydralazine-induced ANA positivity and DIL, but is less important in procainamide- and isoniazid-associated DIL, and does not appear to influence the risk of DIL due to other drugs or idiopathic SLE. There are few genetic associations with DIL. Only HLA-DR4 has been suggested to be linked with hydralazine-induced lupus.

Pathology: CNS and renal findings are rare in DIL. However, other lupus manifestations and pathology may occur in DIL and be pathologically indistinguishable from SLE, including ANA positivity, LE cells, inflammatory pleuritis, pericarditis, and synovitis.

Demographics: DIL affects a greater percentage of males, whites, and the elderly than does idiopathic SLE (Table 2). For all implicated drugs, the incidence of drug-induced ANA positivity alone is far greater (often 2- to 5-fold more common) than the actual DIL syndrome. Prevalence varies for each drug, and reliable rates have only been reported for the most commonly associated drugs—hydralazine and procainamide. The rates of DIL are dose related for hydralazine and time dependent for procainamide. Between 60 and 90% of patients taking procainamide for more than 12 months develop ANA positivity, and roughly one-third of these develop DIL. Rates of ANA positivity approach 50% for those taking 400 mg/day of hydralazine or more, but only 10% develop DIL. With lower doses of hydralazine, lower percentages are seen. The inci-

Table 1
Agents Implicated in Causing Drug-Induced Lupus[a]

Definite/Common	Probable/Uncommon	Possible/Rare
Procainamide	Phenytoin	Gold salts
Hydralazine	Carbamazepine	Oral contraceptives
Isoniazid	Primidone	Nitrofurantoin
Quinidine	Ethosuximide	Griseofulvin
Sulfasalazine	Propylthiouracil	Interferon (α, γ)
Chlorpromazine	Methylthiouracil	Anti-TNF therapy
Methyldopa	Penicillamine	
	Lithium carbonate	
	Acebutolol	
	Practolol	
	Minocycline	

[a]Drugs are listed according to strength of association and frequency of ANA or DIL.

dence of ANA positivity in those treated with isoniazid, methyldopa, chlorpromazine, or quinidine ranges from 10 to 30%, yet very few develop clinical features of the DIL syndrome. DIL due to minocycline has only been seen after prolonged exposure (>12 months) to the antibiotic.

Cardinal Findings: Most patients present with insidious onset of constitutional features (e.g., low-grade fever, fatigue, anorexia, weight loss, arthralgias, or myalgias. However, the pattern of organ involvement differs from that of idiopathic SLE (Table 2).

—*Renal:* Kidney involvement is rare in DIL and has only been sporadically described with hydralazine-induced lupus. Such findings include sporadic proteinuria, abnormal urinary sediments, impaired creatinine clearance, or biopsy-proven nephritis. Most of these findings tend to resolve with drug withdrawal.

—*CNS:* CNS involvement is very rare in DIL. There are few reports of neuropathy.

—*Skin:* Lupus skin findings (e.g., malar rash, oral ulcers, photosensitivity, alopecia, Raynaud's phenomenon) are uncommon in DIL patients.

—*Musculoskeletal:* As in SLE, articular findings are common. Myalgias and arthralgias are very frequent at presentation and if present, synovitis tends to be symmetric and polyarticular and involves the knees and fingers. Polymyalgia rheumatica has also been described.

—*Pulmonary:* Alveolar infiltrates are common in procainamide-induced lupus but are rarely seen with other implicated drugs (Table 1). Chronic interstitial lung disease has been described, but pulmonary hemorrhage has not.

—*Serositis:* Symptomatic pleural or pericardial effusions are common in DIL, especially in procainamide-induced lupus. LE cells and ANA may be found in serosal fluids.

Table 2
Comparison of Drug-Induced Lupus and SLE

Feature	Hydralazine Lupus	Procainamide Lupus	SLE
Demographics			
Female:male	1.6:1	0.9:1	9:1
Black:white	0.2:1	0.5:1	2.7:1
Mean onset age (years)	50	62	29
Clinical features			
Renal	13%	0	44%
Neurologic	7%	1%	45%
Skin	27%	11%	71%
Articular	86%	82%	92%
Pulmonary	3%	41%	1%
Serosal (pleuropericardial)	18%	46%	46%

Uncommon Findings: CNS, renal, and lupus skin disease are uncommon. There have been uncommon reports of pericardial tamponade and constrictive pericarditis.

Diagnostic Tests: Requisite findings in DIL include lupus clinical features in association with ANA positivity (or a positive LE cell preparation). Patients with DIL have very high titers (e.g., >1:1280) of ANA, often in a diffuse or speckled pattern. Such ANAs are directed toward deoxyribonucleoproteins (i.e., histones). Antihistone antibodies are commonly found in DIL but are also seen in SLE and, therefore, cannot distinguish between the two. Nonetheless, antibodies against specific histone complexes have been identified for procainamide and sulfasalazine (against H2A-H2B), hydralazine (H3-H2A), and quinidine (H1-H2B). Antibodies against double-stranded DNA (dsDNA) and complement levels should be negative or normal. Leukopenia, lymphopenia, and Coombs-positive hemolytic anemia have all been well described in DIL. Elevated ESR may been seen during active DIL. Lupus anticoagulants and antiphospholipid antibodies have frequently been reported, but thromboses and the antiphospholipid syndrome are rare.

Keys to Diagnosis: This diagnosis can be suspected in older adults taking an "implicated" drug who develop lupuslike features described above. Development of ANA alone does not suffice for the diagnosis or for withdrawal of the drug.

Diagnostic Criteria: Most patients meet the American College of Rheumatology criteria for the diagnosis of SLE (see p. 363), although this is not necessary. The diagnosis of DIL can be established if there is (*a*) no history of SLE prior to drug exposure, (*b*) one or more clinical features of SLE in addition to ANA positivity, and (*c*) resolution of symptoms and ultimately the ANA with drug withdrawal. Rechallenge with the offending agent is not necessary.

Therapy: Most patients respond promptly to drug withdrawal and symptomatic therapy. Commonly, patients benefit from rest, analgesics, and possible NSAIDs when treating constitutional, articular, or serosal manifestations. Infrequently, corticosteroids are necessary to treat refractory pleural/pericardial effusions, pericardial tamponade, moderate-to-severe pneumonitis, or symptomatic hemolytic anemia. Pericardiocentesis or surgery is rarely necessary for pericardial tamponade.

Course: The vast majority experience rapid resolution of their symptoms upon drug withdrawal. ANA positivity may persist for 6 to 12 months following cessation.

Comment: Drugs implicated in causing DIL (Table 1) can be safely used in patients with idiopathic SLE without risk. Identification of ANA positivity alone (without clinical features of lupus) is not sufficient reason to withdraw potentially beneficial therapy.

REFERENCES

Cush JJ, Goldings EA. Southwestern Internal Medicine Conference: Drug-induced lupus: clinical spectrum and pathogenesis. Am J Med Sci 1985;290:36–45.

Rich MW. Drug-induced lupus. The list of culprits grows. Postgrad Med 1996;100:299–302.

Yung RL, Richardson BC. Drug-induced lupus. Rheum Dis Clin North Am 1994;10:61–86.

DUPUYTREN'S CONTRACTURE

ICD9 Code: 728.6

Definition: Dupuytren's contracture results from thickening and shortening of the palmar fascia of the hand. Flexion deformities of involved fingers may cause considerable morbidity.

Etiology: The etiology is unknown; it may be familial (autosomal dominant) in up to 10% of patients.

Demographics: Dupuytren's contracture may be seen in 3 to 5% of adults. Men are affected about 5 times more frequently than women, and incidence increases with age. It occurs most commonly in Caucasians, particularly northern Europeans.

Associated Conditions: Dupuytren's contracture is often seen in those with alcoholism, diabetes, epilepsy, hypercholesterolemia, rheumatoid arthritis, or reflex sympathetic dystrophy.

Cardinal Findings: Findings may be unilateral or bilateral. In early disease, painless nodularity of the fascia may be mistaken for local tenosynovial swelling. As the disease progresses, the appearance becomes more classic, with thick cordlike swelling of the fascia that is easily palpable below the thickened and puckered dermis. The fibrotic process can extend to involve the digital fascia. Shortening of the fascia results in flexion contracture of the fingers, particularly the 4th finger, although digits 2 through 5 may also be involved.

Therapy: Physical therapy and local therapies, such as heat, are often recommended for patients with mild contracture. Some authors also recommend intralesional corticosteroids, although such injections have varied success. Patients with more severe cases may require surgical intervention to release the contracture.

REFERENCES

Hill NA. Dupuytren's contracture. J Bone Joint Surg 1985;65A:1439–1443.

EPSTEIN-BARR VIRUS (EBV)-ASSOCIATED DISEASES

Definition: EBV is a DNA herpesvirus responsible for acute and rarely chronic infectious illnesses and occasional rheumatologic manifestations.

ICD9 Code: Infectious mononucleosis, 075.0

Etiology: EBV infects human B lymphocytes and is a potent polyclonal B-cell activator. EBV has been examined as a putative pathogen in certain chronic diseases such as rheumatoid arthritis, Sjögren's syndrome, and the chronic fatigue syndrome. To date, no firm direct associations with chronic inflammatory disorders have been established. Further, no credible scientific data associates EBV infection with chronic fatigue syndrome.

Demographics: Males and females are equally affected. Infectious mononucleosis (IM), caused by EBV, is a disease of adolescents and young adults. Rarely, EBV may cause chronic mononucleosis.

Cardinal Findings: Acute IM is characterized by severe pharyngitis with prominent tonsil enlargement, fever, marked regional and generalized lymphadenopathy, and hepatosplenomegaly. Headache, vomiting, jaundice, and rash are occasionally noted. About 2% of patients with IM develop arthralgias, and at least 20% experience myalgias. Frank monoarticular (particularly a knee or an ankle) or oligoarticular large-joint arthritis have been rarely reported.

Diagnostic Testing: Heterophile antibody or atypical lymphocytosis are very useful to confirm a clinically suspected diagnosis. ESR may be normal to markedly elevated. Hepatocellular liver enzymes are not uncommonly elevated, sometimes markedly. Urinalysis shows proteinuria in about 10% of cases. When arthritis is present, the synovial fluid is typically inflammatory. EBV-specific antibodies include IgG and IgM viral capsid antigen (VCA), early antigen (EA), and Epstein-Barr nuclear antigen (EBNA). The earliest antibody (IgM) response is to VCA, and IgG antibodies persist indefinitely after EBV infection (see p. 143). Antibody response to EA starts 1 month after infection and lasts for 3 to 6 months. EBNA starts to rise approximately 1 month after EA and persists for many years.

Keys to Diagnosis: IM, a febrile illness with severe pharyngitis and marked constitutional symptoms, is confirmed by a positive heterophile test.

Therapy: Supportive therapy with no specific interventions other than analgesics is indicated for the musculoskeletal manifestations and most other IM manifestations. Short courses of corticosteroids are occasionally used for obstructing tonsils and other serious and rare manifestations of EBV infection (e.g., hemolytic anemia, thrombocytopenic purpura, and neurologic or cardiac disease).

REFERENCES

Straus SE, Tosato G, Meier J. Epstein-Barr virus infections: biology, pathogenesis, and management. Ann Intern Med 1993;118:45–58.
Yitteberg SR. Viral arthritis. In: Koopman WJ, ed. Arthritis and allied conditions: a textbook of rheumatology. 13th ed. Baltimore: Williams & Wilkins, 1997:2341–2360.

ENTEROPATHIC ARTHRITIS

Synonyms: Inflammatory bowel disease (IBD)-associated arthritis, Crohn's arthritis; (also see Whipple's disease or intestinal bypass syndrome)

ICD9 Code: 713.1

Definition: Enteropathic arthritis refers to the inflammatory arthritis associated with Crohn's disease or ulcerative colitis. In both, clinical and histologic gut inflammation, altered intestinal permeability, and development of an inflammatory peripheral or axial arthritis may be seen.

Etiology: There is no association between HLA-B27 and colitic peripheral arthritis. However, HLA-B27 is found in 50% of patients with spondylitic colitis. Thus, enteropathic arthritis should be considered in the setting of HLA-B27-negative ankylosing spondylitis.

Pathology: Gastrointestinal (GI) manifestations and pathology may be insidious or subclinical. In ulcerative colitis, mucosal lesions appear in the colon as ulceration, edema, friability, or microabscesses. In Crohn's disease, lesions may be present anywhere in the GI tract, although the terminal ileum and colon are most common. Lesions may be ulcerative (aphthoid), patchy, or transmural, with evidence of granulomas. Synovial biopsy reveals chronic inflammatory changes.

Demographics: Peripheral arthritis affects men and women equally. All age groups are affected. While the onset of arthritis follows established intestinal inflammation in adults, the converse may be seen in children. In contrast with peripheral arthritis, axial disease may precede or coincide with the onset of colitis and is more common in men.

Cardinal Findings: Triad features of Crohn's disease includes abdominal pain, weight loss, and diarrhea. Ulcerative colitis is characterized by diarrhea and intestinal blood loss. Disease onset is sometimes heralded by low-grade fever, painful oral (aphthous) ulcers, or ocular (conjunctivitis, anterior uveitis) or cutaneous manifestations (erythema nodosum, pyoderma gangrenosum). In most cases, GI manifestations antedate or coincide with the onset of arthritis.

Axial arthritis occurs in 10 to 15% of IBD patients and is clinically and radiographically indistinguishable from ankylosing spondylitis. Chronic low back pain/stiffness and limited range of motion are common. The activity of axial disease does not parallel gut involvement.

Peripheral arthritis is seen in nearly 20% of patients. Peripheral arthritis manifests as an inflammatory, nonerosive, asymmetric oligoarthritis or monarthritis affecting large joints (knees, ankles, elbows), especially of the lower extremities. It is usually chronic but may be migratory and resolve in weeks or months. Enthesitis (i.e., heel pain) and "sausage digits" (toes or fingers) may occur. The activity of peripheral arthritis parallels gut inflammation. Peripheral arthropathy more frequently occurs in those with extraintestinal manifestations (erythema nodosum, uveitis, etc).

Uncommon Findings: Clubbing, erosive arthritis, pericarditis, amyloidosis, thrombophlebitis are rarely seen.

Diagnostic Tests: Abnormalities may include increased ESR or CRP, thrombocytosis, and hypochromic anemia. Synovial fluid WBC ranges from 2000 to 50,000 cells/mm^3.

Imaging: Axial disease is radiographically indistinguishable from ankylosing spondylitis. Periostitis and radiographic enthesitis may be present.

Keys to Diagnosis: The presence of spondylitis or a seronegative oligoarthritis along with GI symptom evidence of inflammatory bowel disease may suggest this diagnosis.

Differential Diagnosis: Articular disease may be confused with seronegative rheumatoid arthritis, other spondyloarthropathies, or Behçet's syndrome. GI manifestations may also be seen in patients with the vasculitides, Whipple's disease, intestinal bypass syndrome, scleroderma, amyloidosis, Henoch-Schön-lein purpura, familial Mediterranean fever, postdysenteric reactive arthritis, and lymphoma and in those with GI toxicity related to antirheumatic therapies.

Therapy: Control of colitis may improve the peripheral arthritis but not axial disease. Treatment options are similar to those used in ankylosing spondylitis. NSAIDs tend to be helpful. Rarely NSAIDs exacerbate the enteritis. Corticosteroids are not advised in spondylitis but may be useful in low doses for peripheral arthritis or when injected intraarticularly for uncontrolled mono- or oligoarthritis. Sulfasalazine, methotrexate, and azathioprine should be reserved for those with uncontrolled arthritis, with or without active colitis.

Surgery: Joint surgery is seldom indicated. Bowel surgery may be indicated but not for arthritis alone.

REFERENCES

Mielants H, Veys EM. Enteropathic arthritis: idiopathic inflammatory bowel disease. In: Koopman WJ, ed. Arthritis and allied conditions: a textbook of rheumatology. 13th ed. Baltimore: Williams & Wilkins, 1997:1245–1248.

EOSINOPHILIA MYALGIA SYNDROME (EMS)

ICD9 Code: 710.5

Definition: EMS is considered a variant form of scleroderma. Most cases have been associated with ingestion of L-tryptophan.

Etiology: Ingestion of specific lots of L-tryptophan in 1989 and 1990 resulted in development of large numbers of cases of EMS and was correlated with a trace contaminant due to a change in the manufacturing process for L-trypto-phan. Sporadic cases reported before and after the contaminated L-tryptophan was available may be due to similar trace contaminants in other supplements or to inborn errors of tryptophan metabolism.

Pathology: Full-thickness skin biopsy specimens show thickened fascia with accumulation of collagen in the dermis. Inflammatory infiltrates, which may contain eosinophils, are found in subcutaneous fat (panniculitis) and surrounding small blood vessels or muscle spindles.

Demographics: An epidemic of cases appeared after 1989 and quickly subsided after the suspect preparation was recalled. Most of the epidemic-associated patients were female.

Cardinal Findings: Myalgias are severe and may be debilitating. A minority of patients show muscle enzyme elevations. Skin induration is most commonly seen on the trunk, generally sparing the extremities and face. Central nervous system involvement, manifested by difficulty with memory or other cognitive problems and peripheral neuropathy, occurs in most patients.

Uncommon Findings: Cardiac involvement with functional impairment is rare but may contribute to conduction changes and, possibly, sudden death.

Diagnostic Tests: Peripheral eosinophilia is seen in most patients. A full-thickness skin biopsy, including deep fascial tissue, is important for establishing a diagnosis.

Keys to Diagnosis: Skin thickening and severe myalgias should suggest the diagnosis; rare cases may not be associated with ingestion of L-tryptophan.

Differential Diagnosis: The skin changes of EMS resemble eosinophilic fasciitis. However, eosinophilic fasciitis does not usually exhibit cognitive dysfunction and myalgias. Localized forms of scleroderma and underlying malignancies should be also considered.

Diagnostic Criteria

1. Eosinophil count $> 1 \times 10^9/L$
2. Generalized myalgias that limit activity
3. Absence of underlying malignancy

Therapy: Acute symptoms respond to treatment with glucocorticoids, but late symptoms, including cognitive dysfunction, are relatively resistant to therapy.

Surgery: Surgery is not generally indicated except diagnostic skin biopsy.

Prognosis: A chronic phase develops in at least half of patients, with muscle cramps and CNS abnormalities that may impair normal daily activity.

REFERENCES

Pincus T. Eosinophilia-myalgia syndrome: patient status 2–4 years after onset. J Rheumatol 1996;23:19–25.
Winkelmann RK, Connolly SM, Quimby SR, et al. Histopathologic features of the L-tryptophan-related eosinophilia-myalgia syndrome. Mayo Clinic Proc 1991;66:457–463.

EOSINOPHILIC FASCIITIS

ICD9 Code: 728.89

Synonyms: Schulman's syndrome, diffuse fasciitis with eosinophilia

Definition: Eosinophilic fasciitis is considered a variant form of scleroderma. Skin tightening is limited to the extremities and spares the face. Onset is often abrupt and may be preceded by vigorous exercise.

Etiology: Most cases are sporadic and of unknown cause. Exposure to organic solvents has been implicated as causative in isolated patients. Skin fibroblasts secrete excessive amounts of collagen, which may be cytokine-driven.

Pathology: Full-thickness skin biopsy specimens show collagen accumulation in the dermis, with panniculitis and a cellular infiltrate, often containing significant numbers of eosinophils.

Demographics: Onset is usually in middle age. Equal numbers of males and females are affected.

Cardinal Findings: Skin of the extremities is thickened with a corrugated or dimpled (*peau d'orange*) appearance. If periarticular areas are involved, joint contractures may develop. The face and distal extremities are usually spared, Raynaud's phenomenon is absent, and nailfold capillaroscopy is normal, distinguishing this syndrome from scleroderma.

Uncommon Manifestations: Pulmonary hypertension, thromboembolic disease, and liver abnormalities have been reported.

Diagnostic Tests: A full-thickness skin biopsy that must include deep fascial tissue is necessary to establish the diagnosis.

Keys to Diagnosis: Peripheral eosinophilia and hypergammaglobulinemia are usually present. Serologic tests for ANA and RF are negative. Skin biopsy specimens may show skin thickening accompanied by tissue eosinophilia.

Differential Diagnosis: Rare cases of this syndrome develop in association with underlying malignancies. Eosinophilia-myalgia syndrome associated with ingestion of L-tryptophan more commonly shows muscle, CNS, and visceral involvement. Other localized forms of scleroderma should be considered.

Therapy: Treatment with prednisone benefits most patients. Hydroxychloroquine, penicillamine, and methotrexate may also be beneficial.

Surgery: Surgery is not generally indicated except diagnostic skin biopsies.

Prognosis: Most patients respond to medical therapy and show significant improvement. Spontaneous remissions have been reported.

REFERENCES

Claw DW, Crofford LJ. Eosinophilic rheumatic disorders (review). Rheum Dis Clin North Am 1995;21:231–246.
Silver RM. Variant forms of scleroderma. In: Koopman WJ, ed. Arthritis and allied conditions: a textbook of rheumatology. 13th ed. Baltimore: Williams & Wilkins, 1997:1465–1480.

ERYTHEMA NODOSUM

Synonym: Panniculitis (see p. 289)

ICD9 Code: 695.2

Definition: Erythema nodosum is an acute, usually self-limited, septal panniculitis characterized by tender subcutaneous nodules, typically on the anterior tibial surface.

Etiology: Half of cases have an underlying associated condition (Table 1). Pathogenesis is unknown but may be related to circulating immune complexes. There is an association with HLA-B8.

Pathology: Acute (neutrophilic) and chronic (granulomatous) septal inflammation is seen in subcutaneous adipose tissue and around blood vessels.

Demographics: Women are predominantly affected, with a M:F ratio of 1:3. It is most common in those between the ages of 25 and 40 years. Incidence has been reported to be 2 to 3 cases per 100,000 population.

Cardinal Findings: There is sudden onset of one or more tender, erythematous nodules on the anterior tibial surface, rarely over the thighs or forearms. Lesions are deep nodules, 1 to 10 cm in diameter, which evolve into softer, ecchymotic lesions and usually heal in 6 to 8 weeks without scar formation. In dark-skinned individuals, lesions are usually hyperpigmented. Symptoms such as fever and arthralgia are usually those of the associated condition. Synovitis may involve the knees or ankles. *Loefgren's syndrome*, a specific variant of sarcoidosis, describes the triad of bilateral hilar adenopathy, erythema nodosum, and polyarthralgia or polyarthritis. Inflammatory bowel disease has been associated with erythema nodosum, and lesions tend to parallel disease activity.

Uncommon Findings: Cutaneous ulceration is extremely rare. Migratory and chronic forms have been described.

Diagnostic Tests: A careful clinical search to identify associated conditions should be undertaken. The ESR is usually elevated. Additional investigations may include pharyngeal culture (for group A β-hemolytic streptococci), chest radiography (to look for bilateral hilar adenopathy, pulmonary tuberculosis, or deep fungal infections), intradermal tests (for tuberculosis and deep fungi), or stool cultures (for *Yersinia* and *Salmonella* infections).

Keys to Diagnosis: Look for tender, erythematous, subcutaneous nodules on anterior tibial surface.

Differential Diagnosis: Erythema nodosum may be confused with vasculitis with nodular lesions, Weber-Christian disease, or panniculitis associated with pancreatitis.

Therapy: Treat any underlying condition. Symptomatic management includes

Table 1
Disorders Commonly Associated with Erythema Nodosum

Category	Associated Condition	Diagnostic Test(s)
Infections	Streptococcal pharyngitis	Pharyngeal culture
	Tuberculosis	CXR, skin tests
	Deep fungal infections	CXR, skin tests
	Enteric infections	Stool culture, serology
	Leprosy	Skin biopsy, acid-fast stain
Drugs	Sulfonamides	Drug withdrawal
	Oral contraceptives	Drug withdrawal
	Penicillin	Drug withdrawal
Systemic disorders	Pregnancy	β-HCG
	Sarcoidosis	CXR
	Inflammatory bowel disease	Endoscopy
Idiopathic		

bed rest, cold compresses, and NSAIDs. A short course of systemic corticosteroids or potassium iodide can be very helpful.

Prognosis: Erythema nodosum is usually self-limited, with resolution in 6 to 8 weeks. Prognosis may be determined by the associated disorder, if any.

REFERENCES

Callen JP. Miscellaneous disorders that commonly affect both skin and joints: panniculitis. In: Sontheimer RD, Provost TT, eds. Cutaneous manifestations of rheumatic diseases. Baltimore: Williams & Wilkins, 1996:266–268.

FAMILIAL MEDITERRANEAN FEVER (FMF)

Synonyms: Periodic fever, periodic disease, familial recurrent polyserositis

ICD9 Code: 277.3

Definition: FMF is an intermittent febrile disorder with inflammatory serositis, arthritis, and rash.

Etiology: FMF is an autosomal recessive disorder of unknown etiology. The genetic defect has been localized to the short arm of chromosome 16. This may account for an inherited deficiency of the inhibitor to the chemotactic anaphylatoxin C5a, which may in turn contribute to the enhanced neutrophil chemotaxis. Heterozygous carriers of this gene are asymptomatic.

Pathology: Synovial biopsy shows nonspecific inflammation. Skin lesions show dense dermal infiltration with neutrophils and no evidence of vasculitis.

Demographics: Eastern Mediterranean persons (especially Armenians,

Arabs, Turks, and Sephardic Jews) are most frequently affected. It is uncommon in other Mediterranean populations. In Iraqis and Sephardic Jews, the prevalence of FMF is between 1:250 and 1:1000. The prevalence in Ashkenazi Jews is 1:73,000. Male:female ratio is 3:2. Less than half have a family history of FMF.

Cardinal Findings: Acute, recurrent, unpredictable attacks of fever, serositis (e.g., peritonitis, pleuritis), arthritis, and an erysipelas-like rash are seen. Over 80% of attacks begin before age 20, and initial attacks are very rare after age 40. Although fever and serosal attacks usually last 12 to 72 hours, arthritis may last for several weeks. Disease-free intervals may last days or months. Attacks may be precipitated by menses, stress, or physical exercise.

—*Fever:* The magnitude of fever varies.

—*Serositis:* Nearly all patients (>95%) have abdominal attacks at some time. Peritoneal attacks manifest as localized or generalized pain, abdominal distention, or signs of peritoneal inflammation. Constipation or diarrhea may accompany the attack. Pleural attacks occur in 25 to 50% of patients and tend to be unilateral and associated with a pleural rub and effusion or chest x-ray.

—*Arthritis:* Seen in up to 75% of patients, arthritis tends to be acute, very painful, and monarticular, and typically affects the knee, ankle, and hip. Synovial effusion is usually detectable. Persistent synovitis is uncommon but may last for weeks or months. Such patients may have x-ray evidence of osteopenia or joint damage. Febrile myalgias may also be intense and last for weeks.

—*Erysipelas-like rash:* Seen in 20 to 46% of patients, rash may occur with fever, is usually on the anterior lower extremity, and may be uni- or bilateral. Lesions are sharply demarcated, erythematous, tender, and sometimes swollen. Purpura is less common.

Uncommon Findings: Pericarditis is rare. Scrotal edema and pain have been described.

Complications: Amyloidosis develops in 10 to 40% and is unrelated to severity or frequency of FMF. Such patients may exhibit proteinuria, renal failure, or intestinal malabsorption. Less than 5% of children manifest Henoch-Schönlein purpura. FMF may coexist with polyarteritis nodosa.

Diagnostic Tests: Leukocytosis, elevated ESR, and inflammatory synovial fluid are usually seen. A normochromic, normocytic anemia may be found. Transient albuminuria and microscopic hematuria may be seen during the febrile attacks. Sterile exudative peritoneal or pleural fluid, with a neutrophil predominance, is common. C5a-inhibitor and interleukin-8 may be decreased in serosal or joint fluid (these tests are not routinely available).

Differential Diagnosis: Acute appendicitis, porphyria, hereditary angioedema, systemic juvenile arthritis (Still's disease), rheumatic fever, septic arthritis, and endometriosis or pelvic inflammatory disease in women should be considered.

Therapy: Symptomatic relief is the goal of therapy. Corticosteroids are ineffective. Colchicine prophylaxis (0.6 mg b.i.d. or t.i.d.) reduces the frequency of attacks, protects against amyloidosis, and stabilizes or lessens the proteinuria. Intravenous colchicine should be avoided.

REFERENCES

Kastner DL. Intermittent and periodic arthritis syndromes: familial Mediterranean fever. In: Koopman WJ, ed. Arthritis and allied conditions: a textbook of rheumatology. Baltimore: Williams & Wilkins, 1997:1280–1287.

FELTY'S SYNDROME

ICD9 Code: 714.1

Definition: Felty's syndrome is defined as the triad of erosive deforming arthritis, splenomegaly, and leukopenia. Felty's syndrome is now considered to represent a rare subset of patients with severe rheumatoid arthritis (RA).

Risk Factors: Felty's syndrome occurs almost exclusively among patients with severe, erosive, deforming arthritis who have high titers of rheumatoid factor (RF) in their serum. Furthermore, genetic studies have demonstrated that patients with Felty's syndrome commonly have the HLA-DR alleles associated with disease severity in RA (e.g., DR-4). Patients with Felty's syndrome also commonly have other extraarticular manifestations of RA, such as nodules, rheumatoid vasculitis, episcleritis, and pericarditis.

Etiology: The cause of Felty's syndrome is unknown. Neutropenia may result from splenic sequestration of granulocytes. Defective granulocytic phagocytosis and chemotaxis may contribute to the susceptibility to infection.

Demographics: Felty's syndrome is rare. It is predominantly seen in Caucasian RA patients.

Cardinal Findings: Although patients with Felty's syndrome have evidence of deforming erosive RA, active synovitis may not be present at the time of diagnosis. Patients often display other extraarticular manifestations (e.g., rheumatoid nodules, Sjögren's syndrome) and may have evidence of weight loss, leg ulcers, recurrent infections, and splenomegaly. Splenomegaly may not be detected in all patients with extraarticular manifestations of RA and leukopenia. However, splenomegaly in Felty's syndrome may be massive.

Diagnostic Tests: The leukopenia of Felty's syndrome is typically a neutropenia ($<2000/mm^3$). Although lymphocyte numbers may be depressed in some patients, a number of patients with Felty's syndrome have an increased number of large granular lymphocytes (LGL) in the circulation. It is not known whether or how these LGLs relate to the pathogenesis of Felty's syndrome.

Platelet counts are usually within normal limits, despite splenomegaly. As expected with severe RA, most patients are anemic. However, the anemia of patients with Felty's syndrome has been suggested to be more severe than otherwise expected for the anemia of chronic disease. Despite being leukopenic and neutropenic, most patients with Felty's syndrome do not seem more susceptible to infection than other patients with severe RA. Thrombocytopenia is rarely seen. Rheumatoid factor is uniformly present and may be accompanied by other autoantibodies (e.g., ANA, pANCA).

Differential Diagnosis: Splenomegaly is uncommon in RA without evidence of Felty's syndrome or neutropenia. Other causes of splenomegaly in RA patients should be considered, including drug reactions, myeloproliferative diseases, lymphoma, amyloidosis, tuberculosis, and other chronic infections.

Therapy: Treatment of Felty's syndrome parallels the treatment of severe RA. Many patients are treated with low-dose corticosteroids, at least initially. Most patients with Felty's syndrome receive a second-line agent or DMARD. Currently, methotrexate is often the initial DMARD chosen, although injectable gold salts have a long history of use in this condition. Splenectomy is not routinely recommended in Felty's syndrome, as it does not appear to correct the other clinical manifestations consistently. Splenectomy may be considered in those with massive splenomegaly or recurrent infections. Patients with significant neutropenia and fever or documented infection may benefit from administration of colony stimulating factors (e.g., G-CSF), although such agents may exacerbate the synovitis of RA.

REFERENCES

Rosenstein ED, Kramer N. Felty's and pseudo-Felty's syndromes. Semin Arthritis Rheum 1991;21:129–142.

FIBROMYALGIA

Synonyms: Fibrositis, myofascial pain syndrome, neurasthenic pain syndrome

ICD9 Codes: 729.0

Definition: Fibromyalgia (formerly called fibrositis) is a very common pain syndrome of unknown origin that is characterized by widespread soft tissue pain, identified as localized tender areas called "trigger points."

Etiology: The cause is unknown. Numerous studies have speculated on contributory role(s) for trauma, stress, depression, poor cardiovascular fitness, abnormalities of the hypothalamic-pituitary-adrenal axis, and loss of non-REM (stage IV) sleep.

Pathogenesis: Although most of the pain arises from nociceptors in muscle, numerous muscle studies (e.g., histopathology, electromyography, exercise testing, NMR spectroscopy) have failed to identify consistent abnormalities. Central mechanisms may underlie these heightened pain responses. Sleep EEG studies have documented alpha wave intrusion during delta (stage IV) sleep and a reduction in rapid eye movement (REM) sleep. Recent studies using SPECT scans demonstrate lower cerebral blood flow in the thalamus and caudate nucleus of fibromyalgia patients than in normal controls. Such studies are not diagnostic of fibromyalgia, but they do suggest that central mechanisms may play a key role.

Demographics: Fibromyalgia is estimated to affect between 3 and 6 million, or as many as 2% of Americans. Population studies suggest that the prevalence of widespread pain ranges from 10 to 23% and increases with age. Most reported series show that 80% or more of fibromyalgia patients are female. The average age at presentation is between 30 and 50 years, although fibromyalgia has been uncommonly described in children and is probably underreported in the elderly. Racial and ethnic associations have not been described, and in fact, the pattern of age and gender is remarkably constant in studies from countries around the world. Fibromyalgia often accompanies other rheumatic disorders, where it is referred to as "secondary fibromyalgia." Nearly 30% of RA and SLE patients and up to 50% of Sjögren's syndrome patients have been reported to have secondary fibromyalgia.

Cardinal Findings: All patients exhibit widespread pain affecting the upper and lower torso and both sides of the body. Asymmetric or focal areas of soft tissue pain and spasm may be referred to as the "myofascial pain syndrome." Patients typically complain of axial pain affecting the neck, interscapular area, and low back. Others may initially present with focal joint pains (e.g., shoulder, elbow, or hip), only to demonstrate other evidence of widespread pain on examination. In addition to arthralgias and myalgias, patients complain of prominent fatigue, malaise, and morning stiffness, often lasting hours. Gel phenomenon and activity-induced articular pains are common. Articular symptoms often wax and wane and may be related to exacerbating factors. Many patients complain of joint swelling, although objective evidence of effusion or synovial proliferation is lacking.

Sleep disturbance occurs in the vast majority of patients, with difficulty falling asleep, staying asleep, frequent awakening, restlessness, or early morning awakening. Most patients admit to only sleeping for short intervals throughout the night and feeling worse or tired upon wakening. This results in loss of the normal progression of sleep stages, and it is thought that loss of slow or delta wave (stage IV) sleep is especially disturbed. Few patients have an underlying sleep apnea syndrome, most of whom are males.

Tender trigger points, some of which may not be apparent to the patient, are required for the diagnosis. Trigger points are defined as a focal painful response elicited by 4 kg of digital pressure (enough to blanch a thumbnail) over specific locations (Fig. 1). The physical examination should test all 18 trigger points. For purposes of disease classification, the American College of Rheumatology requires that at least 11 of these points be tender to have the diagnosis and be included in clinical trials.

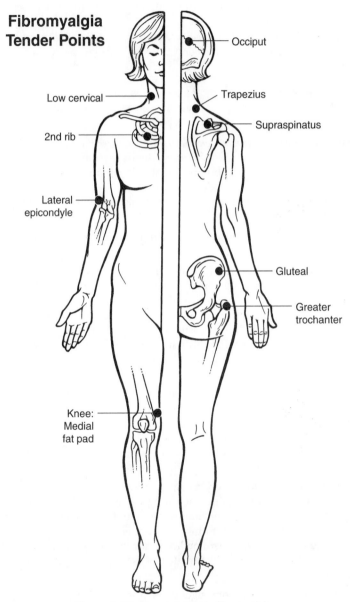

Figure 1. Trigger point sites in fibromyalgia.

Commonly associated disorders include migraine headache, irritable bowel syndrome, premenstrual syndrome, chronic fatigue syndrome, depression, and multiple drug allergies,

Numerous psychiatric disorders have been associated with fibromyalgia, but less than 20% of patients exhibit major depression. Anxiety, panic attacks, and inadequate coping mechanisms have all been found in a minority of patients.

Uncommon Findings: Atypical chest pains (often with chest wall tenderness), TMJ pain, Raynaud's phenomenon, restless leg syndrome, memory loss, and cognitive dysfunction have been reported.

Diagnostic Tests: *Extensive laboratory testing is rarely indicated*, and wide batteries of tests should be avoided. Although there are patients with secondary fibromyalgia, the diagnosis of fibromyalgia should not prompt additional testing to identify an associated or underlying disorder. Use of the ANA or thyroid function tests should be predicated on symptoms that suggest SLE or hypothyroidism, respectively.

Imaging: MRI and CT scans are normal and should not be performed unless otherwise indicated.

Keys to Diagnosis: Several clues should strongly suggest the diagnosis of fibromyalgia. Most common is the presentation of a patient who claims widespread and impressive musculoskeletal symptoms whose history is not substantiated by physical findings or abnormalities (e.g., no joint swelling). This should prompt a search for soft tissue trigger points and supportive features such as a sleep disturbance. Patients who present with musculoskeletal symptoms and a past history of psychiatric disorders (e.g., depression) should be evaluated for fibromyalgia.

Diagnostic Criteria: Diagnostic criteria based entirely on these clinical features have been developed primarily for use in clinical studies (Table 1). These criteria may be instructive in establishing a diagnosis of fibromyalgia in individual patients, but in clinical practice it is not necessary that 11 or more trigger points be present. The diagnosis should be considered for someone with multiple tender trigger points, evidence of widespread pain, and a sleep disturbance.

Differential Diagnosis: Many rheumatic disorders manifest prominent soft tissue pain during the onset period or during disease flares. Disorders that may masquerade as fibromyalgia include hypothyroidism, psychogenic rheumatism, hypochondriasis, somatoform pain disorder, chronic fatigue syndrome, drug-induced myopathy, hypermobility syndrome, polymyalgia rheumatica, or the onset/flare of a connective tissue disease (e.g., SLE, polymyositis, vasculitis, spondyloarthropathy).

Therapy: Patients with fibromyalgia differ from each other in the scope and severity of symptoms. Therefore, treatment approaches should be tailored to the individual patient and are best coordinated by a single physician who knows the patient well. Therapeutic modalities are in three main areas. Components from each area may be combined for a more effective, multifaceted approach.

Table 1
The American College of Rheumatology 1990 Criteria for the Classification of Fibromyalgia[a]

1. History of widespread pain

    Definition. Pain is considered widespread when all of the following are present: pain in the left side of the body, pain in the right side of the body, pain above the waist, and pain below the waist. In addition, axial skeletal pain (cervical spine or anterior chest or thoracic spine or low back) must be present. In this definition, shoulder and buttock pain is considered as pain for each involved side. "Low back" pain is considered lower segment pain.

2. Pain in 11 of 18 tender point sited on digital palpation

    Definition. Pain, on digital palpation, must be present in at least 11 of the following 18 tender point sites:

    Occiput: bilateral, at the suboccipital muscle insertions

    Low cervical: bilateral, at the anterior aspects of the intertransverse spaces at C5–C7

    Trapezius: bilateral, at the midpoint of the upper border

    Supraspinatus: bilateral, at origins, above the scapula spine near the medial border

    Second rib: bilateral, at the second costochondral junctions, just lateral to the junctions on upper surfaces

    Lateral epicondyle: bilateral, 2 cm distal to the epicondyles

    Gluteal: bilateral, in upper outer quadrants of buttocks in anterior fold of muscle

    Greater trochanter: bilateral, posterior to the trochanteric prominence

    Knee: bilateral, at the medial fat pad proximal to the joint line

    Digital palpation should be performed with an approximate force of 4 kg

    For a tender point to be considered, "positive," the subject must state that the palpation was painful; "tender" is not to be considered "painful"

[a]For classification purposes, patients will be said to have fibromyalgia if both criteria are satisfied. Widespread pain must have been present for at least 3 months. The presence of a second clinical disorder does not exclude the diagnosis of fibromyalgia.

—*Pharmacologic agents:* Most useful are drugs that target pain, muscle tension, and abnormal patterns of sleep. Analgesic medications may be used to decrease pain. Commonly used agents include acetaminophen (3–5 g/day), NSAIDs, or the nonnarcotic analgesic, tramadol (50–100 mg b.i.d. or t.i.d.). Attempts to control pain with these agents alone are uniformly unsuccessful. Thus, the clinician should avoid the temptation to escalate NSAID use (with resultant gastrointestinal risks) or to resort to chronic narcotic analgesic use to control recalcitrant pain. Tricyclic antidepressants are useful adjuncts and should also be considered as first-line therapy. These drugs tend to normalize sleep patterns while providing muscle relaxing and analgesic effects. Bedtime amitriptyline (10, 25, or 50 mg) or trazodone (50 or 100 mg) are commonly used agents in this category. Doses may be escalated to optimize nighttime sleep without causing attendant daytime drowsiness. Trazodone may be less sedating than amitriptyline (see Appendix D, p. 513). Newer antidepressant agents that inhibit serotonin reuptake, such as sertraline and fluoxetine, may benefit some patients. However, there is less experience with these drugs in fibromyalgia than with the tricyclic antidepressants, and the expense is generally greater. Muscle relaxants such as cyclobenzaprine, carisoprodol, or orphenadrine may benefit patients with muscle spasm as a predominant symptom. Drowsiness during daytime hours may be undesirable, so these agents may be given at bedtime only, either with or instead of tricyclic antidepressant sleep aids.

—*Physical modalities:* Supervised therapy or exercise is important in the overall therapeutic plan in fibromyalgia. Physical therapists who perform the technique of myofascial release are helpful in treating patients with significant muscle spasm or muscle tension. Some patients benefit from conventional massage therapy, but this is usually temporary unless combined with a more sustained program. Supervised therapy in a pool (aquatherapy) may allow patients with pain or weakness to exercise with less discomfort than is the case outside of water. For maximum comfort and to minimize posttreatment muscle spasm, both the water and the surrounding room should be relatively warm. Exercises that emphasize stretching, such as some types of yoga, may be useful and should be done at least initially under supervision. In some studies, a program of conditioning aerobic exercise has improved symptoms in some patients. This finding may relate to the observation that most patients have less aerobic capacity than normal sedentary individuals. A supervised program of exercise starting at a low level thus may be of benefit as part of the treatment plan.

—*Psychologic approaches:* Many patients with fibromyalgia exhibit symptoms of psychologic stress, including anxiety and depression. Treatment of these related problems may include cognitive-behavioral therapy. Such a program can include training in relaxation and coping skills as well as guidance in reinforcing positive behaviors. Successful application of these techniques under the guidance of a trained therapist may help reduce pain and enhance functional status.

Monitoring: The frequency of monitoring is determined by the medications used and response to therapy. At each follow-up visit, the clinician should assess the magnitude of the patient's pain, the quality and quantity of sleep, any limitations on activities of daily living, and the number of tender trigger points.

Prognosis: Longitudinal studies suggest that the duration of disease is often many years and that only a minority of patients (10–20%) improve over time. However, the number of patients requesting disability benefits is increasing. Fibromyalgia is a significant cause of long-term disability and given the high prevalence of this condition and relatively young age of most patients, the economic and social impact of this disorder is profound. One Canadian study has estimated that the cost in terms of long-term disability payments may be $200 million/year. In many, disability can be avoided by vocational counseling, modification of work schedule and activities, and avoidance of exacerbating factors (e.g., trauma, stress, poor sleep, depression, arthritis).

REFERENCES

Bennett RM, Clark SR, Goldger L, et al. Aerobic fitness in patients with fibrositis. A controlled study of respiratory gas exchange and 133 xenon clearance from exercising muscle. Arthritis Rheum 1989;32:454–460.

Forseth KO, Gran JT. The prevalence of fibromyalgia among women aged 20–49 years in Arendal, Norway. Scand J Rheumatol 1991;21:74–78.

McCain GA, Bell DA, Mai FM, Halliday PD. A controlled study of the effects of a supervised cardiovascular fitness training program on the manifestations of primary fibromyalgia. Arthritis Rheum 1988;31:1135–1141.

McCain GA, Cameron R, Kennedy JC. The problem of long-term disability payments and litigation in primary fibromyalgia: the Canadian perspective. J Rheumatol 1989;16:174–176.

Moldofsky H, Scarisbrick P. Induction of neurasthenic musculoskeletal pain syndrome by selective sleep stage deprivation. Psychosom Med 1976;38:35–44.

Wolfe F, Ross K, Anderson J, et al. The prevalence and characteristics of fibromyalgia in the general population. Arthritis Rheum 1995;38:19–28.

Wolfe F, Smythe HA, Yunnus MB, et al. The American College of Rheumatology 1990 criteria for the classification of fibromyalgia: report of the Multicenter Criteria Committee. Arthritis Rheum 1990;33:160–172.

FROSTBITE

ICD9 Code: Multiple sites, 991.3; hand, 991.1; foot, 991.2

Definition: Frostbite injury to the extremities can result in vascular damage and thrombi with associated chondrocyte damage. As a result, patients suffering frostbite may develop osteoarthritis months or even years after exposure.

Cardinal Findings: Frostbite injury tends to occur in the distal extremities, particularly in the hands and feet. Findings of osteoarthritis related to frostbite may resemble primary (e.g., Heberden's and Bouchard's nodes) or erosive osteoarthritis. In children, frostbite exposure may result in premature closure of the epiphyses and impaired growth, usually of the fingers.

Imaging: Typical radiographic findings include demineralization, periostitis, subchondral (juxtaarticular) cysts, joint space narrowing, and formation of osteophytes.

Therapy: Because the signs and symptoms of frostbite arthritis develop some time after exposure, there is no specific therapy for this condition. Therapy is comparable to that for idiopathic osteoarthritis (see p. 277).

REFERENCES

Glick R, Parhami N. Frostbite arthritis. J Rheumatol 1979;6:456–460.

FUNGAL ARTHRITIS

ICD9 Codes: Arthropathy associated with mycoses, 711.8 (code underlying disease first: sporotrichosis, 117.1; *Candida* arthritis, 112.9; coccidioidomycosis, 114.9; blastomycosis, 116.0; cryptococcosis, 117.5; histoplasmosis, 115.9)

Demographics: With the exception of those with sporotrichosis and histoplasmosis, most individuals with serious bone or joint involvement from fungal organisms are immunocompromised hosts who have systemic illnesses such as HIV disease, malignancy, chronic inflammatory disorders requiring corticosteroid therapy, or other chronic disease such as diabetes mellitus.

Specific Infections (also see Appendix F, p. 517)

Sporotrichosis: Osteoarticular infections may be caused by *Sporothrix schenckii*, which has worldwide distribution. Exposure is through the skin, often secondary to plant thorn injury in gardeners and agricultural or other outdoor workers. Infection begins in the skin as a painful skin nodule. Indolent unifocal arthritis most commonly involves the knee but also can affect the wrist, hand, ankle, or elbow. Tenosynovitis is also possible. Polyarticular arthritis is rarely seen in disseminated skin and bone infection occurring in immunocompromised hosts. Diagnosis is made by culture from skin, synovial fluid, or bone. Amphotericin B is being superseded by oral itraconazole for lymphocutaneous, articular, and osseous disease, with 70 to 100% cure rates. Surgical resection is sometime necessary.

***Candida* Arthritis:** Commonly caused by *Candida albicans,* infection is due to direct seeding of a joint or by hematogenous spread, often from an indwelling transcutaneous catheter. It manifests as a monoarthritis in 60 to 75% of patients, most commonly affecting the knee. Diagnosis is established by culture of synovial fluid and/or blood. The preferred treatment is systemic amphotericin B. Prognosis is poor, and mortality rates are high because of comorbidities and frequent, concurrent candidemia.

Coccidioidomycosis: Infection with *Coccidioides immitis* is commonly seen in the western and southwestern United States, with a higher incidence in summer months. Primary respiratory infection occurs after inhalation of spores and may be associated with constitutional and systemic manifestations, including erythema nodosum and migratory arthritis. Disseminated infection is rare (except in immunocompromised hosts) and is associated with frequent bone involvement and monarthritis, particularly of the knee. It can progress to an indolent arthritis with pannus. Histologic examination reveals noncaseating granulomas with fungal spores. Diagnosis is suggested by a positive skin test result that is seen in 80% of patients within 1 to 3 weeks of infection. Synovial fluid culture is difficult but occasionally positive. Serologies are positive in diffuse disease. Chest radiographs may also be abnormal. Treatment options include itraconazole or fluconazole for limited-to-moderate disease. Amphotericin B is recommended for disseminated infection.

Blastomycosis: *Blastomyces dermatitidis* causes an uncommon infection in the Mississippi and Ohio river valleys and Middle Atlantic states of the United States. Primary respiratory infection occurs after inhalation of spores. Acutely, arthralgias and myalgias are common. Uncommonly, there is lymphatic or hematogenous dissemination to bone, joints, and skin. Joints are less commonly involved than bone and may be due to direct extension from adjacent osteomyelitis. Skeletal involvement is occasionally asymptomatic. Long bones, ribs, and vertebrae are most commonly affected and appear osteolytic on radiographs. Soft tissue or vertebral abscesses may occur. Fungi may be detected in synovial fluid after KOH preparation. Culture on Sabouraud's media is confirmatory. Serologic tests are available, sensitive, but nonspecific and are not routinely recommended. Itraconazole may be effective with mild-to-moderate disease. Amphotericin B is reserved for severe infection in immunocompromised hosts.

Cryptococcosis: Infection with Cryptococcus neoformans is seen worldwide, especially in the immunocompromised host. Primary respiratory infection occurs after inhalation of spores (ubiquitous, found in pigeon droppings). Bone involvement is uncommon (<10% of cases), and infectious arthritis is rare. The latex agglutination test for cryptococcal antigen is generally positive. Limited disease may be treated with fluconazole alone. Amphotericin B with 5-fluorocytosine is recommended for severe cases.

Histoplasmosis: Infection with *Histoplasma capsulatum* is most commonly seen in the Mississippi and Ohio river valleys of United States but is also found worldwide. Primary respiratory infection is usually asymptomatic. Spores tend to grow and persist in soil contaminated with avian or bat excreta. Histoplasmosis is usually a benign, self-limited, respiratory illness. Acute infections may be heralded by erythema nodosum, arthralgia, or acute oligo- or polyarthritis. Chronic infection very rare. The diagnosis is confirmed by histopathology (caseating granulomas) or by culture. Itraconazole is indicated for mild-to-moderate disease. Amphotericin B, with or without surgical debridement, may be necessary with severe disease or if the host is severely immunocompromised.

REFERENCES

Kauffman CA. Newer developments in therapy for endemic mycoses. Clin Infect Dis 1994;19(Suppl 1):S28.

Mahowald ML, Messner RP. Arthritis due to mycobacteria, fungi, and parasites. In: Koopman WJ, ed. Arthritis and allied conditions: a textbook of rheumatology. 13th ed. Baltimore: Williams & Wilkins, 1997:2305–2320.

Terrell CL, Hughes CE. Antifungal agents used for deep-seated mycotic infections. Mayo Clin Proc 1992;67:69.

GANGLION CYSTS

ICD9 Code: 727.40

Definition: Ganglions are cystic masses that arise in proximity to joint capsules or tendon sheaths but do not communicate with the joint cavity. They are most common with repetitive strain or overuse, trauma, or inflammatory arthritis.

Pathology: Ganglia are formed by a dense capsule of mesenchymal connective tissue that encloses one or more cavities. These cavities are thin-walled and contain a viscous, mucinous fluid.

Cardinal Findings: Ganglia arise most commonly on the dorsal aspect of the wrist; however they also occur on the volar aspect of the wrist, the medial and lateral aspects of the knee, the dorsum of the foot, and the anterior aspect of the lower leg. Although most ganglia are asymptomatic, symptoms may relate to their location and impingement on adjacent structures (e.g., restriction of motion or paresthesias). They may become painful if traumatized. Recently formed ganglia are easily compressible; with chronicity, they may become more indurated and nodule-like.

Therapy: Patients with ganglia may seek medical therapy for symptoms related to tendinous, neural, or vascular impingement or for cosmetic reasons. Ganglia may resolve spontaneously and recur over time. Treatment varies according to duration and symptoms. Ganglia of only a few months duration may be treated by firm compression. This can be accomplished with a firm object such as a padded coin secured by an elastic bandage for several weeks. Alternatively, the mucinous fluid can be removed with a large-bore needle. Corticosteroid injection may also be used. Chronic or recurrent ganglionic cysts may require excision.

REFERENCES

Soren A. Clinical and pathologic characteristics and treatment of ganglia. Contemp Orthop 1995;31:34–38.

GOODPASTURE'S SYNDROME

Synonyms: Anti–glomerular basement membrane antibody disease

ICD9 Code: 446.2

Definition: Goodpasture's syndrome is an autoimmune disorder characterized by pulmonary hemorrhage and rapidly progressive glomerulonephritis (RPGN) in association with antibodies to alveolar and glomerular basement membrane (GBM).

Etiology: The cause of Goodpasture's syndrome is unknown. Some patients have had antecedent respiratory infections such as influenza, while others appeared to have developed the syndrome after toxic lung injury. Rarely, patients have developed Goodpasture's syndrome as an adverse effect to the antirheumatic drug D-penicillamine. The pathogenesis of Goodpasture's syndrome is related to anti-GBM antibodies. Such antibodies are a sensitive diagnostic test, as they occur in more than 95% of patients. Moreover, they are specific, and they are rarely seen in normal persons or in patients with other pulmonary/renal syndromes (see also p. 53, pulmonary/renal syndromes).

Pathology: Support for the pathogenic role of anti-GBM antibodies in Good-pasture's syndrome comes from histopathologic studies. Immunofluorescent staining of biopsy specimens from the lungs and kidneys of patients with Good-pasture's syndrome reveals a characteristic linear pattern of antibody deposition. The specific antigenic epitopes recognized by anti-GBM antibodies were recently shown to be present on the α3 chain of type IV collagen. Type IV collagen is the major component of basement membranes and provides structural support. Although other chains of type IV collagen occur widely throughout the body, the α3 chain has more limited expression. This provides an explanation for why end-organ involvement of Goodpasture's syndrome is typically limited to the lungs and kidneys.

Demographics: Goodpasture's syndrome characteristically affects Caucasian men in their third decade, although males and females of all races and ages can be affected. It is a rare disorder.

Cardinal Findings: Overall, approximately 75% of those with Goodpasture's syndrome have both pulmonary and renal involvement; the remainder have only RPGN. Isolated pulmonary disease is rare, although some patients with biopsy-proven Goodpasture's syndrome may appear to have minimal renal involvement as evidenced by routine laboratory studies such as serum creatinine and urinalysis. Hemoptysis is the initial complaint in most patients, and alveolar infiltrates may be seen on chest radiographs. Other symptoms include cough and dyspnea. Renal manifestations generally lag behind pulmonary signs and symptoms.

Diagnostic Tests: Laboratory studies often reveal an anemia that may be related to both anemia of chronic disease and iron deficiency, depending upon the severity and chronicity of the pulmonary hemorrhage. Patients may also be hypoxic. Less than half of patients demonstrate renal insufficiency at initial evaluation, but more than 80% eventually display azotemia or proteinuria. Hematuria is very common. Anti-GBM assays are performed by ELISA in a number of reference laboratories, and anti-GBM is present in more than 95% of patients with Goodpasture's syndrome (see p. 80).

Imaging: Chest roentgenograms usually reveal diffuse, extensive alveolar infiltrates.

Differential Diagnosis: Various other pulmonary/renal syndromes, such as SLE, cryoglobulinemia, and several types of vasculitis must be distinguished.

Keys to Diagnosis: The diagnosis of Goodpasture's syndrome may be secured by demonstrating linear antibody staining of the basement membrane of renal or pulmonary biopsy specimens. However, patients are often quite ill during the initial course of the disease, making biopsy more difficult. Tests for serum anti-GBM antibodies are most commonly used to diagnose Goodpasture's syndrome because of their widespread availability and high sensitivity and specificity.

Therapy: Goodpasture's syndrome used to be associated with a poor prognosis and high associated mortality. Recently, the prognosis has improved, in part because of the availability of diagnostic tests and advances in immunomodulatory interventions, although improvements in the intensive care of critically ill persons have no doubt contributed. Because most patients present in extreme distress (hemoptysis, hypoxia, etc.) large boluses of corticosteroids (e.g., 1 g of methylprednisolone intravenously for 3–4 days) are commonly used. Plasmapheresis appears to benefit many patients and is also commonly used. Many patients are treated with cytotoxic drugs, such as daily oral cyclophosphamide, in conjunction with plasmapheresis. In contrast to some other pulmonary renal syndromes, such as SLE, production of anti-GBM antibodies is usually self-limited. Thus, these aggressive immunomodulatory therapies may often be stopped when the patient has demonstrated significant clinical improvement.

REFERENCES

Gravelyn TR, Lynch JP. Alveolar hemorrhage syndromes. IM Intern Med Special 1987;8:63–83.

Johnson JP, Whitman W, Briggs WA. Plasmapheresis and immunosuppressive agents in antibasement membrane antibody-induced Goodpasture's syndrome. Am J Med 1978;64: 354–359.

Turner N, Mason PJ, Brown R, et al. Molecular cloning of the human Goodpasture antigen demonstrates it to be the α3 chain of type IV collagen. J Clin Invest 1992;89:592–601.

GOUT

ICD9 Codes: Gouty arthritis, 274.0; gouty nephropathy, 274.1; uric acid nephrolithiasis, 274.11

Definition: Gout is a syndrome caused by an inflammatory response to tissue deposition of monosodium urate (MSU) crystals. Several descriptive terms are often used in association with gout:

—*Acute gout:* single or recurrent attacks of inflammatory mono- or oligoarthritis.

—*Tophaceous gout:* accumulation of crystalline MSU aggregates in soft tissues; nodular aggregates are referred to as "tophi"

—*Hyperuricemia:* serum level of uric acid above which supersaturation of MSU in extracellular fluids theoretically occurs ($\geq$6.8 mg/dL)

—*Asymptomatic hyperuricemia:* the state in which the serum uric acid level is abnormally high (>7.0 mg/dL in men, >6.0 mg/dL in postmenopausal women) but no symptoms of gout or nephrolithiasis have occurred

—*Primary gout:* gout resulting from abnormalities in purine metabolism or from idiopathic decreased renal excretion of urate

—*Secondary gout:* gout resulting from increased serum uric acid levels resulting from an associated disorder (e.g., neoplasms, lymphoproliferative disease, chronic renal failure) or drug therapy (e.g., diuretics, ethanol, cytotoxics)

Etiology: The common denominator of gout is hyperuricemia. Uric acid, the product of purine degradation, is synthesized mainly in the liver. Two-thirds of the uric acid pool is excreted by the kidney, with the remainder secreted into the intestine. The causes of hyperuricemia can be divided into disorders of over-production and disorders of decreased renal clearance of urate (Table 1). Most cases of gout (90%) are due to underexcretion of uric acid; overproduction due to inherited enzyme defects (hypoxanthine-guanine adenine phosphoribosyl-transferase [HGPRT] deficiency or overactivity of 5-phosphoribosyl 1-py-rophosphate [PRPP] synthestase) accounts for less than 1% of cases.

The pathogenesis of acute gout involves the response of polymorphonu-clear leukocytes to formation of MSU crystals. Acute gout is thought to result from formation of new crystals rather than from release of crystals from pre-formed MSU synovial deposits or tophi. Crystals are coated with IgG which re-acts with Fc receptors on polymorphonuclear cells that phagocytose the crys-tals. Intracellularly, the crystals are stripped of their protein coats and disrupt the cell, releasing a variety of inflammatory mediators.

Factors provoking episodes of acute gouty arthritis include trauma, surgery, alcohol ingestion, starvation, overindulgence in purine-rich foods, and drugs that raise urate concentrations (Table 1). Alcohol (ethanol) increases serum lactate levels, which blocks renal excretion of urate.

Pathology: The most frequent sites of MSU deposition are cartilage, epiphy-seal bone, periarticular structures, and the kidney. Deposition in other sites is rare. Crystal aggregates cause a foreign body reaction. A tophus is composed of MSU crystals, a proteoglycan-rich intercrystalline matrix, and surrounding fi-brous tissue. Affected joints may develop cartilage degeneration, erosion of marginal bone, and synovial proliferation. In the kidney, crystal deposition causes arteriosclerosis and interstitial fibrosis.

Demographics: The prevalence of *asymptomatic hyperuricemia* in adult Ameri-cans is 5 to 8%. The prevalence of gout is estimated to be 13 cases per 1000 men and 6.4 cases per 1000 women in North America. The risk of developing gout in-creases with higher uric acid levels: the annual incidence in relation to serum uric acid concentration is 0.1% for those with a serum uric acid level below 7.0 mg/dL); 0.5% for levels between 7.0 and 8.9 mg/dL; and 4.9% for levels above 9.0 mg/dL.

Over 90% of patients with primary gout are men. Women rarely develop the disorder before menopause, as estrogen is thought to enhance uric acid ex-cretion. The peak incidence for men is in the fifth decade. Primary gout is often associated with obesity, hyperlipidemia, diabetes mellitus, hypertension, and atherosclerosis. Secondary gout may be associated with alcoholism and myelo-proliferative and lymphoproliferative disorders. Gout is more prevalent among patients of African descent, largely because of the prevalence of hypertension. Lead poisoning is an important environmental risk factor, most often occurring as "Saturnine gout" caused by moonshine.

Table 1
Causes of Hyperuricemia

Overproducers: increased purine synthesis or urate production
  Idiopathic
  Inherited enzyme defects
    Hypoxanthine-guanine phosphoribosyltransferase (HGPRT) deficiency
      Complete (Lesch-Nyhan syndrome)
      Incomplete
    Phosphoribosylpyrophosphate synthetase (PRPP) overactivity
  Diseases with purine overproduction
    Lympho- and myeloproliferative disorders
    Hemolytic disorders
    Malignant diseases
    Obesity
    Drugs and diet
      Ethanol
      Cytotoxic drugs
      Warfarin
      Purine-rich diets
Underexcreters: decreased renal clearance of urate
  Primary idiopathic uric acid underexcretion
  Secondary uric acid underexcretion
    Chronic renal failure
    Hypertension
    Dehydration
    Obesity
    Hyperparathyroidism
    Hypothyroidism
    Drugs
      Ethanol
      Diuretics
      Low-dose salicylate
      Cyclosporine
      Ethambutol
      Pyrazinamide
      Levodopa

Cardinal Findings

—*Acute gout:* Acute gouty arthritis is the most common early clinical manifestation of gout. The metatarsophalangeal (MTP) joint of the first toe is the commonest site (often referred to as *podagra*) of involvement, affecting 75 to 90% of patients at some time in the course of their disease, with 50% experiencing their first attack of acute gout in this joint. Approximately 80% of initial attacks are monoarticular, typically involving joints of the distal lower extremity: the MTPs, ankle, and knee. Less common initial sites of involvement include the wrist, fingers, and elbows. Onset is usually abrupt, often waking the patient at night. The affected joints may be warm, swollen, and tender, with diffuse periarticular erythema that is often confused with cellulitis or thrombophlebitis. Fever may occur. Attacks may be associated with impressive soft tissue pitting edema. Early attacks generally subside spontaneously over 3 to 10 days, even in the absence of treatment. Postinflammatory desquamation of the skin overlying the joint may occur. Patients are typically symptom free after an acute attack. Subsequent episodes may occur more frequently, involve more joints, and persist longer. Trivial episodes of pain lasting a few hours may precede the first dramatic attack of acute gout. Although affected joints usually recover completely, erosions may develop in those with repeated attacks. Polyarticular attacks may also occur in those with established, poorly controlled disease. Such attacks may display a migratory pattern or involve periarticular structures such as tendons and bursae.

—*Intercritical gout:* The interval between acute gouty attacks is termed the *intercritical period.* If necessary, MSU crystals can be recovered from previously affected joints in this symptom-free period. The duration of this period varies; most untreated patients experience a second episode within 2 years. A minority evolve into chronic polyarticular gout without pain-free intercritical periods. At this stage, the clinical picture can be confused with rheumatoid arthritis, especially if tophi are mistaken for rheumatoid nodules.

—*Chronic tophaceous gout:* This form of gout is characterized by the deposition of solid urate (tophi) in connective tissues, including articular structures, with an eventual destructive arthropathy. Tophaceous gout may be associated with early age of onset, long duration of active untreated disease, frequent attacks, high serum urate levels, upper extremity involvement, and polyarticular disease. Such patients often have multiple causes of hyperuricemia. Organ transplant recipients treated with cyclosporine or diuretics are also at increased risk for accelerated development of chronic tophaceous gout. Although the helix of the ear is a classic location for tophi, they are seldom found. More-common sites include the olecranon and prepatellar bursae, ulnar surface of the forearm, and Achilles tendons. Deposits on the hands may be particularly large protuberances with crippling joint destruction. The skin overlying such deposits is often shiny and may ulcerate, with excretion of a white chalky material composed of MSU crystals. Tophi typically progress insidiously, with the patient reporting increasing stiffness and pain in affected joints.

—*Renal disease:* Renal disease includes *urolithiasis, urate nephropathy* (deposition of MSU crystals in the interstitium), and *uric acid nephropathy* (deposition of MSU crystals in the collecting tubules). Uric acid stones account for 5 to 10% of all renal stones. The prevalence of *urolithiasis* is 22% in primary gout and 42% in secondary gout, and renal stones antedate arthritis in 40% of cases. Serum uric acid levels are directly related to the incidence of urolithiasis (found in nearly 50% of patients excreting more than 1100 mg of uric acid daily). Urate nephropathy and uric acid nephropathy are difficult to differentiate clinically, and they are often referred to as *gouty kidney*. Uric acid nephropathy may present acutely in patients with malignancy treated with chemotherapy or radiation. Urate nephropathy is slowly progressive and associated with hypertension and proteinuria. A causal relationship between renal dysfunction in gout and hypertension is equivocal.

Uncommon Findings: Uncommon sites of initial involvement are the hands, shoulders, sternoclavicular joints, hips, spine, and sacroiliac joints. Initial presentation of gout may be polyarticular, especially in women. Aseptic necrosis of the hip has been reported as a manifestation of gout. Tophaceous involvement of the axial skeleton has been rarely noted. Tophaceous involvement of parenchymal organs, although rare, has been also been reported. Uncommonly, gout arises in "nodal" osteoarthritis with acute inflammatory swelling affecting the Heberden's or Bouchard's nodes. Such patients tend to be elderly females with renal insufficiency, often treated with diuretics.

Diagnostic Tests: At initial presentation, serum uric acid levels are usually elevated, although they are normal in up to 40% of patients experiencing an acute gouty attack. Nonetheless, the vast majority of patients with gout demonstrate an elevated uric acid level at some time. The serum creatinine level should be determined, as it may influence subsequent therapy. During an acute attack there is frequently leukocytosis, thrombocytosis, and elevated acute-phase reactant (ESR, CRP) levels.

—*Joint fluid:* Synovial fluid in acute gout is inflammatory, with high leukocyte counts (>2000 cells/mm^3; WBC differential >75% neutrophils); occasionally, synovial leukocyte counts are very high (>50,000 cells/mm^3). MSU crystals are identified with the polarized light microscopy. Needle-shaped crystals, 5 to 25 μm, can be seen against a dark background. These are best identified with polarizing lenses and a red compensator, which reveals characteristic negatively birefringent crystals that appear yellow against a lilac background when parallel to the plane of the red compensator and blue when at right angles to it. In acute gout, urate crystals are usually intracellular (within neutrophils); between attacks, urate crystals may still be seen, but they tend to be extracellular. Only one or two drops of synovial fluid are necessary for crystal examination. Needle-shaped MSU crystals can also be seen under plain light microscopy. Demonstration of MSU crystals does not exclude pseudogout or septic arthritis, as these conditions may coexist with gout. If septic arthritis is considered, gram staining and culture should be performed. Exudate from gouty tophi can be examined for MSU crystals in a similar manner.

—*Urine tests:* A 24-h collection for uric acid determination is useful for assessing the risk of renal stones and for planning therapy (if use of a uricosuric agent is contemplated).

Imaging: Radiographic examination in acute gout is most valuable in excluding other types of arthritis (e.g., septic arthritis, fracture). Roentgenographic abnormalities seen in longstanding gout are an asymmetric, erosive arthritis with characteristic "punched-out" marginal erosions with sclerotic borders and often an overhanging shelf of cortical bone. Periarticular osteopenia is absent, and the joint space is preserved until late in the disease.

Keys to Diagnosis: A history of podagra, dramatic onset of arthritis, history of episodic or prior arthritis with spontaneous resolution in 3 to 10 days, and the presence of tophi should all suggest a diagnosis of gout. For the diagnosis of acute gout, serum uric acid concentrations are neither sensitive (often not raised in acute attacks) nor specific. Definitive diagnosis rests on demonstration of MSU crystals within leukocytes in affected joints. A key radiographic finding is a sharply "punched-out" marginal joint erosion with sclerotic borders and an overhanging margin in the absence of periarticular osteopenia (helps differentiate gout from rheumatoid arthritis).

Differential Diagnosis: The differential diagnosis depends upon the stage of gout encountered.

—*Acute gout:* The differential diagnosis of acute gout is essentially that of acute inflammatory monarthritis and includes septic arthritis, pseudogout, Reiter's syndrome, acute rheumatic fever, and other crystalline arthropathies. Fever, leukocytosis, and localized erythema may lead to erroneous consideration of cellulitis or thrombophlebitis (when the distal lower extremity is involved).

—*Chronic tophaceous gout:* The differential diagnosis of chronic tophaceous gout includes other destructive arthropathies, rheumatoid arthritis (RA), chronic calcium pyrophosphate dihydrate (CPPD) crystal deposition disease, seronegative spondyloarthropathies, and erosive osteoarthritis. Tophi are often mistaken for rheumatoid nodules because of their appearance and location. Coexistence of gout and RA is exceedingly rare.

Therapy: The goal of therapy is to treat the acute attack of gout and prevent recurrent attacks and the complications of untreated gout. There is usually no justification for treating asymptomatic hyperuricemia. However, some physicians make exceptions when serum urate levels are very high (e.g., >12 mg/dL) and the risk of nephrolithiasis is substantial. In addition, allopurinol therapy may be indicated in the setting of malignancy, when the anticipation of tumor lysis results in acute overproduction of urate. Treatment options vary with the stage of gout encountered (Fig. 1).

—*Acute gout:* NSAIDs, corticosteroids (locally or systemically), or oral colchicine may be used (Fig. 1). The choice of therapy is often determined on an individual basis, weighing considerations of efficacy and toxicity. NSAIDs are the preferred modality in acute gout, as they have a rapid clinical effect

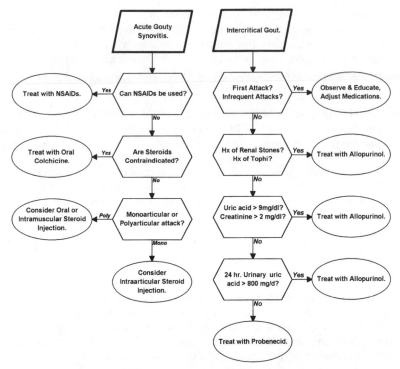

Figure 1. Treatment of acute gout and intercritical gout.

and are usually well tolerated when used for 3 to 14 days or until the attack subsides. Nonetheless, NSAIDs may be associated with acute gastritis and renal toxicity and should be avoided in those with a history of gastrointestinal intolerance, renal insufficiency, congestive heart failure (CHF), ascites, bleeding diathesis, or chronic anticoagulant therapy. Indomethacin (1–2 mg/kg/day) is historically the most widely used NSAID for treatment of acute gout. Antiinflammatory doses of other NSAIDs may also be used. When NSAIDs are contraindicated, corticosteroids are usually effective. They may be particularly useful in the elderly, in persons with renal insufficiency or CHF, and in organ transplant recipients—all situations in which NSAIDs and colchicine may be relatively contraindicated. Intraarticular preparations (e.g., methylprednisolone acetate) are particularly efficacious in monarticular gout. Oral and parenteral steroids (e.g., ACTH, 40–80 IU IM) are also effective in the treatment of monarticular and polyarticular gout. Historically, colchicine therapy has been used to control acute attacks. However, unacceptable GI toxicity (i.e., nausea, diarrhea) and delayed onset of action makes this option least favored in acute gout. In patients with normal renal function, colchicine can be administered orally with a dose of 1.2 mg initially, followed by 0.6 mg every 2 hours, until abdominal discomfort or diarrhea develops or a total dose of 8 mg has been administered. Most patients have some relief of arthritic symptoms by 18 hours, with joint inflammation subsiding in 48 hours. Colchicines effect relates to the inhibition of microtubule formation and neutrophil chemotaxis. Intravenous colchicine should not be used (see "Comments" below). Antihyperuricemic measures (i.e., allopurinol) should not be initiated or continued until the acute attack is resolved, since the duration of joint inflammation may be prolonged.

—*Intercritical gout:* Once the acute attack has resolved, attention is directed at prevention and prophylaxis. The decision to initiate chronic pharmacotherapy is made in accord with the patient's wishes (Fig. 1). Those suffering one or few attacks may prefer to wait and treat the attack, when and if it arises. Those with multiple attacks should be offered the opportunity to prevent attacks with medical therapy. Prevention can be achieved by correcting hyperuricemia, either by eliminating identifiable causes of hyperuricemia (diuretic therapy) or by administering drugs that lower uric acid production or enhance its excretion. Complete avoidance of purine-rich foods (meats, yeast, alcohol, legumes, spinach, asparagus, cauliflower, and mushrooms) is impractical, ineffective, and rarely adhered to in clinical practice. Gout can be prevented or diminished by lowering serum uric acid levels with uricosuric agents (probenecid, sulfinpyrazone) or by inhibiting production of uric acid (allopurinol). Indications for pharmacologic lowering of serum uric acid include inability to reverse secondary causes of gout, recurrent attacks of gout arthritis, chronic tophaceous gout, and an increased risk of nephrolithiasis. In general, use of uricosuric agents is limited to persons with normal renal function, decreased urinary urate excretion (<800 mg/day on a normal diet), and no evidence of tophi. They are contraindicated in the presence of renal stones and have no benefit in persons with low urinary volumes (<1 mL/min) and renal insufficiency (creatinine clearance < 50 mL/min). Uricosuric agents carry the risk of developing urolithiasis, which can be decreased by ensuring high urinary volumes and by addition of sodium bicarbonate, 1 g three to four times per day. Two agents are available: probenecid (1–2 g/day) and sulfinpyrazone (50–400 mg twice daily). Dosage should be gradually increased until serum uric acid levels are below 6.0 mg/day. Therapy may be unsuccessful in some patients. Allopurinol effectively lowers uric acid levels in both overproducers and underexcreters of urate and is indicated in persons with overproduction of uric acid, renal stones, tophi, renal insufficiency, and extreme elevation of uric acid and those in whom uricosuric agents are contraindicated or are ineffective. Allopurinol is also indicated in the prophylaxis of tumor lysis syndrome. The usual dose of 300 mg/day must be reduced in the presence of renal insufficiency (200 mg/day for a creatinine clearance below 60 mL/min, 100 mg/day for a creatinine clearance below 30 mL/min). Beginning with small doses reduces the likelihood of precipitating an attack of acute gout. The chief side effect of allopurinol is a rash that develops in up to 2% of patients and can occasionally be life threatening if exfoliative dermatitis develops (1 in 1000 cases). Chronic colchicine therapy (0.6–1.2 mg/day) may also be prophylactic against gouty attacks. Dosage must be adjusted for renal insufficiency. Neuromyopathy is a rare side effect strongly associated with renal insufficiency.

Prognosis: Untreated, gout progresses over several years from the initial attack of acute gout, through a period of intercritical gout, to chronic tophaceous gout. More-rapid progression may be seen in the presence of severe renal insufficiency. Early intervention can interrupt this progression. Tophi can regress completely with prolonged treatment. Occasionally, gout is difficult to manage, often because of multiple factors such as compliance, alcoholism, renal insufficiency, and the need for continued diuretic therapy.

Comment: The clinician should refrain from using intravenous colchicine to treat acute gout because of the risk of acute bone marrow suppression and hepatic, renal, and central nervous system toxicity, especially in those with renal impairment. While the intravenous preparation is available in the United States, it is banned on many formularies and in many other countries, including the U.K. and Australia.

REFERENCES

Emmerson BT. The management of gout. N Engl J Med 1996;334:445–451.

HEMOCHROMATOSIS

ICD9 Code: 275.0

Definition: Hemochromatosis is a common hereditary disorder of excessive iron absorption and deposition causing tissue damage and organ dysfunction.

Etiology: Hemochromatosis is caused by an autosomal recessive mutant HLA-H gene on chromosome 6 that has age-related incomplete penetrance and varied clinical expression. The defect causes increased intestinal absorption of iron, resulting in increased saturation of serum transferrin, elevated serum ferritin concentrations, and deposition in the liver, heart, certain endocrine organs, and joints. Heterozygotes have increased iron stores but rarely develop clinical disease.

Demographics: Although present from birth, the peak age of symptom onset is 40 to 60 years. Female:male ratio is 1:5. Prevalence is 30 to 60/10,000. It is mostly seen in northern European populations; 10% of Caucasians are heterozygous for the mutation.

Cardinal Findings: Multiple organ systems may be affected.

—*Liver:* Transaminases are elevated, with occasional hepatomegaly and tenderness and eventual cirrhosis.

—*Endocrine:* Diabetes is usually a late manifestation. Hypogonadism (loss of libido, impotence, testicular atrophy, gynecomastia) and skin pigmentation (related to increased melanin) are often seen.

—*Heart:* Cardiac involvement is uncommon but may present as a cardiomyopathy.

—*Arthropathy:* This may be a presenting feature. Joints typically involved include the second and third metacarpophalangeal (MCP) and proximal interphalangeal (PIP) joints, hips, knees, or spine. Joints may be mildly tender, swollen, or clinically resemble osteoarthritis; 50% have chondrocalcinosis. Iron deposition may cause pseudogout.

Diagnostic Tests: Screen with transferrin saturation (100 × serum iron/total iron binding capacity); if above 50%, measure serum ferritin—in hemochromatosis, serum ferritin exceeds 200 ng/mL in males and 100 ng/mL in females. Ferritin behaves as an acute-phase reactant and levels may increase in the presence of inflammatory disease elsewhere. Diagnosis should be confirmed with liver biopsy. Noninvasive imaging with CT or MRI may be useful. Screen first-degree relatives because early detection and treatment can prevent clinical disease.

Keys to Diagnosis: Consider hemochromatosis in all cases of "transaminitis" and chondrocalcinosis and when an osteoarthritis-like disease is seen in men in their fourth and fifth decades.

Therapy: Weekly phlebotomy is administered to deplete iron stores; maintenance phlebotomy should occur 3–6 times per year to keep the hematocrit below 40%. The arthropathy is usually not reversible. Arthritis should be treated symptomatically.

REFERENCES

Schumacher HR Jr. Ochronosis, hemochromatosis, and Wilson's disease. In: Koopman WJ, ed. Arthritis and allied conditions: a textbook of rheumatology. 13th ed. Baltimore: Williams & Wilkins, 1997:2193–2194.

Smith LH. Overview of hemochromatosis. West J Med 1990;153:296–308.

HEMOPHILIA

Synonyms: Hemophilia A (factor VIII deficiency), hemophilia B (factor IX deficiency)

ICD9 Code: Hemophilia A, 286.0; hemophilia B, 286.1; hemarthrosis, 719.10

Definition: Hemophilia A and B are congenital, X-linked recessive disorders of the coagulation cascade that manifest with hemorrhage into weight-bearing joints, muscle, or soft tissues. Hemophilia A and B are clinically similar; hemophilia A accounts for more than 80% of cases. Disease severity is based upon the amount of factor present (<2% is severe, 2–5% is moderate, and 5–25% is mild). Factor levels above 25% are rarely associated with hemorrhagic events.

Etiology: Hemophilia is caused by congenital deficiency of factors VIII or IX. Acquired deficiencies have been reported.

Pathology: Intraarticular blood does not coagulate because of the lack of pro-thrombin, fibrinogen, and tissue thromboplastin. RBCs may incite inflammation and may lead to synovial proliferation (without inflammatory cells), pannus, and cartilage damage. Hemosiderin is found in synovium and chondrocytes.

Demographics: Hemophilia A affects 1 in 10,000 males. Females are asymp-tomatic. Males are commonly affected and the first episode of bleeding often oc-curs before the age of 5 years.

Cardinal Findings: Acute hemarthrosis may begin as stiffness or warmth that is followed by intense pain. Low-grade fever may occur. Intraarticular he-morrhage commonly affects the knees, ankles, and elbows and manifests as an acute, erythematous, warm mono-or oligoarthritis. Involvement of small joints (fingers, wrist, sternoclavicular) is unusual and should suggest other diagnoses. Repetitive hemarthrosis may cause secondary osteoarthritis, deformity, or less commonly a chronic synovitis (with or without effusion). Other common sites of bleeding include muscle (resulting in myonecrosis or compartments syn-drome), bone, CNS, or kidney (manifest as hematuria).

Complications: Transfusions and factor VIII therapy has resulted in HIV positivity, AIDS, hepatitis B or C infection, and chronic liver disease. Septic arthritis rarely accompanies hemarthrosis. Nonetheless, staphylococcal, pneu-mococcal, and salmonella septic arthritis have been well described in hemo-philia.

Diagnostic Tests: Activated partial thromboplastin time (PTT) is prolonged; prothrombin time and platelet counts are normal. Assays for factor VIII are commonly available, and titers are low during bleeding episodes. Synovial fluid shows a predominance of RBCs and neutrophils.

Imaging: Radiographs may show soft tissue swelling, juxtaarticular osteope-nia, joint space narrowing, and subchondral cyst formation. Marginal erosions may be seen with chronic disease. Widening of the femoral intercondylar notch is said to be characteristic of hemophilia.

Keys to Diagnosis: Look for a positive family history or antecedent diagno-sis of hemophilia associated with hemorrhage into joints or soft tissues.

Differential Diagnosis: Hemorrhagic joint effusions may also be due to von Willebrand's disease, vitamin K deficiency, platelet disorders, crystal-induced arthritis, trauma, fracture, ligament tear (cruciate), neuropathic arthritis, and pigmented villonodular synovitis. Acute hemophiliac hemarthrosis must be distinguished from septic arthritis, HIV-related arthropathies, and crystal-in-duced arthritis.

Therapy: Chronic aspirin and NSAIDs should be avoided. Acute bleeding can be treated with sufficient recombinant factor VIII to elevate levels to 40 to 50%. The dose is calculated from the patient's weight and factor VIII level. Ice, rest, analgesia, and joint extension (to avoid contractures) is advised. Do not attempt invasive procedures (e.g., arthrocentesis) until factor VIII levels are above 50%. Arthrocentesis is indicated if infection is suspected. Septic arthritis may accompany an acute hemarthrosis. The therapeutic value of arthrocentesis to remove blood and RBCs that may exacerbate inflammation is controversial. Intraarticular steroids should not be used. Major bleeding (e.g., CNS) requires chronic factor VIII levels above 50% until resolved. Prophylactic administration of factor VIII (3 times weekly) has been advocated for patients with recurrent or severe bleeding. Although seldom used, reports suggest that chronic inflammatory synovitis may benefit from penicillamine or gold therapy.

Surgery: Arthroscopic synovectomy is seldom required for chronic synovitis. Surgical procedures (e.g., total joint replacement) can be cautiously performed with adequate factor replacement.

REFERENCES

Steven MM, Yogarajah S, Madhok R, et al. Haemophilic arthritis. Q J Med 1986;58:181–197.

HENOCH-SCHÖNLEIN PURPURA

Synonyms: Anaphylactoid purpura, allergic purpura

ICD9 Code: 287.0

Definition: Henoch-Schönlein purpura (HSP) is a systemic, small-vessel vasculopathy affecting the skin (lower extremities), gut, and kidneys. HSP is classically characterized by the triad of nonthrombocytopenic purpura, arthralgia, and abdominal pain.

Etiology: The cause of HSP is unknown; it is labeled as "allergic" because peak onset is in the spring, often following upper respiratory infection (URI) by viruses or streptococci. It is sometimes a consequence of certain drugs (e.g., ampicillin, penicillin, erythromycin, quinidine, or quinine).

Pathology: Biopsies demonstrate leukocytoclastic vasculitis (venulitis) in skin or GI tract. IgA deposition, found in 70% of skin and 90% of renal lesions, is diagnostic. Renal biopsy may show mesangial hypercellularity and segmental necrotizing glomerulonephritis.

Demographics: Age of onset is bimodal. Most cases affect children, usually between the ages of 2 and 11 years. The mean age of onset is 43 years for adults (range, 30–70 years). Males are affected more than females.

Cardinal Findings: Onset is usually heralded by persistent or intermittent palpable purpura or petechiae involving the lower extremities and buttocks, sometimes with dependent edema. Lesions often progress from red to purple to brown. They may coalesce to form large ecchymoses. Fever is seen in 50%, and musculoskeletal manifestations (arthralgia/arthritis of ankles or knees) are present in 75% of patients. Intestinal disease (diarrhea, cramping) is more common in children and manifests as cramping, GI bleeding, hematemesis, melena, or rarely intussusception. IgA nephropathy is more common in adults than children. Renal insufficiency is typically brief but may develop in 3 to 15% of patients.

Uncommon Manifestations: Skin involvement of face, upper extremities, or torso; ulcerative lesions; bleeding gums; bowel perforation; renal insufficiency; headache; neuropathy; seizures; orchitis; hemoptysis; and cardiac arrhythmias have been reported.

Diagnostic Tests: Anemia, leukocytosis, elevated ESR, and abnormal urinalysis (hematuria, casts, proteinuria) are common.

Keys to Diagnosis: Consider the diagnosis of HSP with lower extremity palpable purpura and/or evidence of leukocytoclastic vasculitis and IgA deposition in skin, gut, or kidney.

Differential Diagnosis: Cryoglobulinemia, polyarteritis nodosa, Wegener's granulomatosis, bacterial endocarditis, SLE, or lymphoma should be considered.

Diagnostic Criteria: The ACR requires two of the following four criteria: age below 20 years at onset; palpable purpura; acute abdominal pain; or biopsy evidence of granulocytes in walls of venules or small arterioles (leukocytoclastic vasculitis).

Therapy: Most patients (especially children) require only (*a*) supportive care (bed rest, hydration), (*b*) treatment of suspected infection, or (*c*) removal of the offending drug. ASA or NSAIDs are usually ineffective. Corticosteroids tend not to be effective with skin or renal disease and are reserved for CNS, testicular torsion, intestinal bleeding, or severe abdominal or joint pain. Treatment of renal disease is controversial.

Surgery: Surgery is reserved for those with uncontrolled abdominal hemorrhage and perforation.

Prognosis: Most patients show spontaneous improvement in 4 to 16 weeks. Relapse is seen in 5 to 10%. Prognosis depends on renal outcome. Mortality rate is 2%.

REFERENCES

Gay RM Jr, Ball GV. Vasculitis: Henoch-Schönlein purpura. In: Koopman WJ, ed. Arthritis and allied conditions: a textbook of rheumatology. 13th ed. Baltimore: Williams & Wilkins, 1997:1511–1512.

Szer IS. Henoch-Schönlein purpura. Curr Opinion Rheumatol 1994;6:25–31.

HEPATITIS: MUSCULOSKELETAL MANIFESTATIONS

ICD9 Codes: Hepatitis A, 070.1; hepatitis B, 070.30; acute hepatitis C, 070.51; chronic hepatitis C, 070.54; lupoid hepatitis, 571.49; chronic active hepatitis, 571.49; drug-induced hepatitis, 573.3

Definition: A variety of musculoskeletal disorders may be associated with hepatitis caused by hepatitis A virus (HAV), hepatitis B virus (HBV), or hepatitis C virus (HCV).

Etiology: The arthritis associated with acute HBV infection involves a serum sickness syndrome, with formation of circulating immune complexes. Immune complexes are deposited in joints and other parts of the body when the quantity of viral antigens approximates that of the antiviral antibodies. This is often transient, occurring as antigen levels fall and antibody levels rise, typically in the prodromal phase of clinical infection. In addition to arthritis, maculopapular rash, urticaria, and renal disease may result from formation of circulating immune complexes. In chronic HBV and HCV infections, formation of cryoglobulins (especially HCV) or induction of polyarteritis nodosa can further lead to arthritic symptoms. Intermittent viremia may be responsible for chronic arthritis reported in both HBV and HCV infection. A direct viral cytopathogenic effect on the synovium has also been postulated in HBV infection.

Demographics:

—*HAV:* Infection is transmitted enterally. Precise numbers of cases not known; 30,000 cases/year are reported by the CDC. Actual numbers are likely much higher, since the illness is frequently subclinical (30–50% of adults have serologic evidence of past exposure to HAV, but only 3–5% recall a clinically compatible acute illness). Transient arthralgia has been reported in 10% of patients and is twice as frequent in icteric patients. Arthritis rarely occurs in HAV infection.

—*HBV:* Transmitted parenterally, sexually, and vertically, 200,000 cases of HBV occur annually in the United States, with 6 to 10% becoming chronic. Most cases occur in young adults, especially in high-risk groups like parenteral drug users and certain immigrant groups from endemic regions. Arthralgias develop in 25% of patients and frank arthritis in 10%; there is a slight male preponderance (1.5:1 M:F ratio).

—*HCV:* Antibodies to HCV are detected in 1.4% of the U.S. population. Prevalence is higher in developing countries. Transmission is primarily via contaminated blood. Risk factors include parenteral drug use, tattooing, blood transfusions, and hemodialysis. In 40 to 50% no risk factors can be identified. Persistent infection occurs in 50 to 60% of patients. HCV-associated arthritis is rare. Arthritic syndromes associated with type II cryoglobulinemia are relatively more common.

Cardinal Findings

—*HAV:* Transient arthralgias may occur in acute infection. A transient serum sickness–like syndrome uncommonly occurs.

—*HBV:* The most common rheumatic syndrome in acute HBV infection is abrupt onset of a severe, symmetric polyarthritis in the prodromal phase. Simultaneous joint involvement is the usual pattern; occasionally a migratory or additive pattern is observed. The arthritis and rash are often short-lived and typically disappear with the onset of jaundice. Urticaria, petechiae, and maculopapular eruptions commonly accompany the arthritis. A similar syndrome, following HBV vaccination, has been reported. In 1% of cases of chronic HBV infection, polyarteritis nodosa (PAN) may occur with necrotizing vasculitis, mononeuritis multiplex, and fever. HBV-associated glomerulonephritis is a variant of this condition.

—*HCV:* Acute arthritis is a rare phenomenon. Mixed cryoglobulinemia (type II cryoglobulins) has been strongly associated with chronic HCV infection (30–90%) with associated membranoproliferative glomerulonephritis. Sjögren's syndrome has also been associated with chronic HCV infection. Chronic and intermittent arthritis, in both oligoarticular and polyarticular patterns, have also been reported in HCV infection.

Uncommon Findings

—*HAV:* Rarely, cryoglobulinemia may occur with purpura and arthritis.

—*HBV:* Cryoglobulinemia may occur. In persistent HBV infection, chronic polyarthritis may occur.

—*HCV:* Anti-HCV antibodies have been detected in 14% of patients with PAN.

Diagnostic Tests: See p. 116 for more information on serologic tests for hepatitis.

—*HAV:* HAV accounts for approximately 20% of cases of acute viral hepatitis in the United States. Anti-HAV IgM is found in acute HAV infection. Anti-HAV IgG indicates prior exposure to HAV. Serum transaminases rise in the prodromal phase and peak by the time jaundice develops. Other findings include leukopenia. In the icteric phase, many liver function abnormalities are noted, including hyperbilirubinemia and a prolonged prothrombin time, depending on the severity of the illness.

—*HBV:* HBV causes approximately 60% of cases of acute viral hepatitis in the United States. HBsAg is the first serologic marker to appear; anti-HBsAg follows. In chronic HBV infection, HBsAg is detectable; anti-HBsAg is not. Serum transaminase levels vary and are often less than twice normal. Hyperbilirubinemia, if present, is usually mild.

—*HCV:* HCV causes approximately 20% of cases of acute viral hepatitis in the United States (but HCV is responsible for 90% of posttransfusion hepatitis). IgG anti-HCV antibody is usually not seen until 2 to 6 months following acute infection. Biochemical abnormalities are typically mild; transaminase levels often wax and wane. More-sensitive assays for HCV infection include enzyme-linked immunosorbent assays (ELISA), recombinant immunoblot assays (RIBA), polymerase chain reactions (PCR), and branched DNA assays (bDNA).

Differential Diagnosis

—*Acute arthritis:* Since arthritis occurs in the prodromal preicteric phase of hepatitis, clues to the correct diagnosis are few. Serum transaminases are frequently elevated, but the diagnosis is often made retrospectively, after jaundice develops. Nonetheless, acute polyarthritis, especially when accompanied by a serum sickness–like syndrome, should raise suspicion of acute viral hepatitis. Other viral infections presenting in a similar manner include rubella, mumps, parvovirus B19, herpesviruses, human immunodeficiency virus, enteroviruses, and a variety of arboviruses. At the outset, acute HBV infection may be mistaken for RA, SLE, rheumatic fever, gonococcal arthritis, or Reiter's syndrome.

—*Cryoglobulinemia:* Detection of cryoglobulins should prompt testing for viral hepatitis (HBV, HCV). Other causes of cryoglobulinemia include connective tissue diseases and myeloproliferative and lymphoproliferative disorders.

—*Polyarteritis nodosa:* Ten to 25% of cases of classic PAN are associated with chronic HBV or HCV infection.

Keys to Diagnosis: The availability of sensitive and specific assays for viral hepatitis has greatly simplified diagnosis. A high index of suspicion, especially when such risk factors for viral hepatitis as household exposure, blood transfusion, hemodialysis, and parenteral drug use are present, is the main key to establishing the correct diagnosis.

Therapy

—*Acute arthritis:* Short-lived, acute arthritis is managed symptomatically with analgesics or NSAIDs.

—*Cryoglobulinemia:* Interferon α (IFN-α) has been used successfully in the management of HCV infection. In patients with HCV-associated cryoglobulinemia, IFN-α can decrease the cryocrit and improve purpura, but symptoms often rebound after discontinuation of therapy. Purpura and arthritis can be managed with NSAIDs. If visceral organs such as the kidney and lung are involved, corticosteroids and cyclophosphamide may be required. Plasma exchange also has a role as a supplementary measure with fulminant disease especially. Liver transplantation may be indicated in selected patients with chronic HCV infection.

—*Polyarteritis nodosa:* PAN associated with HBV infection is often problematic to treat, since interferon α has immunostimulatory effects and glucocorticoid therapy can exacerbate HBV infection. Corticosteroids are often used initially for rapid control of the most life-threatening manifestations of polyarteritis nodosa. This can be followed by antiviral regimens of vidarabine or interferon α combined with cyclophosphamide, with plasma exchange playing a supplementary role.

Prognosis

—*HAV:* Arthritis is usually transient and self-limited.

—*HBV:* Arthritis is usually self-limited but may occasionally become chronic with persistent HBV infection. HBV-associated PAN, when treated, had an 83% survival rate in one series, compared with an untreated 5-year survival rate of 13%.

—*HCV:* Arthritis is usually transient; rarely, it is chronic. HCV-associated cryoglobulinemia has a 70% 10-year survival rate overall; it is lower in patients who develop renal disease.

REFERENCES

Sharara AI, Hunt CM, Hamilton JD. Hepatitis C. Ann Intern Med 1996;125:658–668.

HUMAN IMMUNODEFICIENCY VIRUS (HIV): MUSCULOSKELETAL MANIFESTATIONS

ICD9 Code: HIV, 042.0

Definition: A variety of rheumatic syndromes may be associated with HIV-1 infection.

Etiology: Some rheumatic syndromes (e.g., septic arthritis and pyomyositis) may result from immunodeficiency secondary to CD4 T cell depletion. Others such as the lymphocytic infiltrative syndromes are a consequence of the host response to chronic antigenic stimulation by HIV-1. The diffuse infiltrative lymphocytosis syndrome (DILS) has been associated with certain human leukocyte antigens (HLA): HLA-B45, HLA-B49, HLA-B50, HLA-DR5, and HLA-DR6. Infection with HIV-1 causes immune dysregulation manifest as abnormal cytokine production, which may be responsible for inflammatory arthritis. CD8-dependent diseases such as Reiter's syndrome and psoriasis seem to have a more aggressive course in HIV-1 infection.

Demographics: Patients manifesting musculoskeletal disorders usually have evidence of, or recent progression to, the acquired immunodeficiency syndrome (AIDS). Epidemiologic studies on those with Reiter's syndrome and psoriasis have yielded conflicting data. In general, rheumatic syndromes in the HIV population seem to occur with the same frequency as in immunocompetent populations, although they may be more aggressive or demonstrate atypical features.

Clinical Subsets: Several distinct syndromes have been reported in HIV-positive patients.

—*Inflammatory arthritis:* A rheumatoid-factor-positive symmetric, erosive polyarthritis can occur in HIV-1 infection, despite CD4 T cell depletion. There are anecdotal reports of RA patients developing HIV infection with improvement of synovitis. However, this occurrence is rare, and the relationship between RA activity and HIV infection remains unresolved.

—*Reiter's syndrome and psoriatic arthritis:* Onset is usually heralded by urethritis or enteritis and is later followed by skin and joint disease. Uveitis and sacroiliitis are rare. Cutaneous disease (psoriasis or keratoderma blenorrhagica) is very prominent. Keratoderma blenorrhagica, a papulosquamous eruption that occurs on the palms, soles, and penis, may be indistinguishable from pustular psoriasis. Oligoarticular arthritis (involving the knee or ankle), dactylitis, and enthesitis is common.

—*Diffuse infiltrative lymphocytosis syndrome (DILS):* DILS, a disorder resembling Sjögren's syndrome, is caused by CD8 T-cell infiltration with bilateral parotid gland enlargement (often massive), sicca symptoms (often minor), and prominent extraglandular sites of lymphocytic infiltration (lung, muscle, lymph nodes). CD8 T-cell infiltration of the lung causes a lymphocytic interstitial pneumonitis presenting with dyspnea and can progress to fibrosis. DILS is associated with a very slow progression to AIDS.

—*Myopathy:* CD8 T cell infiltration may cause a myopathy indistinguishable from idiopathic polymyositis, with elevated serum creatine kinase levels, proximal muscle weakness, and occasionally skin lesions characteristic of dermatomyositis (heliotrope, Gottron's papules, periungual erythema). HIV therapy with zidovudine (AZT) can cause a myopathy similar to polymyositis but with less inflammatory infiltrate.

—*Vasculitis:* Sporadic reports in the literature describe HIV associated with hypersensitivity vasculitis (often a drug reaction), polyarteritis nodosa, granulomatous angiitis, or primary angiitis of the central nervous system.

—*Musculoskeletal infections:* As in normal individuals, *Staphylococcus aureus* infection accounts for over 70% of cases of nongonococcal septic arthritis. Such patients often present with an acute monarthritis with systemic symptoms. Pyogenic sacroiliitis, primarily occurring in intravenous drug users, is also usually due to *S. aureus*. With advanced CD4 T cell depletion, fungal (e.g., cryptococcal) and mycobacterial septic arthritis have been reported. The arthritis is generally monarticular and more indolent, with subtle inflammation. Juxtaarticular osteomyelitis is not an uncommon complication. Pyomyositis, or deep muscle abscess, typically presents with acute muscle pain (often in the thigh), with woody induration, swelling, and erythema; it is usually caused by *S. aureus*.

Diagnostic Tests: Abnormalities vary with the clinical picture. HIV-positive patients may have a low incidence of low-titer ANA and rheumatoid factor. Others have been described with antiphospholipid antibodies and cryoglobulins.

—*Arthritis:* Monoarthritis or oligarthritis with systemic features (e.g., fever) should prompt consideration of diagnostic arthrocentesis, synovial fluid analysis with cell count, and stains and cultures for bacteria, fungi, and mycobacteria. Blood cultures may also be indicated in such cases. HLA-B27 testing is rarely needed to diagnose Reiter's syndrome.

—*Myopathy:* Serum creatine kinase, urine toxicology screen (i.e., cocaine), and withdrawal of zidovudine (if applicable) with repeat serum creatine kinase assay in 4 to 6 weeks should be considered. Persistent unexplained serum creatine kinase elevation should be investigated with EMG or muscle biopsy for evidence of inflammatory myositis. In pyomyositis, imaging studies (ultrasonography, CT, or MRI) are necessary for diagnosis and can be used for diagnostic aspiration, gram stain, and culture.

—*Suspected vasculitis:* Biopsy of the most accessible or involved tissue (e.g., skin, nerve, liver, kidney) or angiography may be required to document vasculitis.

—*DILS:* Exocrine involvement can be documented by minor salivary gland biopsy or noninvasively with gallium[67] scans.

Therapy: Many patients with HIV infection can be safely treated with corticosteroids and a few selected agents detailed below. However, certain immunosuppressive medications (e.g., methotrexate, azathioprine, cyclosporine, cyclophosphamide) should be avoided, as they may further immunosuppress the patient.

—*Infectious musculoskeletal disease:* Antimicrobial therapy should be tailored to the causative organism. Septic joints should be serially aspirated. Inaccessible joints like the sacroiliac require imaging-guided aspiration.

—*Reiter's syndrome or psoriatic arthritis:* Initially, optimize antiretroviral therapy. Consider using sulfasalazine (2–3 g/day in divided doses). Both indomethacin (75–150 mg/day) and hydroxychloroquine (400 mg/day) have proven beneficial and have anti-HIV effects as well. Effective treatment with etretinate has been reported.

—*Polymyositis:* Often, polymyositis can be safely treated with prednisone (0.5–1.0 mg/kg/day for 3 months and quickly tapered to minimum effective dose). Refractory patients may respond to intravenous gamma globulin therapy.

—*DILS:* Frequently, DILS responds to antiretroviral therapy alone. Prednisone (20–40 mg/day) will rapidly decrease salivary gland size and improve lymphocytic interstitial pneumonitis. Taper to minimum effective dose. Patients seem to tolerate low-dose prednisone well.

—*Vasculitis:* High-dose corticosteroids may be necessary for those with systemic necrotizing vasculitis. Advanced HIV infection often precludes immunsuppressive therapy, but it has been used in some patients with life-threatening vasculitis.

Prognosis: HIV stage often determines the prognosis. Patients with advanced HIV infection generally have poorer response to therapy. Patients with DILS generally respond well and are typically long-term nonprogressors. Vasculitis in HIV-1 has a poor prognosis. The protease inhibitors (relatively new, powerful antiretroviral drugs) can, in some instances, dramatically reverse clinical disease.

REFERENCES
Itescu S. Rheumatic aspects of acquired immunodeficiency syndromes. Curr Opinion Rheumatol 1996;8:346–353.
Kazi S, Cohen PR, Williams F, et al. The diffuse infiltrative lymphocytosis syndrome. Clinical and immunogenetic features in 35 patients. AIDS 1996;10(4):385–391.

HYPERTROPHIC OSTEOARTHROPATHY (HOA)

Synonyms: Acropachy, familial idiopathic hypertrophic osteoarthropathy, pachydermoperiostosis, Marie-Bamberger syndrome, secondary hypertrophic osteoarthropathy, HOA

ICD9 Code: 731.2

Definition: HOA is a syndrome characterized by proliferation of skin and bone in the distal extremities. The complete HOA syndrome includes clubbing of the fingers and toes, periostitis (with new bone formation on long bones) and arthritis. Not all patients have all manifestations.

Etiology: The primary form is of unknown etiology, but most likely has a genetic basis. Secondary forms are associated with pulmonary (cystic fibrosis, pulmonary fibrosis, cancer, chronic infection), cardiac (cyanotic congenital heart disease, patent ductus arteriosus, bacterial endocarditis), gastrointestinal (inflammatory bowel disease, cancer, cirrhosis), or malignant disorders (lymphoma). Pathogenic mechanisms for these associations are not known.

Pathology: Long bones show various stages of new bone formation on cortical surfaces. Clubbed digits show increased numbers of fibroblasts, and collagenous tissue and synovial membranes may have proliferative features.

Demographics: The primary genetic form appears in children or young adults. Secondary forms are more likely to be seen in older patients.

Cardinal Findings: Clubbed digits (fingers and toes) have been described as having a drumstick-like appearance, with softening and mobility of the nail bed. Involvement of long bones may produce severe, incapacitating, or "deep" bone pain. Areas affected by periostitis are often painful and may be associated with overlying warmth or edema. Arthralgias or arthritis is often symmetric and involves the MCP, wrist, elbow, knee, and ankle joints. Joints may be warm and swollen with an effusion.

Uncommon Findings: Thickening of the skin (pachydermia) may alter facial features and produce coarse or "leonine" features. Pachydermia is uncommon in the secondary forms of HOA. Thyroid acropachy, a rare manifestation of hyperthyroidism, may be associated with exophthalmos and pretibial myxedema.

Diagnostic Tests: Laboratory tests are not specific for HOA but may reflect the underlying malignant or infectious disorder. The ESR is often elevated in secondary HOA. Synovial fluid is often noninflammatory (WBC < 2000 cells/mm^3).

Imaging: Radiographs of long bones show new bone formation (periostitis), especially in the extremities. Periostitis is common in the distal tibia or fibula, radius, or ulna. It is less common in the phalanges. Acro-osteolysis may be seen; joint space narrowing or erosions are absent. Bone scanning may be useful.

Diagnostic Criteria: Digital clubbing and periostosis of tubular bones are required for the complete syndrome. Three incomplete forms are also defined: (*a*) clubbing alone; (*b*) periostosis without clubbing but with any of the systemic illnesses associated with HOA; and (*c*) pachydermia associated with any of the minor manifestations, including synovial effusions.

Differential Diagnosis: Skin changes may resemble scleroderma. Numerous disorders may be associated with periostitis (see p. 292).

Therapy: Clubbing alone requires no specific treatment. Secondary forms respond to removal or treatment of underlying thoracic disease. NSAIDs are used to treat painful bone lesions.

Prognosis: In secondary forms, the outcome is dictated by the underlying disorder.

REFERENCES

Altman RD. Hypertrophic osteoarthropathy. In: Koopman WJ, ed. Arthritis and allied conditions: a textbook of rheumatology. 13th ed. Baltimore: Williams & Wilkins, 1997: 1751–1758.

Martinez-Lavin M, Matucci-Cerinic M, Jajic I, Pineda C. Hypertrophic osteoarthropathy: consensus on its definition, classification, assessment and diagnostic criteria. J Rheumatol 1993;20:1386–1387.

IMMUNODEFICIENCY

Synonyms: Common variable (CVID) immunodeficiency; severe combined (SCID) immunodeficiency; X-linked immunodeficiency

ICD9 Codes: Immunodeficiency, 279.3; common variable, 279.06; severe combined, 279.2

Definition: Immunodeficiency diseases are a diverse group of disorders that result from quantitative or qualitative defects in specific parts of the immune system. They may be categorized as primary or secondary (Table 1).

Table 1
Immunodeficiency Diseases

Selected primary immunodeficiencies
  B cell (antibody/immunoglobulin) defects
    X-linked (Bruton's) agammaglobulinemia
    Common variable immunodeficiency (CVID)
    IgA deficiency
  Combined B cell and T cell defects
    Severe combined immunodeficiency (SCID)
    Wiskott-Aldrich syndrome
  T cell defects
    DiGeorge syndrome
  Phagocyte defects
    Chronic granulomatous disease
  Complement deficiencies
Selected causes of secondary immunodeficiency
  Pharmacologic/therapeutic
    Corticosteroids
    Chemotherapeutic drugs
    Plasmapheresis
    Irradiation
  Lymphoproliferative disease
    Lymphoma/leukemia
  Infectious diseases
    HIV-1, HIV-2
    Influenza
  Systemic inflammatory diseases
    SLE
    RA
  Other diseases
    Protein-losing nephropathy/enteropathy
    Diabetes mellitus
    Solid tumors
    Malnutrition

Etiology: Primary immunodeficiencies often relate to focal defects in enzyme systems, cell surface molecules, or other factors critical to development or function of immunocompetent cells. Secondary immunodeficiencies represent impairments in the immune response related to use of immunosuppressive medications, systemic infections, and other conditions.

Demographics: The incidence of primary immunodeficiencies ranges from 1 in 10,000 to 1 in 100,000 population. They typically arise in children, and approximately 85% of cases are found in persons 15 years of age or younger. Because many of the primary immunodeficiencies are X-linked, boys substantially outnumber girls. Secondary immunodeficiencies are much more common than primary; in addition, they occur most commonly among older adults.

Cardinal Findings: The clinical hallmark of immunodeficiency is increased susceptibility to infection. However, some immunodeficiencies are associated with a variety of autoimmune and musculoskeletal manifestations. This is particularly true for antibody- or immunoglobulin-deficiency syndromes, which have been associated with increased incidence of arthritis, SLE, immune thrombocytopenia, autoimmune hemolytic anemia, dermatomyositis, and vasculitis. The most common musculoskeletal manifestation is arthritis, which may occur in 35% of untreated patients with immunoglobulin deficiency. The arthritis is usually oligoarticular and affects the larger joints such as the knee. However, some patients have joint involvement resembling that of rheumatoid arthritis. In some patients, the arthritis may be related to infection with mycoplasma. The presumed infectious etiology of the arthritis in these patients is supported by a decreased incidence among patients receiving therapy with gamma globulin.

Diagnostic Tests: The diagnosis of an immunodeficiency is established by demonstrating defects in particular components of the immune response. For immunoglobulin deficiencies, one should initially determine the serum immunoglobulin (IgG, IgA, IgM) levels (see p. 122). In rare cases, more elaborate testing may be required.

Keys to Diagnosis: Key to the diagnosis of an underlying immunodeficiency is a high degree of clinical suspicion. Patients typically have a history of recurrent infections that may also be excessively severe, respond poorly to therapy, or be caused by unusual organisms.

Therapy: Therapy of antibody deficiency syndromes consists of gamma globulin, typically administered intravenously at 4-week intervals. This has almost entirely replaced such older forms of therapy as intramuscular gamma globulin or prophylactic antibiotics.

Prognosis: With appropriate treatment, the prognosis of those with antibody deficiency diseases improves substantially and approaches normal.

REFERENCES

Cassidy JT, Burt A, Petty R, Sullivan D. Selective IgA deficiency in connective tissue diseases. N Engl J Med 1969;280:275–279.
Huston DP, Kavanaugh AF, Rohane PW, Huston MM. Immunoglobulin deficiency syndromes and therapy. J Allergy Clin Immunol 1991;87:1–19.
Rosen FS, Cooper MD, Wedgwood JP. The primary immunodeficiencies. N Engl J Med 1995;333:431–440.

INCLUSION BODY MYOSITIS

Definition: Inclusion body myositis (IBM) is a form of idiopathic inflammatory myositis (IIM) (see p. 301). IBM has distinct differences from the more common forms of IIM, polymyositis (PM) and dermatomyositis (DM).

Etiology: Unknown.

Pathology: Histopathologic analysis is the key differentiating feature between IBM and other forms of IIM. On light microscopic analysis, there is an endomysial accumulation of mononuclear cells, particularly CD8+ T cells (similar to the findings in PM). Other characteristic findings in muscle include vacuoles lined with basophilic granules, eosinophilic inclusions, abnormal microtubular filaments in nuclear and cytoplasmic inclusions, and "ragged red" fibers.

Demographics: Affected patients are usually over 50 years old. The male:female ratio is 2:1 or higher. IBM represents 15 to 30% of IIM cases, which have a prevalence of 5 to 10/million population.

Cardinal Findings: Symmetric proximal muscle weakness is typically present. Weakness is often slowly progressive and painless. In contrast to PM/DM, distal muscle weakness and asymmetric involvement are more commonly seen in IBM. In addition, 30% of patients may have an associated axonal neuropathy.

Diagnostic Tests: Muscle enzymes (e.g., CK) are elevated in IBM as they are in other IIMs, but usually less so in IBM (up to 10 times normal) than in PM/DM (up to 50 times normal). EMG shows a myopathic pattern (similar to that of PM/DM). Nonetheless, muscle biopsy with electron microscopic analysis is required to make a diagnosis of IBM.

Keys to Diagnosis: Often the diagnosis of IBM is made when patients with presumed PM or DM either do not respond to steroid therapy or display atypical manifestations (e.g., asymmetry, distal muscle weakness, or peripheral neuropathy). In such instances, IBM should be suspected, and muscle biopsy repeated or reviewed with emphasis on electron microscopic findings.

Differential Diagnosis: The differential diagnosis of IBM includes other types of IIM as well as other endocrinologic, metabolic, infectious, and toxic etiologies (see p. 57 and p. 261).

Diagnostic Criteria: Diagnostic criteria for IBM have been proposed, but not validated (Table 1).

Table 1
Proposed Diagnostic Criteria for IBM

Pathologic criteria
  Electron microscopy
    1. Microtubular filaments in the inclusions
  Light microscopy
    1. Lined vacuoles
    2. Intranuclear and intracytoplasmic inclusions
Clinical criteria
    1. Proximal muscle weakness (insidious onset)
    2. Distal muscle weakness
    3. EMG evidence of generalized inflammatory myopathy
    4. Elevation of muscle enzyme levels (CK, aldolase)
    5. Failure of muscle weakness to improve with steroids
Definite IBM = pathologic electron microscopic criterion and clinical criterion 1 plus 1 other clinical criterion.
Probable IBM = pathologic light microscopic criterion 1 and clinical criterion 1 plus 3 other clinical criteria.
Possible IBM = pathologic light microscopic criterion 2 plus any 3 clinical criteria

Therapy: Patients are treated like patients with PM/DM. However, because of the poor response to corticosteroid or immunosuppressive therapies, many physicians do not pursue aggressive or alternative therapies in IBM patients with little or no response to corticosteroids.

Prognosis: IBM patients are less likely to respond to therapy than those with other types of IIM. Approximately 50% of patients have no response to corticosteroids; rare patients have a complete response.

REFERENCES

Sayers ME, Chou SM, Calabrese LH. Inclusion body myositis: analysis of 32 cases. J Rheumatol 1992;19:1385–1389.
Wortmann RL. The dilemma of treating patients with inclusion body myositis. J Rheumatol 1992;19:1327–1329.

INFECTIVE ENDOCARDITIS

Synonyms: Infective endocarditis, subacute bacterial endocarditis (SBE)

ICD9 Code: Infective endocarditis, 421.0; prosthetic valve endocarditis, 996.61

Definition: Infective endocarditis implies infection of valvular or mural endocardium. Endocarditis is an uncommon cause of fever, arthralgia, and low back pain.

Etiology: Most infections occur over abnormal valves or damaged endocardial surfaces, where abnormal blood flow patterns lead to development of platelet-thrombin clots that serve as foci for infections. Some cases occur in intravenous drug abusers and are caused by more highly virulent organisms such as *Staphylococcus aureus*, which can severely damage normal endocardium and valves. Acute endocarditis is commonly caused by staphylococcus and streptococcus. Subacute endocarditis may be caused by α-hemolytic streptococci, *Streptococcus bovis*, and enterococci. Endocarditis with intravenous drug abuse may be caused by *S. aureus, Pseudomonas* spp., gram-negative species, and *Candida*.

Pathology: Infections are usually formed over areas of sterile vegetations consisting of platelets and fibrin. Most occur in high-pressure areas, usually on the left side of the heart. Underlying valves may show thickening from previous damage.

Demographics: Those at risk include older individuals, those with rheumatic and other forms of valvular disease, prosthetic valves, intravenous drug abuse, indwelling intravenous catheters, and those with bacteremia.

Cardinal Findings: Most patients have fever (with or without "night sweats") and a cardiac murmur. Tender nodules on the fingertips (Osler's nodes) and splinter hemorrhages under the fingernails may be seen. Anorexia, weight loss, arthralgias, frank arthritis, low back pain, and splenomegaly are common. Back pain may be caused by bacteremia or septic emboli resulting in septic discitis.

Uncommon Findings: A small number of patients develop septic arthritis due to seeding with the causative organism. Multiple joints may be involved.

Complications: Congestive heart failure, ruptured valve cusp or chordae tendineae, abscesses (myocardial, aortic root, brain), or infarction (lung, spleen, bowel, or myocardium) from emboli may be seen. Renal failure from glomerulonephritis has been described.

Diagnostic Tests: Positive blood cultures are diagnostic, but a significant minority of patients remain culture negative. Previous antibiotics may alter culture results. Elevated levels of acute-phase reactants (ESR, CRP) are expected. In subacute endocarditis, an anemia of chronic disease, low complement levels, and positive rheumatoid factor may be seen.

Imaging: Echocardiography, including transesophageal approaches, is useful for detecting the smallest vegetations.

Keys to Diagnosis: Fever with other systemic complaints and a heart murmur should prompt repeated blood cultures.

Differential Diagnosis: Patients may present with fever of unknown origin. Splinter hemorrhages and Osler's nodes may suggest a systemic vasculitis (e.g., PAN, Churg-Strauss angiitis, cryoglobulinemia). Multiple swollen joints and inflamed joints might suggest gout or Reiter's syndrome. Some patients are transiently positive for rheumatoid factor, so polyarthritis might be mistaken for RA. Other possibilities include osteomyelitis, rheumatic fever, and tuberculosis.

Therapy: Definitive therapy requires an extended course of appropriate antibiotics. Subsequent antibiotic prophylaxis is recommended for all invasive procedures.

Surgery: Heart valve replacement may be required.

Prognosis: Long-term outcome is dictated by the severity of the underlying heart disease or drug addiction or development of complications.

REFERENCES

Churchill MA, Geraci JE, Hunder GG. Musculoskeletal manifestations of bacterial endocarditis. Ann Intern Med 1977;87:754–759.

Roberts-Thomson PJ, Rischmueller M, Kwiatek RA, et al. Rheumatic manifestations of infective endocarditis. Rheumatol Int 1992;12:61–63.

INTESTINAL BYPASS SYNDROME

Synonyms: Arthritis-dermatitis syndrome

Definition: Arthritis and dermatitis may develop in less than 30% of patients following intestinal (jejunoileal or jejunocolonic) bypass surgery for the treatment of morbid obesity.

Etiology: Symptoms result from "blind loop" bacterial overgrowth; treatment with antibiotics tends to alleviate symptoms. This may represent a form of reactive arthritis. The significance of circulating cryoglobulins and immune complexes is unknown.

Demographics: Women are more often affected than men.

Cardinal Findings: Acute onset occurs 1 to 30 months after bypass surgery. Patients may complain of intermittent diarrhea, bloating, cramping, low-grade fever, and malaise. Patients may have episodic or migratory arthralgias or nondeforming symmetric polyarthritis involving large and small joints. Joint effusions tend to be mildly inflammatory. Tendinitis and myalgias are common. Joint symptoms and GI symptoms do not run a parallel course. Cutaneous findings (66–80%) often accompany arthritis and manifest as vesiculopustular lesions over the extremities or trunk. Less common are erythematous macules, urticarial or erythema nodosum–like lesions.

Uncommon Findings: Sacroiliitis, spondylitis, conjunctivitis, episcleritis, retinal vasculitis, serositis, Raynaud's phenomenon, dysarthria, hemolytic anemia, and thrombocytopenia can be seen.

Diagnostic Tests: CBC is normal or reveals mild leukocytosis. ESR is modestly elevated (20–60 mm/h). Cryoglobulins and circulating immune complexes are found in some patients.

Imaging: Radiographs may reveal only soft tissue swelling.

Differential Diagnosis: Gonococcal arthritis, Sweet's syndrome, erythema nodosum, ulcerative colitis, reactive arthritis, Behçet's syndrome, and Whipple's disease should be considered.

Therapy: Some patients respond to antibiotic therapy (tetracyclines, clindamycin, or metronidazole). Most require NSAIDs or low-dose corticosteroids (5–15 mg prednisone per day). Nonresponsive patients may respond to dapsone or may require corrective surgery (sphincteroplasty or reanastomosis).

REFERENCES

Mielants H, Veys EM. Enteropathic arthritis: intestinal bypass arthritis. In: Koopman WJ, ed. Arthritis and allied conditions: a textbook of rheumatology. 13th ed. Baltimore: Williams & Wilkins, 1997:1251.

JUVENILE ARTHRITIS (JA)

Synonyms: Juvenile rheumatoid arthritis (JRA); juvenile chronic arthritis (JCA)

ICD9 Codes: JA, 714.3; systemic JA, 714.3; polyarticular JA, 714.31; pauciarticular JA, 714.32

Definition: JA comprises a group of inflammatory arthropathies that affect children under the age of 16 years. JA may be divided into 4 subsets that differ in their presentation and outcomes: pauciarticular JA, juvenile spondylitis, polyarticular JA, and systemic-onset JA (Table 1).

Etiology: The cause of JA is unknown. Disordered immunoregulation has been reported, and some have suggested a role for latent viral infection, especially rubella. Increased numbers of JA patients are seen among those with IgA deficiency and hypogammaglobulinemia.

Pathology: Synovial tissue shows inflammatory changes similar to those seen in rheumatoid arthritis (RA).

Demographics: JA may affect children of any age from birth to 16 years. Onset is usually before the age of 9 years. Incidence rates are roughly 12 to 20 cases

Table 1
Comparison of Juvenile Arthritis Subsets

	Pauciarticular-Onset JA	Juvenile Spondylitis	Polyarticular-Onset JA	Systemic Onset JA
Frequency	50%	10%	30%	10%
Onset age (years)	1–10	9–16	3–16	3–16 yrs
Female:male	5:1	1:4	4:1	1:1
Joint pattern	Mono- or pauciarticular	Sacroiliitis or asymmetric oligoarthrtis	Polyarticular, symmetric	Polyarticular
Extraarticular features	Rare	Psoriasis, enthesitis, inflammatory bowel disease	Rheumatoid nodules, weight loss	Fever, rash, lymphadenopathy, serositis, hepatosplenomegaly
Uveitis	10–50%	10%	Rare	Rare
Laboratory findings	RF(−), 85% ANA(+)	50% are HLA-B27(+)	80% RF(−), 20% RF(+), 40% ANA(+)	Leukocytosis, ESR > 50 mm/h, anemia, increased LFTs, negative ANA & RF
Prognosis	Excellent for joints: guarded for eyes	? Risk of spondylitis and uveitis	Severe erosive arthritis in 50% of RF(+) and 20% of RF(−) patients	50% develop chronic arthritis; 20% severe erosive arthritis

per 100,000 population. Females are more commonly affected than males, with the exception of juvenile spondylitis (males predominate) and systemic JA (equally affected) (Table 1).

Cardinal Findings: Disease subsets are classified on the basis of arthritis and pattern of disease observed in the first 6 months. Presentations and manifestations vary with each disease subset.

—*Pauciarticular JA:* This is the most common variety of JA, accounting for more than 50% of cases. Onset is usually before age 6 years. Monarthritis or oligoarthritis (2–4 joints) is seen in the first 6 months. The knee is most commonly and hip least commonly affected. Most achieve remission. However, there is a serious risk of uveitis in this subset. Blindness occurs in less than 10% of patients and can be prevented by early detection and treatment. Most patients are ANA positive.

—*Juvenile spondylitis:* This is also known as late-onset pauciarticular disease. Males are more commonly affected than females, and onset is usually between 9 and 16 years of age. Onset is typically characterized by pauciarthritis affecting the knee, ankle, or hip. Some patients have a family history of psoriasis or a spondyloarthropathy (SpA). Extraarticular features of an SpA rarely antedate and usually follow the onset of arthritis. HLA-B27 positivity is seen in nearly half, and sacroiliitis may be clinically or radiographically evident. Between 20 and 50% of these patients go on to develop a chronic SpA (see p. 355).

—*Polyarticular JA:* Nearly 30% of patients have involvement of five or more joints, often in a symmetric distribution similar to that seen in adult RA. Rheumatoid factor positivity is seen in 20 to 30%, and ANA positivity is seen in 40% of polyarticular patients. Constitutional features of low-grade fever, weight loss, lymphadenopathy are occasionally seen. Rheumatoid nodules are only seen in RF(+) patients. This subset tends to have a chronic course and significant disability. More than 20% develop severe, erosive JA that is indistinguishable from seropositive adult RA.

—*Systemic-onset JA:* Also known as Still's disease, this subset accounts for 10% of cases. Manifestations include daily spiking (quotidian) fevers of 102°F or higher; an evanescent, salmon-pink rash; arthritis; generalized lymphadenopathy; serositis; hepato- or splenomegaly; weight loss; myalgias; neutrophilic leukocytosis; anemia; increased ESR (often >50 mm/h); negative serologic tests for ANA and RF; and nonspecific elevations of hepatic enzymes. Systemic disease is seldom life threatening (i.e., pericardial tamponade or disseminated intravascular coagulation (DIC)), and prognosis is most often determined by the arthritis. Severe erosive, chronic, disabling arthritis develops in more than 20%. This subset is identical to adult-onset Still's disease (see p. 152), with the exceptional lack of a prodromal sore throat in juveniles.

Uncommon Findings: Patients with polyarticular disease are at risk for micrognathia and growth retardation. Systemic JA patients may develop pleuritis, pericarditis, myocarditis, DIC, amyloidosis, or salicylate hepatotoxicity.

Complications: Chronic nongranulomatous uveitis (see p. 379) occurs in 10 to 50% of pauciarticular patients. There is a questionable association of uveitis with ANA positivity. Most patients are asymptomatic, but some manifest pain and altered vision. It tends to be bilateral, chronic, and progressive and may can lead to band keratopathy, posterior synechiae, cataracts, glaucoma, visual loss, or blindness. All patients with pauciarticular and polyarticular JA should undergo slit-lamp examinations every 3–6 months to identify early inflammatory lesions.

Cervical arthritis, especially C2–C3 apophyseal fusion, may be seen in patients with pauciarticular, polyarticular, or systemic disease.

Diagnostic Tests: There is no diagnostic laboratory test for JA. Extreme elevations of the WBC and ESR are typical in the systemic subset. RF positivity is seen in a minority of polyarticular patients. ANA positivity is common in both pauciarticular and RF(+) polyarticular patients. HLA-B27 assay (see p. 118) is seldom necessary to establish a diagnosis of juvenile spondylitis.

Imaging: Early radiographic changes may include soft tissue swelling, juxtaarticular osteopenia, or periostitis. Stunted or accelerated bone growth may be seen. With chronicity, loss of joint space and marginal erosions may develop. Fusion of cervical zygoapophyseal joints (especially C2–C3) may be seen. Atlantoaxial (C1–C2) subluxation is less common than in RA.

Keys to Diagnosis: JA should be suspected with development of a chronic (≥6 weeks) inflammatory arthritis in a child. The diagnosis is further established by identifying the pattern of arthritis and associated extraarticular features.

Diagnostic Criteria: American College of Rheumatology criteria are shown in Table 2.

Differential Diagnosis: Other disorders may affect children in a similar fashion, including SLE, reactive arthritis, Lyme disease, dermatomyositis,

Table 2

American College or Rheumatology Classification Criteria for the Diagnosis of Juvenile Rheumatoid Arthritis

1. Age at onset younger than 16 years
2. Arthritis in one or more joints: defined as swelling or effusion or at least 2 of the following:
   Limitation of range of motion
   Tenderness or pain on motion
   Increased heat
3. Duration of disease ≥ 6 weeks
4. Type of onset of disease during the first 6 months, classified as
   a. Polyarthritis: 5 joints or more
   b. Oligoarthritis: 4 joints or fewer
   c. Systemic disease with arthritis and intermittent fever
5. Exclusion of other forms of juvenile arthritis

Kawasaki disease, rheumatic fever, infantile-onset multisystemic inflammatory disease, and the vasculitides. Acute-onset inflammatory mono- or oligoarthritis should raise the possibility of septic arthritis, toxic synovitis of the hip, especially staphylococcal, streptococcal, or gonococcal arthritis. Arthritis may be the initial manifestation of neoplasia (e.g., leukemia, neuroblastoma) in children.

Therapy: A comprehensive approach to treatment must be initiated from the time of diagnosis and must involve the patient and family. Ongoing patient/family education should be interspersed with assessments by the physical therapist, ophthalmologist, dentist, and orthopaedist, if necessary. Patients should be enrolled in a program of active exercise, passive stretch, and periods of rest when the disease is most active. The goal of drug therapy is to reduce pain and inflammation, maintain optimal function, and avoid drug toxicity. This is particularly important with regard to corticosteroids, which should be avoided in children, as growth retardation may be an unfortunate consequence.

—*NSAIDs:* Aspirin (ASA) has historically been used to treat JA. Doses of 80 to 100 mg/kg/day are used to achieve serum levels between 18 and 25 mg/dL. Due to the risk for Reye's syndrome, ASA should not be used in children suspected of having influenza, varicella, or other active viral infections. ASA and NSAIDs do not alter the course of disease but are effective in ameliorating joint pain and stiffness. JA children may be at increased risk for salicylate hepatotoxicity. In recent years a variety of NSAIDs have gained popularity, and few are FDA approved for use in JA. Commonly used NSAIDs are dosed according to body mass and include ibuprofen (30–50 mg/kg/day) q.i.d., tolmetin (15–30 mg/kg/day) q.i.d., naproxen (10–20 mg/kg/day) b.i.d., and indomethacin (1–3 mg/kg/day) t.i.d. These agents are dosed on the basis of body mass. Less than 50% of patients respond to NSAIDs alone. Multiple NSAIDs should not be used contemporaneously, as this increases the risk of serious GI toxicity.

—*DMARDs (disease modifying antirheumatic drugs):* Methotrexate (10–15 mg/m^2/week) or intramuscular gold (5 mg test dose, then 0.75–1.0 mg/kg/week) is most commonly used in the treatment of chronic poly- or pauciarticular JA unresponsive to NSAID therapy and other conservative measures. Alternative DMARDs include hydroxychloroquine (5–7 mg/kg/day), D-penicillamine (5–10 mg/kg/day), auranofin (0.1 mg/kg/day), sulfasalazine (30–50 mg/kg/day), and cyclosporine. Patients with intractable systemic-onset arthritis (i.e., fever, rash, etc.) may benefit from chronic methotrexate therapy. Alternatively, patients may receive hydroxychloroquine, azathioprine, or cyclosporine to control their systemic manifestations.

—*Corticosteroids:* Systemic steroids should be avoided unless absolutely indicated. Prednisone doses of 5 mg/day or more may result in growth retardation. Corticosteroid therapy should be reserved for intractable systemic disease, life-threatening pericarditis or pericardial tamponade, and visual compromise due to iridocyclitis. Patients with refractory monarthritis or new joint contracture due to synovitis may benefit from intraarticular corticosteroid injection(s).

—Eye Disease: Inflammatory uveitis may respond to topical corticosteroid eye drops and mydriatics. Systemic administration is seldom necessary. Secondary glaucoma may also require treatment.

REFERENCES

Emery HM, Bowyer LS, Sisung CE. Rehabilitation of the child with rheumatic disease. Pediatr Clin North Am 1995;42:1263–1283.

Giannini EH, Cawkwell GD. Drug treatment in children with juvenile rheumatoid arthritis. Past, present and future. Pediatr Clin North Am 1995;42:1099–1125.

Peterson LS, Mason T, Nelson AM, et al. Juvenile rheumatoid arthritis in Rochester, Minnesota 1960–1993. Is the epidemiology changing? Arthritis Rheum 1996;39:1385–1390.

Schaller JG. Juvenile rheumatoid arthritis. Pediatr Rev 1997;18:337–349.

KAWASAKI DISEASE

Synonym: Mucocutaneous lymph node syndrome

ICD9 Code: 446.1

Definition: Kawasaki disease is an acute febrile illness of children.

Etiology: While a variety of infectious organisms and other environmental agents have been proposed to be of etiologic relevance, none has been conclusively implicated. However, there is evidence of restricted clonality of T cells in patients with Kawasaki disease, strongly suggesting an immune response to an as yet unidentified antigen.

Demographics: Most affected patients are under 5 years old, with many cases arising in infancy. There is a slight (approximately 1.4:1) female preponderance. While considered an uncommon disease, it may constitute nearly 5% of inflammatory rheumatic diseases among children.

Cardinal Findings: Typically, Kawasaki disease presents acutely. After a few days of intermittent or consistent fever, affected patients usually develop conjunctival injection, erythema, and swelling of the lips and mucous membranes of the mouth, cervical lymphadenopathy, and rash. Skin lesions may occur on the trunk or limbs, where they are usually erythematous macules; they also may arise on the hands and feet, where they may be accompanied by diffuse swelling. The skin lesions may resolve with desquamation. The most feared sequela of Kawasaki disease is aneurysm of the coronary arteries. During the first few weeks of disease, aneurysms can be demonstrated by echocardiography in approximately 40% of patients. The prevalence of these lesions decreases to approximately 20% at 1 month, 10% at 2 months, and 5% at 1 year. Aneurysms of more than 8-mm diameter are less likely to regress than smaller lesions. Potential sequelae of coronary arterial involvement with Kawasaki disease include rupture and myocardial infarction, which largely account for the observed mortality rate of approximately 0.1%.

Diagnostic Testing: Common abnormalities include leukocytosis, thrombocytosis, elevated transaminases, C-reactive protein and ESR. EKG abnormalities are common.

Diagnostic Criteria: Diagnostic features include (*a*) fever for 5 days or longer; (*b*) erythema of the palms or soles with edema or desquamation in the convalescent stage; (*c*) polymorphous truncal rash; (*d*) bilateral conjunctival injection; (*e*) erythema of lips, strawberry tongue, or oral mucosa injection; and (*f*) acute nonpurulent cervical lymphadenopathy. A diagnosis of Kawasaki disease requires that five of the six criteria be fulfilled or that four criteria be present with evidence of coronary aneurysm by echocardiogram or angiography.

Therapy: Treatment is directed primarily at preventing development or progression of coronary aneurysms. The current standard therapy consists of high-dose intravenous gamma globulin (2 g/kg IgG; administered as either a single dose or in split doses, e.g., 400 mg/kg × 5 days) in conjunction with aspirin (30–100 mg/kg/day). Aspirin may be continued in patients with persistent aneurysms until the lesions resolve.

REFERENCES

Kato H, Ichinose E, Kawasaki T. Myocardial infarction in Kawasaki disease: clinical analysis in 195 cases. J Pediatr 1986;108:923–927.
Newburger JW, Takahashi M, Beiser AS, et al. A single intravenous infusion of gamma-globulin as compared with four infusions in the treatment of acute Kawasaki syndrome. N Engl J Med 1991;324:1633–1639.

LIVEDO RETICULARIS

ICD Code: 782.61

Definition: Livedo reticularis is a lacy erythematous to purplish discoloration of the skin overlying the trunk and extremities, exaggerated by cold exposure. It may be associated with connective tissue disorders, vasculitis, Raynaud's phenomenon, fibromyalgia, atheromatous disease, hyperviscosity syndrome, thrombotic conditions, and exposure to cold or heat.

Etiology: Livedo reticularis results from vasospasm or sluggish blood flow through the deep dermal arterioles. Thickening of the dermal capillary walls can ultimately result in ischemia or infarction of affected tissues.

Demographics: Livedo is common (and usually not associated with disease) in infants and fair-skinned children, especially at times of cold exposure. Livedo reticularis is sensitive but not specific for connective tissue disorders. When it occurs in SLE or Raynaud's phenomenon it is highly correlated with antiphospholipid antibodies. Sneddon syndrome is the historical association of livedo reticularis, a false-positive VDRL (a type of antiphospholipid antibody), and stroke in young women.

Diagnostic Testing: Antiphospholipid antibodies or vasculitis autoantibodies (i.e., ANCA) may be sought if warranted by the overall clinical presentation.

Keys to Diagnosis: Cutaneous findings are characteristic. A careful history, physical examination, and selected laboratory evaluation may disclose evidence of underlying cause. In cutaneous polyarteritis nodosa, patchy livedo reticularis is associated with skin nodules.

Therapy: Therapy is directed toward any underlying illness. Few patients will require specific therapy for livedo reticularis.

REFERENCE

Picascia DD, Pellegrini JR. Livedo reticularis. Cutis 1987;39:429–432.

LYME DISEASE (LD)

ICD9 Code: 088.81

Definition: LD is a spirochetal tick-borne infection with acute and chronic sequelae capable of affecting the skin, heart, joints, and nervous system.

Etiology: The spirochete *Borrelia burgdorferi* causes LD and is transmitted by a variety of ticks. Transmission occurs after tick bites in about 10% of cases. *Ixodes* species of "deer ticks" facilitate transmission in the endemic areas of the northeastern United States (*Ixodes dammini* and *I. scapularis*) and in the pacific cost of the U.S. (*I. pacificus*). In the mid-Atlantic United States and Texas, the lone star tick (*Amblyomma americanum*), and in endemic areas of Europe, the sheep tick (*Ixodes ricinus*) are vectors. The white-footed mouse is an intermediate reservoir host for immature stages of the tick.

Pathology: There is evidence that both persisting infection and parainfectious (reactive) etiologies contribute to the pathogenesis of LD. Perhaps secondary to molecular mimicry, persistence of the spirochete in tissues (CNS) leads to an intense inflammatory reaction. Patients with HLA-DR4 and -DR2 are at higher risk than others to develop a chronic, erosive arthropathy mimicking seronegative rheumatoid arthritis. *B. burgdorferi* has been isolated by polymerase chain reaction from synovial fluid in untreated or partially treated disease. However, it is unclear whether chronic arthritis is due to persistent infection or a reactive immunologic mechanism.

Demographics: In the United States, most LD cases have been reported in the northeast and around the Great Lakes (particularly in northern Wisconsin and Minnesota). LD is seasonal and determined by the feeding patterns of the tick nymphs, which are most active in the late spring and early summer. LD is distributed worldwide, with cases reported in Europe, China, Australia, Russia, and Sweden.

Cardinal Findings: Three stages of LD have been described (Fig. 1). However, many patients do not follow an orderly progression of disease manifesta-

Clinical Features of Lyme Disease

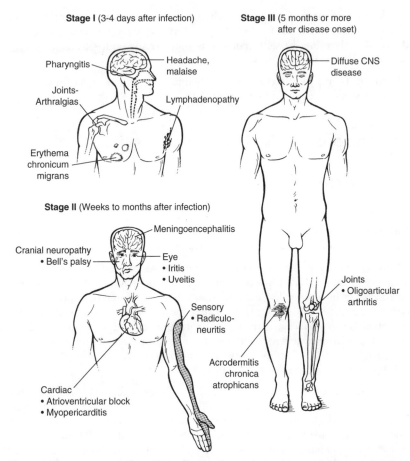

Figure 1. The protean manifestations of Lyme disease (symptoms and signs are sketched in appropriate locations based on early and later LD manifestations).

tions. Some patients may have overlapping features or skip stages entirely. The stages of LD serve only as a guideline to approximate a time course for the most common clinical symptoms.

—*Stage 1 (3 days–4 weeks postinfection):* Constitutional symptoms of malaise, fatigue, and fever predominate. The hallmark manifestation of early LD is the rash of erythema chronicum migrans (ECM). ECM commonly occurs on an extremity or near an intertriginous zone (thigh, groin, axilla) at the site of the tick bite. ECM has a central zone of partial clearing surrounded by an annular area of erythema with an expanding margin that can enlarge up to 20 cm. Lesions may last up to a month and can be asymptomatic, be painful, or occasionally be indurated. Secondary annular skin lesions may also develop in other locations. Diffuse arthralgias or myalgias are early musculoskeletal manifestations. Other nonspecific early symptoms may include headache, pharyngitis, conjunctivitis, regional lymphadenopathy, and testicular swelling.

—*Stage 2 (weeks to months postinfection):* Approximately 8% of people develop cardiac sequelae including atrioventricular heart block (first degree, Wenckebach, or complete), myopericarditis, and rarely cardiomyopathy. Neurologic features occur in 15% of patients and include meningoencephalitis, cranial neuropathies (in particular, Bell's palsy), and radiculoneuritis. Migratory myalgias, arthralgias, and bone or tendon pain may also be detected. Anterior and posterior uveitis, and panophthalmitis have been rarely reported.

—*Stage 3 (>5 months postonset):* In the United States, episodic oligoarticular arthritis predominantly of the lower extremities is the most common late LD manifestation, occurring in 50 to 70% of patients. Knees frequently have large effusions and occasional popliteal cysts. Chronic neurologic sequelae may result in diffuse CNS symptoms that resemble organic brain syndromes. Demyelinating encephalopathy and chronic radiculoneuropathy are other late neurologic complications. Acrodermatitis chronica atrophicans (a sclerotic or atrophic skin change resembling morphea) is a late cutaneous manifestation seen in Europe but rarely in the United States.

Diagnostic Testing: Serologic studies for Lyme disease have been fraught with considerable difficulties and should only be done when LD is strongly suspected. Serologic diagnosis is suspected with a rise in IgG antibodies against *B. burgdorferi* and/or a specific IgM. Serologic increases do not begin until 2 to 4 weeks after infection. ELISA is the current standard for LD serology, with most confirmatory tests performed by Western blot. Significant intra- and interlaboratory variation in serologic assays coupled with substantial false-positive and false-negative results hinder interpretation of this test. Early antibiotics may abort or curtail antibody production. Additionally, significant cross-reactivity exists with *Treponema pallidum* and other spirochetes. In early LD, microscopic hematuria/proteinuria and elevated liver enzymes may be detected in addition to nonspecific indicators of acute inflammation such as an increased ESR and mild anemia. Inflammatory synovial fluid with an average of 25,000 WBCs/mm^3 (mostly neutrophils) is commonly seen. In the setting of CNS LD, lymphocytic pleocytosis and mildly elevated CSF protein are commonly noted. *B. burgdorferi* antibodies may be greater in the CSF than serum in patients with neuroborreliosis. Skin biopsy of the leading edge of ECM uncommonly reveals spirochetes.

Keys to Diagnosis: The characteristic ECM rash (antedated by a tick bite) is most helpful diagnostically. Unfortunately, only 50% of afflicted individuals recall a tick bite, and ECM may be missed or not occur at all. LD is a clinical diagnosis with laboratory confirmation.

Differential Diagnosis: Early LD should be distinguished from other causes of febrile arthritis syndromes with rash, including viral arthritis, acute rheumatic fever, SLE, and adult-onset Still's disease. The LD rash may be mistaken for erythema multiforme. Later stages of LD may be confused with other causes of oligoarticular arthritis such as the seronegative spondyloarthropathies. The migratory nature of LD arthritis and involvement of tendons also may suggest gonococcal arthritis. Polyarthritis may be confused with RA. In the northeast, ehrlichiosis and babesiosis may be coinfections with overlapping clinical manifestations. Severe chronic fatigue and myalgias are occasionally consistent with fibromyalgia rather than chronic LD.

Therapy: Primary prevention of tick bites includes appropriate protective clothing, use of insecticides, and prompt tick removal. The value of preventive antibiotics following a tick bite in an endemic area versus removal of the tick followed by cautious surveillance is controversial. Preventive antibiotic therapy may be cost effective if the risk of LD is greater than 1% after tick bite. Therapeutic recommendations based on the stage of LD and particular disease manifestations are shown in Table 1. Early manifestations without cardiac or neurologic symptoms may be appropriately managed with oral agents such as

Table 1
Treatment of Lyme Disease

Disease Manifestations	Therapeutic Intervention
Early disease (stage I)	
Erythema chronicum migrans	Oral antibiotics for 3 weeks (except as noted)
	Doxycycline 100 mg p.o. b.i.d.[a] OR
	Amoxicillin 500 mg p.o. t.i.d. OR
	Cefuroxime axetil 500 mg b.i.d. OR
	Clarithromycin 500 mg b.i.d.[b] OR
	Azithromycin 500 mg/day for 1 week[b]
Carditis (stage 2)	
Mild (PR interval ≤ 0.30 sec)	Doxycycline 100 mg p.o. b.i.d. for 3 weeks OR
	Amoxicillin 500 mg p.o. t.i.d. for 3 weeks
Moderate or severe	Intravenous therapy for 2 weeks
	Ceftriaxone 2.0 g i.v. q.d. OR
	Cefotaxime 2.0 g q. 4 h i.v. OR
	Pen G 24 million units q.d. i.v.
Isolated Bell's palsy (stage 2)	If lumbar puncture negative consider oral regimens (as above)
Meningitis (stage 2)	Ceftriaxone 2.0 g i.v. q.d. for 3 weeks OR
	Pen G 24 million units q.d. i.v.
Arthritis (stage 3)	Doxycycline 100 mg p.o. b.i.d. for 4 weeks OR
	Amoxicillin with probenecid, both at 500 mg p.o. q.i.d. for 4 weeks OR
	Ceftriaxone 2.0 g i.v. q.d. × 2 weeks

[a]Avoid in pregnant women and in children.
[b]Azithromycin or clarithromycin are not FDA approved for use in Lyme disease.

doxycycline. Mild cardiac disease, limited neurologic involvement (Bell's palsy), and early arthritis may be effectively managed with oral antibiotic therapy. Significant joint, heart, or neurologic involvement requires intravenous therapy, most commonly with ceftriaxone. Significant arthropathy may also respond to intraarticular therapy with corticosteroids and rarely synovectomy. Transient use of cardiac pacing is indicated for symptomatic heart block. A clinical conundrum exists when patients, particularly those who have already received appropriate LD antibiotic therapy, experience chronic arthralgias and fatigue. Intravenous antibiotics are not cost effective in patients with positive serology whose only manifestations are myalgias and fatigue. Work on vaccine strategies is under way. In addition, there appears to be no value to prophylactic antibiotics for asymptomatic individuals, even in endemic areas.

Prognosis: With appropriate antibiotic therapy within 4 weeks of disease onset, LD is a potentially curable infectious illness that may not result in chronic complications. Delayed recognition and therapeutic failure can result in persisting constitutional symptoms, arthralgias, and neurologic complications in up to 34% of cases. An increasing number of late neurologic complications of LD have been reported. More-sustained musculoskeletal impairment and a higher prevalence of verbal memory loss have been associated with late disease. Active persistent infection, particularly after appropriate antibiotic therapy, is an unlikely explanation for these findings. Careful clinical evaluation of these patients shows a high proportion with fibromyalgia or a poorly characterized chronic pain syndrome.

REFERENCES

Lightfoot RW, Luft BJ, Rahn DW, et al. Empiric parenteral antibiotic treatment of patients with fibromyalgia and fatigue and a positive serologic result for Lyme disease: a cost effectiveness analysis. Ann Intern Med 1993;119:503–509.

Shadick NA, Phillips CB, Logigian EL, et al. The long-term clinical outcomes of Lyme disease: a population-based retrospective cohort study. Ann Intern Med 1994;121:560–567.

Sigal LH. Persisting complaints attributed to chronic Lyme disease: possible mechanisms and implications for management. Am J Med 1994;96:365–374.

Steere AC, Levin RE, Molloy PJ, et al. Treatment of Lyme disease. Arthritis Rheum 1994;37: 878–888.

MILWAUKEE SHOULDER SYNDROME

ICD9 Code: 712.0

Definition: Milwaukee shoulder syndrome is an apatite-associated large-joint destructive arthropathy.

Etiology: Milwaukee shoulder syndrome is caused by basic calcium phosphate (apatite or hydroxyapatite) crystal deposition. Predisposing factors include joint instability, trauma, overuse, disorders causing neuropathic joints, and chronic renal failure. It is idiopathic in one-third.

Pathology: Apatite crystal deposition may be seen in association with calcific tendinitis or bursitis, acute synovitis, or osteoarthritis or lead to a destructive arthropathy (Milwaukee shoulder syndrome). Crystal deposition may result in synovial cell activation and release of collagenase and neutral proteinase that can induce rapid chondrolysis. This may lead to extensive joint destruction and damage to periarticular structures (e.g., lysis of the rotator cuff and intrasynovial portion of the long head of the biceps).

Demographics: It is predominantly seen in elderly women; mean age is 72 years (range, 50–90); the female:male ratio is 4.5:1.

Cardinal Findings: Onset is usually slow. Shoulder involvement is most typical, often with a large cool effusion. The dominant shoulder is most commonly affected, but it is often bilateral. Pain is variable and often worse at night. Joint effusion, swelling, stiffness, and loss of function are common. Symptomatic knee involvement occurs in 40%, usually affecting the lateral compartment. Finger, wrist, and hip involvement may occur.

Diagnostic Tests: Synovial fluid analysis usually yields a low leukocyte count and may be hemorrhagic. Basic calcium phosphate (apatite) crystals (see p. 89) are generally not identifiable by light microscopy. Their presence is suggested by the clinical picture and may be confirmed with alizarin red S staining for calcium in synovial fluid spun sediments.

Imaging: Radiographically, there is severe joint destruction, especially on both sides of the glenohumeral joint. Other findings include upward subluxation of the humeral head or soft tissue calcification.

Keys to Diagnosis: Look for an elderly female with unilateral dominant shoulder pain, swelling, and loss of function; bloody synovial fluid with apatite crystals; and radiologic joint destruction.

Therapy: Use repeated joint aspiration and NSAIDs. Some patients need surgical arthroplasty to relieve pain and restore function.

REFERENCES

Halverson PB, McCarty DJ. Basic calcium phosphate (apatite, octacalcium phosphate, tricalcium phosphate) crystal deposition diseases; calcinosis: Milwaukee shoulder/knee syndrome. In: Koopman WJ, ed. Arthritis and allied conditions: a textbook of rheumatology. 13th ed. Baltimore: Williams & Wilkins, 1997:2131–2137.

MIXED CONNECTIVE TISSUE DISEASE

Synonyms: MCTD, undifferentiated connective tissue disease (UCTD), or overlap syndrome

ICD9 Code: 710.8

Definition: As initially described, MCTD is defined as having (*a*) a combination or overlap of clinical symptoms that are characteristic of systemic sclerosis, systemic lupus erythematosus (SLE), and inflammatory myositis (i.e., dermatomyositis or polymyositis) and (*b*) high titers of serum antibodies that react with nuclear ribonuclear proteins (nRNP, or U1-RNP). While MCTD was originally considered a unique disease state, that concept has come under question. Although such patients may have similar symptoms early in their disease, when followed over time MCTD patients evolve into a single identifiable rheumatic condition, most commonly scleroderma. Thus, the reason for designating these patients as undifferentiated, or UCTD. In addition, MCTD patients do not seem to have a unique prognosis or disease course, and antibodies to RNP are not unique to MCTD; they are detectable in more than half of SLE patients as well as in those with other autoimmune diseases. Few MCTD patients will meet ACR criteria for more than one disorder.

Cardinal Findings: Probably more useful than the concept of a single MCTD is the appreciation that many patients have an overlap of signs and symptoms resembling several rheumatic diseases. Overlapping symptoms common to classically described MCTD and several rheumatic diseases include arthritis, dactylitis ("sausage digits"), Raynaud's phenomenon, sclerodactyly, dysphagia, inflammatory myositis, pleuritis/pericarditis, and interstitial lung disease.

Diagnostic Tests: Although such patients are uniformly positive for antinuclear antibodies and often have very high titers of U1-RNP antibodies, neither is specific for MCTD or other connective tissue diseases. Complement levels are normal, and no antibodies to native, double-stranded DNA are detected. Blood counts may reveal leukopenia or thrombocytopenia.

Keys to Diagnosis: Overlap in symptoms among the various rheumatologic conditions may lead to diagnostic uncertainty, particularly early in the disease course. It has been estimated that a third of patients initially presenting with clear rheumatologic complaints cannot be diagnosed with a definitive rheumatologic disease. Such patients may initially be designated as having UCTD (term preferred to MCTD). Careful observation over time usually discloses whether the dominant disorder is scleroderma, SLE, or an inflammatory myopathy.

Therapy: Patients with an undifferentiated disease should be treated according to the symptoms or features present. Thus many patients may be managed with NSAIDs or analgesic agents for their musculoskeletal complaints. In some, therapy is guided by more serious end-organ involvement. For example, patients with severe myositis may require high-dose corticosteroids, whereas those with chronic polyarticular synovitis may be treated according to a paradigm similar to that used for RA.

REFERENCES

Sharp GC, Irwin WS, Tan EM, et al. Mixed connective tissue disease—an apparently distinct rheumatic disease syndrome associated with a specific antibody to extractable nuclear antigen (ENA). Am J Med 1972;52:148–159.

MULTICENTRIC RETICULOHISTIOCYTOSIS

Synonyms: Lipoid dermatoarthritis, normocholesterolemic xanthomatosis
ICD9 Code: 272.8

Definition: Multicentric reticulohistiocytosis (MRH) is a rare disorder characterized by infiltration of lipid-laden histiocytes into various tissues. The typical clinical picture includes skin nodules and a chronic destructive polyarthritis.

Etiology: Although the cause is unknown, infectious agents such as mycobacteria have been suspected as an etiologic agent; none has been conclusively implicated. There are no known genetic associations.

Pathology: MRH is characterized by accumulation of histiocytes and multinucleated giant cells at affected sites.

Demographics: MRH is a rare disorder. While it has been reported in childhood, middle-aged women appear to be affected predominantly.

Cardinal Findings: Because it often presents with a chronic, symmetric, polyarthritis affecting the PIP or DIP joints of the hands, MRH may mimic rheumatoid arthritis (RA) and be associated with joint destruction, particularly of the DIPs. Other joints less commonly involved include the shoulders, knees, wrists, and hips. The skin lesions associated with this disorder include nodules on the hands and elbows that resemble rheumatoid nodules. Nodules may also occur on the ears, chest, face, and mucosal surfaces (e.g., lips, tongue, gingiva). Other skin lesions seen in MRH (but not typical of RA) include small papules that occur in beadlike clusters about the nailfolds, and xanthelasma.

Complications: A minority of patients may be tuberculin positive or have an associated malignancy.

Diagnostic Tests: Less than one-third of patients have an elevated ESR or hypercholesterolemia. Patients are seronegative for RF and ANA. Synovial fluid findings are variable and may reveal inflammatory or noninflammatory fluid.

Keys to Diagnosis: The diagnosis of MRH is made by biopsy of affected synovium or skin lesions. Multinucleated giant cells in these lesions characteristically contain large amounts of PAS (periodic acid-Schiff) staining material, indicating lipid accumulation. There are no diagnostic laboratory tests. X-Rays may reveal destruction of affected joints but are not specific for the disease. In addition to RA, other chronic inflammatory polyarthritides such as psoriatic arthritis should be included in the differential diagnosis of this disorder.

Therapy: Therapeutic agents that have been used for this disorder include corticosteroids and cytotoxic drugs such as cyclophosphamide. The small number of affected patients precludes large therapeutic trials. While spontaneous remission has been reported, particularly among children, most patients suffer a progressive course.

REFERENCE

Krey PR, Comeford FR, Cohen AS. Multicentric reticulohistiocytosis: fine structural analysis of the synovium and synovial fluid cells. Arthritis Rheum 1977;17:615–633.

MULTIPLE SCLEROSIS (MS)

ICD9 Code: 340.0

Definition: MS is a immunologically mediated disease characterized by demyelination within the central nervous system (CNS). The typical clinical presentation is neurologic events separated in time (recurrent or relapsing) and space (arising from distinct parts of the brain, brainstem, and spinal cord).

Demographics: MS occurs predominantly among Caucasians of northern European descent. The prevalence of MS varies dramatically with longitude. MS occurs in approximately 20/100,000 persons living in the southern United States and increases as one moves north; the prevalence exceeds 125/100,000 Canadians. While there is a small genetic predisposition to MS (monozygotic twins have a concordance of approximately 25%), environmental exposure to an unidentified antigen at a young age appears to be important. The peak age of onset of MS is 20 to 40 years. Women are affected twice as often as men.

Cardinal Findings: The characteristic clinical presentation of MS is neurologic defects separated in space and time. Most defects arise acutely, with 75% occurring within a few days. Typically, the defects persist for 6 to 8 weeks, and many resolve spontaneously. In most patients, this is followed by a recurrence of neurologic defects. The most common presenting symptoms include weakness in one or more limbs (50%), numbness in the limbs (45%), optic neuritis (20%), unsteady gait or ataxia (15%), and diplopia (10%). A useful clinical clue to the diagnosis of MS is that the symptoms reflect involvement of the white matter of the CNS. Thus, symptoms seen primarily with gray matter damage in the CNS (e.g., loss of consciousness, seizures, syncope, dementia, muscle atrophy, and pain) are uncommon. Physical examination may reveal evidence of optic (e.g., internuclear ophthalmoplegia) or spinal cord involvement (e.g., a positive Babinski reflex, dysfunctional sphincter).

Diagnostic Tests: Standard laboratory and serologic tests are of little value. CSF studies (see p. 98) may reveal normal cell counts or show a mild mononuclear pleocytosis, mildly increased CSF protein, increased CSF IgG index or synthetic rate (90%), or evidence of CSF oligoclonal bands or myelin basic protein (>85%). In addition, visual evoked potentials or brainstem evoked potentials may help confirm the diagnosis of MS.

Imaging: The diagnosis of MS may be supported by imaging studies. Perhaps the most important advance has been the availability of MRI. Areas of demyelination, or "plaques," are readily revealed by MRI. However, some patients (e.g., those with predominant spinal cord involvement) may have entirely normal scans. While consistent with MS, white matter lesions on MRI may also be seen in other conditions, including hypertensive vasculopathy, SLE with CNS involvement, and various infections (Lyme disease, HIV, HTLV-1, etc).

Therapy: Conservative measures should include evaluation by physical and occupational therapy. Because it has been recognized as an immunologically mediated disorder, treatment of MS has long included such immunomodula-tory agents as corticosteroids (for acute attacks) and chemotherapeutic drugs such as azathioprine, cyclosporine, and cyclophosphamide. More recently, in-terferon-β_{1b} has been approved for use in some MS patients.

REFERENCES

Rolak LA. The diagnosis of multiple sclerosis. Neurol Clin 1996;14:27–43.

MYASTHENIA GRAVIS

ICD9 Code: 358.0

Definition: Myasthenia gravis (MG) is an autoimmune disorder of the neuro-muscular junction. It is characterized clinically by muscle weakness and im-munologically by autoantibodies directed against the postsynaptic acetyl-choline (ACh) receptor. These autoantibodies are pathogenic, causing increased turnover and decreased surface expression of the ACh receptor, which results in decreased muscle depolarization and weakness.

Etiology: While most cases of MG are idiopathic, some patients have associ-ated thymomas or thymic hyperplasia. MG may also occur as a rare reaction to D-penicillamine therapy.

Demographics: MG is rare, with a prevalence of approximately 14/100,000, and has a bimodal distribution. There is a slight female predominance among patients with disease onset in the second and third decades, and a male pre-dominance among patients over 50 years old. There is a genetic predisposition, partly related to expression of the HLA-B8 and DR3 alleles.

Associated Conditions: Many MG patients, particularly those with younger onset of disease, have associated thymomas (10% of patients) or thymic hyper-plasia (70%). MG is also associated with other autoimmune diseases, including thyroid disease (15% of patients), rheumatoid arthritis (4%), and SLE (2%).

Cardinal Findings: The characteristic clinical picture of MG is muscle weak-ness that worsens with repetitive use and improves with rest. Ocular muscle in-volvement is most common, and 2/3 of patients present with symptoms such as ptosis and diplopia. Symptoms typically worsen after strain and at the end of the day. About 15% of patients have MG that remains limited to the ocular muscles. For the remainder, the disease progresses to involve the oropharyn-geal (i.e., dysphagia, dysphonia, dysarthria) and limb muscles. When it affects the respiratory muscles, MG can be fatal. For about 2/3 of patients, maximum muscle weakness occurs in the first year of disease. Exacerbations may be asso-ciated with various factors such as emotional stress, infection, and thyroid dis-ease. In addition, medications that affect neuromuscular transmission (e.g., aminoglycoside antibiotics, neuromuscular blockers, class I antiarrhythmics) may also exacerbate MG.

Diagnostic Tests: The diagnosis of MG may be accomplished by several means. Pharmacologic testing or the "Tensilon test" uses a short-acting acetylcholinesterase inhibitor (e.g., edrophonium) and may reveal dramatic improvement in muscle strength. Pharmacologic testing may be falsely negative in some MG patients, particularly children.

Increased serum concentrations of antibodies directed against the ACh receptor are seen in approximately 65% of patients with MG limited to ocular musculature and 85% of patients with more generalized MG. Anti–ACh receptor antibody tests are available from reference laboratories. The presence of anti-ACh receptor antibodies is relatively specific, although false-positive results may be seen in patients with SLE and among healthy relatives of MG patients.

Finally, electrophysiologic studies may aid diagnosis of MG by demonstrating characteristic abnormalities (e.g., decremental responses on repeated muscle stimulation).

Differential Diagnosis: MG may be mistaken for Eaton-Lambert syndrome (commonly a paraneoplastic syndrome that affects the presynaptic segment of the neuromuscular junction), inflammatory myositis (i.e., polymyositis, dermatomyositis, and inclusion body myositis), other myopathies, multiple sclerosis, and chronic fatigue syndrome.

Therapy: MG therapy must be individualized. Long-acting anticholinesterase drugs (e.g., pyridostigmine) are the mainstay of therapy for most patients. Thymectomy is indicated in many patients with MG, particularly those with thymoma. Thymectomy may not be advisable for those for whom the risks of surgery may outweigh the potential benefit, including the elderly and those with purely ocular muscle involvement. Various immunomodulatory agents also have a role as therapeutic agents for MG patients. Corticosteroids, often used initially at high doses (e.g., 1 mg/kg), achieve a response in about 75% of patients. Other immunomodulatory therapies that have been used include intravenous gamma globulin, plasma exchange, azathioprine, cyclosporine, and cyclophosphamide.

REFERENCES

Drachman DB. Myasthenia gravis. N Engl J Med 1994;330:1797–1803.
Finley JC, Pascuzzi RM. Rational therapy of myasthenia gravis. Semin Neurol 1990;10:70–85.

MYOPATHY

Synonyms: Metabolic diseases of muscle, metabolic myopathies

ICD9 Codes: Myopathy, 359.9; alcoholic, 359.4; amyloid, 277.3; toxic, 359.4

Definition: Myopathy is a generalized term applied to a heterogeneous group of disorders that affect muscle. Inflammatory muscle disease is considered elsewhere (see p. 301). The differential diagnosis of weakness and myopathy is expansive (see pp. 57, 306). The metabolic myopathies include a variety of muscle disorders caused by alterations in biochemical pathways involving lipids, glycogen, or high-energy phosphate compounds.

Etiology: Most of these disorders have a genetic basis and show an autosomal recessive pattern of inheritance.

Hypokalemic periodic paralysis is an autosomal dominant disorder.

Mitochondrial myopathies show a maternal pattern of transmission, since all mitochondrial DNA is derived from the mother.

A small number of cases are acquired and are attributable to other underlying disorders such as cirrhosis, renal failure, or other causes of metabolic derangements.

Pathology: Light microscopic examination of the muscle biopsy specimen may demonstrate lipid deposition (shown on oil red O stain) in lipid storage myopathies. Mitochondrial abnormalities may also be seen on routine microscopic examination, and the presence of irregular, "ragged-red" fibers suggests a mitochondrial disorder. On electron microscopic examination, increased collagen deposition may be observed in patients with glycogen storage diseases. However, biopsy specimens from some patients may appear normal on microscopic examination.

Demographics: Most primary inherited cases become apparent by early adulthood, but patients presenting as old as 70 years have been reported.

Cardinal Findings: Most patients show muscle weakness. Some are able to perform normal daily activities without problems but become symptomatic at higher levels of exercise.

—*McArdle's disease:* Caused by a myophosphorylase deficiency. McArdle's disease manifests as exercise-induced muscle pain, fatigue, cramps, weakness, or myoglobinuria. Symptoms begin between 10 and 30 years of age. Muscle enzymes may be elevated at rest or only with exercise. Diagnosis is suggested by the forearm ischemic exercise test.

—*Tarui's disease:* Caused by a phosphofructokinase deficiency, Tarui's disease has features similar to those of McArdle's disease, but can also cause hemolytic anemia. Most patients are diagnosed as adults.

—*Acid maltase deficiency:* An autosomal recessive disease, acid maltase deficiency may manifest as Pompe's disease with infantile weakness, hypotonia, heart failure, and early death. Another variety begins in early childhood with proximal and respiratory muscle weakness. An adult subset may begin in the 3rd or 4th decade, with muscle weakness and a pattern indistinguishable from polymyositis. Acid maltase deficiency causes a vacuolar myopathy, and biochemical studies are necessary to prove the diagnosis.

—*Carnitine deficiency:* Deficient transfer of long-chain free fatty acids to the mitochondria results from carnitine deficiency. Muscle weakness begins in childhood and may be associated with myalgias, myoglobinuria, cardiomyopathy, increased CPK, and increased lipid in muscle.

—*Carnitine palmityltransferase deficiency:* An autosomal recessive disorder, carnitine palmityltransferase deficiency typically affects males, with myalgias, cramps, stiffness, and myoglobinuria. Attacks are triggered by exercise or fasting. CPK and ischemic exercise tests are usually normal. Diagnosis is based on biochemical analysis of enzyme activity in muscle. Some of these patients develop rhabdomyolysis and renal failure, which is reversible if appropriately treated.

—*Mitochondrial myopathies:* Mitochondrial myopathies include a variety of disorders that result in alterations of mitochondria structure, number, or size. These may arise in children as limb myopathy, with or without ophthalmoplegia. Patients exhibit exercise intolerance, proximal or extraocular muscle weakness, hypermetabolism, salt craving, or peripheral neuropathy. Mitochondrial myopathies may arise in the adult as exercise intolerance, generalized or proximal weakness, and normal or elevated CPK levels.

Diagnostic Tests: Serum potassium, magnesium, and creatine kinase should be measured. Some, but not all, metabolic myopathies are associated with elevated CPK levels; normal values do not exclude these disorders. Defects in the glycogenolytic pathway such as myophosphorylase deficiency may be detected with the forearm ischemic exercise test (absence of the normal increase in postexercise serum lactate levels is diagnostic). Myoglobin should be measured in urine if rhabdomyolysis is a possibility.

Biopsy: A muscle biopsy may be required to establish the diagnosis. Some metabolic syndromes are associated with elevated levels of muscle enzymes, but many do not show any abnormality or have findings only during episodes of rhabdomyolysis; in these cases, measurement of enzymatic activities in the biopsy specimen is usually required. Special handling of tissues is necessary to achieve accurate enzymatic determinations, and consultation with the pathology laboratory that will perform the analysis is essential to ensure that the specimen is collected correctly. The amount of tissue required for enzymatic analysis necessitates an open, rather than a needle, biopsy.

Keys to Diagnosis: Muscle biopsy and measurement of muscle enzyme levels are usually required to establish the diagnosis in a patient with episodic or exercise-induced weakness or rhabdomyolysis. Secondary cases might be detected by routine blood and urine testing for metabolic imbalances.

Therapy: Specific treatments are not always required. However, since the patient may be advised to modify diet and exercise to minimize problems, establishing the diagnosis is very important. For example, patients with carnitine palmityltransferase deficiency should be advised to avoid fasting and strenuous exercise; carbohydrate loading prior to moderate exercise may be useful. Carnitine deficiency may be treated by dietary supplements (carnitine up to 4 g/day), and anecdotal reports suggest the utility of L-carnitine, coenzyme Q_{10}, or menadione in patients with mitochondrial myopathies.

Acute rhabdomyolysis, which may occur in some of these syndromes, constitutes a medical emergency, requiring aggressive hydration and mannitol for urine dilution to avoid permanent renal damage.

Prognosis: Most patients can pursue normal daily activities and do not develop progressive problems. Precautions regarding diet and exercise are an important component of a successful outcome.

REFERENCES

Wortmann RL. Metabolic diseases of muscle. In: Koopman WJ, ed. Arthritis and allied conditions: a textbook of rheumatology. 13th ed. Baltimore: Williams & Wilkins, 1997:2169–2187.

NEUROPATHIC ARTHRITIS

Synonyms: Charcot arthritis

ICD9 Code: 713.5 (diabetic, 250.6; syphilitic, 094.0; syringomyelic, 336.0)

Definition: Neuropathic joint disease (Charcot arthritis) is a chronic, exaggerated form of degenerative arthritis caused by loss of proprioception to involved joints.

Etiology: Loss of proprioception leads to repetitive trauma to unprotected joints and subsequent osteoarthritic change. Alternatively, sympathetic neurovascular reflexes may lead to hyperemia and active bone resorption. Common causes include diabetic neuropathy, tabes dorsalis (syphilis), and syringomyelia. Other causes include calcium pyrophosphate deposition disease (CPPD), recurrent intraarticular steroids, alcoholic neuropathy, amyloidosis, congenital indifference to pain, meningomyelocele, yaws, and spinal dysraphism. Up to one-third of patients have no demonstrable neurologic disorder.

Pathology: Pathologic changes are similar to those of osteoarthritis. Pannus may be seen. There may be coincident and dramatic bony disintegration and new bone formation.

Demographics: Demography depends on the underlying condition. Neuroarthropathy occurs in 0.1 to 0.5% of diabetics, 4 to 10% of patients with tabes dorsalis, and over 30% of those with syringomyelia.

Cardinal Findings: Two modes of presentation have been described:
There may be a large joint effusion, synovitis, joint instability, dislocation, and bony fragments with marked crepitus. Progression is variable.

1. Acute neuropathic arthropathy (atrophic/resorptive form) is rare and manifests as acute-onset inflammatory monarthritis of non-weight-bearing joints, with associated swelling, warmth, and pain. It may be misdiagnosed as infectious or crystal-induced arthritis.
2. Chronic neuropathic arthropathy is the more commonly recognized form. There is often an insidious chronic history of joint problems, usu-

ally involving weight-bearing joints. Joints are typically swollen from effusion or exaggerated osteoarthritic changes. Joints are usually not painful and there is a loss of deep tendon reflexes.

Patterns of joint involvement differ according to etiology.

—*Diabetic neuroarthropathy:* The tarsometatarsal joint is commonly affected (less commonly, the ankle and MTP joint). Overlying soft tissue swelling and ulceration may be seen. The pain is often less than expected for the degree of deformity and osseous change.

—*Tabes dorsalis:* The knee and hip are most commonly affected, often with a genu varum deformity. A large unstable knee may be accompanied by an Argyll Robertson pupil or an absent knee jerk reflex. Axial disease has been described.

—*Syringomyelia:* This degenerative condition affects the spinal cord, resulting in weakness and atrophy of the upper extremities with loss of reflexes and thermal anesthesia. Neuroarthropathy may affect the shoulders, elbows, and cervical spine.

Complications: Spontaneous fractures, dislocation, and osteomyelitis may occur.

Diagnostic Tests: Laboratory tests reflect the underlying disorder. Synovial fluid is either noninflammatory or hemorrhagic. Inflammatory effusions are uncommon and should prompt a search for other causes (e.g., crystal arthritis).

Imaging: During the acute phase, changes are nonspecific and include soft tissue swelling. Early changes resemble osteoarthritis. Later, large osteophytes, new bone formation, bony fragmentation, dislocation, and subluxation may occur. Damage to periarticular structures may lead to malalignment and may contribute to subluxation and deformity. Bone scans show markedly abnormal uptake but are seldom required for diagnosis. Bone scan and MRI may be useful in diagnosing coexistent osteomyelitis or occult fracture.

Keys to Diagnosis: Diagnosis should be suspected in (*a*) diabetics with foot pain; (*b*) patients with exaggerated severe osteoarthritis of the knee; (*c*) spontaneous fracture after little or no trauma; and (*d*) severe scoliosis with destructive x-ray changes (search for syringomyelia or syphilis).

Therapy: The underlying disorder should be treated, which may prevent further damage. Weight reduction, immobilization, and use of orthotics may be helpful. Pain medication and NSAIDs are not required in most. Intraarticular steroids are contraindicated.

Surgery: Arthrodesis and joint replacement have a high failure rate and are generally contraindicated. Amputation may rarely be necessary for advanced disease complicated by infection.

REFERENCES

Ellman MH. Neuropathic joint disease (Charcot joints). In: Koopman WJ, ed. Arthritis and
    allied conditions: a textbook of rheumatology. 13th ed. Baltimore: Williams & Wilkins,
    1997:1641–1659.
Gupta R. A short history of neuropathic arthropathy. Clin Orthop Rel Res 1993;296:43–49.

NEUROPATHY

ICD9 Code: 356.9

Classification: Several patterns of peripheral neuropathy are relevant to
rheumatologic disorders: (*a*) mononeuropathy—involvement of one nerve; (*b*)
mononeuritis multiplex—sequential peripheral nerves are affected usually in
an asymmetric fashion; and (*c*) polyneuropathy—symmetric involvement of
multiple sensory and/or motor nerves.

Etiology: Rheumatologic diseases most commonly associated with peripheral
neuropathy include the vasculitides (particularly polyarteritis nodosa), cryoglobulinemia, rheumatoid arthritis, systemic lupus erythematosus, Sjögren's syndrome, and amyloidosis. Vasculitis leading to mononeuritis multiplex, for example, commonly results in a mixed sensorimotor axonal neuropathy. Lyme disease
may lead to a facial nerve (Bell's) palsy and, less commonly, a sensory radiculoneuritis. Peripheral neuropathy may also result from compression, trauma, or
injury of a nerve root as it emerges from the spinal cord (radiculopathy), in the
brachial plexus (plexopathy), or more distally (focal nerve entrapment) (Table 1).
Entrapment neuropathies are often due to noninflammatory mechanical trauma
but may also be due to abnormal nerve compression, such as median nerve
mononeuropathy (carpal tunnel syndrome) in a patient with wrist synovitis (e.g.,
RA) or progressive degenerative conditions (e.g., diabetes mellitus).

Table 1
Entrapment Neuropathies

Syndrome Name/Site	Nerve Involved	Common Noninflammatory Causes
Carpal tunnel	Median	Repetitive trauma, pregnancy, hypothyroidism, acromegaly
Cubital tunnel	Ulnar	Excessive leaning on elbows (i.e., patients with severe COPD)
Saturday night palsy	Radial	Postanesthesia, sleeping upon an improperly positioned arm while intoxicated
Meralgia paresthetica	Lateral cutaneous nerve of thigh	Obesity, pregnancy, rapid weight gain/loss, tight pants
Head of fibula	Common peroneal	Diabetes, habitual leg crossing
Tarsal tunnel	Posterior tibial	Severe foot deformity, trauma

Pathology: Mononeuritis multiplex results from vasculitis and vascular ischemia of the vessels supplying the nerve (vasa nervorum). In amyloidosis, polyneuropathy is believed to be due to amyloid deposition in or around nerves that alters nerve conduction. Sensory polyneuropathy sometimes seen in Sjögren's syndrome may be caused by small vessel vasculitis and dorsal root ganglionitis. Entrapment neuropathy results from nerve compression, leading first to sensory and then motor deficits.

Cardinal Findings: Painful burning dysesthesia and motor weakness are the hallmark symptoms of peripheral neuropathy. Muscle atrophy, paresthesia, and frank sensory deficits may follow. Foot drop (lower extremity symptoms occur more commonly than upper extremity ones) or wrist drop in a patient who is systemically ill with multiple organ disorder may indicate mononeuritis multiplex due to polyarteritis nodosa or another form of systemic vasculitis.

Diagnostic Testing: Electrodiagnostic evaluation by electromyography (EMG) (see p. 112) and sensory/motor nerve conduction studies (see p. 131) helps pinpoint the areas affected and may elucidate the specific type of abnormality. In peripheral neuropathy, EMGs usually show fibrillation potentials and positive sharp wave due to muscle denervation. Nerve conduction studies show reduced amplitudes with relatively normal sensory and motor conduction velocity. In mononeuritis multiplex, biopsy of the sural nerve is often performed to look for evidence of vasculitis in the vasa nervorum. The nerve itself may show axonal degeneration and, occasionally, patchy demyelination. Other laboratory studies potentially helpful in confirming the cause of an underlying inflammatory disorder should be dictated by the history and physical examination. Useful studies may include CBC, serum creatinine, urinalysis, chest x-ray, ANA, rheumatoid factor, cryoglobulins, hepatitis serology, immunoelectrophoresis, or ANCA.

Keys to Diagnosis: A comprehensive neurologic examination with particular attention to the sensory components of the examination is essential. Diminished vibratory and position sense are sensitive indicators of early peripheral neuropathy.

Therapy: If the neuropathy is due to an active inflammatory process (e.g., a vasculitis), then systemic corticosteroids alone or in combination with immunosuppressive agents are frequently indicated, with dosage dictated by the specific disorder and its severity. Compressive lesions such as carpal tunnel syndrome may respond well to local measures (e.g., splinting) or surgical release. Physical modalities and rehabilitative services, including appropriate use of splints, braces, and occupational and physical therapy, are frequently very appropriate. Infrequently, agents such as tricyclic antidepressants or carbamazepine are used to alleviate neuropathic pain.

Prognosis: The course and prognosis are highly influenced by the underlying pathologic mechanisms and systemic response to antiinflammatory therapy, if indicated.

REFERENCES

Alexander EL. Neurologic disease in Sjogren's syndrome: mononuclear inflammatory vasculopathy affecting central/peripheral nervous system and muscle. Rheum Dis Clin
North Am 1993:19:869–908.

Hadler NH. Nerve entrapment syndromes. In: Koopman WJ, ed. Arthritis and allied conditions: a textbook of rheumatology. 13th ed. Baltimore: Williams & Wilkins, 1997:1859–
1866.

Sigal LH. The neurologic presentation of vasculitic and rheumatologic syndromes. Medicine
(Baltimore) 1987;66:157–180.

Tervaert JWC, Kallenberg C. Neurologic manifestations of systemic vasculitides. Rheum Dis
Clin North Am 1993:19:913–940.

Nonarticular Disorders (Bursitis, Tendinitis, Enthesitis)

Synonyms: Soft tissue rheumatism; overuse syndrome; bursitis; tendinitis; enthesitis

ICD9 Codes: Bursitis 727.3; tendinitis 726.9; Achilles tendinitis 726.71; enthesitis 726.39

Definition: The term *nonarticular disorders* refers to pain and dysfunction attributed to structures that surround and support joints and by their proximity are often mistaken for arthritis. Pain originating in nonarticular structures is perhaps the
most frequent musculoskeletal complaint seen in general practice. Nonarticular
structures include the numerous bursae, tendons, and ligaments present throughout the body. In many cases, injury secondary to repetitive overuse or trauma may
cause inflammation and pain. However, some of these structures can become inflamed secondary to a systemic condition such as rheumatoid arthritis or gout.

—*Bursae:* Numerous bursae (>150) are present throughout the body. They
are typically located between muscles or between muscle and bone and contain scant amounts of synovial-like fluid. Their function is to allow smooth
gliding between adjacent surfaces and to provide some buffer against injury.
Inflammation of a bursa, or bursitis, usually results from trauma (particularly, repetitive trauma), overuse, or other types of direct injury. Bursitis may
also be associated with systemic diseases (e.g., gout, pseudogout, RA). An inflamed or injured bursa often enlarges with fluid and can become a source of
pain. Bursae can also become infected, usually with organisms (e.g., *Staphylococcus aureus*) introduced from overlying skin.

—*Tendons:* Tendons can be a source of pain typically related to such biomechanical causes as overuse or repetitive injury. As is true for bursae, when *tendinitis* is the origin of pain, tenderness can usually be elicited by palpation and
specific range-of-motion testing on physical examination. A number of tendons travel through a fibrous tube or sheath. Inflammation of the lining of this
sheath is known as tenosynovitis. Tenosynovitis may result from direct
trauma, repetitive-use injury, systemic inflammatory diseases, or infection.
Stenosis and/or inflammation of a tendon sheath may interfere with smooth

movement of the tendon. A "trigger finger" occurs when the flexor tendons of the hand cannot pass smoothly through the fibrous tunnels of the fingers and become caught. Other conditions of pain and entrapment related to tenosynovial involvement include de Quervain's tenosynovitis (p. 188), carpal tunnel syndrome (p. 177), and tarsal tunnel syndrome (p. 371). When tendon injury or inflammation becomes chronic, rupture of the tendon may result.

—*Ligaments:* Ligaments attach one bone to another and thereby provide structural integrity to the skeleton. Injury to ligaments usually results from excessive force being applied. Such "sprains" range in severity from mild partial tears to complete disruption of the ligament with resultant laxity.

—*Entheses:* The place where ligaments and tendons insert into bone (the enthesis) may also be the site of inflammation. *Enthesitis* may result from trauma, but may also be associated with systemic inflammatory diseases such as the seronegative spondyloarthropathies (e.g., ankylosing spondylitis).

Etiology: Most forms of nonarticular pain are caused by direct trauma, repetitive-use injury, systemic inflammatory diseases, or infection.

Demographics: Tendinitis, bursitis, and overuse syndromes are very common, affecting young, middle-aged, and older adults. Traumatic conditions are more common in young adults. Males are slightly more often affected than females. The prevalence of bursitis is estimated to be 2%.

Cardinal Findings: Often, a focused history and physical examination can readily pinpoint the specific cause of the patient's complaint. However, it may sometimes be difficult to differentiate these soft tissue syndromes from arthritis or other processes. Often tendinitis, bursitis, or enthesitis can be identified as producing "point tenderness" and may exhibit pain on active, but not passive, motion. Numerous examples of nonarticular pain are presented below.

—*Subacromial (subdeltoid) bursitis.* The subacromial bursa, the largest bursa in the body, lies between the deltoid muscle and the rotator cuff musculature of the shoulder (see shoulder pain, p. 22). It may become inflamed in association with rotator cuff dysfunction or independently. Diagnosis of subacromial bursitis is usually made by demonstration of tenderness on direct palpation (to find the bursa, "walk" the examining fingers along the spine of the scapula, where they will come to the edge of the acromion process; the bursa lies immediately below).

—*Bicipital tendinitis:* Bicipital tendinitis often presents with pain localized to the anterior aspect of the shoulder. Pain often derives from the proximal end of the long head of the biceps, which runs through a tendon sheath in the bicipital groove of the humerus at the shoulder (see p. 22). Direct palpation of an inflamed tendon often generates pain. Pain may also be elicited by forced supination and flexion of the forearm against resistance. Rupture of the tendon of the long head of the biceps results in appearance of a bulge in the upper arm.

—*Olecranon bursitis:* The olecranon bursa lies directly over the olecranon process at the elbow. Olecranon bursitis is a common condition, particularly among older persons. While it may be associated with conditions such as RA, gout, pseudogout, and infection with *S. aureus* (septic bursitis), most cases are idiopathic or result from minor repetitive trauma to the area. Tenderness on palpation and swelling due to effusion are the key findings on physical examination. A useful clue to help differentiate olecranon bursitis from elbow synovitis is that pain related to olecranon bursitis increases as the forearm is fully flexed against the upper arm (which stretches the bursa) and diminishes with the elbow in full extension. By contrast, with true elbow synovitis, patients often hold the elbow in the neutral position (i.e., about 30° of flexion); full flexion or full extension both increase pressure within the synovium and cause pain.

—*Tennis elbow:* Inflammation of the common tendon of the extensor muscles of the forearm as it inserts on the lateral epicondyle of the humerus is known as "tennis elbow." This form of lateral epicondylitis often results from overuse (e.g., repetitive pronating or supinating of the wrist, in extension, against force). Physical examination often revels tenderness over the lateral epicondyle.

— *Medial epicondylitis:* Sometimes referred to as golfer's elbow, medial epicondylitis is less common than lateral epicondylitis. Pain over the insertion of the common flexor tendon at the medial epicondyle is the key to diagnosis. In addition to these conditions, other causes of elbow pain include synovitis of the elbow joint and ulnar nerve entrapment (with tenderness on palpation of the ulnar nerve groove and signs of ulnar neuropathy).

—*Wrist tenosynovitis:* Common in patients with RA, wrist tenosynovitis may be difficult to distinguish from synovitis of the underlying radiocarpal joint. Unilateral tenosynovitis may be seen in patients with disseminated gonococcal infection or gout.

—*de Quervain's tenosynovitis:* Inflammation of the abductor pollicis longus or extensor pollicis brevis on the radial aspect of the wrist is referred to as de Quervain's tenosynovitis (see pp. 23, 71).

—*Trochanteric bursitis:* There are several bursae in the area of the greater trochanter of the femur. These bursae are positioned between the trochanter (the bony prominence felt on the lateral aspect of the upper thigh), the gluteus medius and minimus muscles, and the fascia lata. Trochanteric bursitis is a common cause of pain in the region of the hip (see hip pain, p. 30). It occurs mostly among older persons and is more common in women. It may be associated with other conditions that can affect gait, such as osteoarthritis of the hip, knee, or lumbar spine; leg length discrepancy; and obesity. The typical presentation is chronic, intermittent pain over the lateral aspect of the hip. The pain may radiate inferiorly or superiorly and may be confused with hip pain of other causes. The diagnosis is usually established by demonstration of excessive tenderness on palpation over the trochanter. In addition to NSAIDs and local corticosteroid injections, therapy directed at correcting associated conditions may provide relief.

—*Ischial bursitis:* Inflammation of the ischial bursa presents as pain over the ischial tuberosity (the bony prominences beneath the gluteal muscles) that is exacerbated by prolonged sitting on hard surfaces (see p. 31). Ischial bursitis was previously referred to as "weaver's bottom." *Iliopsoas bursitis* presents with groin pain just anterior to the hip joint and lateral to the femoral vessels.

—*Meralgia paresthetica:* Compression neuropathy of the lateral femoral cutaneous nerve commonly presents with burning pain in the anterolateral aspect of the hip and thigh (see p. 31). It is commonly seen in patients who are pregnant, diabetic, or obese.

—*Anserine bursitis:* The anserine bursa is located just inferior and medial to the knee (see knee pain, pp. 34, 68). Anserine bursitis is common, particularly among overweight women. Pain can be elicited by palpation directly over the bursa and is often exacerbated by stair climbing. Other bursae are located below the medial and lateral collateral ligaments and may be a source of pain.

—*Prepatellar bursitis:* Often manifesting swelling and tenderness superficial to the patella, prepatellar bursitis (known previously as "housemaid's knee") is associated with trauma to the front of the knee, as with kneeling. Tendinitis of the patellar tendon may also produce anterior knee pain. It is typically aggravated by athletic activities and has been referred to as "jumper's knee." In children, particularly 10- to 16-year-old boys, pain over the insertion of the patellar tendon into the tibia may indicate Osgood-Schlatter disease (avulsion of the tibial tubercle).

—*Chondromalacia patellae:* Characterized by knee pain, crepitus, and degenerative cartilage changes on the underside of the patella, chondromalacia patellae occurs primarily in young adults, particularly women. The pain of chondromalacia patella is exacerbated by knee flexion against force, for example with stair climbing. Such movements pull the patella close against the femoral condyles. In addition, patients may complain of pain and stiffness with prolonged inactivity that is relieved with motion. Pain attributable to chondromalacia patella can often be elicited by pushing the patella against the femur, particularly at the lateral aspect. This condition is also known as "patellofemoral pain syndrome" and "patellofemoral tracking abnormality." Relative weakness of the medial thigh muscles that allows lateral drift of the patella and abnormal tracking movements may contribute to the pathophysiology. Furthermore, in addition to NSAIDs and avoidance of overuse, exercises aimed at strengthening the medial thigh muscles (e.g., bicycling) may be a useful therapeutic intervention. In more severe or refractory cases, surgical intervention (e.g., release of the lateral retinaculum, realignment of the vastus medialis oblique muscle) may be indicated in some patients.

—*Baker's cyst:* Patients with synovitis of the knee may develop Adams-Baker's cysts (also known as Baker's cysts or popliteal cysts). In this condition, fluid accumulates within the posterior compartment of the knee. Although effusion and swelling may be asymptomatic initially, continued accumulation often causes pain. In addition, the fluid may dissect inferiorly, between the muscles of the calf. This may result in a clinical presentation resembling deep venous thrombosis, and ultrasound may be necessary to differentiate the two. Various conditions (RA, OA, mechanical derangement of knee) are associated with popliteal cysts. Synovial fluid accumulation in the cyst is caused by a "ball-valve" mechanism, whereby synovial fluid is forced from the anterior to the posterior aspect of the knee and cannot freely flow back. This may be the result of proliferative synovium (e.g., in rheumatoid arthritis or other forms of inflammatory arthritis), a torn meniscus, or a fold of synovium (known as a plica). Therapy is directed at the appropriate underlying condition. Inflammatory conditions can sometimes be treated, and the cyst resolved, by local injection of corticosteroids into the joint rather than the cyst.

—*Achilles tendinitis:* The Achilles tendon may become painful from a variety of causes, including direct trauma (e.g., with improper footwear), repetitive overuse (e.g., with athletic activity), and systemic inflammatory diseases (e.g., ankylosing spondylitis, Reiter's syndrome). Pain on palpation is often appreciated at the bony insertion of the tendon. With chronicity, the tendon can become "bumpy" with irregular swellings and have crepitus with motion. There are also bursae superficial to and deep to the Achilles tendon that can become inflamed and be a source of pain. Although not typically associated with pain, xanthomas or rheumatoid nodules along the Achilles tendon can be seen in patients with hypercholesterolemia or RA, respectively.

—*Plantar fasciitis:* Plantar fascia can be a source of substantial pain. Plantar fasciitis (see p. 294) may be associated with trauma, and some patients have an associated spur on x-ray. This condition is also associated with the spondyloarthropathies.

—*Costochondritis:* Pain may arise from the costochondral junctions. The term *Tietze's syndrome* is commonly used to describe cases of costochondritis in which there is not only substantial tenderness on examination, but also swelling. The first and second costochondral junctions are most commonly affected.

Diagnostic Tests: Laboratory tests are seldom useful, as these diagnoses are often made on clinical findings alone.

Imaging: In general, roentgenograms are of limited value in patients with tendinitis and bursitis. As these soft tissue injuries become chronic, they may be associated with local deposition of calcium, resulting in conditions such as calcific tendinitis and periarthritis.

Keys to Diagnosis: Nonarticular pain should be suspected when there is a history of trauma or repetitive movement associated with the onset of symptoms. "Joint" pain without abnormalities localized to the joint on examination should lead the clinician to search for nonarticular (periarticular) sources of "joint" pain.

Differential Diagnosis: The site of involvement determines the differential diagnosis. In general, a careful history and physical examination are necessary to distinguish true arthritis from tendinitis, bursitis, and enthesitis. Whenever inflammatory findings exist, infectious, crystal-induced, and inflammatory conditions should be considered.

Therapy: Therapy for local soft tissue injuries typically involves several modalities. NSAIDs are commonly used, either at their lower, analgesic doses or at higher, antiinflammatory dosages. Topical therapies (e.g., local heat and/or cold) may offer some benefit. Physiotherapy is an important part of the treatment of these conditions. Because many relate to overuse, rest and protection of the affected area is often beneficial acutely. Subsequently, physiotherapy is aimed at preventing recurrence of the condition by optimizing range of motion, improving flexibility, and maximizing the strength of the surrounding musculature. In some cases, local injection of corticosteroids can effectively ameliorate the inflammation and thus decrease pain.

REFERENCES

Biundo JJ, Mipro RC, Fahey P. Sports-related and other soft-tissue injuries, tendinitis, bursitis and occupation-related syndromes. Curr Opinion Rheumatol 1997;9:151–154.

NSAID GASTROPATHY

ICD9 Codes: Gastritis, 535.5; Gastroesophageal reflux disease, 530.81

Definition: The use of NSAIDs is associated with several important adverse effects in the gastrointestinal (GI) tract, particularly gastric ulceration. NSAID-associated GI side effects are the most frequently reported adverse drug effect in the United States.

Etiology: NSAIDs inhibit cyclooxygenase (COX), the enzyme that converts arachidonic acid into prostaglandin (PG). Inhibition of PG, which normally protects the gastric mucosa, is the major mechanism underlying NSAID gastropathy. Most NSAIDs are also acidic compounds and accumulate at high local concentrations in the gastric mucosa; this potentiates their effects. Other mechanisms may also be involved.

Risk Factors: Important patient risk factors for NSAID gastropathy include (a) past history of peptic ulcer disease (PUD), (b) past history of any GI bleeding, (c) serious comorbid disease (e.g., functionally compromised cardiopulmonary disease), and (d) advanced age (>60 years old). Other risk factors include anticoagulation (e.g., warfarin) and the use of corticosteroids (although apart from NSAIDs, corticosteroids are not a clinically significant cause of GI toxicity). In some series, patients with dyspeptic symptoms (e.g., heartburn) and those self-medicated with over-the-counter antacids were also at increased risk for NSAID gastropathy.

Several risk factors for gastropathy relate to the NSAID itself, including dose (higher doses and multiple NSAID use confers a greater risk), duration of therapy (longer treatment is associated with higher risk), and choice of NSAID. NSAIDs can be roughly ranked in order of the risk of gastropathy, from somewhat higher risk (aspirin, piroxicam, indomethacin, naproxen, sulindac) to somewhat lower risk (diclofenac, etodolac, ibuprofen, nabumetone). Differences in the propensity to cause NSAID gastropathy may relate to differential inhibition of the two isoenzymes of COX (see below). Nonacetylated NSAIDs (e.g., salsalate) are inefficient COX inhibitors (100 fold less than aspirin); they are rarely associated with gastropathy.

Demographics: The prevalence of NSAID gastropathy increases with age and in association with the risk factors outlined above. The prevalence and significance of NSAID gastropathy can be analyzed in several ways. Studies have shown that within the first 3 months of treatment with NSAIDs, 10 to 20% of patients develop a new gastric ulcer (GU), and 4 to 10% develop a new duodenal ulcer (DU). Because these were endoscopic studies and the ulcers seen were sometimes quite small, this may be an overestimate of clinically significant problems. In the United States, NSAID gastropathy results in approximately 70,000 hospitalizations and 7,000 deaths each year. Between 20 and 40% of all patients who present with upper GI bleeding have been found to be taking NSAIDs chronically. Symptomatic GI ulceration occurs in 2 to 4% of patients taking a NSAID for more than 1 year. However, this may be an underestimate, because most NSAID gastropathy is asymptomatic, which makes estimation of its true prevalence difficult. In addition, the widespread use of NSAIDs ($>13 \times 10^6$ people in the United States use NSAIDs chronically) underscores this serious health problem.

Cardinal Findings: NSAID-related GU occurs twice as commonly as DU. In addition to frank ulceration, erosions may also be seen. Asymptomatic bleeding is a substantial problem, as more than 50% of patients with NSAID gastropathy are asymptomatic (compared with approximately 25% of non-NSAID-related gastropathy patients). Esophagitis may be related to, or exacerbated by, NSAID use. Anorexia, unexplained weight loss, dizziness, or anemia may be early signs of occult NSAID-induced GI bleedimg.

Complications: Bleeding is the most common complication. Because many ulcers are asymptomatic, it may be unexpected. Ulcers can be severe, leading to complications such as perforation or cardiovascular collapse due to blood loss.

Differential Diagnosis: Idiopathic PUD is now considered to be secondary to infection with *Helicobacter pylori*. In a patient taking NSAIDs, it may be difficult to distinguish idiopathic from NSAID-related gastropathy. This is particularly true among older persons; advanced age is a risk factor for both NSAID gastropathy and *H. pylori* (the prevalence of this infection exceeds 50% in patients >60 years old). Several characteristics of *H. pylori*–related PUD may allow it to be differentiated from NSAID gastropathy: (*a*) most patients with *H. pylori* have DU rather than GU; (*b*) gastritis is seen; and (*c*) recurrence is very common unless the infection is treated. Nonetheless, patients found to have PUD are often tested for *H. pylori*, even if the PUD is suspected of being related to NSAID use. Such patients are usually treated to eradicate the infection in addition to receiving antiulcer treatment.

Keys to Diagnosis: Patients receiving NSAIDs who have GI symptoms should be suspected of having gastropathy. Because many patients with gastropathy are asymptomatic, a high degree of clinical suspicion is needed, particularly in patients with one or more risk factors for NSAID gastropathy.

Diagnostic Tests: Upper GI radiographic studies are used in patients with symptoms and in asymptomatic patients with evidence of bleeding. Regular testing of the stool for occult blood is a reasonable health maintenance procedure for patients receiving NSAIDs, although it is seldom positive in those with significant GI bleeding. Endoscopy allows definitive assessment of esophagogastroduodenal pathology. CBC may reveal significant blood loss.

Therapy: NSAID gastropathy therapy usually involves NSAID discontinuation. In patients with dyspepsia who do not have PUD or other serious GI pathology, it may be possible to relieve the symptoms by lowering the NSAID dose, switching to a different NSAID, or adding antacids such as H2-histamine blockers (e.g., ranitidine, cimetidine, famotidine). In patients with PUD, the NSAID should be stopped, and treatment with H2 blockers instituted. The healing rate for NSAID-related PUD after stopping NSAIDs approximates that of idiopathic PUD; 95 to 100% of GU and DU are healed within 8 weeks of therapy with H2 blockers. If it is considered necessary to continue NSAIDs, healing of ulcers becomes slower and less complete (80 to 90% healed with 12 weeks of H2-blocker therapy). In such patients, proton pump inhibitors (e.g., omeprazole, lansoprazole) are more effective. The size of the ulcer is a major factor in healing; larger ulcers (>0.5 cm) heal more slowly and less completely than smaller ones.

Prevention of NSAID gastropathy is an important consideration. First, NSAIDs should be avoided unless absolutely required for disease control. While it is not cost-effective to treat all patients receiving NSAIDs, patients with one or more important risk factors for NSAID gastropathy may be offered treatment for long-term prevention of PUD. The standard preventive agent is the prostaglandin analogue misoprostol. In high doses (200 mg q.i.d.), misoprostol is very effective at preventing GU (reducing the incidence of ulcers from 12 to 0.7%) as well as DU (reduction from 4.6 to 0.6%). In addition to preventing endoscopically detected ulcers, misoprostol also decreases the occurrence of serious events related to NSAID gastropathy (e.g., perforation, massive bleeding). Unfortunately, at these high doses, misoprostol may be poorly tolerated as it commonly causes GI symptoms such as diarrhea, and it is also relatively inconvenient (q.i.d. dosing). Other regimens (e.g., misoprostol 100 mg q.i.d. or 200 mg b.i.d.) are better tolerated but slightly less effective at preventing PUD. H2-blockers may be somewhat effective at preventing DU related to NSAID use, but commonly used regimens have not been shown to be effective for long-term prevention of GU. Proton pump inhibitors (e.g., omeprazole), which are effective at treating NSAID-related PUD even when the NSAIDs are continued, have also been shown to be effective in long-term prevention of NSAID gastropathy.

Future Directions: COX has been found in two isoforms: COX-1 and COX-2. COX-1 is constitutively expressed in tissues such as the gastric mucosa, kidney, platelet, and megakaryocyte. PGs produced by COX-1 are important in "housekeeping" functions, such as protection of the gastric mucosa, maintenance of renal function, and platelet aggregation. COX-2 is inducible and is expressed by macrophages and other cells after stimulation. PGs produced by COX-2 are active during inflammation. Theoretically, a NSAID that blocked only COX-2 (not COX-1) would provide antiinflammatory benefit yet would not cause side effects such as gastropathy. This is an area of intense research and product development. NSAIDs currently available show some correlation between their relative selectivity for COX-2 versus COX-1 and adverse effects (NSAIDs that inhibit COX-2 more than COX-1 may be associated with less NSAID gastropathy). COX-2 selective NSAIDs will soon be available, and the prevalence of NSAID gastropathy may diminish.

REFERENCES

Fries JF. NSAID gastropathy: the second most deadly rheumatic disease? Epidemiology and risk appraisal. J Rheumatol 1991;(Suppl 28)18:6–10.

Hawkey CJ, Kanasch JA, Szczeparski L, et al. Omeprazole compared with misoprostol for ulcers associated with nonsteroidal antiinflammatory drugs. N Engl J Med 1998;338: 727–734.

Koch M, Dezi A, Ferrario F, Capurso L. Prevention of nonsteroidal anti-inflammatory drug-induced gastrointestinal mucosal injury; a meta-analysis of randomized controlled clinical trials. Arch Intern Med 1996;156:2321–2332.

Rodriguez LAG, Jick H. Risk of upper gastrointestinal bleeding and perforation associated with individual nonsteroidal anti-inflammatory drugs. Lancet 1994;343:769–772.

OSTEITIS CONDENSANS ILII

ICD9 Code: 733.5

Definition: Osteitis condensans ilii refers to an increase in bone density (sclerosis) located on the inferior-medial aspect of the ilium adjacent to the sacroiliac joint. It is often bilateral, symmetric, and triangular. Sacroiliac and spinal abnormalities (i.e., erosions) are not found.

Etiology: The cause is unknown. It may be due to increased mechanical stress across the sacroiliac joint during pregnancy. It is usually associated with pregnancy, but has also been reported in those with hydroxyapatite crystal deposition disease.

Demographics: It is primarily seen in young multiparous women, but has been reported in men.

Cardinal Findings: Only rarely are the radiographic findings symptomatic with pain.

Imaging: Ill-defined ilial sclerosis varies in size. Radiographic findings may resolve or persist.

Differential Diagnosis: Sacroiliitis and ankylosing spondylitis characteristically affect the sacroiliac joint with erosions, pseudowidening, or ankylosis. Degenerative changes in the sacroiliac joint may be confused with osteitis condensans ilii.

Therapy: None is indicated.

OSTEOARTHRITIS

Synonyms: Osteoarthritis (OA); degenerative joint disease (DJD), osteoarthrosis

ICD9 Codes: 715.9 (multiple sites); hand, 715.4; hip, 715.5; knee, 715.6; spine, 721.90.

Definition: OA is the most common arthropathy seen in adults. This noninflammatory condition arises from degenerative changes and progressive loss of cartilage with resultant hypertrophic changes in surrounding bone.

Etiology: Cause is unknown. Mechanical (e.g., trauma, repetitive stress), biochemical, and inflammatory factors contribute to pathogenesis. A genetic predisposition exists for women with OA of the DIP joints (Heberden's nodes).

Pathology: Biochemical changes in cartilage result in a loss of water content, loss of proteoglycan and collagen, and a decreased number of chondrocytes, changes that soften cartilage and make it more prone to damage. Grossly, there is evidence of cartilage damage, with fissuring, pitting, ulceration, and (eventually) denuded bone. Adjacent to cartilage loss is development of reactive or hypertrophic bone—most often manifest as osteophyte (or "spur") formation. Underlying subchondral bone may remodel and show sclerosis or bony cysts. The synovium in OA may be normal or show mild-to-moderate inflammatory changes, similar to that seen in rheumatoid arthritis, although not as intense. It is possible that intermittent inflammatory synovial disease may further contribute to degeneration of articular cartilage.

Demographics: OA has a prevalence of 12% in the U.S. population and is most common in those over the age of 65 years. Radiographic changes of DJD are seen in more than 80% of those over age 75 years. OA is most common in women. Isolated hip OA is most common in men. All races are affected.

Risk Factors: OA is either primary/idiopathic or secondary. Secondary causes of OA include trauma, obesity, congenital disorders, metabolic disorders (Wilson's disease, alcaptonuria, hemochromatosis), inflammatory arthritis (i.e., RA, gout, septic arthritis), neuropathic arthritis, and hemophilia. Obesity increases the risk of knee OA (especially in women) but does not increase risk of hand or hip OA. There is no added risk of OA in long-distance runners. There is an inverse relationship between OA and bone mass.

Cardinal Findings: Most patients note the insidious onset of pain in affected joints. This mechanical or degenerative pain is worsened by activity and improved with rest and is maximal at the end of the day or during the night and may interfere with sleep. Stiffness tends to be minor in the morning, yet it recurs during periods of sedentary rest throughout the day and is best described as a "gel phenomenon." Inflammatory swelling or effusions are unusual. Instead, bony swelling (or hypertrophy) may develop and interfere with normal range of motion. Bony hypertrophy is most obvious in the DIP joints (Heberden's nodes), PIPs (Bouchard's nodes), and first CMC joints, often in a symmetric fashion. Heberden's nodes are primarily found in women. Interestingly, once the hypertrophic changes have fully evolved in the DIP, PIP, or MCP joints, the pain often subsides. Beyond the hand, asymmetric joint disease is most common and typically affects the hip, knees, MTPs, and cervical and lumbar spine. Shoulders, elbows, ankles, and tarsal joints tend to be spared unless traumatic or occupational events predispose the patient to degenerative changes in these joints. For example, tarsal osteoarthritis is a common finding in ballerinas. Coarse crepitus may be felt in joints with moderate-to-severe OA.

—*Primary generalized OA (Nodal OA):* Occurring predominantly in middle-aged women, primary generalized OA affects the DIP, PIP, first CMC, knee, MTP, hips, and spine.

—*Chondromalacia patellae:* Chondromalacia patellae is a form of degenerative arthritis that affects the patellofemoral joint and is often due to malalignment of the patella within the intercondylar groove. The underside of the patellar cartilage develops degenerative features and manifests with pain that is worsened by walking, running, squatting, or climbing stairs. Such patients are often treated conservatively with NSAIDs, analgesics, and quadriceps-strengthening exercises.

—*Inflammatory OA:* Erosive or inflammatory OA typically affects postmenopausal women with inflammatory changes and erosions at "nodal" sites, the PIP or DIP joints. Medial or lateral subluxation at the PIP or DIP joint is common in this variant of OA. Radiographic changes include loss of joint spaces, sclerosis, and osteophytes, with erosions and occasional ankylosis. In the fingers, these central erosions and peripheral osteophytes may give rise to a "seagull" sign on radiography. Inflammatory OA must be distinguished from psoriatic arthritis. Uncommonly, inflammation arising in Heberden's or Bouchard's nodes may be due to gout. This is usually seen in elderly women with renal insufficiency who are taking diuretics.

Uncommon Findings: OA uncommonly affects the MCP (usually the 2nd and 3rd) joints and may be idiopathic or secondary to trauma or hemochromatosis (see p. 266).

Diagnostic Testing: Laboratory tests (e.g., CBC, ESR, SMA12) tend to be normal for age. Serologic testing for ANA and RF is not necessary. Synovial fluid is usually amber, clear, and noninflammatory (WBC < 2000 cells/mm^3), with normal viscosity.

Imaging: Conventional radiography may help in establishing OA as a diagnosis. Typical radiographic changes include loss of joint space, subchondral sclerosis, bony cysts, and reactive osteophytes. Articular erosions and osteoporosis are rare. It is important to note that radiographic findings do not correlate with clinical symptoms.

Keys to Diagnosis: Two primary patterns should be sought: (*a*) patients with Heberden's and Bouchard's nodes (with or without first CMC hypertrophy) or (*b*) patients with a noninflammatory asymmetric oligo- or monarthritis affecting the hip, knee, MTPs, or spine. The diagnosis is supported by radiography.

Differential Diagnosis: Disorders commonly confused with OA include psoriatic arthritis, Reiter's syndrome, hemochromatosis, osteonecrosis, gout, pseudogout, or hydroxyapatite deposition disease.

Therapy: The primary goals of therapy are to relieve pain and maintain function. The initial approach to treatment should always include patient and family education regarding the nature of the disorder and the prognosis. Physical and occupational therapy should be periodically encouraged to maintain optimal joint protection, mobility, and function. Use of weight loss, splinting, ambulatory assist-devices, and vocational counseling should also be considered where appropriate.

Several studies have shown that regular low-impact aerobic exercise (i.e., stationary bicycling, swimming) and isometric exercise can substantially reduce pain, increase mobility, and (in some patients) even retard progression to joint replacement surgery.

Initial pharmacologic attempts at pain control should rely upon the use of safe therapies, such as nonnarcotic analgesics (e.g., acetaminophen), topical therapies (e.g., ice, heat, capsaicin cream), and nonacetylated salicylate (e.g., salsalate). Low-dose NSAIDs may be used if not contraindicated. Patients who do not respond well to these conservative measures may try other or higher-dose NSAIDs, add other analgesic agents (e.g., propoxyphene, tramadol, or nightly tricyclic antidepressants), or be considered for intraarticular injection. Use of strong narcotics and oral corticosteroids should be discouraged.

Intraarticular corticosteroid injection may provide temporary or sustained relief of pain. Intraarticular injection of hyaluronate (weekly for 5 weeks) has also been shown to be clinically effective in treating OA of the knee. Due to equivocal results, joint lavage is not routinely recommended for the treatment of knee OA.

A variety of metalloproteinase inhibitors and chondroprotective agents is currently undergoing investigation in OA.

Surgery: For those with advanced disease, joint replacement surgery may dramatically improve the quality of life. Surgery should be considered for patients who experience intractable/refractory pain, loss of function or mobility, and radiographic evidence of advanced degenerative changes in the joint. Arthroplasty (joint replacement surgery) is routinely recommended for advanced OA involving the hip or knee. Over 150,000 knee and over 200,000 hip replacements are performed yearly in the United States. Relative contraindications to arthroplasty include obesity, multiple medical disorders (that impart a high perioperative risk of death), and a lack of motivation or inability to participate in a postoperative rehabilitation program.

REFERENCES

Bradley JD, Brandt KD, Katz BP, et al. Comparison of an antiinflammatory dose of ibuprofen, an analgesic dose of ibuprofen and acetaminophen in the treatment of patients with osteoarthritis of the knee. N Engl J Med 1991;325:87–91.

Felson DT. The epidemiology of knee osteoarthritis: results from the Framingham Osteoarthritis Study. Semin Arthritis Rheum 1990;20:42–50.

Hochberg MC, Altman RD, Brandt KD, et al. Guidelines for the medical management of osteoarthritis. Part I: Osteoarthritis of the hip. Part II: Osteoarthritis of the knee. Arthritis Rheum 1995;38:1535–1540, 1541–1546.

Peyron JG. Intraarticular hyaluronan injections in the treatment of osteoarthritis: state-of-the-art review. J Rheumatol 1993;39(Suppl):10–15.

OSTEOMYELITIS

ICD9 Codes: Acute osteomyelitis, 730.0; chronic osteomyelitis, 730.1

Definition: Osteomyelitis is infection of bone and bone marrow.

Etiology: Most cases occur by either hematogenous or contiguous spread from local soft tissue infections or by direct inoculation (e.g., trauma). The highly vascular metaphysis (in children) or diaphysis (in adults) is a frequent site of hematogenous spread. Contiguous spread is more likely to occur in areas of vascular compromise. Acute hematogenous osteomyelitis is commonly caused by *Staphylococcus aureus, Streptococcus* spp., and *Haemophilus influenzae*. Cases caused by contiguous spread may involve mixed aerobic and anaerobic organisms. Infections due to prosthetic devices may be caused by coagulase-negative staphylococci, *S. aureus*, or gram-negative bacteria.

Pathology: In acute osteomyelitis, involved bony tissues show suppurative infiltrates, vascular congestion, edema, and thrombosis. Chronic osteomyelitis involvement shows devitalized bony tissues or fibrotic replacement.

Demographics: In infants and children, almost all cases are due to hematogenous spread. Adults may develop infection from hematogenous dissemination or local spread. Local extension is more likely to involve bone in individuals with significant comorbidity such as diabetes or RA.

Risk Factors: Diabetes, RA, sickle cell disease, intravenous drug use, hemodialysis, trauma, recent fractures, prosthetic implants, and vascular insufficiency are risk factors.

Cardinal Findings: Acute signs of inflammation, such as erythema, swelling, and pain may be localized over affected areas. However, many patients lack localizing signs and present instead with deep bony pain that may be referred some distance from the lesion. Contiguous spread to bone should be suspected around chronic soft tissue infections that may have draining sinuses. Fever is common but not universal. Single or multiple sites may be involved; children usually have multiple lesions. Tubular bones are commonly affected in children, and the vertebral column is frequently involved in adults.

Diagnostic Tests: Bone biopsy and culture are required for definitive diagnosis; cultures of sinus tracts do not reliably indicate the causative organism. Blood cultures can be useful but are positive in only a minority of cases. Leukocytosis and elevated ESR and C-reactive protein levels may be seen.

Imaging: Radiographs may show soft tissue swelling, periosteal elevation, cortical lucencies (with or without surrounding sclerosis), and destruction or erosion of the metaphysis, epiphysis, or diaphysis. Chronic osteomyelitis may be suggested by areas of osteolysis, periostitis, or sequestration. Scintigraphy and MRI may be used to define the extent of the osteomyelitis and are most useful in assessing chronic osteomyelitis.

Key to Diagnosis: Bone pain or radiographic abnormalities in patient with localized infection or possible bacteremia should suggest consideration of osteomyelitis. Osteomyelitis is more likely to occur in immunosuppressed hosts or those with comorbid risk factors.

Differential Diagnosis: Chronic soft tissue infections (cellulitis, abscesses) can be present without bone involvement. In such cases, radionuclide imaging studies (early) or plain radiographs (late) can be useful to suggest whether underlying bone is abnormal. Osteonecrosis and other causes of bony infarcts may be mistaken for osteomyelitis.

Therapy: If the organism is identified by bone biopsy/culture or blood culture, treatment with the appropriate antibiotic, administered parenterally, is required for 4 to 6 weeks.

Surgery: Surgical treatment may be required in chronic osteomyelitis for debridement of nonvital tissues or to drain abscesses. Hyperbaric oxygen therapy is a useful adjunct in cases of vascular insufficiency.

Prognosis: Outcome depends greatly on the time to diagnosis and the comorbidity. Children may recover completely; at the other end of the spectrum, adults with limb infections may require amputation.

REFERENCES

McGuire JH. Osteomyelitis and infections of prosthetic joints. In: Isselbacher KJ, Braunwald E, Wilson JD, et al., eds. Harrison's principles of internal medicine. 13th ed. New York: McGraw-Hill 1994:558–560.

OSTEONECROSIS

Synonyms: Avascular necrosis (AVN), aseptic necrosis, ischemic necrosis of bone

ICD9 Code: 733.40

Definition: Osteonecrosis is the ischemic death of bone and bone marrow, clinically manifest as bone pain with distinctive radiographic sequelae.

Etiology: Although a variety of states predispose to osteonecrosis, it may be idiopathic. Underlying mechanisms may include disruption in normal osseous blood flow, thrombosis, fat emboli, endothelial injury, hypercoagulability, increase in intraosseous pressure, and local alterations in tissue architecture (i.e., trauma) or bone stock (osteomalacia).

Risk Factors: Numerous associations have been described, including (in decreasing order of frequency) trauma (with or without adjacent fracture), high-dose corticosteroids, chronic alcoholism, renal failure, organ transplantation, SLE and other connective tissue diseases (e.g., polymyositis), thrombotic states (e.g., sickle cell anemia, hemoglobinopathies), radiation injury, pancreatitis, gout, pregnancy, hyperlipidemia, and caisson disease (decompression sickness in divers).

Pathology: Sequence of events includes cell death, eosinophilic reticulated necrosis, mesenchymal and capillary ingrowth, resorption of bone, collapse, and deposition of new woven bone upon ischemic/necrotic trabecular bone.

Demographics: The underlying condition or cause determines the demographics. Osteonecrosis may account for nearly 10% of total hip replacements (more than 500,000) done in the United States each year. Most commonly seen in 3rd to 6th decades of life, osteonecrosis is more common in men than women (perhaps due to trauma or alcohol).

Cardinal Findings: Osteonecrosis most commonly affects the proximal femoral head (men), more so than the distal femoral condyles (women). Less common sites include the proximal humeral head, talus, lunate bone of the wrist (Kiembock's disease), and tarsal bones. Once clinically recognized, the symptoms and radiographic changes are progressive.

Diagnostic Tests: Laboratory tests have value only in documenting an underlying cause of osteonecrosis.

Imaging: Plain radiographs usually suffice to make a diagnosis. Table 1 demonstrates the correlation between symptoms and typical imaging changes in the course of osteonecrosis. Common early findings on radiographs include alteration in the normal trabecular pattern, with lytic or sclerotic change. Later findings include a "crescent sign" (subchondral crescent-shaped lucency), collapse, loss of joint space, secondary osteoarthritic changes (osteophytes). Scintigraphy (bone scan) using technetium-99m may show asymmetric changes, whose nature depends on the stage of disease. The early, infarctive stage shows no uptake or a "cold" spot that may be present before the radiographs change. Later, during the reparative stages, the bone scan may show increased areas of uptake. MRI may be more sensitive than bone scanning in picking up earlier lesions, but may yield a false-negative result in the first 2 to 3 weeks. The earliest finding is nonspecific marrow edema, later followed by marrow necrosis with changes in cortical bone.

Keys to Diagnosis: Complaints of vague bone pain (at the ends of long bones), possibly worse at night, in patients with an identifiable risk factor (e.g., steroid use) should suggest osteonecrosis. Remember that clinical symptoms

Table 1
Staging of Osteonecrosis of the Femoral Head

Stage	Symptoms	X-ray	Other Imaging
0	No pain	Normal	Normal bone scan, MRI
1	Minimal or no pain	Normal	Abnormal MRI or bone scan
2	Minimal pain, night pain	Sclerosis or cysts formation; no collapse, normal joint space	Abnormal MRI and bone scan
3	Intermittent groin/thigh pain, limitation of motion	Early subchondral collapse (crescent sign), no flattening, normal joint space	Unnecessary
4	Increasing pain, antalgic limp	Flattening of femoral head, normal joint space	Unnecessary
5	Increasing pain, severe loss of motion	Flattening of femoral head, joint space narrowing and acetabular changes	Unnecessary

precede radiographic evidence of osteonecrosis by months. The earliest and most reliable diagnosis is made by MRI.

Differential Diagnosis: Monarticular osteoarthritis, fracture, transient osteoporosis of the hip, osteoidosteoma, sickle-cell crisis, osteomyelitis, and primary or metastatic tumor should be considered.

Therapy: Treatment varies according to the stage of disease and whether an underlying cause is identified. For instance, abstinence from alcohol, lowering or discontinuing corticosteroid therapy, lipid-lowering therapy, or avoidance of sickle cell crises may benefit some.

Conservative measures should be aimed at maintaining strength, avoiding contractures or debility (with the assistance of physical and occupational therapy), and pain management.

Pain can be managed with analgesic agents (e.g., acetaminophen) or NSAIDs. Intraarticular steroids are not advisable. Pain may be alleviated with ambulatory assist devices (crutches, cane, or walker).

Surgery: Early stages may benefit from debridement of necrotic bone with subsequent bone grafting. Core decompression, with or without biopsy, is controversial and may be indicated in osteonecrosis of the femoral head when applied early. Joint replacement may be indicated for intractable pain with moderate-to-severe radiographic changes.

Total joint replacement, unilateral endoprosthesis, and rotational osteotomy have been used to treat advanced painful disease.

Prognosis: Although some patients with osteonecrosis do not progress to bony collapse, most exhibit progressive pain, debility, and radiographic change and may require surgical intervention. Joint replacement surgery for osteonecrosis is less successful than that for other disorders because of a younger population and other comorbid conditions that may result in weaker bone stock.

REFERENCES

Chang CC, Greenspan A, Gershwin ME. Osteonecrosis: current perspectives on pathogenesis and treatment. Sem Arthritis Rheum 1993;23:47–69.
Mankin HJ. Nontraumatic necrosis of bone (osteonecrosis). N Engl J Med 1992;326:1473–1479.

OSTEOPOROSIS

ICD9 Codes: Generalized 733.0; postmenopausal 733.1

Synonyms: Osteopenia

Definition: Osteoporosis is a reduction in bone density, or osteopenia, that affects all skeletal components. Altered bone density results in increased fragility and may lead to fractures with minimal trauma.

Etiology: Many causes have been identified (Table 1) including excess of glucocorticoids (Cushing's or iatrogenic), deficiencies of sex steroids in men and women, lack of gravitational force (immobilization or space flight), or nutritional deficiencies (calcium, vitamin D), which may result from dietary lack or malabsorption. Estrogen deficiency mediates enhanced bone loss through production of cytokines including interleukin-1.

Pathology: Bone mineral and organic phases are structurally normal and present in normal proportions. The primary defect is in the total quantity of bone, such that trabeculae and cortical areas show decreased thickness.

Demographics: Nearly 25 million Americans are affected by osteoporosis. Postmenopausal women represent the largest patient group. Men over the age of 60 years may show decreasing bone density, although increased fracture risk does not appear until after age 70. Patients of all ages who are treated with glucocorticoids have accelerated bone loss. The risk of vertebral compression fracture and hip fracture in postmenopausal Caucasian women is nearly 20%. Black individuals tend to have greater bone density and are thus at a much lower risk for osteoporotic fractures.

Cardinal Findings: At the outset, osteoporosis is clinically silent. In later stages, fracture may occur in the vertebral bones, with resulting wedge-shaped deformities that can cause radiating pain and contribute to formation of an exaggerated kyphosis, known as the "dowager's hump." Other sites at risk for fracture include the forearm (Colles' fracture) and the hip. Fractures in osteoporotic ribs may be induced by coughing and can cause considerable pain. Cortical bone stress fractures may occur in the lower extremities or feet.

Table 1
Risk Factors for Development of Osteoporosis

Age
Female gender
Hypogonadal (both sexes)
Postmenopausal (females)
Small skeletal mass
Caucasian race
Lifestyle habits: Tobacco, alcohol, lack of exercise, malnutrition
Medications: Glucocorticoids, phenytoin, thyroid preparations, heparin
Comorbid conditions: hyperparathyroidism, hyperthyroidism, diabetes mellitus,
    malabsorption syndromes, Cushing's syndrome, rheumatoid arthritis

Uncommon Manifestations: Vertebral fractures can rarely cause spinal cord compromise.

Diagnostic Tests: Osteoporosis may be suspected or diagnosed on the basis of routine conventional radiography, although these are insensitive measures of bone density. Nonetheless, fractures can be seen on standard radiographs. Bone densitometry (e.g., DEXA scan) measurements are diagnostic (see p. 110). Tests should include two sites: hip and lumbar spine. Measurement of serum calcium and phosphate levels and liver/renal chemistries are important to determine underlying conditions. Elevated serum calcium or unexpectedly low densitometry measurements should be followed by measurement of PTH and, possibly, an endocrinologic evaluation. The need for additional endocrine testing, such as thyroid function tests, depends on the clinical picture.

Keys to Diagnosis: An early diagnosis can be made (before fractures occur) if an individual from the at-risk population (Table 1) is identified and routinely assessed by bone densitometry or radiographic studies.

Differential Diagnosis: Fractures should be distinguished from pathologic fractures and their underlying abnormalities (i.e., bony metastases). Primary hyperparathyroidism causes accelerated bone loss in primarily cortical bone, especially the hip. Osteomalacia may be associated with low levels of 25-hydroxy-vitamin D and phosphate. Bone biopsy may be required for definitive diagnosis of osteomalacia. Heritable disorders of connective tissue—including Marfan's and Ehlers-Danlos syndromes—are often associated with osteoporosis.

Therapy: The primary goal of therapy should be prevention of fractures.

—*General measures:* Lifestyle adjustments should include cessation of tobacco use and of excessive intake of alcohol. Weight-bearing exercise is recommended. Frail and elderly patients with high fracture risk should have a living situation that does not require use of stairs, and ambulation aids should be used if necessary.

—*Drugs:* In postmenopausal women, long-term hormone replacement with conjugated estrogens (with or without progesterone) is an effective treatment. However, estrogen tolerance may be an issue in some women. Estrogen clearly has osseous and cardiovascular benefits, but there may be an associated low risk of uterine or breast cancer. Other options include the use of bisphosphonates (i.e., alendronate, etidronate, etc.) and calcitonin (available as a nasal spray or subcutaneous injection). Calcitonin has the added benefit of analgesic properties, which may be useful for treatment of painful fractures. Calcium (1000–1500 mg/day) and vitamin D supplementation are recommended for all. The use of sodium fluoride is controversial.

The 1997 American College of Rheumatology guidelines on steroid-induced osteoporosis suggest

1. Use the lowest effective steroid dose
2. Use topical or inhaled steroids when possible
3. An adequate intake of calcium ≥1500 mg/day
4. Vitamin D (800 IU/day or 50,000 IU three times weekly) or calcitriol (0.5 μg/day)
5. Quit smoking
6. Limit alcohol consumption
7. Begin daily weight-bearing exercise program
8. Use calcium, vitamin D, and hormone replacement therapy (HRT) unless contraindicated
9. When HRT is contraindicated or refused, use bisphosphonates or calcitonin
10. Patients on steroids with osteoporotic fracture and normal bone mineral density (BMD) should be evaluated for other causes of fracture
11. BMD should include assessment of lumbar spine and femoral neck—if only one site, use the lumbar spine in men and women under 60 years of age and the femoral neck in those over 60 years of age
12. Repeat BMD in 6–12 months
13. Educate the patient

Surgery: Surgery is rarely required except to stabilize fractures. Bone biopsy is occasionally required to confirm that other conditions (osteomalacia, hyperparathyroidism, Paget's disease, and metastatic disease) are not present.

Prognosis: Fractures (especially hip fractures) in elderly patients are associated with significant morbidity and mortality. Improved awareness and a wide range of available treatments for osteoporosis may significantly change the course of this disease.

REFERENCES

Krane SM, Holick MF. Metabolic bone disease. In: Isselbacher KJ, Braunwald E, Wilson JD, Martin JB, Fauci AS, Kasper DL, eds. Harrison's principles of internal medicine. 13th ed. New York: McGraw-Hill, 1994:2172–2183.

Lane NE, Jergas M, Genant HK. Osteoporosis and bone mineral assessment. In: Koopman WJ, ed. Arthritis and allied conditions: a textbook of rheumatology. 13th ed. Baltimore: Williams & Wilkins, 1997:153–171.

OSTEOSARCOMA

Synonyms: Osteogenic sarcoma

ICD9 Code: M9180/3

Definition: Osteosarcoma is a primary bone malignancy characterized by proliferating sarcomatous spindle cells producing osteoid.

Demographics: Incidence approaches 2 cases per million population. Osteosarcoma predominately affects children and adolescents. Males are more commonly afflicted than females. Adults with Paget's disease (<1%) or those who have received prior bone irradiation are also at increased risk.

Cardinal Findings: Intermittent pain progresses to chronic, deep pain in an affected extremity. Firm, fusiform swelling of an extremity is accompanied by loss of movement in the adjacent joint. Primary tumor develops in the metaphyseal region of long bone. Approximately half of cases involve the distal femur or proximal tibia. Lung is the most common site of metastasis.

Keys to Diagnosis: Nonarticular extremity pain and swelling in an older child should suggest osteosarcoma.

Imaging: Plain radiography shows mixed sclerotic and lytic lesions with periosteal reaction and soft-tissue mass. Occasionally a "sun burst" pattern of new bone formation is seen.

Therapy: Amputation or limb-sparing surgery with pre- and postoperative chemotherapy is used most commonly. Osteosarcoma is radioresistant.

Prognosis: Despite an aggressive disease course with a high risk for metastasis, 5-year relapse-free survival as high as 40 to 80% has been reported in some series. Poor prognosis occurs with axial involvement, lesions larger than 15 cm, marked elevations of LDH and alkaline phosphatase, males, and those under 10 years of age. Best prognosis occurs with proximal tibial involvement, age above 20 years, and females.

REFERENCES

Clark CR, Bonfiglio M. Orthopaedics: essentials of diagnosis and treatment. New York: Churchill Livingstone, 1994.

PAGET'S DISEASE

Synonyms: Osteitis deformans

ICD9 Code: 731.0

Definition: Paget's disease is a focal bone disorder in which the bone turnover rate is increased. It can affect single bones or multiple bones simultaneously.

Etiology: No cause is known, although a viral etiology has been postulated.

Pathology: In the earliest stage, increased bone resorption produces a purely lytic picture. This is followed by an intermediate stage in which active bone resorption and new bone formation (reactive sclerosis) occur in close proximity. Bony trabeculae may show thickening. Late in the disease, static sclerotic bony changes occur without further remodeling.

Demographics: The prevalence of Paget's disease is approximately 3% in those over the age of 40 years. Some studies have suggested a higher prevalence in more temperate climates.

Cardinal Findings: With the widespread use of automated laboratory test profiles, most patients are detected in the asymptomatic stage by the finding of an elevated alkaline phosphatase. Bone pain and deformities can occur, whose distribution depends upon the specific skeletal elements that are involved. Pain is described as deep, constant, and worse at night and may be aggravated by heat. Deformities include elongation of the long bones, causing bowing of the legs. The skull may also increase in size with resultant frontal bossing. Unstable pagetic bone may result in pathologic fractures following minimal trauma.

Uncommon Findings: Because of the high blood flow through newly formed bone, skin overlying the affected area may be warm. In severe cases, heart failure or decreased mentation may occur because of the high-output state. Hearing loss or vertigo may accompany impingement on the eighth cranial nerve. There is a small increased risk of giant cell tumors and osteogenic sarcoma.

Diagnostic Tests: Elevated alkaline phosphatase level suggests the diagnosis. Urinary excretion of hydroxyproline is increased and may be useful in following disease activity. Bone biopsy is rarely indicated to exclude the presence of bone tumor.

Imaging: If bone pain is present, radiographs of these areas may be diagnostic. Long bones show the various stages of the disease from osteolysis to excessive bone formation. Thickening of the cranial bones may be seen on a skull film. Since the lumbar spine and sacrum are commonly affected, radiographs of these sites may be useful even in the absence of symptoms. Radionuclide bone scanning helps to determine the extent of skeletal involvement.

Keys to Diagnosis: Isolated elevation of alkaline phosphatase in an older in-

Table 1
Paget's Disease—Key Points

- Alkaline phosphatase is high
- Calcium level is normal
- Urine hydroxyproline is high
- Decreased/increased bone on x-ray
- Treatment with bisphosphonates, calcitonin

dividual suggests Paget's disease. Bone films are then indicated, especially if pain is present.

Differential Diagnosis: Some of the lytic lesions may suggest metastatic disease. Bony changes associated with hyperparathyroidism might be considered, but in Paget's disease the serum calcium levels are usually normal.

Therapy: Asymptomatic patients require no treatment. Bony pain, spinal involvement, deformities, or uncomfortable warmth are indications for medical therapy. Bisphosphonates (e.g., etidronate, alendronate, and pamidronate) are useful in reducing bone turnover and exert relatively long-lasting effects. Hyperphosphatemia is a possible side effect that can be corrected by lowering the dose. Bisphosphonates must be taken on an empty stomach to facilitate absorption. Calcitonin, another useful agent, is available as a nasal spray. Pain control may be better with calcitonin than with diphosphonates, but effects of this agent are short-lived. Thus, flares are more frequent when the drug is stopped.

Surgery: Correction of deformities, including total joint replacements, appears to have the same success rate as in patients without Paget's disease.

Prognosis: Medications that alter the disease course make cures possible in some patients.

REFERENCES

Hamdy RC. Clinical features and pharmacologic treatment of Paget's disease. Endocrinol Metab Clin North Am 1995;24:421–433.

Kanis JA. Treatment of Paget's disease—an overview. Semin Arthritis Rheum 1994;23:254–255.

Klein RM, Norman A. Diagnostic procedures for Paget's disease: radiologic, pathologic, and laboratory testing. Endocrinol Metab Clin North Am 1995;24:437–449.

PANNICULITIS

Synonyms: Erythema nodosum, Weber-Christian disease

ICD9 Code: 729.30

Definition: Panniculitis is inflammation within subcutaneous fat.

Etiology: Panniculitis can be caused by a variety of systemic diseases and is classified according to histopathologic criteria in four major groups: *septal, lobular, mixed,* and *with vasculitis* (Table 1). Panniculitis seldom occurs in association with hypersensitivity vasculitis or polyarteritis nadosa. The pathogenesis involves a dynamic process of inflammation evolving from a neutrophilic infiltrate to eventual fibrosis.

Pathology: Skin/fat biopsy findings reflect the age of the lesion. Neutrophils are seen early, followed by macrophage infiltration and the formation of granulomata. Fibrosis is seen late.

Demographics: Panniculitis is rare; prevalence is less than 1/100,000. It occurs in the 3rd to 5th decades (Table 1).

Table 1
Major Types of Panniculitis

Disease	Histologic Subtype	Peak Age	M:F Ratio	Key Features
Erythema nodosum	Septal	None	1:3	Acute process, anterior tibia; resolves without scarring
Weber-Christian disease	Lobular	37	3:7	Fever, multiple sites, visceral involvement
Lupus panniculitis (lupus profundus)	Mixed	27	1:9	Lesions on face, upper arms, buttocks, breasts; may ulcerate with scarring

Cardinal Findings: Features common to all panniculitides include tender subcutaneous nodules (Table 1). Associated phenomena are common and depend on the underlying clinical syndrome. In *erythema nodosum* (see p. 203), tender nodules appear on the anterior tibial surface and evolve into ecchymotic lesions that typically regress in 4 to 6 weeks without scarring. *Weber-Christian disease* is characterized by multiple recurrent subcutaneous nodules, fever, arthralgia, myalgia, and occasional abdominal pain; eventually fibrosis occurs. *Lupus erythematosus panniculitis (lupus profundus)* is seen in less than 3% of SLE patients, with tender nodules that may ulcerate occurring on the face, arms, buttocks, or breasts. In polyarteritis nodosa, small vessel vasculitis may cause panniculitis. Some patients with pancreatic disease develop subcutaneous fat necrosis (lobular panniculitis) with polyarthritis. Lobular panniculitis has also been associated with α_1-antitrypsin deficiency.

Keys to Diagnosis: Panniculitis should be suspected with tender subcutaneous nodules that are often red and may turn violaceous. Fibrosis is seen in late cases. Ulceration is rare.

Diagnostic Tests: Choice of tests depends on the clinical picture but may include pharyngeal culture for streptococcal infection, chest radiograph, skin test for tuberculosis, and serum tests for amylase, lipase, and α_1-antitrypsin. Skin/fat biopsy is usually not necessary to diagnose erythema nodosum but may be helpful in other forms of panniculitis.

Therapy: Therapy is directed at underlying disease, if detected. In idiopathic cases, management is symptomatic: bed rest and elevation of extremity (if involved). NSAIDs may be useful, and oral corticosteroids are effective in most. Immunosuppressive agents are reserved for recurrent/recalcitrant disease.

Prognosis: Prognosis depends on underlying disease. Most cases of erythema nodosum resolve in 4 to 6 weeks. Weber-Christian disease is typically chronic, with death in 10 to 15% of cases. In lupus profundus, the course often does not follow systemic disease activity.

REFERENCES

Callen JP. Miscellaneous disorders that commonly affect both skin and joints: panniculitis. In: Sontheimer RD, Provost TT, eds. Cutaneous manifestations of rheumatic diseases. Baltimore: Williams & Wilkins, 1996:266–273.

PARVOVIRUS B19

Synonym: "Fifth's disease" or erythema infectiosum

ICD9 Code: Fifth's disease, 057.0; arthropathy associated with viral diseases, 711.5

Definition: Human parvovirus B19 is the most common viral cause of arthralgias and symmetric polyarthritis in adults. Fifth's disease is seen in children.

Pathology: Parvovirus has tissue tropism for red blood cell progenitors. Parvovirus B19 has been isolated from bone marrow and synovium of affected individuals by molecular biologic techniques. This suggests viral persistence as a possible explanation for the chronic arthropathy that is sometimes seen.

Demographics: Parvovirus B19 is nearly endemic among school children. Up to 60% of adults in the United States demonstrate serologic evidence of past infection. Periodic outbreaks occur most commonly in late winter and spring. Young to middle-aged adult women are at highest risk for parvovirus B19 arthropathy.

Cardinal Findings: Children typically manifest a bright red "slapped cheek" rash and may be diagnosed with erythema infectiosum. Less commonly, a lacy erythematous eruption may be seen on the torso or extremities. The rash may be accompanied by mild constitutional symptoms and low-grade fever. Some children may be asymptomatic.

Adults infected with B19 develop a flulike illness. A mild maculopapular rash of the extremities may be seen. Arthralgia or arthritis is seen in 20% of patients. Joint symptoms are more frequent in adults and usually manifest as arthralgias with morning stiffness. An acute polyarthritis is less common, but well described, and may persist for weeks to months in some. Knees, PIPs, wrists, and/or ankles are most often affected in a symmetric distribution. The symmetric polyarthritis of parvovirus closely resembles early RA.

Uncommon Findings: Chronic arthropathy is a rare result of parvovirus B19 infection. Reports of subsequent RA and SLE after B19 infections exist, but no causal relationship is established. Other complications of parvovirus B19 infection include aplastic crises, chronic hemolytic anemia, bone marrow suppression in patients with an underlying immunodeficiency state, and hydrops fetalis.

Keys to Diagnosis: Abrupt-onset symmetric polyarthritis in young women exposed to children infected with erythema infectiosum should suggest parvovirus B19 infection.

Diagnostic Testing: Anemia may result from diminished RBC production. High-titer anti-IgM antibodies on ELISA help to confirm the diagnosis. However, IgM is only elevated for approximately 2 to 3 months following an attack. Positive B19 IgG antibody is consistent with prior exposure but does not help establish a diagnosis because of the high prevalence of seroconversion in the general population. Rheumatoid factor and ANA are usually absent or transiently detected in low titer. Radiographic erosions are uncommon.

Therapy: Analgesics are given for joint pain in adults. NSAIDs may occasionally be helpful. Temporary supportive care is required for many because infection is self-limiting. For rare patients with persistent polyarthritis, therapy is similar to that used for RA.

Prognosis: In most patients, symptoms resolve within a couple of weeks. A subset of individuals develop protracted or intermittent musculoskeletal symptoms that may last months. Many patients meet classification criteria for RA at some point in the disease course.

REFERENCES

Foto F, Saag KG, Scharosch LL, et al. Parvovirus B19–specific DNA in bone marrow from B19 arthropathy patients: evidence for B19 viral persistence. J Infect Dis 1993;167:744–748.

Gran JT, Johnsen V, Myklebust G, et al. The variable clinical picture of arthritis induced by human parvovirus B19: report of seven adult cases and review of the literature. Scand J Rheumatol 1995;24:174–179.

Naides SJ, Scharosch LL, Foto F, Howard EJ. Rheumatologic manifestations of human parvovirus B19 infection in adults: initial two-year clinical experience. Arthritis Rheum 1990;33:1297–1307.

PERIOSTITIS

ICD9 Code: 730.30

Definition: Periostitis refers to radiographic elevation of the periosteum in response to injury, inflammation, or infection.

Pathology: Periostitis is often associated with increased vascularity and local blood flow. Early round cell infiltration into the outer or fibrous layer is followed by deposition of new bone on the original cortical bone. Periosteal new bone is less dense pathologically and radiographically.

Associated Disorders: Hypertrophic pulmonary osteoarthropathy (primary or secondary), osteomyelitis, thyroid acropachy, psoriatic arthritis, rheumatoid arthritis, Reiter's syndrome, juvenile arthritis, diffuse idiopathic skeletal hyperostosis, syphilis, lymphoma, plasma cell dyscrasias, neurofibromatosis, hypervitaminosis A, fluorosis, or venous stasis may be associated with periostitis.

Cardinal Findings: Periostitis may be asymptomatic or painful. It tends to be painful during the early or acute stage. Pain may be described as deep, aching, or burning, or be associated with palpable tenderness. Periostitis may also produce local warmth or swelling, with or without associated pitting edema.

Diagnostic Tests: Radiographic changes are diagnostic.

Imaging: Periostitis is best imaged by conventional radiography but may be identified by scintigraphy or CT. Periosteal elevation is frequently found near (in decreasing frequency) the diaphysis, metaphysis, or epiphysis of long bones, especially the tibia, fibula, radius, metacarpals, or metatarsals.

Therapy: Treat the underlying disorder. Limb elevation, local ice, or NSAIDs may be effective in managing pain.

REFERENCES

Resnick D, Niwayama G. Enostosis, hyperostosis and periostitis. In: Resnick D, Niwayama G, eds. Diagnosis of bone and joint disorders. 2nd ed. Philadelphia: WB Saunders, 1988:4073–4139.

PIGMENTED VILLONODULAR SYNOVITIS (PVNS)

ICD9 Code: 719.2

Definition: PVNS is a benign tenosynovial or articular neoplasm, frequently containing hemosiderin-laden cells.

Etiology: A nonmalignant tumor of unknown etiology, PVNS is thought to be related to an aberrant inflammatory response to lipids, blood, or an as-yet unidentified microbe. It may be preceded by trauma in up to 50% of cases.

Demographics: The diffuse articular form is rare, with equal sex distribution. A localized tenosynovial form is slightly more common, with a female predominance.

Cardinal Findings: Diffuse PVNS often presents insidiously as monarthritis of a lower extremity, especially the knee; it may mimic a meniscal lesion. Long-standing discomfort and swelling may be confused with chronic inflammatory arthropathies. Localized tenosynovial PVNS occurs as a painless nodular lesion, often next to a finger joint, and may be confused with giant cell tumor of the tendon sheath.

Diagnostic Testing: Routine hematologic and chemistry studies are all normal. Synovial fluid of diffuse articular PVNS is frankly bloody or xanthochromic. Plain radiographs of diffuse disease show cartilage loss with cystic erosive changes in the bones. T2-weighted MRI shows a diminished signal in areas of PVNS. Definitive diagnosis may be established by synovial biopsy or at the time of surgical resection. Diffuse PVNS has coarse villi and is locally invasive to the bone. Grossly, the diffuse lesion is yellow to dark brown.

Keys to Diagnosis: Diffuse PVNS has bloody synovial fluid with characteristic appearance on MRI imaging.

Therapy: Surgical resection is used in most cases; 30 to 50% recur. External and intraarticular irradiation has met with varying success.

REFERENCES

Bentley G, McAuliffe T. Pigmented villonodular synovitis. Ann Rheum Dis 1990;49:210–211.
Canoso JJ. Tumors of joints and related structures. In: Koopman WJ, ed. Arthritis and allied conditions: a textbook of rheumatology. 13th ed. Baltimore: Williams & Wilkins, 1997:1868–1871.

PLANTAR FASCIITIS

Synonyms: Subcalcaneal heel pain, calcaneal bursitis

ICD9 Code: 728.71

Definition: Plantar fasciitis is acute or chronic pain from the plantar surface of the heel and plantar fascia, worsened by weight bearing or local manual pressure. Often there are associated calcaneal spurs or bursitis.

Etiology: Plantar fasciitis may be idiopathic or post-traumatic with resultant inflammatory change due to overuse or reinjury. It may result from athletic activity, prolonged walking, improper shoes, structural instability, obesity, or direct trauma to the heel. Plantar fasciitis may also be associated with spondyloarthropathies.

Pathology: There is local degenerative change in the origin of the plantar fascia with traction periostitis of the medical calcaneal tubercle. With repetitive stress, microtears develop, resulting in inflammation involving the bursa, plantar fascia, and enthesis (attachment sites on the calcaneus).

Demographics: Plantar fasciitis is most common between 40 and 60 years of age. Most patients have calcaneal spurs or history of trauma. In young patients, suspect trauma or a spondyloarthropathy.

Cardinal Findings: Intense, sharp, aching or burning heel pain tends to be unilateral and worse in the morning; it may improve with time and ambulation. However, pain may be exacerbated by prolonged standing or walking. Tenderness can be elicited by palpation over the inferior calcaneus near the insertion of the plantar fascia. Pronation (eversion) may worsen pain.

Associations: Inflammatory conditions (spondyloarthropathies, RA, SLE), structural abnormalities (pes valgus, flexible flat foot), overuse (long distance running, prolonged standing, aerobic dance, obesity), poor footwear, diabetes, calcaneal spurs, Dupuytren's contracture, Achilles tendinitis, or metabolic bone disease may be associated with plantar fasciitis.

Diagnostic Tests: No laboratory tests are indicated.

Imaging: Radiographic calcaneal spurs may not be present. Sharp, demarcated spurs tend to be degenerative. Soft, fluffy, cloudy, ill-defined spurs are typically inflammatory and may indicate a spondyloarthropathy (see p. 355). Periostitis is sometimes seen.

Keys to Diagnosis: Ask about activities that may provoke pain (e.g., running) and examine shoes. Diagnosis is based on history, tenderness on palpation, or radiographic spurs.

Differential Diagnosis: Spondyloarthropathies, fat atrophy of the heel pad, calcaneal stress fracture, tarsal tunnel syndrome, plantar fascia rupture (from local steroid injections), or nerve entrapment of the abductor digiti quinti should be considered.

Therapy: Rest, reduction of activity/ambulation, heel pads or heel cup orthoses, arch supports, analgesics, and NSAIDs are advised and useful. Examine shoes for appropriate heel and arch support, wear, or instability. Referral to physical therapy for stretching exercises for Achilles tendon (dorsiflexion of ankle) and plantar fascia (dorsiflexion of great toe) may be beneficial. Night splint with 5° of dorsiflexion may help. Local injection (may be painful) of corticosteroids (10–20 mg prednisolone) should be tried when conservative measures fail. Surgery (partial plantar fascia release) is rarely necessary.

REFERENCES

Chandler TJ, Kibler WB. A biomechanical approach to the prevention, treatment and rehabilitation of plantar fasciitis. [Review] Sports Med 1993;15:344–352.

Sibbitt WL Jr. Fibrosing syndromes—Dupuytren's contracture, diabetic stiff hand syndrome, plantar fasciitis, and retroperitoneal fibrosis: plantar fasciitis. In: Koopman WJ, ed. Arthritis and allied conditions: a textbook of rheumatology. 13th ed. Baltimore: Williams & Wilkins, 1997:1852–1854.

POEMS SYNDROME

Definition: POEMS syndrome is a rare multisystem disorder seen in association with plasma cell dyscrasias.

Pathogenesis: Pathogenesis is unknown. Elevated serum concentrations of the proinflammatory cytokines IL-1, IL-6, and TNF-α have been shown in POEMS patients.

Demographics: POEMS syndrome is rare.

Cardinal Findings: The acronym POEMS represents the key features, including:

—*Plasma cell dyscrasia with polyneuropathy:* Plasmocytomas often present as sclerotic bony lesions. Neuropathy is uncommon but may manifest as a chronic, severe, sensorimotor inflammatory polyneuropathy.

—*Organomegaly:* Hepatomegaly and lymphadenopathy are present in 67%; splenomegaly is seen in 33% of patients.

—*Endocrinopathy:* Hypothyroidism, hypogonadism with gynecomastia, amenorrhea, impotence, or hyperprolactinemia may be seen.

—*Monoclonal gammopathy:* Patients usually demonstrate an IgG or IgA monoclonal paraproteinemia.

—*Skin changes:* Scleroderma-like skin changes are common, but changes may also include hyperpigmentation, hypertrichosis, hyperhidrosis, and angiomas.

—*Other characteristic features:* Fever, anorexia, and thrombocytosis occur, symptoms suggesting excess cytokine production.

Therapy: Initially, most patients are treated with corticosteroids. Cyclophosphamide and other immunomodulatory agents have been used in refractory cases.

REFERENCES

Gherardi RK, Belec L, Soubrier M, et al. Overproduction of proinflammatory cytokines imbalanced by their antagonists in POEMS syndrome. Blood 1996;87:1458–1465.

POLYARTERITIS NODOSA (PAN)

Synonyms: Polyangiitis, periarteritis nodosa, systemic necrotizing vasculitis (PAN is part of this larger disease spectrum)

ICD9 Code: 446.0

Definition: PAN is a type of systemic necrotizing vasculitis that affects medium and small muscular arteries of the skin, kidneys, muscle, gastrointestinal tract, and peripheral nerves. Microscopic polyangiitis (MPA), a PAN variant, affects smaller-sized arteries. MPA is less severe, predominately affecting the skin, musculoskeletal system, and lungs.

Etiology: PAN is systemic vasculitis of uncertain etiology. Although no infectious cause is known, PAN is associated with hepatitis B antigenemia in populations prone to intravenous substance abuse.

Pathology: Immune complexes deposited in the vascular endothelium activate complement, attracting inflammatory cells. The cellular infiltrate contains both neutrophils and mononuclear cells. Release of proteolytic enzymes and oxygen free radicals results in destruction of the entire vessel wall with fibrinoid necrosis. Eosinophils and granuloma are very rare. New and healed lesions may both be present in a single specimen.

Demographics: PAN is an uncommon disorder, predominately of middle-aged men. Median age is 40 to 60 years, with a 2:1 male predominance.

Cardinal Findings: Significant constitutional symptoms may predominate early and include fever, weight loss, and severe malaise. Arthralgias/myalgias (50%) and severe abdominal pain often herald disease onset. Visceral organ manifestations (in order of decreasing frequency) include:

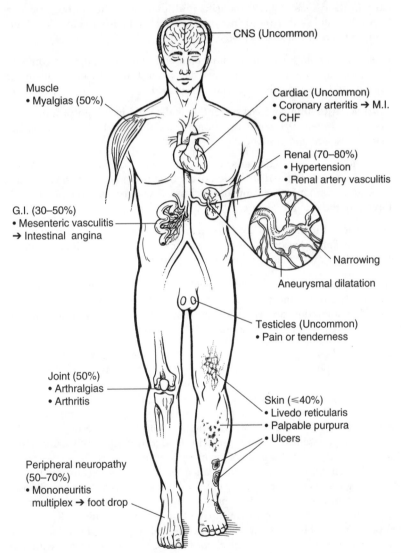

Figure 1. Manifestations of polyarteritis nodosa. Drawing of a visceral angiogram with classic vasculitis findings.

—*Renal* (70–80%): Impaired renal function, proteinuria, and hypertension are secondary to renal artery involvement.

—*Nerve* (50–70%): Peripheral neuropathy is common and often manifests early in the disease as mononeuritis multiplex (vasculitis of the vasa nervorum). Distal sensorimotor polyneuropathy and late CNS involovement leading to encephalopathy also occur.

—*Gastrointestinal:* Severe abdominal pain with intestinal angina is common. GI hemorrhage, perforation, cholecystitis, pancreatitis, intrahepatic aneurysm rupture, and appendicitis have all been reported.

—*Cardiac:* Although coronary vasculitis is detected in a high proportion of cases postmortem, symptomatic coronary vasculitis and PAN-associated cardiac disease are uncommon.

—*Skin* (40%): Livedo reticularis, nonspecific maculopapular eruptions, and large ulcerations in the distribution of major subcutaneous arteries are seen. Subcutaneous skin lesions unusual in classic PAN are more common in PAN limited to the skin (cutaneous PAN).

Uncommon Findings: PAN seldom involves the cerebral or pulmonary vasculature. Palpable purpura is also uncommon. In contrast, MPAN often involves the lung and can lead to pulmonary hemorrhage.

Complications: Infarction of the bowel leading to hemorrhage and/or perforation is one of the most feared complications. Congestive heart failure and myocardial infarction are occasionally seen. MPA can be accompanied by rapidly progressive glomerulonephritis.

Diagnostic Testing: Nonspecific measures of systemic inflammation include elevated acute-phase reactants (ESR or CRP), leukocytosis, anemia of chronic disease, and thrombocytosis. In the setting of renal disease, an abnormal urinalysis with proteinuria, granular or red blood cell casts, and declining creatinine clearance is frequently seen. Hypocomplementemia (low C4, C3) and circulating immune complexes are inconsistently detected; the latter are not recommended because of their poor sensitivity and specificity. Evidence of hepatitis B or C infection should be sought. An angiogram of the mesenteric or renal arteries may strongly suggest PAN if vascular tapering, microaneurysms, and beading are noted. A histologic diagnosis is made by biopsy of a medium-size muscular artery. Biopsies are best performed in areas of documented clinical involvement and may include a sural nerve (with foot drop or neuropathy), a muscle (with myopathy or myalgia), or less preferably, a symptomatic testicle. Renal biopsy is not helpful, as specimens seldom exhibit characteristic abnormalities. MPA is associated with antineutrophil cytoplasmic antibody in the peripheral pattern (p-ANCA).

Keys to Diagnosis: PAN may be a diagnostic challenge. Histopathologic evidence of medium-vessel vasculitis or a pathognomonic angiogram in the appropriate clinical setting confirm a clinical diagnosis.

Diagnostic Criteria: 1990 ACR criteria include (*a*) weight loss of at least 4 kg; (*b*) livedo reticularis; (*c*) testicular pain or tenderness; (*d*) myalgias, weakness, or leg tenderness; (*e*) mononeuropathy or polyneuropathy; (*f*) diastolic blood pressure above 90 mm Hg; (*g*) BUN above 40 mg/dL or creatinine above 1.5 mg/dL; (*h*) hepatitis B virus antigen or antibodies in serum; (*i*) arteriographic abnormalities (e.g., occlusions or aneurysms); and (*j*) small- or medium-sized artery biopsy specimen demonstrating PMN leukocytes. The presence of at least three of these features yields an 82% sensitivity and 87% specificity for the diagnosis of PAN.

Differential Diagnosis: Alternative forms of systemic vasculitis with overlapping features include Wegener's granulomatosis, microscopic polyangiitis, Churg-Strauss angiitis, hypersensitivity vasculitis, and angiitis secondary to amphetamine or cocaine abuse. The vasculitides are compared in Appendix I (see p. 523). Medium-sized vessel arteritis may be a feature of many connective tissue and idiopathic inflammatory disorders (RA, SLE, cryoglobulinemia, and Behçet's syndrome). Occult malignancy, infective endocarditis, cholesterol emboli syndrome, and left atrial myxoma are also in the differential. Hairy cell leukemia has been associated with PAN.

Therapy: In PAN, high-dose corticosteroids are the first line of treatment and are generally begun with at least 1 mg/kg in divided doses. Addition of such cytotoxic agents as cyclophosphamide, and less commonly azathioprine, is often justified, both for steroid sparing and for disease refractory to steroids alone. Some studies suggest improved survival with use of cyclophosphamide. The aggressiveness of therapy is based on the tempo of the disease and the extent of visceral involvement. Addition of plasma exchange to the therapeutic regimen is not of proven benefit. Antiviral therapy with α-interferon should be considered in PAN patients with evidence of active hepatitis B infections. The benign course of limited cutaneous PAN supports conservative therapy for this variant.

Prognosis: PAN is associated with very high morbidity and substantial mortality. Untreated, mortality is over 90%, but with corticosteroids it decreases to 50%. The survival advantages of cytotoxic therapy are controversial. Most mortality is due to renal failure, gastrointestinal perforation/hemorrhage, and cardiac involvement. Patients who survive the initial manifestations of PAN are at high risk of infectious complications because of the potent immunosuppressive therapy necessary to control the disease. Chronic cardiac and/or renal disease are other long-term sequelae.

REFERENCES

Guillevin L, Lhote F. Distinguishing polyarteritis nodosa from microscopic polyangiitis and implications for treatment. Curr Opin Rheumatol 1995;7:20–24.

Jennette C, Falk R, Andrassy K, et al. Nomenclature of systemic vasculitides: proposal of an international consensus conference. Arthritis Rheum 1994;37:187–192.

Lhote F, Guillevin L. Polyarteritis nodosa, microscopic polyangiitis and Churg Strauss syndrome: clinical aspects and treatment. Rheum Dis Clin North Am 1995;21:911–948.

Lightfoot RW, Michel BA, Bloch DA, et al. The American College of Rheumatology 1990 criteria for the classification of polyarteritis nodosa. Arthritis Rheum 1990;33:1088–1093.

POLYMYALGIA RHEUMATICA (PMR)

ICD9 Code: 725.0

Definition: PMR is an inflammatory disorder of older, Caucasian adults that causes pain and stiffness in the proximal musculature.

Etiology: The cause of PMR is unknown. PMR has a strong association with certain HLA markers, especially HLA-DR4. As in rheumatoid arthritis (RA), the genotype HLA-DRB1*04 more commonly occurs in PMR than in the general population. Seasonal clustering of PMR and a preponderance in people of northern latitudes may provide etiopathogenetic clues.

Pathology: No well-defined pathologic lesion has been identified in either muscle or surrounding joints. Arthroscopic synovial biopsy of the shoulders in affected patients has shown low-grade synovitis, suggesting a link with large-joint arthritis.

Demographics: The prevalence of PMR approaches that of RA in older populations. It is almost twice as common in women as in men, and it occurs preferentially in adults of northern European ancestry. It is very uncommon in non-Caucasians. Approximately 85% of PMR patients are over 60 years of age.

Cardinal Findings: Onset before the age of 50 is highly unusual. Symptoms may begin abruptly or insidiously as pain, stiffness, and tenderness in the neck, hip, and shoulder girdle. Prolonged morning stiffness and "gelling" with inactivity is also quite characteristic. Associated constitutional symptoms often include anorexia, weight loss, low-grade fevers, depression, and occasional night sweats. New-onset fatigue, often limiting daily activities, is a significant complaint of many elderly patients and may be influenced by nighttime pain causing disturbed sleep. PMR commonly overlaps with late-onset RA. Synovial swelling may occur in the wrists, knees, and occasionally the small joints of the hands.

Complications: Up to 20% of patients with polymyalgia rheumatica have concurrent temporal arteritis (TA) (see p. 375). This association must be considered because of the risk of sudden blindness and other vascular problems that may be averted with higher doses of corticosteroids. Nonetheless, blind temporal artery biopsies should not be done in PMR patients.

Diagnostic Testing: A moderately to markedly elevated ESR (usually greater than 60 mm/h) or CRP is highly characteristic. Anemia of chronic disease, leukocytosis, reactive thrombocytosis, and decreased albumin are also common. Alkaline phosphatase and hepatic enzymes may be elevated. Factor VIII/von Willebrand factor and other endothelially derived proteins also may be elevated in patients with PMR, but testing is not clinically indicated. Radioisotope scans have identified synovitis in large joints but are not of value clinically.

Keys to Diagnosis: Look for abrupt onset of pain/soreness in the shoulder and hip girdle muscles in association with stiffness, fatigue, and elevated ESR in an older, Caucasian woman or man.

Differential Diagnosis: A myriad of other systemic inflammatory, infectious, and neoplastic disorders can present with similar protean symptoms. Hypothyroidism is a frequent consideration. PMR is differentiated from inflammatory myopathy (dermatomyositis and polymyositis) by the absence of frank muscle weakness or characteristic skin and other nonmusculoskeletal findings. Unlike fibromyalgia, PMR has significant evidence of systemic inflammation, with laboratory abnormalities.

Therapy: Initial treatment with low- to moderate-dose corticosteroid (prednisone, 10–20 mg/day) is highly effective in relieving symptoms. A significant response to prednisone within 2 to 3 days may be diagnostically helpful. Once symptoms are well controlled, corticosteroids may be tapered by approximately 1 to 2 mg/month. Because corticosteroid therapy may frequently be required for more than 2 years, steroid-sparing agents are sometimes considered. Hydroxychloroquine has been successfully used to treat PMR coupled with late-onset RA. NSAIDs may be added to help control mild inflammatory symptoms once the prednisone dose is 10 mg/day or less.

Prognosis: Although it may impose substantial disability, PMR itself is not a life-threatening illness. Nonetheless, considerable morbidity may result from chronic corticosteroid therapy.

REFERENCES

Bird HA, Esselinckx A, Dixon ASJ, et al. An evaluation of criteria for polymyalgia rheumatica. Ann Rheum Dis 1979;38:434–439.

Chuang T-Y, Hunder GG, Ilstrup DM, Kurland LT. Polymyalgia rheumatica: a ten year epidemiologic study. Ann Intern Med 1982;97:672–680.

Weyand CM, Hunder NNH, Hicok KC, et al. HLA-DRB1 alleles in polymyalgia rheumatica, giant cell arteritis, and rheumatoid arthritis. Arthritis Rheum 1994;37:514–520.

POLYMYOSITIS/DERMATOMYOSITIS

Synonyms: Idiopathic inflammatory myopathy, PM/DM, inflammatory myositis

ICD9 Code: Dermatomyositis, 710.3; Polymyositis, 710.4

Definition: Polymyositis (PM) and dermatomyositis (DM) are types of idiopathic inflammatory myopathy (IIM). Other less common causes of IIM, such as inclusion body myositis (IBM; see p. 240), are listed in Table 1. IIM is characterized clinically by proximal muscle weakness, histopathologically by inflammation and damage to skeletal muscle, and serologically by elevated concentrations of muscle-derived proteins (e.g., creatinine kinase (CK)).

Etiology: There is no known cause for these conditions. Somewhat distinct histopathologic findings suggest that DM, PM, and IBM may have different causes. A number of cases of IIM, particularly DM, occur in patients with malignancies (see below).

Table 1
Idiopathic Inflammatory Myopathies

I. Polymyositis/dermatomyositis
  A. Adult polymyositis
  B. Adult dermatomyositis
  C. Dermatomyositis associated with malignancy
  D. Juvenile dermatomyositis (or, less commonly, juvenile polymyositis)
  E. Overlap (i.e., DM or PM associated with another autoimmune disease, particularly
    SLE or scleroderma)
II. Inclusion body myositis
III. Miscellaneous
  A. Dermatomyositis *sine* myositis (amyopathic dermatomyositis; i.e. patients with
    the characteristic DM skin lesions without associated muscle inflammation)
  B. Myositis associated with infection
  C. Focal myositis (e.g. orbital myositis)
  D. Myositis associated with drugs or toxins
  E. Granulomatous myositis (e.g., in sarcoidosis, mycobacterial infection)

Pathology: Histopathologic analysis of muscle tissue shows a mononuclear cell infiltrate, consisting predominantly of lymphocytes that surround or invade muscle fibers. Muscle fiber necrosis, degeneration, phagocytosis, and regeneration are also seen; atrophy, fibrosis, and fat replacement are late findings. In typical PM, the predominant cells are cytotoxic CD8+ T cells that are endomysial in location. In typical DM, the infiltrates are predominantly perimysial and consist of CD4+ T cells and B cells. Deposition of complement fragments (e.g., the membrane attack complex) in the muscle microvasculature causes vascular injury, leading to vasculitis and perifascicular atrophy.

Genetics: Some cases of DM are associated with the MHC alleles HLA-DR3 and DRw52. (*Note:* this genotype is associated with formation of antibodies to aminoacyl-tRNA synthetase; see below.)

Demographics: The overall prevalence of PM and DM is 5 to 10 cases per million population. Whereas PM is more common (1.5:1) than DM in adults, the reverse is true in children. Peak incidence occurs between 40 and 60 years of age. The female:male ratio is 2:1. Familial aggregation is rare (thus, a family history of muscle problems should suggest an alternative diagnosis).

Cardinal Findings: IIM may affect skeletal muscle, skin, and other sites.

—*Muscle:* Most patients present with symmetric, proximal muscle weakness. Involvement of the large muscles of the legs and arms may compromise activities such as climbing stairs, getting in and out of a car, rising from the tub or toilet, and raising arms over the head. Neck weakness may cause difficulty raising the head while recumbent. Less than half of patients complain of myalgia at the onset. Pharyngeal skeletal muscle may be involved, causing upper pharyngeal dysphagia, dysphonia, nasal regurgitation, and the risk of aspiration. Some patients have involvement of the respiratory muscles (e.g., diaphragm or intercostals), which may result in dyspnea, respiratory failure, or even death.

—*Skin:* Patients with several characteristic cutaneous manifestations and inflammatory myositis are said to have DM. *Gottron's papules* are raised, scaly, erythematous or violaceous, nontender lesions commonly seen over the MCPs, PIPs, or knees; they are seen in more than 70% of DM patients. The *heliotrope rash* is a purplish ("violaceous") rash over the eyelids, often accompanied by periorbital edema. An erythematous or *violaceous "V-neck" or "shawl" pattern rash* is often noted in sun-exposed areas, affecting the upper chest, upper back, and base of the neck. *Periungual erythema* and dilated nailfold capillaries may be seen. Nailfold capillaroscopy (see p. 129) may show capillary dilatation or hemorrhage similar to that seen in scleroderma. *"Mechanic's hands"* (hyperkeratosis and scaling over the fingers) and *calcinosis* (soft tissue calcification) are uncommon. Calcinosis is more common in children.

—*Other findings:* Cardiac involvement (e.g., dysrhythmia, ECG changes) may be detected in 50% of patients but is infrequently systomatic. Pulmonary involvement is less common and includes respiratory muscle weakness and interstitial lung disease. Some patients display constitutional symptoms including fever, weight loss, anorexia, and malaise.

Complications: Pulmonary involvement (aspiration pneumonia, interstitial lung disease, respiratory failure) is the most common cause of death. Cardiomyopathy is a rare, but serious complication of PM/DM. Persistently active disease may cause substantial muscle loss and irreversible weakness.

Juvenile Dermatomyositis: DM is much more common (20:1) than PM in children. The peak age of onset is 5 to 14 years, and it is associated genetically with the MHC HLA-B8 and DR-3 alleles. Classically, the DM rash, which closely resembles rashes in the adult, precedes muscle involvement. There are several important differences between adult and childhood DM. Coexistent vasculitis, ectopic calcification of subcutaneous tissue or muscle, and lipodystrophy are more common in children with DM than adults. It has been suggested that measurements of aldolase may be more useful than CK in childhood myositis. In contrast with adult DM, childhood DM is rarely associated with malignancy. With successful therapy, children with DM return to normal strength and function more frequently than adults.

PM/DM and Malignancy: The possible association of IIM with malignancy has been debated in the medical literature for nearly a century. Studies have been hampered by small numbers of patients. Approximately 9% of PM and 15% or more of DM cases are associated with malignancy. The cancer may precede, follow, or be diagnosed concurrently with the myositis. In about 1/5 of DM cases, the tumor behaves as a "paraneoplastic" syndrome, with the activities of the two conditions apparently linked. The cancers observed are the same as those seen in the general population (i.e., in the United States, lung and breast cancer; in Japan, gastric cancer), although it has been suggested that ovarian cancer is seen with greater frequency. Most investigators recommend that only a thorough, directed history, physical, and laboratory evaluation (appropriate for the patient's age and sex) be performed. No evidence supports more extensive testing (imaging studies, tumor markers, etc.); such investigations are expensive and unlikely to yield useful data.

Diagnostic Criteria: See Table 2.

Diagnostic Tests

—*Markers of muscle damage:* Elevation in serum CK reflects skeletal muscle injury; CK is the most commonly used diagnostic test in PM/DM. Its advantages include (*a*) sensitivity (elevations in CK are observed in at least 70–90% of cases); (*b*) relative specificity for skeletal muscle (although CK is also found in brain and myocardium); (*c*) correlation of CK levels with disease activity (increases may be seen weeks before a clinical flare; normalization correlates with successful treatment); and (*d*) dynamic range (increases in CK with PM/DM are often 20–50 times normal). *Note:* Normal CK levels vary with sex (higher in men) and race (higher in blacks). Other tests that reflect muscle injury include aldolase (also relatively specific), LDH, AST, and less commonly ALT.

—*Electromyography:* EMG is very useful for confirming the diagnosis of PM/DM. It is abnormal in more than 90% of patients and can help exclude other potential causes of muscle weakness (e.g., neuropathy). EMG findings characteristic of PM/DM include myopathic motor unit potentials (small units, early recruitment), a myopathic interference pattern (full, low amplitude), and spontaneous and insertional activity (fibrillations, positive sharp waves, com-

Table 2
Diagnostic Criteria for PM/DM (Bohan and Peter)

Criterion	Definition
Muscle weakness	Symmetric proximal muscle weakness (limb girdle muscles and anterior neck flexors) progressing over weeks to months, with or without dysphagia or respiratory muscle involvement
Muscle histology	Inflammatory cellular infiltrate, often perivascular, with myofiber necrosis
Serum enzymes	Elevation in serum of skeletal-muscle enzymes, particularly CK or aldolase; LDH, AST, and ALT may also be elevated
EMG	Electromyographic evidence of low-amplitude polyphasic motor unit potentials, fibrillation, positive sharp waves, insertional activity
Rash (DM)	Gottron's papules, heliotrope rash, erythematous patchy rash on sun-exposed areas

PM or DM is definite when the patient has 4 of 5 criteria; probable when 3 criteria are present; and possible when 2 are present. Patients with DM must have a characteristic rash.

plex repetitive discharges, but not fasciculations). Nerve conduction velocity (NCV) studies should be normal. EMG is also used in longitudinal follow-up of disease activity in PM/DM patients. It can be useful in determining whether new symptoms of weakness relate to recurrence of inflammatory activity or some other cause (e.g., steroid myopathy). Practical considerations for EMG include (a) doing muscle enzyme determinations before EMG, because the procedure may elevate them, and (b) doing EMG unilaterally to allow biopsy on the contralateral side.

—*Muscle biopsy:* Specimens may be required to confirm the diagnosis. Needle biopsies may provide sufficient tissue for examination, but definitive open surgical biopsies are commonly used. The biopsy yield may be improved by prior localization of involved muscle by EMG or MRI (see below). (Histopathologic changes in PM/DM are discussed above). Proper procedures for handling the tissue should be discussed with the pathologist who will receive the specimen.

—*MRI:* Magnetic resonance imaging is a relatively new approach to the evaluation of IIM. T1-weighted images provide detail of muscle anatomy, but T2-weighted images are better for detecting inflammation. Fat-suppressed T2 (STIR) images may also be useful. While MRI seems promising in evaluating PM/DM, it is expensive, and the results have not yet been widely correlated with histopathologic findings; thus, it is not routinely recommended.

—*Autoantibodies:* ANA is positive in 50 to 80% of PM/DM patients (thus it usually does not help in evaluating any single patient). Autoantibodies to certain aminoacyl-tRNA synthetases are characteristic of certain subsets of IIM; for example, anti-Jo-1 (anti-histidyl-tRNA synthetase) and anti-PL-7 (anti-threonyl-tRNA synthetase). These antibodies are found in 25 to 30% of patients (more with PM than DM). Patients with antisynthetase antibodies comprise a distinct clinical subset of myositis patients, with disease characterized by interstitial lung disease, polyarticular arthritis (particularly of the small joints of the hands), Raynaud's, fever, acute onset, and "mechanic's hands" rash.

—*Other tests:* Acute-phase reactants (e.g., CRP and ESR) are elevated in about 50% of cases.

Differential Diagnosis: The differential diagnosis of IIM includes various neuromuscular, metabolic, endocrinologic, infectious, and other causes of muscle weakness (Table 3). The evaluation of weakness (see p. 57) and myopathy (see p. 261) is discussed elsewhere.

Therapy: Early recognition and treatment of PM/DM are critical. Delays in treatment increase the chance of irreversible muscle damage and decrease the likelihood of a full recovery. Glucocorticosteroids are the mainstay of therapy. Initial doses are usually 1 mg/kg or more of prednisone. These high doses are used for weeks to months to achieve disease control and lower serum muscle enzyme levels. Steroids may then be tapered over the next 2 to 3 months while the patient's symptoms (weakness) and muscle enzymes are carefully monitored. The response to steroids is often slow and may take 8 to 12 weeks. About 25% of

Table 3
Differential Diagnosis of PM/DM

Neuromuscular disease
   Myasthenia gravis
   Guillain-Barré syndrome
   Eaton-Lambert syndrome
   Muscular dystrophy
   Mitochondrial myopathy
   Muscle necrosis (e.g., due to trauma, rhabdomyolysis)
Metabolic muscle disease
   Myophosphorylase deficiency (McArdle's disease)
   Lipid storage disease
   Myoadenylate deaminase deficiency
Endocrinopathies
   Hypo- or hyperthyroidism
   Hypercortisolism (Cushing's disease)
   Hypo- or hyperparathyroidism
   Hypokalemia (including periodic paralysis)
   Diabetes mellitus
Toxic myopathy due to drugs
   Ethanol
   Corticosteroids
   Colchicine
   Chloroquine
   Cocaine
   HMG-CoA reductase inhibitors
   Cyclosporine
Drugs associated with IIM
   Zidovudine (AZT)
   D-Penicillamine
Infections
   Viruses
      HIV
      HTLV-1
      Coxsackie
      Picorna
      Influenza
   Bacteria
      Suppurative anaerobic staphylococci and streptococci (tropical pyomyositis)
      Lyme disease
      Clostridial myonecrosis
      Mycobacteria (tuberculosis, leprosy)
   Parasite
      Trichinosis
      Toxoplasmosis
      Cysticercosis
      Trypanosoma cruzi (Chagas' disease)
   Fungi
      Candida

patients have a complete response, 60% a partial response, and 15% no response to an initial prednisone trial. In patients with no response or partial response to prednisone, second-line agents are commonly used to improve outcome and limit exposure to steroids. Methotrexate (15 to 25 mg/week) or azathioprine (1 to 2 mg/kg/day) are most commonly used, often in combination with prednisone initially. High-dose immunoglobulin (intravenous IgG (IVIG), 2 g/kg) has been successful, but response is transient.

—*Steroid myopathy:* Steroids can cause a myopathy, which becomes a consideration in patients receiving chronic therapy with these drugs. EMG or muscle biopsy are often required to distinguish steroid myopathy from active IIM.

—*Physical therapy:* In addition to pharmacologic therapy, treatment of patients with PM/DM may include physiotherapy to improve functional status and facilitate rehabilitation.

REFERENCES

Bohan A, Peter JB. Polymyositis and dermatomyositis (parts 1 and 2). N Engl J Med 1975;292:344–347, 403–407.

Dalakas MC. Polymyositis, dermatomyositis, and inclusion-body myositis. N Engl J Med 1991;325:1487–1498.

Joffe MM, Love LA, Leff RL, et al. Drug therapy of the idiopathic inflammatory myopathies: predictors of response to prednisone, azathioprine and methotrexate and a comparison of their efficacy. Am J Med 1993;94:379–387.

Plotz PH, Rider LG, Targoff IN, et al. Myositis: immunologic contributions to understanding cause, pathogenesis, and therapy. Ann Intern Med 1995;122:715–724.

Sigurgeirsson B, Lindelöf B, Edhag O, Allander E. Risk of cancer in patients with dermatomyositis or polymyositis; a population based study. N Engl J Med 1992;326:363–367.

PSORIATIC ARTHRITIS

Synonyms: Psoriatic spondylitis, arthritis mutilans

ICD9 Code: Psoriatic arthritis, 696.0; cutaneous psoriasis 696.1

Definition: Psoriatic arthritis is an inflammatory arthropathy that occurs in individuals with established cutaneous psoriasis, with or without nail changes. Most patients have mild-moderate, manageable arthritis, but some exhibit progressive, erosive, or disabling arthritis.

Etiology: No etiologic agent or reactive process has been proven, although stress, trauma, heat-shock proteins, and infection with streptococcus or staphylococcus have been implicated. Genetic associations with psoriatic arthritis are heterogeneous. Cutaneous psoriasis is associated with HLA-B13, HLA-B17, HLA-37, and HLA-Cw6. By contrast, HLA-B39 and HLA-B27 have been associated with psoriatic sacroiliitis and spondylitis. HLA-Cw6, HLA-Bw38, HLA-DR4, and HLA-DR7 have been linked with peripheral arthropathy.

Pathology: Histopathology of psoriatic synovitis is similar to that seen in other inflammatory arthritides such as RA. There is usually a lack of intrasynovial immunoglobulin and rheumatoid factor production, and a greater propensity for fibrous ankylosis, osseous resorption, and heterotopic bone formation.

Demographics: Psoriatic arthritis develops in 5% of psoriasis patients. Risk increases with a family history of spondyloarthropathy or extensive nail pitting. Age of onset is usually between 30 and 55 years. Although psoriatic arthritis affects men and women equally, psoriatic spondylitis has a male:female ratio of 2.3:1.

Disease Subsets: Six variants of psoriatic arthritis have been described. These variants are not mutually exclusive, and patients may possess overlapping features.

1. Asymmetric oligoarthritis is seen in 30–40% of patients and involves large and small joints. "Sausage digits" (dactylitis) of the fingers or toes may be present. Skin disease may be minimal or overlooked.
2. Distal interphalangeal (DIP) arthritis is seen in 10 to 15% of patients. A strong association with nail changes (nail pitting) exists.
3. Rheumatoid arthritis–like polyarthritis (25–50% of patients) with symmetric arthritis, but lacks serum rheumatoid factor or nodules.
4. Psoriatic spondylitis is seen in approximately 20% of psoriatic arthritis patients, 50% of whom are HLA-B27 positive.
5. Arthritis mutilans, seen in 5% or less of patients, presents as destructive, erosive, polyarticular arthritis affecting the hands and feet. It often leads to deformity and disability.
6. HIV-associated psoriatic arthritis. The severity of psoriatic arthritis appears to be enhanced by coexistent HIV infection. Such patients often have aggressive cutaneous psoriasis, severe pauciarticular or polyarticular arthritis, impressive enthesitis, and poor correlation with CD4 lymphocyte counts. Spondylitis and uveitis are rare.

Cardinal Findings: Psoriatic arthritis typically has an insidious onset and a progressive course. The arthritis may manifest as axial or peripheral joint stiffness, pain, or swelling. Peripheral arthritis may present as a chronic, asymmetric oligoarthropathy, a symmetric DIP polyarthritis, or a rheumatoid-like (MCPs and PIPs) polyarthrititis. Inflammatory sausage-like swelling of the digits (dactylitis) involving the fingers or toes is common. Psoriatic spondylitis is seen in 20% of patients and manifests as spinal stiffness, pain, or limited range of motion affecting the lumbosacral more than cervical spine. Enthesitis (inflammation where tendon inserts on bone) manifests as pain in the heel, greater trochanter, or anterior iliac crest. Psoriatic arthritis tends to arise in patients with established cutaneous disease. However, in children and young adults, the arthritis may precede the development of psoriasis by months or years. The degree of psoriatic skin disease correlates poorly with the extent of arthritis. A careful examination of the scalp, buttocks, umbilicus, genitalia, and nails (fingers and toes) may reveal psoriatic lesions. Typical nail lesions may include pitting, onycholysis, subungual hyperkeratosis, and transverse ridging. Eye disease (conjunctivitis, iritis, episcleritis, or keratoconjunctivitis sicca) occurs in up to 30% of patients.

Uncommon Findings: Myopathy and aortic insufficiency are rare. A minority of patients have clinical and radiographic features that overlap with Reiter's syndrome.

Complications: This is a risk for limited spinal mobility and spinal fracture in patients with spondylitis and ankylosis. Aortic insufficiency is rarely symptomatic.

Diagnostic Tests: Inflammatory indices with increased ESR or anemia of chronic disease are common. Hyperuricemia may be found and often correlates with the severity of cutaneous psoriasis. Synovial fluid WBC counts range from 2000 to 40000 cells/mm^3, with a neutrophil predominance.

Imaging: Radiographic changes include soft tissue swelling, erosions, and periostitis. DIP disease or arthritis mutilans may develop a typical "pencil and cup" deformity resulting from erosive change and formation of reactive, heterotopic bone in the phalanges. Psoriatic spondylitis is characterized by asymmetric sacroiliitis and spondylitis with asymmetric, nonmarginal, "bulky" syndesmophytes (bridging osteophytes between vertebrae). Acroosteolysis, paravertebral ossification, and pericapsular calcification are uncommon.

Keys to Diagnosis: Look for psoriatic cutaneous or nail changes in association with one of the recognized articular subsets. Carefully examine scalp, ears, buttocks, nails, and umbilicus for psoriatic lesions.

Diagnostic Criteria: None are validated.

Differential Diagnosis: Cutaneous psoriasis should be distinguished from seborrheic dermatitis, fungal infection, exfoliative dermatitis, eczema, Gottron's papules, keratoderma blennorrhagica, and palmoplantar pustulosis. Psoriatic arthritis should be distinguished from erosive osteoarthritis, gout, RA, pauciarticular juvenile arthritis, ankylosing spondylitis, and Reiter's syndrome.

Therapy: Treatment should be aimed at reducing pain, swelling, and stiffness while preserving optimal function and halting disease progression. The foundation of therapy should include patient education, joint protection, a rational program of exercise and rest, physical therapy, occupational therapy, and dietary and vocational counseling. Patients with psoriatic spondylitis should be reminded that lifelong physical therapy is necessary to maintain an erect posture. Treatment of skin disease may include sunlight, topical agents (e.g., corticosteroids), or methoxypsoralen and PUVA. Specific articular therapies may include:

—*NSAIDs:* NSAIDs may modify symptoms in some, but they do not suppress disease progression. All NSAIDs are equally efficacious and possess similar toxicity profiles. However, some advocate indomethacin and diclofenac as having greater efficacy in the spondyloarthropathies. Antiinflammatory (higher) doses may be necessary to control inflammation, although an increased risk of GI and renal toxicity may result.

—*Corticosteroids:* Corticosteroid therapy is infrequently used, but may be used as an intraarticular steroid injection (for uncontrolled mono- or oligoarthritis), intralesional steroid to control enthesitis (i.e., Achilles tendinitis or plantar fasciitis), or topical steroid for treatment of conjunctivitis or uveitis. Use of oral low-dose prednisone (5–10 mg/day) should be reserved for severe, uncontrolled peripheral arthritis. Oral steroids are seldom effective in patients with psoriatic spondylitis. Withdrawal of oral steroids may incite a flare of skin disease and should be avoided in pustular psoriasis.

—*Slow-Acting Antirheumatic Drugs (SAARDs):* SAARDs are indicated when initial NSAID attempts are unsuccessful or contraindicated. Sulfasalazine and methotrexate have been tested and advocated for use in psoriatic arthritis. Placebo-controlled trials of sulfasalazine (2 g/day) indicate greatest efficacy in patients with peripheral arthritis and enthesitis. It is uncertain if patients with longstanding erosive disease, spondylitis, sacroiliitis, or ankylosis will respond to sulfasalazine. Nonetheless, sulfasalazine should be considered in poorly controlled spondylitis patients. The usual dose of sulfasalazine is 2 to 4 g/day.

Methotrexate at doses of 7.5–20 mg/week, orally, subcutaneously, or intramuscularly) is often effective in the treatment of both cutaneous and articular psoriasis. Higher doses and prolonged use have been associated with unacceptable hepatotoxicity and cirrhosis. Unlike RA, liver biopsy should be considered in those receiving a cumulative dose above 1500 mg and those with persistently abnormal hepatic enzymes. Cyclosporine (3–5 mg/kg/day) has a narrow therapeutic window and an increased risk for toxicity (GI, renal, hypertension) but may be very effective in controlling cutaneous and articular disease in patients unresponsive to conventional measures.

Patients have also benefited from treatment with gold salts (i.e., myochrysine), hydroxychloroquine, azathioprine, or etretinate. Sulfasalazine or etretinate should be considered for HIV-associated psoriatic arthritis.

Monitoring: Monitoring is tailored to the disease severity and the medications used. For example, stable psoriatic spondylitis patients receiving indomethacin may need evaluation every 3 to 6 months, while a patient with uncontrolled, severe polyarthritis on methotrexate or cyclosporine may require monthly assessment.

Surgery: Surgery should be considered when pain and immobility markedly interfere with the patient's lifestyle. Total joint replacement is commonly performed in the hip or knee. The success of arthroplasty may be limited by postsurgical heterotopic bone formation. Surgical correction of spinal deformities or fusion is generally not advised.

REFERENCES

Bulbul R, Williams WV, Schumacher HR Jr. Psoriatic arthritis. Diverse and sometimes highly destructive. Postgrad Med 1995;97:97–108.
Clegg DO, Reda DJ, Mejias E, et al. Comparison of sulfasalazine and placebo in the treatment

of psoriatic arthritis: a Department of Veterans Affairs Cooperative study. Arthritis Rheum 1996;39:2013–2020.

Cush JJ, Lipsky PE. The spondyloarthropathies. In: Goldman L, Bennett JC, eds. Cecil textbook of internal medicine. 21st ed. Philadelphia: WB Saunders, in press.

Vasey FB. Seronegative spondyloarthropathies: psoriatic arthritis. In: Schumacher HR Jr, ed. Primer on the rheumatic diseases. Atlanta: Arthritis Foundation, 1996:161–163.

RAYNAUD'S PHENOMENON

Synonyms: Raynaud's disease

ICD9 Code: 443.0

Definition: Raynaud's phenomenon is paroxysmal, reversible vasospasm of small arteries, which may be triggered by cold exposure or stress. When it occurs in the absence of another underlying connective tissue disease, the term *primary Raynaud's syndrome* or *Raynaud's disease* is used.

Etiology: Structural and functional alterations of blood vessels are probably contributory. Arteries are usually narrowed (see "Pathology," below), so even normal vasospastic responses may occlude the lumen. Other data suggest changes in mediators of vascular tone, such as endothelin. Underlying causes for these abnormalities are unknown.

Pathology: Digital arteries show proliferation of subintimal tissues and fibrotic change. Small thrombi may form on the altered intimal surfaces. Luminal narrowing or occlusion can occur in these small vessels as well as in larger arteries. Vasculitis is not present.

Demographics: Females predominate and account for at least 80% of those with Raynaud's phenomenon. Raynaud's disease may appear in younger women than the corresponding syndrome occurring in association with other connective tissue disorders. Almost all patients with systemic sclerosis have Raynaud's phenomenon.

Associated Conditions: Raynaud's phenomenon may be associated with diffuse and limited (CREST) systemic sclerosis, SLE, MCTD, RA, polymyositis, cryoglobulinemia, and Sjögren's syndrome.

Cardinal Findings: The classic "red, white, and blue" changes do not occur in all cases. Initially, severe blanching, or "white," is due to vasospasm and lack of arterial perfusion. This phase is uncommon and is followed by the commonly observed blueness due to venous pooling and tissue cyanosis. On rewarming, reactive painful hyperemia causes redness in the fingers or hand. These changes are usually bilateral and accompanied by pain. The hands are most commonly affected, but feet and the tips of the nose and ears also can be involved.

Patients with primary Raynaud's phenomenon have a normal physical examination and only manifest physical findings in the distal extremities. Such patients usually have normal nailfold capillaries (see p. 129) and a low risk of developing other connective tissue diseases.

Patients with secondary Raynaud's phenomenon clearly demonstrate evidence of the underlying connective tissue disorder (e.g., sclerodactyly, malar rash, arthritis). Nailfold capillaroscopy should be abnormal. The prognosis is guarded.

Uncommon Findings: Distal finger pad ulcerations and scarring are uncommon. In extreme cases, gangrene and autoamputation may develop.

Diagnostic Tests: The diagnosis is made largely on clinical data (history, physical examination). In patients without evidence of an associated connective tissue disorder (e.g., scleroderma or SLE), measurement of ANA may be useful in predicting the risk of developing such disorders.

Imaging: Changes in small capillaries can be viewed by nailfold capillaroscopy (see p. 129), which may provide prognostically important information. Radiographs show osteolysis of distal phalanges. Angiography is rarely required to distinguish Raynaud's phenomenon from occluding blood clots or cholesterol emboli.

Keys to Diagnosis: Cold-induced pain, pallor, or cyanosis of digits is an important clue.

Differential Diagnosis: Atherosclerotic occlusion of small vessels occurs in older individuals, has a male predominance, and is less likely to be symmetric. Thromboangiitis obliterans (Buerger's disease) involves lower extremities more often than the hands and is usually accompanied by claudication. Heavy cigarette smoking can cause symptomatic vasospasm; a careful tobacco use history is important for all patients. Other causes of "blue" digits include cryoglobulinemia, hyperviscosity states, and the antiphospholipid syndrome.

Therapy: The hands and feet should be kept warm with gloves and other coverings that may be required both at night and during the day. Ulcerated finger tips may require protective bandages or guards. Tobacco should be discontinued, and certain medications (e.g., β-blockers, ergotamine, amphetamines) should be avoided. Biofeedback training may be effective. A few pharmacologic agents, such as long-acting forms of nifedipine, are useful and well-tolerated; blood pressure should be closely monitored. Antiplatelet therapy (e.g., ASA or dipyridamole) is advisable in some. Topical nitrates may help with digits, but use may be limited by headaches.

Surgery: Truncal or digital sympathectomy may be attempted if local measures and drugs are ineffective. Digital ischemic ulcers are best treated with local wound care measures rather than with surgical intervention. Gangrenous fingertips should be allowed to self-demarcate whenever possible.

Prognosis: For patients with secondary Raynaud's, outcome is related to the underlying disease. Raynaud's phenomenon has such a high prevalence in scleroderma (see pp. 183, 343) that it does not identify a prognostic subset. Patients may have an increased chance of developing other connective tissue disorders if Raynaud's phenomenon is accompanied by abnormal periungual capillaries, puffy fingers, pitting of the nails, or serum autoantibodies.

REFERENCES

Medsger TA. Systemic sclerosis (scleroderma): clinical aspects. In: Koopman WJ, ed. Arthritis and allied conditions: a textbook of rheumatology. 13th ed. Baltimore: Williams & Wilkins, 1997:1433–1464.

Wigley FM, Flavahan NA. Raynaud's phenomenon. Rheum Dis Clin North Am 1996;22: 765–781.

REFLEX SYMPATHETIC DYSTROPHY (RSD)

ICD9 Code: 733.7

Synonyms: Shoulder-hand syndrome; Sudeck's atrophy; algodystrophy

Definition: Reflex sympathetic dystrophy is diffuse persistent pain, usually in an extremity, often associated with vasomotor disturbances, trophic changes, and limitation or immobility of joints. Causalgia, a different syndrome, refers to a traumatized peripheral nerve with resultant pain along the distribution of that nerve.

Etiology: Many diseases have been associated with RSD: trauma, fractures (especially Colles' fracture), hemiplegia (prevalence of RSD 12–21%), arterial thrombosis, peripheral nerve injury (prevalence, 3%), coronary artery disease (prevalence, 5–20%), painful rotator cuff lesions, herpes zoster with postherpetic neuralgia, and spinal cord disorders. It is idiopathic in 25% of cases. Pathogenesis is obscure. RSD may be a disorder of pain signaling and regulation, as well as a persisting neural injury generating pain signals with reflex neurologic mechanisms involved. It has been proposed that primary afferent nociceptor neurons develop α_1-adrenoreceptors, making them responsive to norepinephrine released by sympathetic nerve terminals. This may in part explain the reduction in pain by α1-antagonists. Central mechanisms of neuronal hyperresponsitivity may also be a factor, especially at later stages of this syndrome.

Pathology: Skin and subcutaneous tissue are usually normal. Affected bone is hyperemic with patchy osteoporosis. There may be synovial proliferation with minimal inflammatory cell infiltrate.

Demographics: In adults, there is a slight female predominance. It is reported in all ages, most commonly between 40 and 60 years. In children, 80% are female, often with lower extremity involvement.

Cardinal Findings: Three overlapping stages have been recognized in RSD, although the validity and usefulness of this approach has been questioned. The *acute stage* lasts 3–6 months and is characterized by intense limb pain, tenderness, swelling, and vasomotor disturbances (cyanosis or erythema, hyperhidrosis). The *dystrophic (or subacute) stage* lasts 6–12 months, during which acute symptoms resolve (often incompletely) while atrophic changes in the skin evolve, and chronic aching or burning pain persists. Skin becomes dry and may be edematous or develop a brawny thickening. In the *atrophic stage*, skin and subcutaneous atrophy and contractures predominate.

—*Site:* RSD is usually unilateral and affects the upper extremity more often than the lower extremity. It may involve the entire hand or foot. RSD may be bilateral in 25% of cases.

—*Pain:* Pain is often constant, burning, and severe early on. Chronic aching pain or myofascial limb pain may be present.

—*Appearance:* There is swelling, trophic skin changes and signs of vasomotor (Raynaud's phenomenon, temperature variation) and sudomotor (sweating) instability. Pitting or nonpitting edema are usually present.

—*Tenderness:* Exquisite tenderness occurs, especially in periarticular tissues. Allodynia (pain induced by light touch) and hyperpathia (persistent pain after light pressure) are characteristic.

—*Neurologic changes:* Tremor, incoordination, weakness, or sensory changes may occur.

Uncommon Findings: Nail changes and segmental involvement (one or two digital rays of the hand or foot) or involvement of knee, hip, portions of bone (zonal), or femoral head can be seen.

Diagnostic Tests: Common laboratory tests (CBC, chemistry, ESR) are not useful.

Imaging: Plain radiography shows patchy or mottled osteopenia; however, this is neither sensitive nor specific. Late cases have a ground-glass appearance. Cortical breaks and crumbling erosion may also be noted. Scintigraphy is the most useful objective test. Three-phase bone scan shows asymmetry in all three phases, increased or decreased blood flow, pool, and uptake phases.

Keys to Diagnosis: Look for pain and swelling in a distal extremity with trophic skin changes and vasomotor instability, often with a history of preceding trauma (especially fracture), myocardial infarction, hemiplegic stroke, or peripheral nerve injury (Table 1).

Therapy: Early diagnosis or prevention is important, especially in high-risk individuals (trauma, myocardial infarction, hemiplegia). Treat the underlying problem, if one is identified. Once RSD is established, initiate therapy early: analgesia, local heat, ice, physical therapy, and stress-loading and desensitization programs. Pharmacologic maneuvers include sympathetic blockage, followed by sympathectomy in those that respond (70–80% improve). Oral α_1-antagonists (phenoxybenzamine, prazosin, terazosin, doxazosin) may be useful. Systemic corticosteroids (e.g., prednisone 20–60 mg/day for 4–6 weeks) may be useful in patients with "hot" bone scans, especially early in the disease. Calcitonin may also be useful. Recalcitrant disease is often managed by the princi-

Table 1
Proposed Diagnostic Criteria for RSD

Definite RSD
1. Pain associated with allodynia or hyperpathia
2. Tenderness
3. Vasomotor and sudomotor changes
    Cool, pallid extremity (vasospasm)
    Warm erythematous extremity (hyperemia)
    Hyperhidrosis or hypertrichosis
4. Dystrophic skin changes
    Shiny skin with loss of normal wrinkling
    Atrophy
    Scaling
    Nail changes (color, friable)
    Thickened palmar/plantar fascia
5. Swelling
Probable RSD
1. Pain and allodynia
2. Vasomotor or sudomotor changes
3. Swelling
Possible RSD
1. Vasomotor or sudomotor changes
2. Swelling

ples of chronic pain management. Rarely, amputation has been resorted to; even this measure may leave the patient with phantom limb pain.

Prognosis: Overall, 50% of patients still have significant pain or disability after 2 years.

REFERENCES

Dhar S, Kleneran L. Reflex sympathetic dystrophy (algodystrophy). Br J Rheumatol 1993;21:2–3.
Kozin F. Painful shoulder and the reflex sympathetic dystrophy syndrome. In: Koopman WJ, ed. Arthritis and allied conditions: a textbook of rheumatology. 13th ed. Baltimore: Williams & Wilkins, 1997:1908–1915.

REITER'S SYNDROME

Synonyms: Reactive arthritis, incomplete Reiter's, sexually acquired reactive arthritis

ICD9 Code: 099.3

Definition: Reiter's syndrome is the most common form of reactive arthritis. Reactive arthritis is an acute inflammatory arthritis occurring 1 to 4 weeks after an infection. Reiter's syndrome and reactive arthritis share a postinfectious onset, asymmetric oligoarthritis, extraarticular sites of inflammation, and an association with HLA-B27. The arthritis is usually self-limited but may be chronic and disabling.

Etiology: HLA-B27 positivity is seen in 75 to 80% of Caucasians with Reiter's syndrome, but only 50% of African Americans. HLA-B27 (see p. 118) is associated with increased disease susceptibility, greater disease severity, and risk of developing spinal disease and uveitis. Several arthritogenic bacteria have been associated with reactive arthritis. There may be molecular mimicry between bacterial antigens and self-proteins. Postdysenteric reactive arthritis may arise in those who are HLA-B27 negative, many of whom have HLA-B7 or other cross reactive antigens.

Pathology: Characteristic findings include inflammatory synovitis, inflammation and erosions at the insertion of ligaments and tendons (entheses), excessive production of heterotopic bone at sites of inflammation, and cutaneous pathology similar to that observed in psoriasis. Subclinical intestinal inflammation of the terminal ileum or colon occurs in 60% of patients and may parallel the clinical status and response to therapy.

Demographics: Reiter's syndrome is the most common cause of inflammatory arthritis in young men. In Minnesota, the age-adjusted incidence rate for males (<50 years) was 3.5 cases per 100,000 men. Recent studies suggest that its frequency is decreasing in the HIV era, possibly because of increased use of condoms. Peak onset is during the third decade, but Reiter's syndrome may also be seen in children. Male:female ratio is 5:1 or 6:1 or above. Women may go undiagnosed because of occult genitourinary disease and less-severe arthritis. Postvenereal Reiter's syndrome is more common in males, yet postdysenteric Reiter's syndrome affects men and women equally. With epidemic dysentery due to arthritogenic strains, 5% of infected individuals, and 20% of infected HLA-B27-positive individuals, develop reactive arthritis.

Infectious Triggers: The most common pathogens known to induce Reiter's syndrome are enteric (*Shigella, Salmonella, Yersinia,* or *Campylobacter*) or urogenital/postvenereal (*Chlamydia, Ureaplasma,* HIV) pathogens. With enteric infections, the diarrheal illness resolves before the onset of arthritis (usually 1–4 weeks later). HLA-B27-negative Reiter's patients may been seen with epidemic dysentery. Between 2 and 6% of patients develop Reiter's syndrome following epidemic dysentery due to *Shigella (S. flexneri)* and *Salmonella (S. typhimurium)*. In most instances, no infectious cause can be identified.

—*Chlamydia trachomatis:* More than 50% of patients with Reiter's syndrome have antibodies to *C. trachomatis*. Rheumatic features of *Chlamydia* infections are similar to those described in classic Reiter's syndrome, except less than 50% are B27 positive, 15% have no urogenital features, and more than 50% develop chronic arthritis. Diagnosis is suggested by persistent mono- or oligoarthritis; genitourinary symptoms; positive serologic tests, cultures, or PCR evidence of chlamydial infection and a response to antibiotic therapy.

—*HIV and reactive arthritis:* Although Reiter's syndrome has been described in AIDS patients, studies have not shown an increased risk for Reiter's syndrome in an HIV-positive population matched for other risk factors. Most AIDS patients with reactive arthritis are HLA-B27-positive and present with incomplete Reiter's syndrome with either (*a*) an additive, asymmetric polyarthritis or (*b*) an intermittent oligoarthritis. Dactylitis, conjunctivitis, urethritis, enthesitis, and fasciitis are common. These patients tend to have severe chronic disease and poor response to NSAIDs. Immunosuppressive drugs (i.e., methotrexate, azathioprine) should be avoided in such patients.

Cardinal Findings: The triad of arthritis, urethritis, and conjunctivitis defines Reiter's syndrome. However, less than 33% manifest the full triad. Most patients present with an acute, additive, lower extremity oligoarthritis. A careful history may reveal antecedent infection or extraarticular features to suggest the diagnosis.

—*Onset (within 1 to 4 weeks of exposure):* Onset is heralded by extraarticular features. Genitourinary involvement may manifest as dysuria, urethral discharge, prostatitis, cervicitis, or vaginitis. Fever, anorexia, malaise, fatigue, weight loss, and ocular symptoms are also common during onset.

—*Arthritis:* Typically an acute, asymmetric, additive, and ascending inflammatory oligoarthritis, involvement of the lower extremity (knees, ankles, and toes) is most common. The toes or fingers may be affected by dactylitis, resulting in a "sausage digit." RA-like polyarthritis is uncommon.

—*Axial disease:* Symptomatic inflammatory back pain is present in approximately 50% of individuals. However, radiographic changes are seen in less than 20% of affected individuals. Sacroiliitis and spondylitis are seen in those with chronic disease.

—*Enthesitis:* Inflammation at the insertion sites of tendon or ligament onto bone is called enthesitis. These sites are often painful and may be swollen. Common sites of enthesitis include the heel (insertion of Achilles tendon and plantar fascia), "sausage digits," symphysis pubis, ischium, iliac crest, and greater trochanter. Enthesitis may cause chest pain due to inflammation at the serratus anterior attachments to the anterolateral ribs.

—*Mucocutaneous:* A sterile urethritis (in <33% of patients) may be transient in men and asymptomatic in women. Genitourinary symptoms are seen in postdysenteric or postvenereal reactive arthritis. Common findings also include circinate balanitis, cervicitis, and painless lingual or palatal oral ulcerations. Circinate balanitis is painless and may present as vesicles, shallow ulcerations, or plaques on the glans or shaft of the penis. Keratoderma blennorrhagica appears as painless, papulosquamous lesions on the soles or palms. Nail changes typically manifest as onycholysis, yellowish discoloration, or subungual hyperkeratosis.

—*Ocular:* Conjunctivitis, uveitis, or keratitis is seen in most patients. Conjunctivitis tends to be bilateral or unilateral, recurrent, and painful; it lasts days rather than weeks. Nongranulomatous uveitis (see p. 379) often occurs with established disease and may folow a chronic or relapsing course.

Uncommon Findings: Cardiac conduction disturbances, myocarditis, aortitis, aortic regurgitation, amyloidosis, central nervous system involvement, serositis, and pulmonary infiltrates are rarely seen.

Diagnostic Tests: Most patients exhibit elevated ESR and C-reactive protein levels. Thrombocytosis, leukocytosis, hypoproliferative anemia, and elevated hepatic enzymes may also be seen. The synovial fluid is inflammatory, with a predominance of neutrophils.

Culture of arthritogenic organisms is uncommon. Culture or serologic proof of infection is not necessary but may indicate the need for antibiotic therapy in *Yersinia*- or *Chlamydia*-induced arthritis. HIV testing is not routinely recommended; it should be reserved for those engaged in high-risk behavior.

HLA-B27 testing is seldom necessary. Only a small number of B27-positive individuals develop Reiter's syndrome. Thus, HLA-B27 has a low predictive value as a screening test. HLA-B27 may prove useful in patients with early incomplete features of Reiter's syndrome.

Imaging: Radiographs may show soft tissue swelling, joint space narrowing, or erosions in the small joints of the feet, hands, knees, and sacroiliac joints. Formation of reactive new bone is characteristic and may result in periostitis, enthesitis, or poorly defined intraarticular erosions. Radiographic changes are often most striking in the foot, ankle, and knee. Heel spurs are found at the insertion of the plantar aponeurosis, associated with erosive or proliferative osseous changes with poorly defined outlines.

Axial involvement most often manifests as sacroiliitis. In chronic Reiter's syndrome, 40 to 60% have radiographic evidence of bilateral, asymmetric, or unilateral sacroiliitis. Ileal sclerosis and ankylosis are late findings. Asymmetric paravertebral ossification with nonmarginal syndesmophytes (bulky osteophytes) is common.

Bone scan, CT scan, and MRI are sensitive in detecting occult sacroiliitis but are rarely indicated.

Keys to Diagnosis: An asymmetric, inflammatory oligoarthritis with enthesitis (heel pain), genitourinary, or ocular findings should lead one to suspect Reiter's syndrome.

Diagnostic Criteria: ACR criteria require peripheral arthritis of more than 1 month's duration and association with urethritis or cervicitis. These criteria show a sensitivity of 84.3% and specificity of 98.2%.

Differential Diagnosis: Reiter's syndrome should be distinguished from septic (especially gonococcal) arthritis, gout, sarcoidosis, erythema nodosum, seronegative RA, and acute rheumatic fever. Distinguishing Reiter's syndrome from the other spondyloarthropathies (see p. 355) (e.g., ankylosing spondylitis, psoriatic arthritis, or enteropathic arthritis) and other reactive arthritides (e.g., *Yersinia, Chlamydia*) may be difficult. Patients have been described with overlapping features of Reiter's syndrome and psoriasis or enteropathic arthritis.

Therapy: General therapy should be aimed at joint protection, maintenance of function, patient education, relief of pain, suppression of inflammation, and, when appropriate, eradication of infection. Inactivity and immobilization should be discouraged, and stretching and range-of-motion exercises should be encouraged.

Treatment with NSAIDs improves symptoms but does not alter the course of chronic inflammatory disease. Indomethacin, sulindac, naproxen, diclofenac, enteric-coated salicylate, and phenylbutazone are approved by the Food and Drug Administration for use in ankylosing spondylitis or Reiter's syndrome. Phenylbutazone is no longer available, primarily because of the risk of aplastic anemia. Indomethacin, in antiinflammatory doses (2–3 mg/kg), is commonly used in the treatment of Reiter's syndrome. The sustained-release form is effective in the treatment of morning stiffness. Other NSAIDs also have been used. Chronic NSAID therapy is indicated as long as clinical evidence of inflammation persists.

Corticosteroids are relatively ineffective in the routine management of Reiter's syndrome. However, intraarticular or perilesional (tendons or entheses) injections or topical corticosteroids may benefit some patients.

DMARD therapy is indicated in patients with chronic Reiter's syndrome unresponsive to NSAIDs. Azathioprine, methotrexate, and sulfasalazine have shown efficacy in uncontrolled trials. Methotrexate appears to be effective at doses of 7.5 to 20 mg/week. Sulfasalazine was effective in uncontrolled trials and may also resolve the subclinical intestinal inflammation associated with active disease. In a multicenter, placebo-controlled trial, sulfasalazine (2 g/day) was effective in treating the peripheral arthritis of Reiter's syndrome.

Antibiotic therapy may be indicated in patients with culture or serologically proven *Yersinia*- or *Chlamydia*-induced arthritis. Several reports suggested more than 3 months of antibiotic therapy (doxycycline or lymecycline) for patients with *Chlamydia*-induced arthritis. Reactive arthritides due to salmonella and shigella do not respond to antibiotic therapy. Thus, most patients with idiopathic Reiter's syndrome will not benefit from antibiotic therapy.

Prognosis: In most patients, the initial episode of arthritis is self-limiting and lasts weeks to months. Many patients experience recurrent attacks, often after prolonged disease-free intervals. Less than 30% of patients exhibit a chronic arthritis. Severe disability occurs in less than 15% of patients and may be secondary to persistent lower extremity arthritis, aggressive axial involvement, or blindness. Death is rare and is usually from cardiac complications or amyloidosis.

REFERENCES

Arnett FC. Seronegative spondyloarthropathies. Bull Rheum Dis 1987;37:1–12.

Clegg DO, Reda DJ, Weisman MH, et al. Comparison of sulfasalazine and placebo in the treatment of reactive arthritis (Reiter's syndrome): a Department of Veterans Affairs cooperative study. Arthritis Rheum 1996;39:2021–2027.

Cush JJ, Lipsky PE. Reiter's syndrome and reactive arthritis. In: Koopman WJ, ed. Arthritis and allied conditions: a textbook of rheumatology. 13th ed. Baltimore: Williams & Wilkins, 1997:1209–1227.

Thomson GTD, DeRubeis DA, Hodge MA, et al. Post-salmonella reactive arthritis: late clinical sequelae in a point source cohort. Am J Med 1995;98:13–21.

Wordsworth BP. Should we treat postvenereal Reiter's syndrome by antibiotics? J Rheumatol 1993;20:907.

RELAPSING POLYCHONDRITIS

ICD9 Code: 733.99

Definition: Relapsing polychondritis is a rare disease characterized by inflammation and destruction of the cartilage. It affects auricular cartilage in 85% of patients and may also affect nasal cartilage (50% of patients), laryngotracheal cartilage (50% of patients), and other organ systems.

Etiology: Although the etiology is unknown, there is both cellular and humoral immune reactivity to cartilage, particularly types IX and XI. In addition, CD4+ T cells play an important role in the disease process, and the prevalence of HLA-DR4 is higher in patients than in controls.

Demographics: Relapsing polychondritis is a rare disorder. While it has been described in many age groups, its incidence peaks in the fifth decade. There is no sexual predominance, and Caucasians are most commonly affected.

Cardinal Findings: Ear pain and swelling, which may occur after minor trauma, is the initial complaint in nearly half of affected patients. While the pinna of the ear may be grossly inflamed, the lower ear lobule is unaffected because it lacks underlying cartilage. Persistent or recurrent inflammation can lead to complete destruction of the cartilage, leaving a floppy or scarred pinna. Inflammation may also cause occlusion of the external auditory canal and hearing loss (~30% of patients). Up to a third of patients may experience auditory or vestibular abnormalities secondary to vasculitis of the internal auditory artery.

Nasal and laryngotracheal cartilage may be affected (both ~50% of patients). Nasal cartilage destruction may result in a "saddle nose" deformity. A saddle nose deformity may also be seen in Wegener's granulomatosis, syphilis, or leprosy. Laryngotracheal involvement, which may present as hoarseness, stridor, or local tenderness, may be life threatening if the airway is involved.

Other organ involvement includes ocular (50%; iridocyclitis, retinal vasculitis, extraocular muscle paresis, periorbital edema, scleritis, episcleritis, conjunctivitis), articular (50%; chronic, seronegative, nonerosive, inflammatory oligoarthritis), vascular (10%; vasculitis of arteries of all sizes), and renal (10%; segmental proliferative glomerulonephritis).

Uncommon Findings: Aortic insufficiency, aortitis, and coexistent connective tissue disorders (e.g., vasculitis, JRA, SLE, Sjögren's syndrome, Reiter's syndrome) may occur. The overlap of Behçet's syndrome and relapsing polychondritis has been termed the *"MAGIC" syndrome* (*m*outh *a*nd *g*enital ulcers with *i*nflamed *c*artilage).

Diagnostic Testing: There is no diagnostic test for relapsing polychondritis. Supportive, nonspecific findings include increased ESR, anemia of chronic disease, and hypergammaglobulinemia. Antibodies to type II collagen are found in 50% of patients. Pulmonary function tests, including flow volume curves, should be performed for baseline assessment and with respiratory symptoms.

Imaging: Tomograms and CT may help determine the presence and severity of laryngotracheal involvement.

Keys to Diagnosis: Diagnosis is based on the constellation of appropriate clinical findings. Biopsy is often not needed but may be done in atypical cases. Histopathologic confirmation of cartilage inflammation and destruction supports the diagnosis and may help exclude other diagnoses.

Differential Diagnosis: Wegener's granulomatosis, infection (e.g., fungal, mycobacterial, spirochetal), vasculitis, and malignancy should be considered.

Treatment: Therapy depends on the severity and extent of disease. In a minority of patients, NSAIDs and mild analgesics may suffice. Patients with more severe or refractory disease often require corticosteroids. Some patients, for example, those with severe vasculitis, renal, or respiratory disease, may require high-dose oral corticosteroids or immunosuppressives (methotrexate, cyclophosphamide, cyclosporine). Laryngotracheal involvement associated with airway compromise may require surgical intervention such as excision or stenting.

Prognosis: The severity of involvement in particular organ systems determines the prognosis. Overall, 5-year survival has been reported as 74%. Death is usually due to infection, vasculitis, malignancy, or airway collapse.

REFERENCES

Isaak BL, Liesegang TJ, Michet CJ. Ocular and systemic findings in relapsing polychondritis. Ophthalmology 1986;93:681–689.

Michet CJ, McKenna CH, Luthra HS. Relapsing polychondritis: survival and predictive role of early disease manifestations. Ann Intern Med 1986;104:74–78.

REMITTING SERONEGATIVE SYMMETRIC SYNOVITIS WITH PITTING EDEMA (RS3PE)

Definition: Remitting inflammatory arthritis of hands and feet affecting primarily the elderly.

Etiology: The etiology is unknown. The association with HLA-B7, infrequent sacroiliitis, and rheumatoid-like presentation has suggested that RS3PE is a variant of RA or spondyloarthropathy.

Demographics: Males over 50 years of age (mean age, 71 years) are preferentially affected.

Cardinal Findings: Abrupt onset of marked dorsal swelling of the hands with pitting edema, wrist synovitis, and flexor tendinitis of fingers is common. Ankles and feet can be similarly involved. Most cases remit in a year; a minority develop into RA or spondyloarthropathy. Few cases of malignancy have been described.

Diagnostic Tests: Rheumatoid factor (RF) is absent; ESR is usually elevated, and noninflammatory synovial fluid is typical. Radiographic joint destruction is absent.

Keys to Diagnosis: Onset of a symmetric polyarthritis with pitting edema in older males is characteristic.

Therapy: Rapid response to low-dose prednisone is typical. NSAID and hydroxychloroquine have also been necessary in some.

REFERENCES

McCarty DJ, O'Duffy JD, Pearson L, Hunter JB. Remitting seronegative symmetrical synovitis with pitting edema. RS3PE syndrome. JAMA 1985;254:2763–2767.
Olive A, del Blanco J, Pons M, Vaquero M, Tena X. The clinical spectrum of remitting seronegative symmetrical synovitis with pitting edema. The Catalan Group for the Study of RS3PE. J Rheumatol 1997;24:233–236.

RHEUMATOID ARTHRITIS

ICD9 Code: RA 714.0; Felty's syndrome 714.1; rheumatoid vasculitis 447.6; rheumatoid nodules 729.89

Definition: Rheumatoid arthritis (RA) is a chronic, progressive, systemic inflammatory disorder in which the joints are the primary target. The classic presentation of RA is a symmetric polyarthritis, particularly of the small joints of the hands and feet. Arthritis is often accompanied by constitutional symptoms such as fatigue.

Etiology: The etiology of RA is unknown. The pathophysiology of RA is presumed to relate to a persistent immunologic response of a genetically susceptible host to some unknown antigen, possibly an infectious agent. Over the past 100 years, many viruses and bacteria have been suggested as the cause of RA (including mycobacteria, streptococci, mycoplasma, *Yersinia*, rubella, Epstein-Barr virus). Despite the resemblance of RA to known infectious arthritides (e.g., Lyme disease) and extensive investigations, no agent has been conclusively implicated.

Genetics: Family studies demonstrate a genetic predisposition to development of RA. The concordance rate for monozygotic twins is approximately 25% (i.e., if one twin has RA, there is a 1/4 chance the other will develop RA). First-degree relatives of RA patients develop RA at a rate about four times that of the general population. The most clearly defined genetic association with RA is with particular alleles of the class II major histocompatibility complex (MHC) genes. Certain HLA-DR molecules (e.g., HLA-DR4, HLA-DR1, which are currently designated HLA-DRB1*0401, 0101, 0404, etc.) are associated with the development and severity of RA.

Pathology: The most characteristic pathologic changes in RA occur in the joints. RA can affect any diarthrodial joint (i.e., joints having cartilage overlying bone, and a joint cavity lined by a synovial membrane that contains synovial fluid). With the onset of arthritis, the normally thin synovial lining layer hypertrophies and becomes infiltrated with leukocytes and other cells. Below the synovial layer are organized accumulations of mononuclear cells, predominantly CD4+ "helper" T cells and antigen-presenting cells (dendritic cells and macrophages). Lymphoid follicles and germinal centers are also seen; in these areas, large amounts of immunoglobulin, including rheumatoid factor, are produced. Substantial vascular changes (e.g., angiogenesis) reflect activation of the endothelium of the synovial blood vessels. Fibroblast activity is reflected by increased synthesis of extracellular matrix components. This swollen, hypertrophied synovium projects into the joint space, erodes into subchondral bone, and destroys cartilage. Such alterations in the synovium are not pathognomonic of RA and may be seen in other types of inflammatory arthritis. However, the intensity of such changes is characteristic of RA. The synovial fluid in RA reflects the inflammatory nature of the arthritis, typically containing large numbers of neutrophils. Rheumatoid nodules show palisading histiocytes arrayed about an area of central necrosis. Although uncommon, vasculitis of small or medium-sized vessels has been reported.

Immunologically, several components of the immune system contribute to the pathogenesis of RA. Several lines of evidence indicate that CD4+ "helper" T cells orchestrate the immune response in RA. Supporting this are the consistent infiltration of the synovium with these cells and the HLA-DR association of RA. In addition to T cells, cells of the monocyte/macrophage lineage play an important role, both by interacting with T cells and by elaborating inflammatory cytokines. B cells secrete immunoglobulin, including rheumatoid factor (immunoglobulin, usually of the IgM isotype, that binds to the Fc portion of IgG). Many manifestations of RA derive from the effects of proinflammatory cytokines, particularly IL-1, TNF-α, and IL-6.

Demographics: The prevalence of RA is remarkably consistent; throughout the world it affects approximately 1% of the population. Exceptions include the scarcity of RA in rural sub-Saharan Africa and a higher prevalence of RA (>5%) among certain Native American populations. In all populations, women are affected about three times as often as men. The prevalence of RA increases with age, and sex differences diminish among older patients. RA develops most commonly during the fourth and fifth decades of life. Peak onset age (80% of cases) occurs between 35 and 50 years.

Risk Factors: The greater prevalence of RA among women argues for an effect of sex hormones on the disease. This is supported by the tendency of RA to improve during pregnancy and with oral contraceptive use. Historical evidence supports some environmental exposure as a risk factor for RA. Thus, unlike other types of arthritis such as osteoarthritis and gout, it does not appear that RA existed prior to the industrial age.

Cardinal Findings: RA is a clinical diagnosis, easily made by history and examination.

—*Onset:* For about 2/3 of patients, onset of RA is insidious; symmetric arthritis develops over the course of weeks to months. About 10 to 15% of patients have a fulminant onset of polyarticular arthritis, and the diagnosis of RA is established more easily. Arthritis is often accompanied by prolonged morning stiffness affecting the joints that typically lasts an hour or more. Many patients also have constitutional symptoms such as fatigue, anorexia, and low-grade fever.

—*Joints:* Although the cardinal signs of inflammation (pain, swelling, erythema, warmth) may be seen early in the disease course or during flares, erythema and warmth may be absent in chronic RA. *Warmth* is often a subtle finding and *erythema* may be short-lived. *Pain* referred to the joint originates predominantly from the joint capsule, which is abundantly supplied with pain fibers and is exquisitely sensitive to distention. Factors that contribute to *swelling* of the joint include accumulation of synovial fluid and hypertrophy of the synovium. *Loss of function* of the joints relates primarily to loss of motion. Initially, the patient may voluntarily restrict motion in response to pain. With progression of disease, tendon shortening and destruction of periarticular supporting structures may cause irreversible joint deformities (e.g., swan-neck deformity). Bony ankylosis (destruction of joints with collapse and bony overgrowth) tends to occur in some joints, particularly the wrist and ankle. Loss of function is critical to the patient, as it is associated with substantial morbidity (e.g., interference with the ability to perform activities of daily living).

While RA can affect any diarthrodial joint, there is a distinct predilection for certain joints, such as the small joints of the hands (Table 1). Certain joints may be of particular concern to patients; for example, arthritis of the hands and wrists interferes substantially with daily life and often prompts patients to seek medical advice.

—*Deformities:* Damage to articular and periarticular (i.e., tendons, ligaments) structures may result in deformities (Fig. 1), including swan-neck deformity (manifest as hyperextension at the PIP joints and flexion at the DIP joints of the fingers); boutonnière deformity (flexion at the PIP joint and hyperextension at the DIP joint); ulnar drift (deviation of the MCP joint and fingers ulnarly); piano-key deformity (with manual compression, prominent up and down movement of the ulnar styloid, caused by damage at the radioulnar joint); bent-fork deformity of the wrist (due to collapse of the carpal bones with subluxation at the carpometacarpal joints, which results in a stepdown appearance over the dorsum of the wrist); and hallux valgus (valgus deformity affecting the first MTP joints, with medial displacement at the MTP and lateral deviation of the first toe bilaterally).

Table 1
Joint Involvement in RA

Involved Joint	Frequency of Involvement (%)
Metacarpophalangeal (MCP)	85
Wrist	80
Proximal interphalangeal (PIP)	75
Knee	75
Metatarsophalangeal (MTP)	75
Ankle (tibiotalar + subtalar)	75
Shoulder	60
Midfoot (tarsus)	60
Hip	50
Elbow	50
Acromioclavicular (AC)	50
Cervical spine	40
Temporomandibular (TMJ)	30
Sternoclavicular (SC)	30

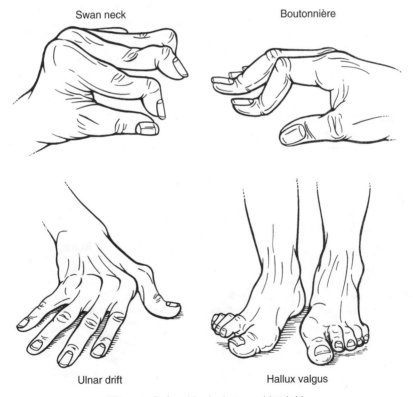

Figure 1. Deformities in rheumatoid arthritis.

—*Extraarticular manifestations:* Although arthritis may be its most prominent clinical feature, RA is indeed a systemic disease. Many patients have a variety of extraarticular manifestations (Table 2). Extraarticular manifestations tend to occur in patients with high titers of rheumatoid factor in the serum. Some manifestations, for example, subcutaneous rheumatoid nodules (see p. 331), are common (30% of RA patients) but usually do not require specific intervention. Rheumatoid nodules are commonly seen over the ulna, olecranon, fingers, and Achilles tendon or in the olecranon bursa. Rheumatoid nodules are only seen in patients with rheumatoid factor (often in high titers). Pulmonary manifestations of RA are also common (some pathologic changes may be seen almost universally at autopsy) but infrequently become clinically apparent. Some extraarticular manifestations (e.g., vasculitis, Felty's syndrome) are rare but often require specific therapy (see "Rheumatoid Vasculitis," p. 332 and "Felty's Syndrome," p. 331).

Complications: Joint destruction and deformities are the most common complications of RA. These changes can substantially impair the patient's mobility as well as the ability to perform activities of daily living (e.g., preparing food, bathing, dressing). Extraarticular manifestations of RA may also cause complications (e.g., symptomatic pleural or pericardial effusion, vasculitic damage). Subluxation of upper cervical vertebrae is commonly seen on radiographs but is usually asymptomatic. Rarely, C1–C2 subluxation results in spinal cord compression with permanent neurologic deficit.

Table 2
Extraarticular Manifestations of RA

Organ System	Manifestations
Constitutional	Fever, anorexia, fatigue, weakness, lymphadenopathy
Cutaneous	Rheumatoid nodules, vasculitis
Ocular	Sjögren's syndrome (keratoconjunctivitis sicca), scleritis, episcleritis
Cardiovascular	Pericarditis, pericardial effusion
Pulmonary	Pleuritis, pleural effusion, interstitial fibrosis, rheumatoid nodules in the lung, Caplan syndrome (nodular pulmonary infiltrates in RA patients with pneumoconiosis)
Hematologic	Anemia of chronic disease, thrombocytosis, eosinophilia, Felty' syndrome (RA associated with neutropenia and splenomegaly)
Gastrointestinal	Sjögren's syndrome (xerostomia), amyloidosis, vasculitis
Neurologic	Entrapment neuropathy, myelopathy/myositis
Renal	Amyloidosis, renal tubular acidosis, interstitial nephritis
Metabolic	Osteoporosis

Diagnostic Tests: No laboratory or other test is diagnostic for RA; rather, the presence of various findings on laboratory and other tests provides support for a diagnosis suspected on clinical grounds.

Rheumatoid factor (RF) is the laboratory test most closely associated with RA. RF (see p. 136) is an autoantibody (usually IgM) that binds to the Fc portion of IgG and is present in 75 to 85% of patients with RA. Thus, nearly 20% of patients with RA are seronegative for RF. Moreover, by definition, 5% of the general population test positive for RF, and nearly 20% of healthy elderly persons may be RF positive. In addition, RF is seen in a number of conditions other than RA, including Sjögren's syndrome, cryoglobulinemia, SLE, bacterial endocarditis, mycobacterial disease, hepatitis, and lymphoproliferative malignancies. Because RA is present in approximately 1% of the population, random screening using RF would be expected to generate a large number of false-positive results. In patients with RA, high-titer RF is associated with aggressive disease, as evidenced by development of bony erosions, extraarticular involvement, and functional disability.

Other laboratory tests that can be useful in supporting the diagnosis of RA include synovial fluid analysis, measurement of acute-phase reactants (ESR and CRP), and the CBC. In RA, synovial fluid is expected to be inflammatory with negative results on microbiologic culture and crystal analysis. Elevations in the ESR or CRP level provides a surrogate measure of active inflammation and may be useful in establishing a diagnosis, estimating the prognosis, and gauging the response to therapy. The most common abnormality in the CBC in RA patients is a normochromic, normocytic anemia (anemia of chronic disease). Thrombocytosis may also be seen with uncontrolled inflammation.

Imaging: Several imaging studies are used in assessing patients with RA. Early in the disease course, plain radiographs may show only soft tissue swelling or joint effusion. As the disease progresses, more abnormalities appear. Juxtaarticular osteopenia is characteristic of RA and other chronic inflammatory arthritides. Loss of articular cartilage and bony erosions may develop after months of active disease. Nearly 70% of patients will develop bony erosions within the first 2 years of disease. Erosions may be seen in virtually any joint but are most common in the MTP, MCP, and wrist joints. Plain radiographs are useful in helping to establish prognosis, in assessing joint damage longitudinally, and when surgery is considered. MRI may demonstrate erosions much earlier than conventional x-ray and offers superior detail in depicting the articular structures. However, its cost precludes widespread use in routine assessment of patients.

Keys to Diagnosis: Because it is the most common type of chronic inflammatory arthritis, RA should be a major consideration in patients with such a presentation. A large number of joints involved, a symmetric pattern to the arthritis, prominent involvement of the small joints of the hands and feet, and the presence of constitutional symptoms, subcutaneous nodules, or serum RF add support to the diagnosis.

Table 3
1987 Revised Criteria for the Classification of Rheumatoid Arthritis

1. Stiffness in and around the joints lasting 1 hour before maximal improvement
2. Arthritis of three or more joint areas, simultaneously, observed by a physician
3. Arthritis of the proximal interphalangeal (PIP), metacarpophalangeal (MCP), or wrist joints
4. Symmetric arthritis
5. Rheumatoid nodules
6. A positive test for serum rheumatoid factor (RF)
7. X-ray changes characteristic of RA (erosions and/or periarticular osteopenia in hand and/or wrist joints)

A person can be classified as having RA if 4 or more criteria are present at any time
Criteria 1 through 4 must be present for at least 6 weeks
Criteria 2 through 5 must be observed by a physician

Diagnostic Criteria: Classification criteria for RA are shown in Table 3. Note that patients do not have to have a positive test for RF to be diagnosed with RA. However, seronegative patients must have a very characteristic clinical presentation to be diagnosed with RA.

Differential Diagnosis: Acutely, RA is often confused with reactive arthritis, Reiter's syndrome, viral arthritis (e.g., parvovirus B19, EBV, hepatitis B), Lyme disease, or the articular onset of other connective tissue disorders (e.g., polymyositis, scleroderma, SLE). Chronically, RA needs to be distinguished from other forms of chronic, polyarticular, inflammatory arthritis: SLE, Lyme disease, psoriatic arthritis, polyarticular gout or pseudogout, Reiter's syndrome, reactive arthritis, enteropathic arthritis, erosive/inflammatory osteoarthritis, scleroderma, rheumatic fever, and inflammatory myositis. There is a negative association between RA and gout.

Prognosis: Until the 1980s, RA was considered predominantly a benign disease; it was thought that many patients would go into spontaneous remission. This was based on population studies that included large numbers of arthritis patients who would not currently be considered to have RA. Now it is realized that RA is a chronic, progressive disease associated with substantial morbidity and accelerated mortality. Patients with severe RA have been shown to have a limited survival, comparable to that of patients with three-vessel coronary disease or advanced Hodgkin's disease. This has had important implications for the approach to therapy of RA. Several factors are associated with a worse outcome for RA patients (Table 4), and several of these are linked. For example, patients with certain genotypes (e.g., HLA-DR4) are more likely to have high titers of RF and extraarticular manifestations.

Therapy: The goals of therapy for patients with RA are (*a*) relief of pain, (*b*) preservation of functional status, (*c*) reduction of inflammation, (*d*) control of systemic involvement, (*e*) protection of articular and extraarticular structures, (*f*) control of disease progression, and (*g*) avoidance of complications related to therapy.

Table 4
Features of RA Associated with Aggressive Disease

High positive titers of rheumatoid factor (RF)
Elevated acute-phase reactants (e.g., ESR, CRP)
Radiographic evidence of bony erosions
Arthritis of numerous joints (e.g., >20)
Functional disability (inability to perform activities of daily living)
Rheumatoid nodules (and other extraarticular manifestations)
Specific HLA-DR alleles (e.g. HLA-DR4)
Lower socioeconomic status/less education

Table 5
Therapies for Patients with RA

Pharmacologic	Nonpharmacologic
Analgesics	Ambulatory assist devices
Nonnarcotic	Physiotherapy
Antidepressants	Splints/orthotics
Narcotic	Occupational therapy
NSAIDs	Patient education
Topical agents (e.g., capsaicin)	Exercise/rest
Corticosteroids	Orthopaedic surgery
DMARDs	Synovectomy
Methotrexate	Tendon repair
Hydroxychloroquine	Joint reconstruction
Sulfasalazine	Joint fusion (arthrodesis)
Injectable gold salts	Joint replacement
Cyclosporine	
D-Penicillamine	
Azathioprine	
Cyclophosphamide	
Auranofin	
Minocycline	

The types of therapeutic interventions include pharmacologic agents (including oral, parenteral, and topical agents) and nonpharmacologic agents (Table 5).

In previous years, therapy of RA was guided by the "therapeutic pyramid." In this scheme, which was based upon the assumption that RA was predominantly a benign disease with spontaneous remissions, therapy began with NSAIDs. Other agents, such as injectable gold salts, were added in a stepwise fashion as patients clearly failed treatment with NSAIDs. Now that it is recognized that RA is a chronic progressive disease and that damage can occur early in the disease course, therapy of RA has become more aggressive.

A critical decision point in the approach to therapy of patients with RA is an estimation of the severity of disease and its expected prognosis. Patients with several prognostic factors consistent with a worse outcome (Table 4) may be considered to have "aggressive" disease. RA patients lacking these features may be considered as having "slowly progressive" disease. These categories are not static; many patients initially labeled "slowly progressive" may later develop more aggressive disease features and thus fall into the category of "aggressive" RA. Close follow-up and repeated evaluations are crucial for patients with RA. At these follow-up evaluations, the patient should be assessed for (a) activity of the disease, (b) changes in functional status, (c) response to the therapeutic interventions (e.g., control of pain and inflammation), and (d) development of adverse effects related to therapy.

Patients with slowly progressive disease are often treated with NSAIDs (see Appendix A, p. 507). Some patients may require low-dose oral corticosteroids (e.g., prednisone < 10 mg/day) or intraarticular steroids in one to two joints. DMARDs may be used in patients with slowly progressive RA, particularly those with incomplete relief from NSAIDs, analgesics, and nonpharmacologic therapies. Hydroxychloroquine, sulfasalazine, and auranofin are commonly used in patients with slowly progressive disease.

Patients with aggressive RA may also receive NSAIDs; however higher, antiinflammatory doses may be used. Low-dose oral steroids and intraarticular steroid injections are commonly used. DMARDs are used very early in the disease course for patients with aggressive RA. Methotrexate (with concomitant folate) is the most commonly used DMARD in such patients. Other DMARDs have also been used with success in RA (Table 5).

DMARDs form the mainstay of therapy for many patients with RA (see Appendix B, p. 509). The choice of individual agent depends on several factors including (a) the severity and activity of disease, (b) comorbidity in the patient (e.g., methotrexate is not the drug of choice in an alcoholic patient), (c) cost and convenience issues. Many RA patients fail to remain on any given DMARD long term because of either therapeutic inefficacy or development of adverse effects.

Many advocate combination DMARDs therapy in an effort to enhance efficacy while minimizing toxicity. Unfortunately, limited evidence supports this concept. To date, only two combination DMARD regimens (methotrexate plus cyclosporine, and methotrexate plus hydroxychloroquine plus sulfasalazine) have demonstrable utility in patients not responding to more conservative single DMARD regimens. Various experimental therapies are under investigation for patients with RA. Of these, therapies that target inflammatory cytokines (e.g., TNF-α, IL-1) show significant promise and may be available in the near future.

Surgery: A number of orthopaedic surgical interventions have revolutionized the care of the RA patient (Table 5). Surgical outcomes have improved consistently in recent years and offer many patients the chance for substantial improvement in functional status and quality of life. Indications for surgery include (a) impending tendon rupture, (b) marked functional limitation, and (c) severe pain related to extensive joint damage (see p. 501).

REFERENCES

Alarcon GS. Epidemiology of rheumatoid arthritis. Rheum Dis Clin North Am 1995;21:589–604.
Arnett FC, Edworthy SM, Bloch DA, et al. The ARA 1987 revised criteria for the classification of rheumatoid arthritis. Arthritis Rheum 1988;31:315–324.

Brooks PM. Clinical management of rheumatoid arthritis. Lancet 1993;341:286–290.

Cush JJ, Kavanaugh AF. Biologic interventions in rheumatoid arthritis. Rheum Dis Clin North Am 1995;21:797–816.

D'Cruz D, Hughes G. Rheumatoid arthritis: the clinical features. J Musculoskel Med 1993; 10:85–95.

Harris ED. Rheumatoid arthritis: pathophysiology and implications for therapy. N Engl J Med 1990;322:1277–1289.

Pincus T, Brooks RH, Callahan LF. Prediction of long-term mortality in patients with rheumatoid arthritis according to simple questionnaire and joint count measures. Ann Intern Med 1994;120:26–34.

Sewell KL, Trentham DE. Pathogenesis of rheumatoid arthritis. Lancet 1993;341:283–286.

Wolfe F. 50 years of antirheumatic therapy: the progress of rheumatoid arthritis. J Rheumatol 1990(Suppl 22)17:24–32.

Wolfe F, Mitchell DM, Sibley JT, et al. The mortality of rheumatoid arthritis. Arthritis Rheum 1994;37:481–494.

RHEUMATOID NODULES

ICD9 Code: 729.89

Definition: Soft tissue accumulations of inflammatory connective tissue are located in periarticular or peritendinous areas, especially at sites of friction or pressure. Although most cases are associated with seropositive rheumatoid arthritis, nodulosis can occur with other autoimmune diseases or as an isolated entity without other systemic manifestations.

Etiology: Nodules most likely begin as a localized area of vascular inflammation associated with immune complexes containing rheumatoid factors. Some patients treated with methotrexate may also develop numerous small nodules around joints of the fingers. These differ from classic nodules in their small size and peripheral location. The etiology of "methotrexate nodulosis" remains unclear.

Pathology: The characteristic features are a central area of noncaseating necrosis surrounded by palisading histiocytes. Giant cells are absent. Stains for mycobacteria or other infectious agents are usually negative.

Demographics: One-third of patients with seropositive RA have nodules at some time during their disease course. Classic rheumatoid nodules do not occur in patients who are seronegative for IgM rheumatoid factor. As with other extraarticular manifestations of RA, men represent a disproportionate number of nodule-positive patients.

Cardinal Findings: Nodules are most commonly noted over areas of friction such as the elbow, heel (Achilles tendon), hands, or dorsum of the feet. Less common sites can include the sacrum, occiput, pleura (where friction between inflamed serosal surfaces may contribute to development of the nodule), and the pulmonary parenchyma (where the radiographic appearance can suggest metastatic malignancy or infectious granulomata). The palpable nodules have a rubbery texture and are usually not tender. In early stages, they are often fixed to underlying periosteum, but with time, nodules may dissociate from the bone and be freely movable under the skin.

Uncommon Manifestations: Rarely, nodules have been reported in heart valves, where integrity of the valve may be compromised.

Diagnostic Tests: All patients should be IgM-RF positive. Appearance of nodules in the setting of active, seropositive RA usually does not present a diagnostic dilemma, and further evaluation of most such patients is not required. Nodules in the presence of seronegative tests for IgM-RF should suggest the possibility of tophaceous gout, as rheumatoid nodules and gouty tophi may be mistaken for one another and there is negative correlation between RA and gout. In such instances, aspiration or biopsy may be useful.

Differential Diagnosis: Gouty tophi, ganglion cysts, osseous nodules due to osteophytes, tendon xanthomas, or nodules associated with rheumatic fever, leprosy, MCTD, or multicentric reticulohistiocytosis may masquerade as rheumatoid nodules.

Therapy: The underlying arthritis must be treated. Some second-line agents, especially gold salts or penicillamine, can result in diminution or resolution of nodules. Methotrexate-induced nodules may regress with discontinuation of the drug or can be approached by concomitant treatment with another agent (e.g., hydroxychloroquine, colchicine). Local injection with corticosteroids may be effective with obstructive or problematic nodules.

Surgery: If nodules show cutaneous breakdown, present other mechanical problems, or are cosmetically unacceptable, they can be removed. This may be especially useful in feet, where proper fitting of shoes can be significantly compromised. Most patients do not require surgery.

Prognosis: The presence of rheumatoid nodules may be associated with a more aggressive form of RA. Otherwise, the nodules themselves usually do not compromise joint function.

REFERENCES

Bacon PA, Moots RJ. Extra-articular rheumatoid arthritis. In: Koopman WJ, ed. Arthritis and allied conditions: a textbook of rheumatology. 13th ed. Baltimore: Williams & Wilkins, 1997:1071–1088.

RHEUMATOID VASCULITIS

ICD9 Code: 447.6

Definition: Rheumatoid vasculitis is inflammation of blood vessels in patients with rheumatoid arthritis. Vasculitis is considered a serious extraarticular manifestation of RA.

Etiology: Immune complexes, probably containing rheumatoid factors, are passively deposited on blood vessel walls. Although serum IgG-RF is most closely associated with development of vasculitis, all patients manifesting rheumatoid vasculitis have strongly positive titers of IgM-RF. Most of these RF-containing complexes also fix complement, which contributes to tissue damage.

Pathology: Histologic features depend upon the size of the blood vessel involved. In small to medium-sized vessels, the lesion may include an infiltrate consisting of both mononuclear and polymorphonuclear cells, and fibrinoid necrosis. In small vessels of the skin, leukocytoclastic vasculitis may be seen.

Demographics: Rheumatoid vasculitis is usually associated with aggressive and longstanding RA. The incidence in males is somewhat higher than in females. The vast majority of patients are positive for IgM-RF; cases in putatively seronegative patients may be associated with IgG-RF, which is not detected by routine clinical assays. This complication of RA appears to be decreasing in incidence. Limited cutaneous lesions are more common than severe necrotizing complications, which are rare. Autopsy studies suggest that the true incidence of vasculitis is higher, although most cases are subclinical and not detected during life.

Cardinal Findings: Nailfold lesions are most common and include prominent periungual vessels, localized infarction, splinter hemorrhages, and tender macules of the fingertips (which may be dark red or brown). Palpable purpura has been described. Larger vessel involvement often manifests as leg ulcers. Nerve involvement presents most commonly as a mononeuritis multiplex syndrome (e.g., with wrist or foot drop).

Uncommon Manifestations: Involvement of larger arteries, resulting in infarction of the myocardium, bowel, lung, etc. is seen rarely.

Diagnostic Tests: Patients are universally seropositive with high titers of IgM-RF. The diagnosis should be questioned in a seronegative patient. Acute-phase reactants (ESR, CRP) are elevated, sometimes to very high levels. Complement levels (C3, C4) are usually decreased. Leukocytosis, anemia of chronic disease, and cryoglobulinemia may be present. Nerve conduction velocity testing may indicate a mononeuritis multiplex.

Key to Diagnosis: A diagnosis of rheumatoid vasculitis should be questioned if the patient does not have severe seropositive rheumatoid arthritis of longstanding duration. However, the synovitis may be relatively inactive and the degree of active joint inflammation does not correlate with the activity of the vasculitis. In cases of specific organ or tissue involvement such as a mononeuritis syndrome, biopsy of the affected tissue (in this case the nerve) may be very useful in establishing a diagnosis. Skin biopsy should be performed if vasculitis is suspected.

Differential Diagnosis: Clinical and pathologic lesions may resemble those seen in association with subacute bacterial endocarditis, polyarteritis nodosa, Wegner's granulomatosis, or cholesterol emboli syndrome.

Therapy: Aggressive therapy with cyclophosphamide is required for treatment of rheumatoid vasculitis involving medium- to large-sized vessels. Cyclophosphamide may be administered as a daily oral dose or as an intermittent intravenous bolus infusion. Concomitant treatment with moderate doses of prednisone is required. The duration of therapy is unclear, although some require maintenance therapy with therapeutic or subtherapeutic doses for years. Concomitant antibiotic therapy should be given for associated cutaneous infections. Foot and wrist drops are managed with splints.

Surgery: Consultation with a plastic surgeon may be required when cutaneous involvement has left significant soft tissue deficits or debridement is required. No reconstructive procedures such as skin grafts should be attempted before the active disease has been adequately treated.

Prognosis: Outcome depends on the organ system involved. Patients whose vasculitis is limited to fingertip lesions generally do well, whereas involvement of major nerves or arteries in organs such as the heart is associated with a poorer prognosis. The use of cyclophosphamide has had a major impact in reducing associated morbidity and mortality.

REFERENCES

Bacon PA, Kitas GD. The significance of vascular inflammation in rheumatoid arthritis [Review]. Ann Rheum Dis 1994;53:621–623.

Bacon PA, Moots RJ. Extra-articular rheumatoid arthritis. In: Koopman WJ, ed. Arthritis and allied conditions: a textbook of rheumatology. 13th ed. Baltimore: Williams & Wilkins, 1997:1071–1088.

ROTATOR CUFF DYSFUNCTION

Synonyms: Rotator cuff tendinitis, impingement syndrome

ICD9 Code: Rotator cuff tear, 727.61; rotator cuff dysfunction NOS, 726.11

Definition: Rotator cuff dysfunction refers to a spectrum of pathologic changes in the rotator cuff tendons, ranging from mild inflammation or tendinitis through a complete tear. Associated pathologic changes have given rise to names such as "impingement syndrome" and "frozen shoulder." Many patients also have subacromial bursitis in conjunction with rotator cuff dysfunction. Rotator cuff dysfunction is the most common cause of shoulder complaints among the elderly, accounting for more than 75% of cases. This is notable because shoulder problems are the second most common musculoskeletal complaint in general practice.

Anatomic Considerations: Four muscles and their tendons constitute the rotator cuff apparatus. These muscles (the supraspinatus, infraspinatus, subscapularis, and teres minor) originate on the scapula, pass through a tunnel of ligaments on the underside of the acromion process, and insert on the trochanters of the humerus. They function to abduct, internally rotate, and externally rotate the humeral head. This allows free upper extremity movement in many different planes. The rotator cuff tendons also form the roof of the glenohumeral joint, being contiguous with its fibrous capsule. The rotator cuff tendons are separated from the overlying deltoid muscle by the subacromial bursa.

Pathology: Pathologically, it can be demonstrated that the rotator cuff tendons tend to degenerate with advancing age, which provides some explanation for the increasing prevalence of rotator cuff problems with advancing age. Intrinsic degeneration may be exacerbated by chronic overuse (e.g., manual labor involving repetitive shoulder movements against force) or by arthritis in adjacent joints (e.g., RA affecting the acromioclavicular or glenohumeral joints). Rotator cuff dysfunction in many persons represents a continuum of disease. Initial involvement with mild tendinitis may progress, resulting in a complete tear of the rotator cuff tendons. Also, mild tendinitis may cause the patient to favor the affected arm, diminishing movements of the affected muscles. This allows the deltoid to pull the humeral head higher in the glenohumeral fossa, which in turn reduces the area of the space through which the rotator cuff tendons must pass. This may result in "impingement" of the rotator cuff against the acromion, which can cause further pain and worsen the entire process. If this is allowed to become chronic, tendon shortening may ensue, greatly diminishing movement of the shoulder. This "frozen shoulder" syndrome has also been referred to as adhesive capsulitis. However, because adhesions are not typically a part of the pathologic process, "restrictive capsulitis" has become the preferred term.

Demographics: Those at risk include the elderly, those with inflammatory arthritis of the shoulder (e.g., RA), diabetics, alcoholics, athletes with repetitive overhead or throwing movement, carpenters, welders, and painters.

Cardinal Findings: In some cases, particularly in younger persons (e.g., baseball pitchers), injury to the rotator cuff is acute. More commonly, pain related to rotator cuff dysfunction arises insidiously and often becomes chronic.

Patients with rotator cuff dysfunction characteristically complain of shoulder pain. The pain is usually somewhat difficult for the patient to localize more specifically, other than perhaps saying it is "deep." Many patients complain of waking at night because of the pain. It is often worsened by movements that require specific use of the affected muscles. However, patients may compensate and perform movements that normally use the rotator cuff muscles by using other motions. For example, patients may avoid upper extremity abduction while hair brushing. Patients often report pain performing activities that require rotator cuff muscles (e.g., tying an apron behind the back or tucking a shirt into the back of the pants).

Physical examination for rotator cuff function should assess active and passive range of motion of the shoulder and test the muscles individually for pain or weakness. Patients with rotator cuff dysfunction typically have no difficulty with forward flexion or extension of the shoulder. Many have problems with abduction. Normally, the first 15° of abduction is initiated by the deltoid. Abduction from there through 90° depends mostly on the supraspinatus (above 90° there is little further abduction; rather, the trapezius and rhomboid muscles tilt the scapula and bring it toward the midline). Patients with rotator cuff dysfunction frequently have pain on, or limited range of, active abduction. If it is severe, for example in someone with longstanding disease and restrictive capsulitis, passive movements (i.e., done by the examiner) may be limited or result in pain. Some consider patients with impaired range of active motion but normal range of passive motion to have evidence of impingement. The other rotator cuff muscles can also be a source of pain and should be assessed. The subscapularis internally rotates the humeral head. This can be tested by having the patient hold the elbow against the side, with 90° of elbow flexion, and try to move the hand medially against the examiner's resistance. External rotation is mediated by the infraspinatus and teres minor. It can be tested as for internal rotation, except the examiner provides resistance against the patient's attempt to move the hand laterally. In some cases, it may be possible to differentiate tendon inflammation from a complete tendon tear; the former being associated with pain, the latter with both pain and weakness. However, in practicality, it is difficult to differentiate between the two.

Complete tear of the rotator cuff is usually an acute posttraumatic event. Patients also complain of shoulder pain and weakness and may have a positive "drop arm test" (see p. 13).

Diagnostic Tests: No laboratory tests are helpful in diagnosing rotator cuff disease.

Imaging: Imaging modalities, although usually unnecessary to establish rotator cuff dysfunction as the cause of shoulder pain, may be helpful in determining the need for surgery or in unusual cases. Plain x-rays are not usually helpful, as bony abnormalities are not commonly a critical part of the pathology. Commonly, the humeral head appears to be displaced slightly superiorly in the glenohumeral fossa. Some patients have AC joint hypertrophy, which may contribute to impingement. Ultrasound may define abnormalities in the rotator cuff, but the interpretation and utility of the study depends to a large extent on the experience of the ultrasonographer. MRI allows exquisite detail of the relevant tissues. It has replaced arthrography in the diagnosis of complete rotator cuff tendon tears.

Treatment: The treatment of rotator cuff disease may incorporate rest in acute settings. The use of hot packs, ice packs, ultrasound, analgesic agents, or NSAIDs may be helpful in some individuals. However, aggressive physiotherapy with range-of-motion exercises and strengthening of the rotator cuff muscles is a critical component of therapy for all. Injection of the subacromial bursa with corticosteroids can provide substantial relief, particularly in patients with evidence of subacromial bursitis.

Surgery: Surgery is indicated in particular circumstances. For example, in patients with evidence of impingement, acromioplasty can increase the available space and decrease symptoms. In past years, some patients with frozen shoulder underwent surgical "release." However, because this intervention did not appear to affect the ultimate outcome for these patients, most patients are now treated conservatively.

REFERENCES

Bland JH, Merrit JA, Boushey DR. The painful shoulder. Semin Arthritis Rheum 1977;7:21–47.

Chard MD, Hazleman R, Hazleman BL, et al. Shoulder disorders in the elderly: a community survey. Arthritis Rheum 1991;34:766–769.

Dalton SE. The conservative management of rotator cuff disorders. Br J Rheumatol 1994;33:663–667.

Kavanaugh A, Eshagi N, Cush J, Awad R. Rotator cuff dysfunction in patients with rheumatoid arthritis. J Clin Rheumatol 1995;1:274–279.

RUBELLA ARTHRITIS

Synonyms: Rubella is also known as German measles

ICD9 Code: 056.71

Definition: Rubella arthritis is a previously common childhood exanthem that may lead to arthritis in affected adults or children.

Etiology: Chronic rubella arthritis is due to infection with an RNA virus. The rubella virus has been isolated from synovial fluid and peripheral blood. Although viral persistence may be detected, the exact pathogenic mechanism of rubella arthritis remains unclear.

Demographics: Rubella arthritis most commonly affects young women who are exposed to school-age children. It develops in about one-third of natural infections. Arthritis also has been described following rubella vaccination, which uses a live attenuated virus. Prior vaccine strains were more commonly associated with arthropathy than those used currently. Despite widespread vaccination, sporadic outbreaks are reported in hospitals, prenatal clinics, and colleges.

Cardinal Findings: The classic morbilliform rash can precede or accompany joint symptoms. Nonspecific constitutional symptoms may briefly antedate the rash and include malaise, fever, anorexia, upper respiratory tract infection, lymphadenopathy, and eye pain. Symmetric inflammatory arthritis, which occurs more often in adults than children, affects both small and large joints, including the proximal interphalangeal joints, wrist, and knees. Carpal tunnel syndrome or tendinitis occasionally develops. Joint symptoms may be the sole manifestation in adults. Arthropathy generally remits by 1 month but may last up to a year in some. Atypical neurologic sequelae, such as radiculoneuritis affecting an arm or leg, have been described following vaccine administration.

Diagnostic Tests: Diagnosis is confirmed serologically by hemagglutination inhibition, complement fixation, or ELISA. Rheumatoid factor is elevated in less than 25% of patients. Synovial fluid is moderately inflammatory. The virus is occasionally isolated from respiratory secretions.

Keys to Diagnosis: Look for abrupt-onset arthritis with classic rash following exposure to infected children or vaccination and diagnostic confirmation by serologic tests.

Therapy: There is no specific therapy other than analgesics and occasionally NSAIDs. Symptoms are self-limiting except in rare cases. Rubella vaccination has markedly diminished the incidence of acute rubella but has resulted in new cases of postvaccination rubella-like illnesses.

REFERENCES

Smith CA, Petty RE, Tingle AJ. Rubella virus and arthritis. Rheum Dis Clin North Am 1987;13:265.

SAPHO (SYNOVITIS, ACNE, PUSTULOSIS, HYPEROSTOSIS, OSTEITIS) SYNDROME

Synonyms: Palmoplantar pustulosis, sternocostoclavicular hyperostosis, pustulotic arthrosteitis, chronic recurrent multifocal osteomyelitis, acne arthritis or acne-associated spondyloarthropathy, and hidradenitis suppurativa–associated arthritis.

Definition: SAPHO comprises a variety of disorders manifesting reactive osteitis, arthritis, and chronic cutaneous pustular lesions.

Etiology: The cause is unknown. Because of the clinical similarities with the seronegative spondyloarthropathies, these disorders are often considered to be "reactive."

Pathology: Hyperostotic bony lesions, osteitis, and inflammatory synovitis are seen.

Demographics: This very rare disorder affects males and females equally. Most cases are reported in Japan. Far fewer cases are seen in Caucasians, predominantly from Scandinavia and France. Most frequently it affects adults between 20 and 60 years of age.

Cardinal Findings: Painful, nodular swelling of skeletal lesions characterized by development of early erosive and late hyperostotic changes in the joints of the anterior chest wall or axial skeleton. Skeletal disease develops after established pustulosis (i.e., palmoplantar pustulosis, acne conglobata, acne fulminans, hidradenitis suppurativa, or pustular psoriasis). The anterior chest wall and axial skeleton are preferentially targeted. Affected amphiarthroses (saddle joints) of the anterior chest wall include the sternoclavicular, manubriosternal, and sternocostal joints. Peripheral involvement of the hands and feet is uncommon. Spondylodiscitis and enthesitis are sometimes seen. Chronic, relapsing pustular lesions may affect palms or soles (palmoplantar pustulosis), intertriginous areas (hidradenitis), or face, trunk, and extremities (acne).

Diagnostic Tests: Mild-moderate elevation of the acute-phase reactants and increased leukocyte counts are common. Serum rheumatoid factor is usually absent, and HLA-B27 is positive in less than 30% of patients.

Differential Diagnosis: Other spondyloarthropathies, DISH, fluorosis, retinoid therapy, ochronosis, alcaptonuria, and hypoparathyroidism should be considered.

Imaging: Early in the disease, radiographs show erosive changes in the anterior chest wall joints, sometimes accompanied by subchondral sclerosis and periostitis. With chronicity, subchondral sclerosis and hyperostosis ensue. Bony ankylosis is uncommon. Spondylodiscitis is the most common axial finding and is suggested by erosions of the vertebral plates with reactive vertebral sclerosis. Sacroiliitis is seen in up to one-third of patients and may be unilateral or bilateral. Bone scans reveal increased uptake in affected skeletal areas.

Therapy: Topical and systemic therapies are directed at the underlying pustular disorder. The musculoskeletal manifestations are often difficult to treat, although most individuals exhibit some response to systemic antibiotics, NSAIDs, and oral or intraarticular corticosteroids. Sulfasalazine and colchicine have been suggested but not tested extensively.

Surgery: Resection of the proximal clavicular head or synovectomy may be necessary to control pain.

REFERENCES

Cush JJ, Lipsky PE. Reiter's syndrome and reactive arthritis: hyperostotic syndromes associated with cutaneous pustular lesions. In: Koopman WJ, ed. Arthritis and allied conditions: a textbook of rheumatology. 13th ed. Baltimore: Williams & Wilkins, 1997:1222–1223.
Kahn MF, Chamot AM. SAPHO syndrome. Rheum Dis Clin North Am 1992;18:225–246.

SARCOIDOSIS

Synonyms: Boeck's sarcoid, Uveoparotid fever, Lofgren's syndrome

ICD9 Codes: 135.0

Definition: Sarcoidosis is a chronic systemic inflammatory disorder of unknown etiology, characterized by noncaseating granulomata at involved sites.

Etiology: While exposure to an infectious organism or some other environmental agent has long been hypothesized to be etiologically relevant to the disease, none has been conclusively implicated. A variety of infectious agents (particularly intracellular pathogens such as fungi) can induce similar histopathologic changes, but none has been reliably recovered from sarcoid lesions. Similar changes may also be seen in association with malignancy.

Pathology: Based upon histopathologic studies, activated CD4+ helper T cells are considered to play a central role in the orchestration of sarcoid inflammation.

Although commonly considered a pulmonary disorder, the disease process affects many other organ systems. Indeed, about half of sarcoid patients present initially with constitutional symptoms such as fever, or symptoms related to inflammation at extrathoracic sites, including musculoskeletal complaints. Extrathoracic involvement is also common throughout the course of the disease. For example, approximately 10 to 15% of patients with sarcoidosis suffer from arthritis.

Demographics: Sarcoid typically affects young and middle-aged adults. There is a slight female preponderance. Prevalence is highest among African Americans (~40/100,000) and Caucasians of northern European extraction (~60/100,000). It has been suggested that sarcoid patients carrying the HLA-B8 allele may be more prone to develop erythema nodosum and acute arthritis, whereas sarcoid patients positive for HLA-DR3 may be more likely to develop the chronic form of arthritis.

Cardinal Findings: Sarcoid often affects multiple organ systems.

—*Pulmonary:* While some patients may never relate pulmonary symptoms, more than 90% show abnormalities on chest x-rays. Characteristic abnormalities have been classified into three types: type I, bilateral hilar lymphadenopathy, sometimes associated with right paratracheal lymphadenopathy; type II, lymphadenopathy as in type I plus pulmonary infiltrates; and type III, pulmonary infiltrates without lymphadenopathy. Patients with type I chest x-ray findings achieve spontaneous remission much more frequently than those with types II and III and typically require far less therapeutic intervention.

—*Musculoskeletal:* The most common musculoskeletal complaint of sarcoidosis is arthritis, which affects 10 to 15% of patients. Sarcoid arthritis may occur in two distinct patterns, and arthritis arising early in the disease course (e.g., within the initial 6 months) differs from that occurring later. Early arthritis, which is the more common type and may be the initial symptom of sarcoidosis, typically manifests as oligoarthritis of the ankles and, less commonly, the knees. In addition to true arthritis, patients may also have tenosynovitis and periarticular swelling. If joint effusions are present, they are often noninflammatory. Early sarcoid arthritis is often self-limited, lasting for days to months, and the prognosis is excellent. For example, most patients with *Lofgren's syndrome* (acute arthritis, erythema nodosum, and bilateral hilar lymphadenopathy), which occurs in a subset of patients with early disease, achieve spontaneous remission. Late sarcoid arthritis typically occurs more than 6 months after disease onset. Although it may manifest as monoarthritis, it typically presents as an oligoarthritis, with two or three joints involved. In decreasing order of frequency, affected joints include the knees, ankles, and PIPs. In addition to synovitis, patients may have periarticular swelling. When this occurs in the fingers (dactylitis or sausage digit), it may resemble the findings seen in the seronegative spondyloarthropathies, such as Reiter's syndrome. Although it may also be transient, late sarcoid arthritis persists more frequently than does early arthritis, which has implications for the therapeutic approach. Lastly, while joint x-rays in early sarcoid arthritis are typically normal, changes may be noted in late arthritis, including cystic changes in the middle of the phalanges.

—*Dermatologic:* Approximately one-third of sarcoid patients have one of the varied dermatologic manifestations of this disease. Erythema nodosum often occurs early in the disease course and typically remits spontaneously. It is associated with early arthritis, occurring in two-thirds of such patients. Late arthritis is not associated with erythema nodosum but rather with some of the more chronic dermatologic manifestations of sarcoidosis, including plaques, papules, and nodular and scaly lesions.

—*Other:* Other extrathoracic manifestations of sarcoidosis are relevant from a rheumatologic standpoint, as they may mimic various inflammatory diseases. Ocular involvement, especially uveitis, may develop in more than 20% of sarcoid patients. Uveitis is associated with a variety of systemic inflammatory disorders (see p. 379). Sarcoid involvement of the exocrine glands of the head (e.g., parotid, lacrimal) may resemble the findings of Sjögren's syndrome. Sarcoidosis of the skeletal muscles, although it may be asymptomatic, may present with a clinical picture resembling inflammatory myositis. Finally, sarcoid may also affect the liver, the central (Bell's palsy) and peripheral nervous systems, the lymphoid organs, and the kidney, among others.

Diagnostic Testing: No single clinical test is diagnostic of sarcoidosis. Nonspecific findings include leukopenia, lymphopenia, anemia, and increased hepatic enzymes or alkaline phosphatase. Hypercalciuria and hypercalcemia are seen in less than 10% of patients.

—*Kveim test:* Historically, this was used to make a diagnosis. Material obtained from a sarcoid granuloma was injected intradermally, and the patient was assessed for development of a delayed-type hypersensitivity reaction. However, the sensitivity and specificity of this test were disappointing, and it is no longer acceptable to inject tissue from one patient into another for diagnostic purposes. Thus, this test is no longer performed.

—*Angiotensin converting enzyme (ACE):* Serum levels reflect macrophage activity in granulomata and are elevated in approximately 60% of sarcoid patients. However, elevations in ACE levels are not specific for sarcoid as they are seen in other conditions (see p. 75). Moreover, because they reflect macrophage activity, they are most commonly elevated in patients with substantial active pulmonary involvement. Thus ACE levels are a poor screening diagnostic tool for unselected populations and for patients with less typical presentations.

Imaging: Chest x-ray abnormalities are commonly seen. Many investigators feel that the presence of bilateral and right paratracheal lymphadenopathy is both consistent with the diagnosis of sarcoidosis and associated with a benign prognosis to the extent that further diagnostic intervention may not be warranted. Gallium scans may show uptake in chest, lymph nodes, and parotids during periods of active disease.

Keys to Diagnosis: The diagnosis of sarcoidosis is usually achieved by the constellation of clinical findings, exclusion of diseases with similar conditions, and (if indicated) demonstration of noncaseating granulomata in histopathologic specimens.

Differential Diagnosis: Diseases with clinical presentations similar to sarcoidosis include infectious diseases (e.g., mycobacteria and fungi), lymphoproliferative neoplasms, foreign body reactions, Sjögren's syndrome, spondyloarthropathies, and SLE.

Therapy: The therapy of sarcoidosis varies and is usually driven by the most severe organ involvement. In many cases, therapy focuses on pulmonary involvement, although involvement of other organs (e.g., uveitis) sometimes mandates aggressive treatment. Corticosteroids, often at relatively high doses (≥40 mg/day), have been the therapeutic mainstay for severe sarcoidosis.

Early sarcoid arthritis, because it is often self-limited, is usually treated with NSAIDs and simple analgesics. Some cases of late arthritis also respond to such therapy. In refractory cases, a variety of agents have been tried, including colchicine, methotrexate, and other DMARDs. Oral corticosteroids are seldom indicated solely for sarcoid arthritis, but patients treated with steroids for other manifestations may show dramatic improvement in their arthritis. In addition, because sarcoid arthritis is often oligoarticular, intraarticular injection of steroids may be an important therapeutic option.

REFERENCES

FitzGerald AA, Davis P. Arthritis, hilar adenopathy, erythema nodosum complex. J Rheumatol 1982;9:935–938.
Gumpel JM, Johns CJ, Shulman LE. The joint disease of sarcoidosis. Ann Rheum Dis 1967;26:194–205.

SCHMORL'S NODES

Synonyms: Cartilaginous nodes

ICD9 Code: Unspecified, 722.30; lumbar or lumbosacral, 722.32; thoracic, 722.31

Definition: Schmorl's nodes are cartilaginous extrusions of disc material (nucleus pulposus) through the vertebral endplate into the body of the vertebrae. They are often incidental asymptomatic findings on radiographs.

Etiology: Schmorl's nodes may be idiopathic or associated with disorders that weaken or disrupt vertebral endplates or body (e.g., intervertebral osteochondrosis, Scheuermann's disease, trauma, hyperparathyroidism, osteoporosis, infection, and neoplasm).

Demographics: Schmorl's nodes are more common in men than women.

Cardinal Findings: Schmorl's nodes are often asymptomatic but may produce local mechanical pain. They are most frequently found at the lower endplate in the lower thoracic and upper lumbar vertebrae.

Uncommon Findings: Thoracic kyphosis may be seen in young individuals with Scheuermann's disease.

Diagnostic Tests: Conventional radiography is used.

Imaging: On radiographs, vertebral lesions appear as radiolucent (round or irregularly shaped) areas surrounded by sclerosis. They may also be visualized by CT or MRI.

Differential Diagnosis: Intervertebral osteochondrosis, Scheuermann's disease, trauma, hyperparathyroidism, osteoporosis, infection, and neoplasm should be considered.

Therapy: Usually no therapy is required. Analgesic agents may be used for pain.

SCLERODERMA

Synonyms: Progressive systemic sclerosis (PSS); diffuse scleroderma; (CREST syndrome is discussed on p. 183)

ICD9 Code: 710.1

Definition: Scleroderma is a multisystem disorder characterized by skin thickening and vascular abnormalities. In addition to skin, the most commonly affected organs are lung and kidney. Three major disease subsets are recognized, based on the extent of skin disease. Limited disease is defined as skin fibrosis in distal extremities and some areas of the face and neck. Limited disease is also known as the CREST (for calcinosis, Raynaud's, esophageal dysmotility, sclerodactyly, and telangiectasias) syndrome. Diffuse disease includes patients with skin abnormalities extending to the proximal extremities (i.e., above the elbow or knee) and trunk. Localized disease manifests as patches (morphea) or bandlike (linear scleroderma) areas of skin thickening.

Etiology: Causes of scleroderma remain mysterious. Immunologic abnormalities are suggested by the presence of characteristic autoantibodies such as ANA, anticentromere, and anti-Scl-70 antibodies. Early dermal changes include lymphocytic infiltrates consisting primarily of T cells, but the major abnormality is collagen accumulation with fibrosis. In addition, other striking abnormalities are seen in small to medium-sized blood vessels, which show immunologically bland fibrotic change. The theory that the vasculature is the primary target is supported by significant experimental data. In addition to these intrinsic abnormalities, association of scleroderma-like syndromes with epidemic exposures to toxins (e.g., toxic oil syndrome, eosinophilia-myalgia syndrome) suggests that an environmental trigger may start the process in a susceptible individual.

Pathology: Small arteries in skin, lung, and kidney show proliferation of subintimal tissues and fibrotic change. Small thrombi may form on the altered intimal surfaces. Luminal narrowing or occlusion can occur in these small vessels with even small amounts of vasospasm. Increased accumulation of fibrotic tissue, primarily collagen, is seen in the dermis and is accompanied by loss of normal skin appendages such as hair follicles. Skeletal muscle and myocardium may show atrophy of the muscle fibers and replacement by fibrotic tissue. Infrequently, histologic evidence of inflammatory myositis is seen.

Demographics: About 80% of patients are females, and half present before age 40 years. Some studies suggest a higher incidence and severity of disease in black females than in whites. A much higher prevalence is seen in the United States than in northern Europe or in Asia, a difference that at present remains unexplained.

Cardinal Findings: A variety of organ systems may be involved in scleroderma.

—*Skin:* Skin changes are the hallmark of this disease in most patients. Skin thickening is most noticeable in the hands, which in early stages may appear swollen or puffy. The skin is not easily pinched into small folds and may be indurated or bound down to underlying tissues. Normal skinfolds (e.g., over the knuckles) may be obliterated, and hair no longer grows over sclerodermatous skin. In the diffuse form, proximal extremity, truncal, and facial skin thickening is seen. The area around the mouth is often affected, with thinning of the lips and an inability to open the mouth fully. The lack of facial wrinkling may make patients appear younger than their actual age. Skin changes are often accompanied by Raynaud's phenomenon, and fingertips may be cool and dusky, with loss of the usual digital pulp. With time, hyperkeratosis develops under the nails, which may be another clue to Raynaud's phenomenon. Digital pits or scarring of the distal digital pulp are characteristic; some patients may have open ulcerations. Subcutaneous calcinosis can manifest as hard white lesions that uncommonly ulcerate with exudation of chalky material from open ulcers. Rarely, patients are seen without skin changes, but with organ (usually GI) involvement only (*scleroderma sinè scleroderma*).

—*Musculoskeletal:* Arthralgias and joint stiffness are common. Uncommonly, patients may initially display rheumatoid-like synovitis, with subsequent development of sclerodermal skin findings. Palpable tendon friction rubs are best felt over the flexor and extensor surface of the wrists, palms, or knees and produce a palpable grating sensation. Tendon friction rubs are seen early in the course of diffuse disease and are associated with increased incidence of internal organ involvement. Muscle weakness may be from muscle atrophy, fibrosis, or less commonly frank myositis.

—*Gastrointestinal:* Esophageal dysmotility with substernal dysphagia is common. Incompetence of the gastroesophageal sphincter leads to symptomatic reflux esophagitis. Common symptoms are heartburn and a sensation that food or pills are lodged in the chest behind the sternum. Involvement of the small bowel is less common and can produce a malabsorptive or blind loop syndrome. Colon abnormalities may contribute to constipation. Wide-mouthed diverticuli commonly occur in the large intestine.

—*Cardiopulmonary:* Insidious development of interstitial lung involvement is common early in the course of diffuse disease and may lead to a restrictive defect seen on pulmonary function testing. If fibrosis is present, auscultatory dry rales may be appreciated on examination. By contrast, limited scleroderma patients may develop acute-onset pulmonary hypertension late in the disease. Increased pulmonary pressures can contribute to right-sided heart failure.

—*Renal:* Kidney involvement, most common in the diffuse form, is an ominous finding and important cause of death in diffuse scleroderma. Hypertensive crisis may herald the onset of rapidly progressive renal failure. The syndrome includes very high blood pressure, headaches, visual disturbances, and heart failure. Microscopic hematuria may be observed and microangiopathic hemolytic anemia is usually present. Prior to the use of the angiotensin-converting enzyme (ACE) inhibitor class of antihypertensives, this syndrome was uniformly fatal. The more widespread use of ACE inhibitors has dramatically reduced the numbers of renal deaths in diffuse scleroderma. More than half of renal crisis patients do well and avoid long-term dialysis; less than 20% die from this infrequent complication.

—*Eyes/mouth:* Secondary Sjögren's syndrome occurs in a significant number of scleroderma patients, who are usually anti-SSA antibody positive and exhibit dry eyes and dry mouth.

—*Thyroid:* Hypothyroidism, present in about one-fourth of patients, is often clinically unrecognized. The thyroid gland shows fibrotic change. Hyperthyroidism is rare.

Uncommon Manifestations: Exudative pleural or pericardial effusions are rare. Intestinal pseudo-obstruction has been reported. Primary biliary cirrhosis appears to be increased in patients with the limited variant of scleroderma.

Diagnostic Tests: The diagnosis is made largely by history and physical examination. Laboratory information may provide supportive or prognostic information. Over 90% of patients are positive for antinuclear antibodies. The nucleolar ANA pattern is common in patients with diffuse scleroderma and the centromere pattern is characteristic of the limited (CREST) variant. Antibodies to Scl-70 are directed against topoisomerase-1 and are associated with the diffuse form. Patients tend to have either anticentromere (limited disease) or anti-Scl-70 (diffuse disease) antibodies but not both. Nailfold capillaroscopy (see p. 129) should be performed early in patients with Raynaud's phenomenon or suspected scleroderma to help define the prognosis. Periodic pulmonary function testing, including the force vital capacity and diffusion capacity, or DLCO, is indicated in patients with diffuse disease and is an effective measure of interstitial lung disease. Routine hemogram, chemistries, and urinalysis are most often indicated as part of drug monitoring.

Table 1
Proposed Criteria for the Classification of Patients with Scleroderma

A. Major criteria
    Proximal scleroderma: skin thickening/induration proximal to the MCP (or MTP)
    joints, in areas including face, neck, proximal extremities, and trunk
B. Minor criteria
    1. Sclerodactyly
    2. Digital pitting scars or loss of terminal digital pulp
    3. Bibasilar pulmonary fibrosis seen on standard chest radiograph
A diagnosis of scleroderma requires one major or two minor criteria.

Imaging: Chest radiographs should be performed to evaluate pulmonary symptoms and may aid in diagnosis of pulmonary fibrosis. High-resolution CT scans may be used to further evaluate pulmonary fibrosis and may show a "honeycomb" (with pulmonary fibrosis) or "ground-glass" (with alveolitis) appearance. Esophageal studies such as barium swallow with a cinè esophagram can identify lower esophageal dysmotility.

Keys to Diagnosis: Tightening of the skin, especially of the hands (sclerodactyly), associated with Raynaud's phenomenon strongly suggests scleroderma, either limited or diffuse.

Differential Diagnosis: Eosinophilic fasciitis (see p. 201) is a scleroderma variant in which skin tightening is most common in the extremities but spares the hands, feet, and face and is not associated with Raynaud's phenomenon. Tight skin may also be caused by exposure to vinyl chloride, solvents, rapeseed oil, bleomycin, pentazocine and tryptophan. *Pseudosclerodactyly* refers to waxy or tight skin changes seen with diabetes or hypothyroidism. *Scleromyxedema* causes waxy tightening of extremities and trunk. It is often associated with myopathy, monoclonal gammopathy, lymphoma, arthritis, neuropathy, or Sjögren's syndrome. The cause is unknown.

Diagnostic Criteria: A classification schema for scleroderma has been proposed that includes patients with diffuse or limited forms of the disease while excluding other syndromes such as eosinophilic fasciitis (Table 1). However, it is estimated that about 10% of patients in clinical practice who appear to have scleroderma do not fulfill these criteria.

Therapy: Treatment of Raynaud's phenomenon should include care to keep hands and feet warm with gloves or other coverings; these may required at night as well as during the day. Tobacco should be discontinued and β-blockers should be avoided. Biofeedback training or stress reduction techniques may be effective in limiting frequency or severity of the vasospastic episodes. Major dental procedures or appliances present a problem because of limitation of mouth excursion. Gastric reflux measures should be instituted, including elevating the head of the bed and avoiding late evening meals.

—*Raynaud's phenomenon:* Vasodilating agents may be used, especially long-acting calcium channel blockers such as nifedipine. High blood pressure is best treated with ACE inhibitors.

—*Corticosteroids:* In the early stages of diffuse disease, when hands appear puffy or edematous, low doses of prednisone may be useful. However, data suggest that high doses of corticosteroids can lead to renal crisis or failure. Thus steroids should be avoided in most patients.

—*Penicillamine:* Data from several uncontrolled studies show a reduction in skin thickening with use of penicillamine. Beneficial effects on pulmonary and GI abnormalities have also been reported from retrospective studies. Thus penicillamine is generally recommended in patients with early disease who manifest progressive skin changes, pulmonary compromise, or renal disease. A recent study did not show any clinical difference between low-dose (250–750 mg/day) and high-dose (1000–1500 mg/day) penicillamine. Unfortunately, a placebo-treated group was not included.

—*Others:* Use of other immunosuppressive drugs is not promising; no controlled trials suggest their benefit. Some investigators anecdotally advocate use of cyclophosphamide with progressive pulmonary fibrosis and cyclosporine for rapidly advancing early disease. Agents such as chlorambucil, methotrexate, extracorporeal photopheresis, antithymocyte globulin, interferon-α, and Potaba have been tried but remain unproven.

Surgery: Surgery is not generally indicated. Renal transplants have been relatively successful, and few patients have received heart or lung transplants.

Prognosis: Outcome is most closely related to the extent of significant organ involvement, especially lung and kidney. In one study, 5-year survival in patients without organ involvement was over 90%; patients with pulmonary or renal involvement had survival rates of 70% and 50%, respectively. Patients with diffuse skin involvement show shorter survival times than those with limited involvement. Patients with diffuse disease are at risk for early progressive end-organ damage, and those with limited disease are at a small but significant risk of developing pulmonary hypertension or small bowel malabsorption.

REFERENCES

Mayes MD. Scleroderma epidemiology. Rheum Dis Clin North Am 1996;22:751–764.

Medsger TA. Systemic sclerosis (scleroderma): clinical aspects. In: Koopman WJ, ed. Arthritis and allied conditions: a textbook of rheumatology. 13th ed. Baltimore: Williams & Wilkins, 1997:1433–1464.

Masi AT, Rodnan GP, Medsger TA Jr, et al. Preliminary criteria for the classification of systemic sclerosis (scleroderma). Arthritis Rheum 1980;23:581–590.

SEPTIC BURSITIS

ICD9 Code: Bursitis NOS 727.3 (code first underlying infection if present)

Definition: Septic bursitis is a bacterial infection of the bursal space, most commonly involving the olecranon and prepatellar areas.

Etiology: Most cases are due to inoculation of skin flora into the bursal space by local trauma. Certain occupations (e.g., carpetlaying and roofing) may be predisposed to inflammatory or septic bursitis.

Pathology: Changes of acute and chronic inflammation may develop in the bursa and surrounding tissues.

Demographics: Most series have an excess of males, possibly because of occupational hazards. Normal individuals without underlying comorbid conditions can be affected.

Cardinal Findings: The classic presentation is an acute, painful, warm swelling in the periarticular region. Because the joint is not involved, range of motion is usually unaffected. Fever is usually not present.

Diagnostic Tests: Because of the focal acute inflammatory presentation, bursal aspiration should be performed with a large-bore needle (18 or 19 gauge). Cultures of bursal fluid are diagnostic. The bursal fluid WBC can be variable and does not correlate well with the severity of infection. Even relatively low WBC values can be seen with active bacterial infection; thus, cultures are important in all suspected cases. Gram stains may be useful in making the initial antibiotic choices. The fluid is more superficial than synovial fluid, and the aspirating needle should not enter the joint space.

Keys to Diagnosis: Acute onset of periarticular swelling should raise suspicion. Septic arthritis can be diagnosed by bursal aspiration and cultures.

Differential Diagnosis: Septic arthritis should be considered if there is fever and limited range of motion and if movement of the nearby joint accentuates the pain. Cellulitis or tendinitis may mimic bursitis with periarticular pain and overlying erythematous skin changes.

Therapy: Antibiotics should be started soon after the initial bursal aspiration. Oral antibiotic administration is usually adequate. While culture results are pending (usually 24–48 hours), the initial antibiotic should provide coverage for *Staphylococcus aureus* until culture results can further guide therapy.

Surgery: Surgical drainage or removal of the bursal tissue is rarely, if ever, required.

Prognosis: Most patients recover completely without sequelae.

REFERENCES

Ho G, Su EY. Antibiotic therapy of septic bursitis: its implication in the treatment of septic arthritis. Arthritis Rheum 1981;24:905–911.
Pien FD, Ching D, Kim E. Septic bursitis: experience in a community practice. Orthopedics 1991;14:981–984.

SICKLE-CELL DISEASE: MUSCULOSKELETAL MANIFESTATIONS

ICD9 Code: Sickle cell anemia, 282.60

Definition: Musculoskeletal manifestations may occur as a consequence of sickle cell anemia and related hemoglobinopathies.

Etiology: Certain genetic disorders of the hemoglobin molecule, encompassed by the term *sickle cell disease* (sickle cell anemia, sickle cell trait, sickle cell hemoglobin disease, and various sickle cell thalassemia syndromes) are all characterized by varying degrees of chronic hemolysis and acute intermittent crises related to vasocclusion that may lead to end-organ failure. Musculoskeletal disease likely results from vasocclusive infarction of bone marrow and adjacent cortical, subchondral, and trabecular bone. Subsequent inflammatory reaction increases intramedullary pressure, causing pain. Additionally, disease may result from bone marrow expansion, characteristic of the chronic hemolytic anemias. Hyperuricemia from increased red cell turnover may result in clinical gout. The increased susceptibility to bacterial infection (functional asplenia) greatly increases the frequency of osteomyelitis and septic arthritis. Noninflammatory joint effusions and chronic synovitis are probably related to microvascular occlusion.

Demographics: Sickle cell anemia is almost exclusively a disease of African Americans, 0.2% of whom are homozygous (sickle cell anemia) for the sickle cell gene; 10% are heterozygous (sickle cell trait) and rarely have clinical disease. Combinations of sickle cell with other hemoglobinopathies are much less common. Musculoskeletal symptoms are reported in 80% of patients with sickle cell anemia.

Cardinal Findings: A variety of findings have been reported with sickle disease.

—*Joint effusions:* Usually observed in acute crises, joint effusions are often transient or migratory, involving the knees, elbows, and hands. They are often self-limited, resolving within 1 to 2 weeks without permanent deformities.

—*Chronic arthritis:* Severe disabling arthropathy develops in older patients, with repeated bony infarcts near the knee joint, resembling osteoarthritis.

—*Axial skeleton disease:* Expansion of the bone marrow may cause trabecular changes leading to cuplike vertebral body indentations; compression may lead to dorsal kyphosis and lumbar lordosis.

—*Osteomyelitis and septic arthritis:* Osteomyelitis is 100 times more common in sickle cell patients than in normal populations. Infection with salmonella predominates (50%). Multiple sites may be seen. Pain onset is less dramatic and is often confused with painful bony infarcts. Fever and persistent leukocytosis should raise the possibility of osteomyelitis. Septic arthritis is less common.

—*Sickle cell dactylitis:* Also known as "hand-foot syndrome," dactylitis causes painful swelling, erythema, and warmth of the hands and feet in infants and young children. Fever and leukocytosis are common. Swelling lasts

1 to 3 weeks and often recurs. It usually heals without sequelae, but premature epiphyseal fusion may result in shortened digits.

—*Long-bone infarcts:* Diaphyseal infarcts in acute crises may present as excruciating pain, warmth, and swelling, mimicking soft tissue abscesses or osteomyelitis. Chronically, this may appear radiologically as areas of osteosclerosis.

—*Osteonecrosis:* Osteonecrosis of the femoral and humeral heads is directly related to vascular occlusion. It presents insidiously with pain on weight bearing and motion. It commonly causes chronic disability.

Uncommon Findings: Gout may occur, as 40% of persons with sickle cell anemia are hyperuricemic. Acute gout, which may be polyarticular, has been reported. Rheumatoid arthritis has rarely been reported. Myonecrosis is a newly described complication, affecting proximal muscle groups symmetrically with myofascial pain, tenderness and swelling occur. Muscle biopsy reveals acute myonecrosis.

Diagnostic Tests: For those with an acute painful crisis a CBC and reticulocytes should be done to exclude aplastic crisis. Fever, leukocytosis, and prolonged painful crisis suggests osteomyelitis. Radiographs are not helpful at early stages. Joint aspiration may be necessary to exclude septic arthritis. In uncomplicated arthritis, synovial fluid is noninflammatory.

—*Osteonecrosis:* Radiographs normal in early stages of osteonecrosis. MRI very helpful in establishing the diagnosis. In later stages radiographs initially show a radiolucent subcortical line collapse and bony remodeling.

Therapy: Therapy varies with the clinical presentation.

—*Acute painful crisis:* Use aggressive rehydration and control of pain. NSAIDs may suffice for mild-to-moderate pain. Narcotic analgesics are often required. Exchange transfusion is reserved for life-threatening complications such as acute chest syndrome.

—*Osteonecrosis:* Avoid weight bearing; complete bed rest is preferable. Spontaneous healing may occur. Advanced osteonecrosis often requires total hip arthroplasty.

—*Osteomyelitis:* Antibiotic therapy is recommended for 3 months, based on identification of the organism, if possible.

Prognosis: Acute painful crises are generally self-limited. Osteonecrosis of the femoral head is the leading cause of disability. Osteomyelitis occasionally becomes chronic. Sickle cell dactylitis may result in premature epiphyseal closure and shortening of digits.

REFERENCES

Heck LW. Arthritis associated with hematologic disorders, storage diseases, disorders of lipid metabolism: hemoglobinopathies. In: Koopman WJ, ed. Arthritis and allied conditions: a textbook of rheumatology. 13th ed. Baltimore: Williams & Wilkins, 1997:1704–1707.

Porter DR, Stubbock RD. Rheumatologic complications of sickle cell disease. Ballières Clin Rheumatol 1991;5:221–230.

SILICONE-RELATED RHEUMATIC DISEASE

Synonyms: "human adjuvant disease"; silicone synovitis

Definition: Silicone-related rheumatic disease is a highly controversial subject surrounded by a great deal of litigation and poor scientific evidence. A variety of rheumatic syndromes have been anecdotally related to silicone exposure, particularly in individuals receiving silicone gel–filled augmentation mammoplasty, soft tissue silicone injection, or sialastic joint implants.

Etiology: Pathogenesis underlying these complaints is unclear. Silicone has been reported to migrate from breast implants to regional lymph nodes and distant sites and, in some cases, may induce inflammatory or fibrotic change. To date, a few well-done epidemiologic studies have failed to show an association between silicone exposure and connective tissue diseases (e.g., scleroderma, Raynaud's phenomenon, systemic lupus erythematosus, rheumatoid arthritis, inflammatory myositis). Thus, it appears that the occurrence of connective tissue disease in such persons is likely to be coincidental. Women with silicone implants exhibit the same soft tissue rheumatic complaints commonly observed in age- and sex-matched individuals without silicone implants.

Adjuvants are substances designed to augment the potency of immunogens and to prolong their exposure. The earliest reports of musculoskeletal symptoms occurred in those receiving subcutaneous injection of paraffin or silicone gel for breast augmentation. As these symptoms were reminiscent of adjuvant arthritis in rats, the term "human adjuvant disease" was applied to these patients. This term has fallen into disfavor, however, primarily because of the lack of an appropriate clinical definition or identification of a human equivalent to the animal model of adjuvant arthritis.

Demographics: This syndrome has almost exclusively been applied to those receiving silicone gel–filled implants, silicone injection in the breasts, or sialastic joint implants. Thus, most are women, between 30 and 60 years of age. Musculoskeletal symptoms usually arise many years (>10) after exposure to the silicone product. This syndrome has rarely been reported in men.

Cardinal Findings: Symptoms generally develop 10–15 years after the placement of silicone implants. Most patients have clinical features resembling fibromyalgia (see p. 207) or chronic fatigue syndrome: extreme fatigue and widespread muscle and joint pain, often with an associated sleep disturbance. Although rare, the manifestations of a specific connective tissue disease do not differ from those of its idiopathic form. Onset of rheumatic symptoms is not associated with fibrosis, contracture, or rupture of the implant.

—Silicone synovitis: Silicone elastomer is found in numerous sialastic (artificial) joints used during joint replacement. It appears that some of these joints degrade by movement, shearing, microfractures, and the release of microfragments that induce a foreign body reaction. This is an uncommon syndrome seen in those receiving sialastic joint replacement (usually involving

the MCP joints). Intense local synovitis, osteolysis, or erosion of cartilage and bone may be seen. Regional lymphadenitis has been reported.

Complications: Local complications of silicone gel breast implants rarely include local infection, capsular contracture, and capsular rupture.

Diagnostic Tests: No distinctive laboratory tests are correlated with, or diagnostic of, silicone-related musculoskeletal disease. A low, but increased, percentage of ANA positivity is seen in those receiving silicone implants. These autoantibodies are often transient, of low titer, and of uncertain significance, as true SLE is exceedingly rare. Other autoantibodies are usually absent, and the value or reproducibility of antisilicone antibodies is disappointing and should not be used or interpreted as evidence of a silicone-induced disease state. A consistent pattern of immune responses has not been identified and cannot be tested for. Large batteries of immunologic/rheumatologic tests should be discouraged.

Therapy: The goals of therapy are to reassure the patient and provide symptomatic treatment. The exceptional individual found to have a coincidental connective tissue disease should be managed as those with idiopathic forms of these diseases. There are no reliable data to support removal of implants, as this is not likely to improve the patient's musculoskeletal and systemic symptoms. Removal may be indicated for infection, hardening, rupture, or cosmetic reasons.

Comment: Since April 1992, the Food and Drug Administration has banned the use of silicone gel implants in the United States. Research is still needed to establish a causal relationship between silicone implants and rheumatic disease.

REFERENCES

Hochberg MC, Perlmutter DM. The association of augmentation mammoplasty with connective tissue disease, including systemic sclerosis (scleroderma): a meta-analysis. In: Potter M, Rose NR, eds. Immunology of silicones. Current topics in microbiology and immunology, no. 210. Berlin: Springer-Verlag, 1995:411–417.

Silver RM. Variant forms of scleroderma: scleroderma variants associated with exposure to silica and silicone. In: Koopman WJ, ed. Arthritis and allied conditions: a textbook of rheumatology. 13th ed. Baltimore: Williams & Wilkins, 1997:1471–1473.

SJÖGREN'S SYNDROME

Synonyms: Keratoconjunctivitis sicca (KCS); sicca complex

ICD9 Codes: 710.2

Definition: Sjögren's syndrome is a chronic autoimmune syndrome characterized by lymphocytic infiltration of lacrimal glands and salivary glands with consequent dry eyes (xerophthalmia) and dry mouth (xerostomia). When occurring without another autoimmune disorder, it is considered primary Sjögren's disease. Secondary Sjögren's syndrome occurs in patients with preexisting autoimmune disease, most commonly rheumatoid arthritis and scleroderma.

Etiology: The causative trigger is not known, although various viruses including Epstein-Barr virus and HTLV-I have been proposed as candidate agents. The high incidence in females suggests a facilitating role for sex steroid hormones. HLA associations (HLA-B8, -DR3, and -Dw52 in males) have been described, highlighting a genetic predisposition. Sex hormones may play a role, as the condition is more common in women and improved by androgen therapy.

Pathology: Salivary gland biopsies show benign lymphoepithelial infiltration and proliferation in the exocrine (e.g., salivary, lacrimal, parotid) glands (see labial salivary biopsy, p. 124). Adjacent areas of the gland may appear normal. Helper (CD4+) T cells predominate and most likely activate antibody production by infiltrating B lymphocytes, resulting in hypergammaglobulinemia and circulating autoantibodies. Infiltrating lymphocytes mediate destruction and dysfunction of the adjacent glandular tissue.

Demographics: Onset is usually in middle age, with a predominance of females.

Cardinal Findings: Dry mouth and eyes are the predominant presentation. Xerostomia may or may not be noticeable to the patient and may manifest as accelerated dental caries in some. Inadequate saliva production may result in pharyngeal dysphagia. Dry eyes may manifest as redness, conjunctival irritation, or the sensation of "sand" or "grit" in the eye. Patients blink or rub their eyes excessively in response. Parotid gland enlargement is found in a minority of patients.

Musculoskeletal features include fatigue and fibromyalgia in nearly 50% of patients. Fewer patients complain of arthralgias, and frank arthritis is rare.

Uncommon Manifestations: Lymphocytic infiltration into the kidney may result in tubular dysfunction that is usually not clinically significant. Rarely, such patients manifest a renal tubular acidosis with severe potassium wasting, hypokalemia, and muscle weakness. CNS involvement (i.e., polyneuropathy, cranial nerve neuropathy, multiple sclerosis–like symptoms, headaches, or altered mentation) occurs, but is rare. Pulmonary involvement is subclinical in most and rarely symptomatic. Pulmonary features include bronchitis, interstitial fibrosis, and lymphocytic alveolitis. Gastrointestinal features include dysphagia, atrophic gastritis, primary biliary sclerosis or sclerosing cholangitis. A small subset of Sjögren's syndrome patients may go on to develop malignant lymphoma.

Diagnostic Tests: Common laboratory abnormalities include an elevated ESR, polyclonal hypergammaglobulinemia, and an anemia of chronic disease. Antinuclear antibodies and rheumatoid factor are positive in 65–90% of patients, respectively. SS-A antibodies are not specific for Sjögren's syndrome and can be seen in other autoimmune disorders. SS-B antibodies tend to have a greater association with Sjögren's syndrome. Antibodies against SS-A (anti-Ro) are seen in 70–80% of primary and in less than 10% of secondary Sjögren's syndrome patients. Antibodies against SS-B (anti-La) are seen in 50–75% of primary and less than 5% of secondary Sjögren's syndrome patients.

The diagnosis of keratoconjunctivitis sicca can be further established with quantitative measures of tear production. Schirmer's test (see p. 139) uses adsorbent paper strips inserted into the lower palpebral fold to measure the amount of wetting or tear production. Alternatively, the ophthalmologist can facilitate the diagnosis by performing a rose bengal test (see p. 139). Rose bengal is a vital stain that is taken up by dead or dying cells and is used to evaluate corneal abnormalities in patients with symptomatic or suspected keratoconjunctivitis sicca. Biopsy of glandular tissue (i.e., minor salivary gland of the lip or parotid gland) may also reveal the characteristic lymphocytic infiltration diagnostic of Sjögren's syndrome.

Keys to Diagnosis: Xerostomia and xerophthalmia with parotid gland enlargement strongly suggests this diagnosis.

Differential Diagnosis: Infections (i.e., mumps) and infiltrative processes such as sarcoidosis may cause parotid enlargement. Parotid tumors are likely to be unilateral. Drugs (i.e., tricyclic antidepressants) and irradiation may cause dry eyes and mouth. A subset of HIV(+) patients develop xerostomia, parotid swelling, generalized lymphadenopathy, lymphocytic pulmonary infiltrates, and negative tests for anti-Ro or anti-La.

Diagnostic Criteria: Recently proposed European Criteria are shown in Table 1.

Therapy: Sicca symptoms are treated with lubricating eye drops (see p. 401) and avoidance of aggravating factors such as hair dryers or "drying" medications. Wearing glasses outdoors may protect from the drying effects of the wind. Ophthalmic consultation is recommended for most. Punctal occlusion may improve tear retention and flow. Saliva substitutes are available and may be preferred by some patients. The use of sugar-free lemon hard candies may help stimulate salivary flow. Fastidious dental care is extremely important to avoid dental caries. The

Table 1
Preliminary Criteria for the Classification of Sjögren's Syndrome[a]

1. Ocular symptoms: dry eyes, foreign body sensation in eyes, use of lubricants
2. Oral symptoms: dry mouth, swollen salivary glands, frequent fluid intake with food
3. Ocular signs: Schirmer's or rose bengal tests
4. Characteristic histopathologic features: focus score $\geq$ 1 (labial minor salivary gland biopsy)
5. Salivary gland involvement documented by scintigraphy, sialography, or salivary flow
6. Autoantibodies: RF, ANA, or anti-Ro (SSA) or anti-La (SSB)
The presence of 4 of 6 criteria has a sensitivity of 93.5% and specificity of 94%.

[a] Exclusions: lymphoma, AIDS, sarcoidosis, or graft-versus-host disease.

use of humidifiers at home or work may decrease symptoms significantly. NSAIDs and analgesic agents may improve the arthralgias and myalgias. Corticosteroids should not be used for most and are only indicated with vasculitis, pleuropericarditis, or hemolytic anemia. Numerous second-line and immunosuppressive agents (including methotrexate, penicillamine, and cyclosporine) have been tried, and only hydroxychloroquine appears to have minimal benefit in Sjögren's patients. Investigational agents include bromhexine, interferon, and androgens.

Surgery: Diagnostic minor salivary gland biopsy may be performed by an oral surgeon. Parotid biopsy via a posterior approach to the subauricular portion of the gland is preferred to reduce the risk of facial nerve injury.

Prognosis: Most patients do well. Sicca problems may require prolonged eye care. High-grade lymphoma that may be resistant to chemotherapy is rare.

REFERENCES

Silver RM. Variant forms of scleroderma. In: Koopman WJ, ed. Arthritis and allied conditions: a textbook of rheumatology. Baltimore: Williams & Wilkins, 1996:1465–1480.
Vitali C, Bomardieri S, Moutsopoulos HM, et al. Preliminary criteria for the classification of Sjögren's syndrome: results of a prospective concerted action supported by the European Community. Arthritis Rheum 1993;36:340–347.

SPINAL STENOSIS

ICD9 Code: 724.0

Definition: Spinal stenosis refers to a narrowing of the lumen of the spinal canal. It occurs most commonly in the lumbar region but can also occur in the cervical spine. The characteristic clinical symptom of spinal stenosis is *neurogenic claudication*. Although it may be related in rare cases to developmental bony anomalies, the most common cause of spinal stenosis is degenerative change in the vertebrae (these nonspecific degenerative changes are also known as *spondylosis*).

Pathology: In most patients, a combination of factors contributes to the narrowing of the spinal canal. Anteriorly, degenerative changes of the intervertebral disc cause disc protrusion and extrusion into the spinal canal. Posteriorly, osteoarthritic changes of the facet (apophyseal) joints impinge directly on the spinal cord. Facet joint arthritis, very common among older persons, is also associated with hypertrophy of the ligamentum flavum, which is normally thin and lines the spinal canal. This further diminishes the area of the spinal canal. Degenerative changes of the facet joints may result in laxity and movement of one vertebral body in relation to others, either unilaterally (*spondylolysis*) or bilaterally (*spondylolisthesis*). This may result in further impingement of neural structures.

Demographics: Spinal stenosis is most common among the elderly, with a mean age of onset of approximately 60 years of age. Men are affected about twice as frequently as women. Many patients experience symptoms for months or even years before the correct diagnosis is established.

Cardinal Findings: Symptoms of *neurogenic claudication* (or pseudoclaudication) occur in more than 90% of patients. It is commonly described as an aching pain in the buttocks, posterior thigh, or calf (>90%) and is often provoked or aggravated by walking. However, it may also be described as numbness (~65%) or weakness (~40%) and is bilateral in approximately 70% of patients. Of note, the area of the lumbar spinal canal and neural foramina change with position. This space increases with flexion, and patients with spinal stenosis often report relief of symptoms when their backs are flexed; for example, sitting, bending over, or sleeping in the fetal position. This may provide a useful clue to differentiating vascular from neurogenic claudication. Patients with vascular claudication are limited in their walking by vascular supply. Symptoms are relieved by stopping walking, and patients do not necessarily need to sit down or change position. In contrast, patients with neurogenic claudication find relief by sitting down or bending over. They may also have similar pain by standing erect without walking, and they can walk without limit if their spines are flexed (e.g., pushing a shopping cart or lawnmower).

On physical examination, most patients experience pain on straight leg raising. Many also have depressed lower extremity deep tendon reflexes. Muscle weakness or sensory defects are not common. Pulses are generally easily palpable, another potential point distinguishing neurogenic from vascular claudication.

Diagnostic Testing: Hematologic, chemical, and serologic studies are of no value in evaluating patients with spinal stenosis. Electrodiagnostic studies (e.g., nerve conduction velocity testing) may provide useful information. Such tests may exclude other conditions (e.g., neuropathies) and document the severity and extent of neurologic involvement from spinal stenosis.

Imaging: Plain radiographs are commonly used to evaluate patients with back pain, but their utility may be limited, particularly in spinal stenosis. Radiographs typically show degenerative changes of the lumbar spine. However, such changes provide no information regarding neurologic impingement and do not correlate with the severity of symptoms. Bony abnormalities and narrowing of the spinal canal is easily visualized by CT imaging. However, CT imaging must be combined with myelography for clear definition of bony impingement on the spinal cord or nerve roots. MRI, which allows definition of bone as well as soft and nerve tissue, is now the imaging procedure of choice for patients with spinal stenosis.

Differential Diagnosis: Vascular insufficiency, inflammatory spondyloarthropathy (e.g., ankylosing spondylitis), spinal metastases, disc disease, and Paget's disease should be considered.

Therapy: The most appropriate therapy depends upon the extent and progression of symptoms. Conservative measures include physiotherapy (e.g., optimizing low back mechanics, muscle strengthening, enhancing flexibility) and analgesic medications.

Surgery: Patients with cauda equina syndrome (loss of bowel or bladder function, "saddle" [perineal] anesthesia) may require surgical decompression of the stenosed canal. Patients with progression of either neurologic defects (e.g., radiculopathy) or intractable pain likewise may benefit from surgical intervention. The type of surgery depends on the specific pathologic changes considered most responsible for the patient's symptoms. In most patients, laminectomy is the procedure of choice, although a few patients may benefit from foraminectomy or discectomy. Surgery is not required for all patients, and in some series, patients appear to have similar long-term outcomes with or without surgery.

Prognosis: The course of spinal stenosis is variable. For many patients, it is a chronic condition that may improve with intervention. Some patients experience relatively rapid progression from intermittent pain to excruciating persistent pain to neurologic defect.

REFERENCES

Hall S, Bartleson JD, Onofrio BM, et al. Lumbar spinal stenosis. Ann Intern Med 1985;103: 271–275.
Moreland LW, Lopez-Mendez A, Alarcon GS. Spinal stenosis: a comprehensive review of the literature. Semin Arthritis Rheum 1989;19:127–149.
Swezey RL. Outcomes for lumbar stenosis. J Clin Rheum 1996;2:129–133.

SPONDYLOARTHROPATHY

Synonyms: Seronegative spondyloarthropathies (SNSA), incomplete spondyloarthropathy (SpA); HLA-B27-related spondyloarthropathy

ICD9 Codes: Codes for individual disorders: ankylosing spondylitis (AS), 720.0; Reiter's syndrome, 099.3; psoriatic arthritis, 696.1

Definition: Spondyloarthropathy (SpA) is a generic term applied to a constellation of clinical, radiographic, and immunogenetic features shared by a group of disorders that include AS (see p. 156), Reiter's syndrome (RS) (see p. 315), reactive arthritis, psoriatic arthritis (PsA) (see p. 307), and enteropathic arthritis (see p. 198). As only a minority of patients manifest complete or classic findings of one of these individual disorders and most instead demonstrate incomplete or overlapping features, changes in nosology have been adopted to accommodate what is actually seen in clinical practice. This latter group is often designated as having an incomplete spondyloarthropathy or an HLA-B27-related spondyloarthropathy. The term *spondyloarthropathy* has gained popularity since 1990 when more liberal diagnostic criteria were proposed (Table 1).

Etiology: By virtue of their association with HLA-B27 and overlapping clinical and radiographic features, the disorders are presumed to share a similar etiopathogenesis. Most theories relate to unknown antigenic or infectious inciting events occurring in a genetically susceptible host, leading to either molecular mimicry or a chronic, antigen-driven "reactive" condition.

Table 1
Diagnostic Criteria for the Spondyloarthropathies

ESSG Criteria for Spondyloarthropathy	Amor Criteria for the Spondyloarthropathies	Score
1. Inflammatory spinal pain *or* peripheral synovitis (asymmetric or lower limbs)	Lumbar pain at night or AM stiffness	1
	Asymmetric oligoarthritis	2
	Buttock pain (or bilateral or alternating buttock pain)	1
2. Plus 1 or more of the following: Alternate buttock pain		
Sacroiliitis	Sausagelike toe or digit(s)	2
Enthesopathy	Heel pain or enthesitis	2
Positive family history	Iritis	1
Psoriasis	Nongonococcal urethritis/cervicitis within 1 month of onset	
Inflammatory bowel disease		
Urethritis or cervicitis or acute diarrhea occurring within 1 month of the onset of arthritis	Psoriasis, balanitis, or IBD	1
	Sacroiliitis (bilateral grade 2 or unilateral grade 3)	2
	HLA-B27(+) or (+) family history of a spondyloarthropathy	2
	Rapid (<48 h) response to NSAIDs	2
	Diagnosis of a spondyloarthropathy requires a score ≥6	

Demographics: While limited data exist on the incidence of disorders like AS, RS, PsA, and enteropathic arthritis, no reliable demographic data exist on patients diagnosed under the more general term *spondyloarthropathy*. Nonetheless, this more liberally defined population is likely to be more prevalent than the individual subsets they resemble. Like the other disorders, the spondyloarthropathies are more likely to be seen in men. Women may tend to have milder disease that is more difficult to diagnose. Although seen in all age groups, most patients present between the ages of 20 and 50 years.

Pathology: These disorders share a common pathologic profile, which includes a propensity for axial and peripheral inflammatory arthritis and inflammation involving the eye (conjunctivitis, uveitis), skin (psoriasis, nail changes), mucosal surfaces (oral and genital), and tendinous attachments to bone (enthesitis). Synovial membrane shows histologic inflammation similar to that seen with rheumatoid arthritis, with synovial proliferation and prominent infiltration with mononuclear cells in the sublining and perivascular areas. There is a greater propensity for fibrous ankylosis, osseous resorption, and heterotopic bone formation. Skin changes are compatible with keratoderma blenorrhagica or pustular psoriasis.

Cardinal Findings: The spondyloarthropathies share a constellation of characteristic clinical, radiographic, and immunogenetic manifestations that suggest a common or related etiopathogenesis (Table 1). Distinctive features include a propensity for axial arthritis (sacroiliitis and spondylitis); peripheral arthritis (often asymmetric and oligoarticular); inflammation at tendinous, ligamentous, or fascial insertions (enthesitis); and a familial pattern of inheritance based on the presence of the class I major histocompatibility complex (MHC) antigen, HLA-B27. These disorders can manifest extraarticular features that suggest a particular spondyloarthropathy. Extraarticular manifestations may involve periarticular structures (enthesitis), eyes (uveitis), gastrointestinal tract (oral ulcerations, asymptomatic gut inflammation), genitourinary tract (urethritis), heart (aortitis, heart block), skin (keratoderma blennorrhagica), or nails (onycholysis). Occasionally patients with overlapping features of more than one condition or with HLA-B27(+) unclassifiable disease may be encountered. Thus, approaching these conditions as a group of related disorders is important in understanding their pathologic consequences and in diagnosing them accurately.

Diagnostic Criteria: Criteria for the diagnosis of a spondyloarthropathy have been proposed by the European Spondyloarthropathy Study Group (ESSG) (Table 1). The criteria of Amor et al. perform equally well in population studies. These were devised because other disease-specific criteria (e.g., Rome criteria for AS) exclude many spondyloarthropathy patients. Broader definitions used in these criteria allow earlier diagnosis and more liberal inclusion in clinical trials.

Imaging: Radiographic abnormalities are similar to those seen in AS (p. 156) and RS (see p. 315). There is a propensity for sacroiliitis, spondylitis, and peripheral arthritis with soft tissue swelling, juxtaarticular osteopenia, joint space narrowing, or ill-defined erosions. Areas of periostitis, reactive new bone formation, or osteitis are not uncommon.

Therapy: See sections on AS (p. 156) and RS (p. 315) for guidance.

REFERENCES

Amor B, Dougados M, Khan MA. Management of refractory ankylosing spondylitis and related spondyloarthropathies. Rheum Dis Clin North Am 1995;21:117–128.

Arnett FC. Seronegative spondyloarthropathies. Bull Rheum Dis 1987;37:1–12.

Dougados M, van der Linden SM, Juhlin R, et al. The European Spondyloarthropathy Study Group preliminary criteria for the classification of spondyloarthropathy. Arthritis Rheum 1991;34:1218–1227.

Khan MA, van der Linden SM. A wider spectrum of spondyloarthropathies. Semin Arthritis Rheum 1990;20:107–113.

STREPTOCOCCAL REACTIVE ARTHRITIS

Synonyms: Incomplete rheumatic fever, poststreptococcal arthritis

ICD9 Code: 711.0

Etiology: Reactive arthropathy is due to streptococcal infection (groups A and G).

Demographics: Streptococcal reactive arthritis is most common in children and young adults but also reported in adults.

Cardinal Findings: Onset follows streptococcal pharyngitis. Arthropathy (non-migratory oligo- or polyarthritis) occurs within 2 weeks after a documented infection. About one-third manifest episodic arthralgias or arthritis. Many develop systemic manifestations including fever, myalgias, prostration, and serositis.

Uncommon Findings: Very few patients have developed carditis on long-term follow-up.

Diagnostic Tests: Most patients have an elevated antistreptolysin O or DNase B antibody titer.

Keys to Diagnosis: Streptococcal reactive arthritis is distinguished from acute rheumatic fever (ARF) by lack of sufficient features to meet the Jones criteria. Classic cutaneous, cardiac, and neurologic findings of ARF are absent.

Therapy: Therapy is similar to that of ARF, but whether subsequent antibiotic prophylaxis is necessary is controversial.

Course: Characteristically, response to therapy with salicylates or NSAIDs is slow or incomplete. The course is often benign with a good outcome.

REFERENCES

Arnold MH, Tyndall A. Poststreptococcal reactive arthritis. Ann Rheum Dis 1989;48:686–688.
Deighton C. β-Hemolytic streptococci and reactive arthritis in adults. Ann Rheum Dis 1993;
    52:475–482.

SUBSTANCE ABUSE: MUSCULOSKELETAL MANIFESTATIONS

Synonyms: IVDA-associated arthritis, brown heroin syndrome

ICD9 Code: Drug addiction, 304.9; vasculitis, 446.6; arthralgia, 719.4

Definition: A variety of musculoskeletal syndromes are described among substance abuse patients. Symptoms are due to the offending drug or adulterants within the drug. Implicated drugs include stimulants (e.g., methamphetamines, cocaine), narcotics (heroin), and hallucinogens (D-lysergic acid diethylamide [LSD]. Although patients may admit to abusing a particular drug, abuse of multiple drugs is common.

Etiology: Causes vary, including immune complex–mediated disease, foreign body reactions, vessel spasm/toxicity, or other as-yet unidentified mechanisms.

Pathology: Pathology varies, depending on the syndrome. Vascular lesions may be similar to those seen in polyarteritis. Necrotizing angiitis may involve medium-sized or small arteries of various organs (heart, muscle, kidney, liver, brain, lungs, etc). Refractile particles caused by talc or other adulterants may be seen in small vessels by polarized microscopy.

Demographics: Those engaging in substance abuse are at risk.

Clinical Syndromes

—*Drug withdrawal:* Myalgias and arthralgias, with or without fever, may be seen during drug withdrawal.

—*IVDA-induced angiitis:* Polyarteritis-like angiitis has been seen in those abusing methamphetamines, LSD, and cocaine. Patients have been described with fever, weight loss, arthralgia, myalgia, hypertension, abdominal pain, neuropathy, encephalopathy, pulmonary edema, leukocytosis, hemolysis, proteinuria, medium and large vessel vasculitis, and death.

—*Brown heroin:* Musculoskeletal manifestations have been described in those abusing brown heroin. Brown heroin gets its color from adulterants (procaine or papaverine) or impurities of the opium plant during manufacture. Symptoms arise days to months after use of brown heroin. Patients may complain of neck or low back pain, myalgia, or stiffness. Joint pain tends to be periarticular, affecting the knees, ankles, tarsus, wrist, elbow, or shoulder. Inflammatory synovitis is uncommon. Laboratory abnormalities include increased ESR and hypergammaglobulinemia. A minority test positive for ANA, RF, syphilis, or cryoglobulins. Antibiotics are of no value, but ASA or NSAIDs may be effective.

—*Cocaine vasculitis:* Cerebral vasculitis, Raynaud's phenomenon, myositis, rhabdomyolysis, and leukocytoclastic vasculitis have resulted from cocaine abuse. Such patients often have a very high ESR and an abnormal angiogram. Response to corticosteroids or cytotoxic therapy may be disappointing.

—*Barbiturate-related connective tissue disorders:* Patients using or abusing barbiturates (phenobarbital, primidone) are at low risk to develop arthralgias, Dupuytren's contractures, or Peyronie's disease. Bilateral, rather than unilateral, findings are common.

Also see "Infective Endocarditis" (p. 242), "Septic Arthritis" (p. 347), and "Osteomyelitis" (p. 280).

Infectious Associations: Because of nonsterile injection techniques, patients may be at risk for septic arthritis, osteomyelitis, septic thrombophlebitis, local and systemic candidiasis, and subacute bacterial endocarditis. Septic arthritis and osteomyelitis are more commonly caused by gram-positive infections (e.g., *S. aureus, Streptococcus pyogenes*), but gram-negative (e.g., *Pseudomonas, Serratia*) infections are seen. Septic arthritis commonly affects the large joints (e.g., knee), but may also involve the spine or sternoclavicular joint.

Cardinal Findings: Cutaneous needle tracks and other stigmata of substance abuse should be carefully sought. Cellulitis and cutaneous abscesses may be associated with intravenous or subcutaneous drug administration. (See above for clinical presentations.)

Comorbid Conditions: Chronic alcoholism, depression, drug withdrawal, infections (e.g., bacterial sepsis, pneumonia, subacute bacterial endocarditis, hepatitis, candidiasis, tuberculosis, HIV), pancreatitis, schizophrenia are possible comorbid conditions.

Diagnostic Tests: Toxicologic screening may be necessary to identify the offending drug(s). Leukocytosis, with or without eosinophilia, may be seen. Selected visceral angiography may be useful in documenting vasculitis.

Keys to Diagnosis: A high index of suspicion is necessary, especially in those with past or present history of substance abuse.

Therapy: Discontinuation of the offending agent may improve clinical outcome. Analgesics and NSAIDs may be helpful.

REFERENCES

Lohr KM. Rheumatic manifestations of diseases associated with substance abuse. Semin Arthritis Rheum 1987;17:90–111.

Mattson RH, Cramer JA, McCutchen CB, Veterans Administration Epilepsy Cooperative Study Group. Barbiturate-related connective tissue disorders. Arch Intern Med 1989; 149:911–914.

Pastan RS, Silverman SL, Goldenberg DL. A musculoskeletal syndrome in intravenous heroin users: association with brown heroin. Ann Intern Med 1977;87:22–29.

SWEET'S SYNDROME

Synonyms: Acute febrile neutrophilic dermatosis

ICD9 Code: 685.89

Definition: Sweet's syndrome is a multisystem, febrile disorder accompanied by painful papules or plaques (with cutaneous neutrophilic infiltration), arthritis, and leukocytosis. Sweet's syndrome may occur in association with infection, neoplasms, or other systemic inflammatory disorders.

Etiology: The cause is unknown; a hypersensitivity reaction is proposed.

Pathology: Sweet's syndrome exhibits dense dermal infiltration with neutrophils, without vasculitic changes.

Demographics: Most patients are women between the ages of 30 and 60 years.

Cardinal Findings: Onset may follow upper respiratory infection. Systemic features include fever ($>38°C$ in $>80\%$ of patients), malaise, conjunctivitis, episcleritis, iridocyclitis, oral ulcers, proteinuria, arthralgias, myalgias, and arthritis. Skin lesions appear as tender red or violaceous papules, plaques, or pustules, over the face, neck, and arms. Lesions typically resolve in 4 to 8 weeks but may recur. Self-limiting, asymmetric, oligo- or polyarthritis occurs in up to 25% of patients. Arthritis tends to parallel skin lesions and usually affects the hands, wrists, ankles, or knees. Pulmonary features (cough, dyspnea, or pulmonary infiltrates) occur in less than 10% of patients.

Complications: Some 15 to 25% develop a malignancy, particularly acute myelocytic leukemia, multiple myeloma, myelodysplasia, lymphoma, or solid tumors (e.g., prostate, ovarian, testicular, and breast cancer). Nearly 50% have other underlying conditions such as inflammatory bowel disease, pregnancy, or other connective tissue diseases (RA, SLE, relapsing polychondritis, or Behçet's or Sjögren's syndrome).

Diagnostic Tests: Laboratory abnormalities include anemia and elevated ESR, WBC counts, and alkaline phosphatase. Proteinuria is seen in 15%. Positive p-ANCA tests have been reported.

Diagnostic Criteria: Major criteria are (*a*) abrupt-onset painful plaques or nodules and (*b*) neutrophilic infiltrates in the dermis, without leukocytoclastic vasculitis. Minor criteria are (*a*) preceded by fever or infection; (*b*) accompanied by fever, arthralgia, conjunctivitis, or underlying malignant lesion; (*c*) leukocytosis; (*d*) good response to steroids, but not antibiotics; and (*e*) increased ESR. Diagnosis requires that both major and two minor criteria be fulfilled.

Differential Diagnosis: Erythema elevatum diutinum, erythema nodosum, pyoderma gangrenosum, SLE, and adult Still's disease should be considered.

Therapy: Oral steroids (e.g., prednisone 40–60 mg/day) are effective. Steroids should be tapered over 4 to 6 weeks. Other therapies, including aspirin, NSAIDs, dapsone, colchicine, sulfapyridine, and potassium iodide, have had some success.

Comment: Onset of Sweet's syndrome underscores the need for a thorough history and physical examination to exclude an associated malignancy.

REFERENCES

Fett DL, Gibson LE, Su WPD. Sweets syndrome: systemic signs and symptoms. Mayo Clin Proc 1995;70:234–240.

Werth V. Miscellaneous syndromes involving skin and joints: Sweet's syndrome. In: Schumacher HR Jr, ed. Primer on the rheumatic diseases. Atlanta: Arthritis Foundation, 1996:256–257.

SYSTEMIC LUPUS ERYTHEMATOSUS (SLE)

Synonyms: Lupus; lupus erythematosus; SLE

ICD9 Codes: SLE, 710.0; discoid, 695.4; lupus anticoagulant, 286.5; drug induced, 695.4; nephritis, 583.81

Definition: SLE is an autoimmune disease characterized by inflammation in many organ systems. While some SLE patients have relatively mild disease, others suffer severe morbidity and accelerated mortality. The characteristic laboratory finding of SLE is the presence of autoantibodies that react with various components of the cell nucleus, antinuclear antibodies (ANA). The exact pathophysiologic role of most of these autoantibodies remains unknown. Much end-organ involvement in SLE involves deposition of immune complexes. The presence of specific autoantibodies correlates with particular organ involvement and prognosis.

Etiology: Etiology is unknown. Because of the female preponderance of SLE, sex steroids are presumed to play a key role in disease expression. Genetics play some role; monozygotic twins are concordant for SLE in about 30% of cases, while dizygotic twins and other siblings are concordant in 5%. This implies that other environmental risk factor(s) are superimposed on a susceptible genetic background. Certain MHC alleles (e.g., HLA-B8, DR2, DR3) are associated with a slightly greater risk of developing SLE. In addition, many SLE patients have null alleles for complement protein C4. While this may not be reflected in low serum C4 concentrations, it may affect the patient's ability to remove immune complexes effectively. Similarly, allelic differences in cell surface receptors for the Fc portion of IgG correlate with end-organ involvement in SLE.

Demographics: Peak incidence of SLE is between 15 and 40 years of age. In this age group, women are affected approximately 10 times as commonly as men. This female predominance decreases among older patients. There is a racial disparity: patients of African descent have both a greater incidence of SLE and a tendency toward more severe disease. The overall population prevalence of SLE is approximately 25–50/100,000. Among certain high-risk populations (e.g., young black women), the prevalence may be as high as 4/1,000.

Cardinal Findings: Characteristic clinical findings of SLE are shown in Table 1. The frequencies of end-organ involvement between populations and among SLE patients differ substantially. This is relevant to the treatment of SLE, which is often guided by the particular constellation of clinical characteristics and the most severe end-organ involvement for a given patient. Some manifestations of SLE vary with race; for example, discoid skin lesions are more common and photosensitivity is less common among SLE patients of African descent than others. Some manifestations are more typical of patients with particular autoantibodies (e.g., renal disease in patients with anti-DNA antibodies). A number of SLE patients have an "overlap" of signs and symptoms of other connective tissue diseases. Manifestations typical of scleroderma (sclerodactyly, interstitial pulmonary disease, digital vasculitis) and inflammatory myositis are commonly seen among SLE patients.

—*Skin:* Before the widespread availability of immunologic laboratory tests for SLE, dermatologic manifestations were perhaps the most characteristic finding of SLE. Indeed, before the early 1900s, lupus was considered a purely dermatologic disease. The name *lupus erythematosus* refers to the red appearance of the malar rash, which was likened to a wolf bite. The malar rash, also known as the "butterfly rash," is typically a maculopapular rash over the malar area of the cheeks. The rash tends to spare the nasolabial folds, in contrast to seborrheic dermatitis. Histopathologically, biopsy of a lupus rash reveals granular deposition of immune complexes and complement in a bandlike pattern at the dermoepidermal junction (the so-called lupus band test). In "acute" lupus rashes such as the malar rash, clinically uninvolved skin also shows such deposits. In contrast, in discoid lupus skin lesions, immune deposits are only seen in involved skin. Unlike the malar rash and other dermatologic manifestations, dis-

Table 1
Clinical Manifestations of SLE

Constitutional symptoms
- Fever, fatigue, malaise, anorexia, weight loss

Mucocutaneous
- Malar rash
- Discoid rash
- Other rashes
- Photosensitivity
- Oral/nasal ulcerations (typically painless at the onset),
- Xerophthalmia (dry eyes) and/or xerostomia (dry mouth) (these symptoms, sometimes called "sicca symptoms," are consistent with Sjögren's syndrome)
- Alopecia (usually diffuse, in contrast to alopecia areata or male-pattern alopecia)

Musculoskeletal
- Arthritis
- Fibromyalgia
- Arthralgia
- Inflammatory myositis (with increased CPK and proximal muscle weakness)
- Osteonecrosis (particularly with chronic corticosteroid use)

Renal/urologic
- Glomerulonephritis (WHO classification: I, normal; II, mesangial; III, focal proliferative glomerulonephritis; IV, diffuse proliferative glomerulonephritis; V, membranous glomerulonephritis; VI, diffuse sclerosis)
- Tubulointerstitial inflammation
- Lupus cystitis (*Note:* hemorrhagic cystitis is a potential complication of cyclophosphamide therapy)

Hematologic
- Lymphopenia (absolute lymphocyte count $< 1500/mm^3$)
- Leukopenia (WBC $< 4000/mm^3$)
- Thrombocytopenia (platelet count $< 100,000/mm^3$)
- Hemolytic anemia (defined by positive Coombs' test)
- Lymphadenopathy, splenomegaly

Neuropsychiatric
- Headache (particularly refractory migrainelike headaches)
- Seizures
- Psychosis
- Cerebral vascular accidents
- Peripheral neuropathy
- Cranial neuropathy
- Transverse myelitis
- Depression
- Cognitive dysfunction

Serosal
- Pleuritis (exudative pleural effusion)
- Pericarditis (exudative; rarely associated with hemodynamic compromise)
- Peritoneal inflammation (often presents with diffuse abdominal pain)

Vascular
- Raynaud's phenomenon
- Vasculitis
- Vasculopathy (vessel wall abnormalities with minimal inflammation or damage)
- Hypertension

(continued)

Table 1 *(continued)*
Clinical Manifestations of SLE

- Myocarditis
- Endocarditis (e.g., Libman-Sacks lesions)
- Thromboembolic events (particularly in SLE patients with anticardiolipin antibodies or the so-called lupus anticoagulant)

Immunologic laboratory testing
- ANA (and other autoantibodies [see Table 2])
- False-positive nonspecific tests for syphilis (e.g., VDRL), anticardiolipin antibodies
- Elevated serum concentrations of immune complexes
- Evidence of complement consumption (e.g., decreased serum concentrations of complement components C3 and C4, or increased concentrations of complement split products such as C4b, C5a, sC5b-9)

Miscellaneous
- Pulmonary (pulmonary hemorrhage, pulmonary hypertension, interstitial lung disease)
- Ocular (cytoid bodies)
- Gastrointestinal (lupoid hepatitis, pancreatitis)

coid lupus may occur in the absence of systemic involvement. Another distinguishing feature of discoid lupus is that it tends to involve the supporting skin structures, such as hair follicles, and causes follicular plugging. When discoid lesions resolve, they often result in residual scarring or alopecia that can be disfiguring. By contrast, acute lupus lesions or subacute cutaneous lupus erythematosus (SCLE) lesions typically resolve without scarring. SCLE refers to annular or papulosquamous lesions associated with antibodies to Ro (SS-A) and usually occurs in sun-exposed areas of the arms and trunk. Most lupus rashes tend to be exacerbated by sun exposure, and intense sun exposure may also precipitate a flare of systemic disease. The treatment of lupus rashes depends on their severity and extent. For many patients, topical corticosteroid preparations effectively control the lesions. In addition, the antimalarial hydroxychloroquine is effective for such lesions.

—*Renal:* Kidney involvement is very common in SLE and may be associated with substantial morbidity and mortality. Most SLE patients have deposits of immune complexes and complement in the renal mesangium (Table 1). While such lesions may require no specific intervention, they may progress to more serious lesions. Proliferative glomerular lesions, which may be characterized by subepithelial, subendothelial, and intramembranous immune complex deposits and diffuse glomerular inflammation, are of particular importance. Untreated, they often progress and cause renal failure. Membranous lesions that typically manifest with proteinuria may occur alone in combination with proliferative lesions. SLE patients with high titers of antibodies to double-stranded DNA (anti-DNA antibodies) are at greater risk of developing proliferative lupus nephritis. Evidence of active consumption of serum complement proteins (e.g., low concentrations of C3 or C4) is often seen in patients with active nephritis. Careful monitoring of the urine for signs of lupus activity (e.g., proteinuria, cellular casts, hematuria, pyuria) is an important part of the routine evaluation of lupus patients. In addition, quantification of proteinuria (e.g. by a 24-hour urine collection) offers important information on the prognosis and response to therapy. For many patients, deciding how aggressively to treat lupus nephritis depends upon its effects on the patient's renal function. Therefore, it is important to note that the serum creatinine level or the creatinine clearance estimated from a 24-hour collection may overestimate the glomerular filtration rate (GFR) in patients with lupus nephritis. More accurate determinations of GFR (e.g., inulin clearance) may be of value in monitoring lupus nephritis. Therapy for lupus nephritis typically consists of corticosteroids in conjunction with cytotoxic medications. Many patients are begun on high-dose steroids (e.g., 1 mg/kg prednisone) at the time of diagnosis of lupus nephritis. Depending upon the other organ systems involved, this may be tapered relatively rapidly. Occasionally, boluses of steroids (e.g., 1 g of methylprednisolone on 3 successive days) are used to gain rapid control of disease activity. Based on the results of several prospective trials, cytotoxic drugs have become the standard therapy for lupus nephritis. Presently, a typical regimen uses monthly boluses of cyclophosphamide (at a dose of approximately 750 mg/m^2) for 6 months or longer, followed by additional boluses every 2 or 3 months for a total of at least 2 years. Patients treated with shorter courses tend to have relapses of their disease, and the ultimate length of treatment must be individualized on the basis of the response. Treatment with intermittent boluses of cyclophosphamide is generally preferred to daily oral administration because it is associated with fewer adverse effects, particularly hemorrhagic cystitis. Azathioprine has also been used successfully for treatment of lupus nephritis. For lupus nephritis patients with a rapidly progressive course, plasmapheresis is sometimes used in conjunction with cytotoxic therapy. Drugs currently being evaluated for lupus nephritis include cyclosporine and the nucleoside analogue 2-CDA.

—*Neuropsychiatric:* Neuropsychiatric manifestations of SLE are very common, with a prevalence of approximately 50%. Signs and symptoms can be quite varied (Table 1). It is often difficult to pinpoint SLE as the definite cause of many of these symptoms. Thus, an important part of the diagnosis involves excluding other potential causes, including infections (e.g., bacterial meningitis, viral encephalitis), medications (including psychotropic medications, high-dose corticosteroids, and NSAIDs), metabolic causes (e.g., the CNS effects of uremia), other medical conditions (e.g., hypertensive encephalopathy), and primary psychiatric disorders. Confounding the diagnosis of neuropsychiatric SLE is the fact that there are no pathognomonic laboratory or imaging tests. Patients with CNS lupus may have elevated CSF protein (including CSF-derived or oligoclonal immunoglobulins) (see p. 98), elevated CSF cell counts, abnormal EEGs, and various abnormalities on imaging studies (e.g., scattered high-intensity white matter lesions on MRI). While such testing can help exclude other causes and can be consistent with a diagnosis of CNS lupus, no test definitively establishes the diagnosis. Treatment of neuropsychiatric SLE depends upon the particular manifestations. Many patients, particularly those with severe involvement, receive corticosteroids or even cytotoxic agents. In addition, patients may benefit from therapies specific for their particular symptoms (e.g., antipsychotic medications for psychosis, antidepressants for depression, and anticoagulants for thromboembolism).

—*Musculoskeletal:* Musculoskeletal manifestations of SLE affect almost 90% of patients. While most patients have arthralgia, fewer demonstrate an inflammatory synovitis. The arthritis of SLE typically involves the small joints of the hands, wrists, and knees. In contrast to patients with rheumatoid arthritis, the arthritis is usually not associated with bony erosions observed on x-ray. Some SLE patients develop changes in their joints that resemble those found in RA patients (e.g., swan neck deformity). However, unlike RA, in which there is joint destruction and tendon shortening, deformities in SLE patients (known as "Jacoud's arthropathy") are correctable or "reducible" on physical examination. Treatment of arthritis in SLE patients often includes NSAIDs and the antimalarial drug hydroxychloroquine. While patients often respond to corticosteroids, attempts should be made not to use them chronically solely for arthritis. In SLE patients with severe arthritis, treatment is comparable to that for RA, and drugs such as methotrexate may be used. SLE patients with inflammatory myositis often require treatment with corticosteroids and other immunomodulatory drugs. Finally, osteonecrosis (e.g., hip, knee, shoulder) is seen among SLE patients, particularly those treated with corticosteroids at high doses or for prolonged courses.

—*Vascular:* Vascular involvement is exceedingly common in SLE. Hypertension is among the most powerful predictors of patient survival in SLE. In addition, SLE patients have excessive morbidity and mortality from atherosclerotic cardiovascular disease. Vasculitis with leukocytic infiltration and destruction of the involved vessel wall may be seen in skin lesions and in other organ systems. More commonly, a bland vasculopathy is seen. Such lesions have alterations to the vessel wall and impingement of the vessel lumen without frank vasculitic changes. These changes are commonly seen in the CNS and other organ systems. Another factor that may predispose to thromboembolism is the presence of anticardiolipin antibodies (see pp. 85, 161).

Uncommon Findings: A number of distinct clinical syndromes are seen in lupus patients.

—*Drug-Induced Lupus (see p. 193):* Patients treated with certain medications may develop signs and symptoms of SLE. Drug-induced lupus is also associated with development of positive ANAs, particularly with reactivity to histones. Clinical features of drug-induced lupus typically include fever, arthritis, and serositis; lupus nephritis and CNS lupus are distinctly unusual in patients with drug-induced lupus. Agents strongly associated with drug-induced lupus include procainamide, hydralazine, and isoniazid. Others that have been implicated include Dilantin, penicillamine, and quinidine.

—*Neonatal lupus:* Neonatal lupus arises in newborns of mothers with anti-Ro and/or anti-La antibodies. While some mothers have SLE or Sjögren's syndrome, many are asymptomatic. When the antibodies cross the placenta, they may bind cardiac tissue, resulting in heart block or myocarditis. Other manifestations may include rashes and thrombocytopenia. These are typically transient and resolve as the maternal antibody disappears from the infant's circulation.

Diagnostic Tests: Around 1948, the observation of the LE cell (a leukocyte that had engulfed another leukocyte) provided the basis for the ultimate definition of antinuclear antibodies as the laboratory hallmark of SLE. The LE cell, which depended upon the presence of very high titers of ANA, was relatively specific but insensitive for the diagnosis of SLE, and is only of historic interest currently. It was replaced by immunofluorescent tests that looked specifically for the presence of antibodies capable of binding various nuclear constituents. Initially, ANA tests were performed on rodent tissue sections. Of note, some nuclear antigens (e.g., Ro) are absent in rodents, and some organelles (e.g., nucleoli, centromeres) are present in limited numbers in normal tissue. Thus, in years past there were patients who had clinical manifestations characteristic of SLE but were ANA negative. With the replacement of rodent tissues by the human HEp2 tumor cell as the standard substrate for ANA tests, the concept of "ANA-negative lupus" has largely disappeared. While virtually all SLE patients are positive for ANAs, the ANA test is not very specific. Many patients with other connective tissue diseases and even some healthy persons have ANAs, particularly at low titer.

Typically, positive ANA results are reported in terms of both titer and pattern. Higher titers are more consistent with, but not diagnostic of, SLE. Typically, titers of 1:160 and above are considered positive, whereas titers of 1:80 or less are equivocal and often nonspecific. Titers of positive ANAs do not generally correlate with disease activity, and there is little value in repeating an ANA test in a patient known to be positive.

The patterns of immunofluorescence observed may correlate with different antigen reactivity (Table 2). A *speckled* pattern of immunofluorescence is the most common but perhaps least specific. A speckled ANA is associated with various extractable nuclear antigens (ENAs): Ro (SS-A), La (SS-B), Sm (anti-Smith), RNP, Scl-70, Jo-1, and many others. Anti-Ro and anti-La antibodies are also observed in patients with Sjögren's syndrome (hence the designations SS-A and SS-B) and also may result in neonatal lupus. Anti-Sm is relatively specific for the diagnosis of SLE, as it is seen infrequently in other diseases or in normal persons. Along with anti-RNP antibodies, SLE patients with anti-Sm may be more prone to develop interstitial lung disease. Anti-RNP antibodies were also previously associated with mixed connective tissue disease (see p. 256). Anti-Scl-70 antibodies are associated with the diffuse form of systemic sclerosis.

A *nucleolar* pattern of the ANA is seen not only in SLE but also in inflammatory myositis and systemic sclerosis. A *centromere* pattern is associated with the limited form of systemic sclerosis (CREST syndrome). The *homogeneous* ANA is associated with antibodies to histones. Such antibodies are seen in SLE, and reactivity to specific histone proteins is characteristic of drug-induced lupus (see below).

A *rim* pattern of immunofluorescence is associated with antibodies to native or double-stranded DNA. Anti-DNA antibodies are useful for the diagnosis of SLE as they are seen uncommonly in other diseases. In addition, patients with high titers of anti-DNA antibodies are more prone to develop proliferative lupus nephritis. The titer of anti-DNA antibodies may vary with the activity of disease,

Table 2
Correlations between ANA Pattern, Antigen Specificity, and Clinical Disease

ANA Pattern	Antigen	Clinical Correlate
Diffuse	Deoxyribonucleoprotein	Low titer = nonspecific
	Histones	Drug-induced lupus, others
Peripheral	ds-DNA	50% of SLE (specific)
Speckled	U1-RNP	>90% of MCTD
	Sm	30% of SLE (specific)
	Ro (SS-A)	Sjögren's 60%, SCLE
		Neonatal LE, ANA(−)LE
	La (SS-B)	50% of Sjögren's, 15% SLE
	Scl-70	40% of PSS (diffuse disease)
	PM-Scl (PM-1)	Overlap scleroderma + myositis
	Jo-1	Myositis, lung disease, arthritis
Nucleolar	RNA polymerases	40% of PSS
Centromere	Kinetochore	75% CREST (limited disease)
Cytoplasmic	Ro, ribosomal P,	Sjögren's, SLE psychosis
(nonspecific)	Cardiolipin,	Thrombosis, abortion, ↓Plts
	AMA, ASMA,	PBC, CAH
	tRNA synthetases	myositis, lung disease, arthritis

particularly lupus nephritis, and sequential determination of anti-DNA is sometimes used to follow the activity of SLE. Specific determination of anti-DNA antibodies may be performed by several assays, including the *Crithidia lucilae* assay and the Farr test. Results from these various tests are reported in different units, and it is important to be familiar with the laboratory performing these tests.

Diagnosis: Classification criteria for SLE are shown in Table 3. A patient may be classified as having SLE if 4 or more of these 11 criteria are present at any time. Several relevant considerations affect the use of these criteria. First, they were developed to classify patients as having SLE rather than other autoimmune diseases such as scleroderma; therefore, some signs and symptoms that are very common not only among SLE patients but also among patients with other autoimmune diseases (e.g., Raynaud's phenomenon, alopecia) are not included. Second, they were developed in 1982, and certain tests are no longer widely used (e.g., the LE cell preparation). Finally, they are approximately 95% sensitive and specific. Thus, a number of patients who actually have SLE will not have 4 or more of these criteria, and some patients having 4 or more criteria might actually have another disease process. The diagnosis of SLE can sometimes be aided by characteristic histopathologic findings (e.g., from renal or skin biopsy specimens). The most widely used diagnostic test for SLE is the ANA.

Therapy: Treatment depends upon the particular manifestations for a given patient (see above). Patients with arthritis or serositis frequently respond to

Table 3
American College of Rheumatology Criteria for the Classification of SLE[a]

1. Malar rash
2. Discoid rash
3. Photosensitivity
4. Oral ulcers
5. Arthritis
6. Serositis
7. Renal disorder (persistent proteinuria [>0.5 g/day] or cellular casts)
8. Neurologic disorder (seizures or psychosis)
9. Hematologic disorder (hemolytic anemia, leukopenia, lymphopenia, or thrombocytopenia)
10. Immunologic disorder (anti-DNA antibodies, anti-Sm antibodies, positive LE cell preparation)
11. Antinuclear antibody

[a] A patient may be classified as having SLE if 4 or more of the 11 criteria are present at any time.

NSAIDs. Antimalarials, particularly hydroxychloroquine, are effective for these same manifestations and are also used for SLE skin lesions. Despite concern about the adverse effects related to their use, corticosteroids are widely used for many manifestations of SLE. For skin disease, topical steroid preparations may suffice. For minor or moderate disease activity, doses of prednisone (≤0.5 mg/kg) are often of great benefit. For severe manifestations, high-dose steroids (1 mg/kg prednisone) may be required. In all instances, attempts should be made to taper steroids as rapidly as disease activity permits. Boluses of high doses of steroids (e.g., 250–1000 mg of prednisone) have been used to gain rapid control of disease activity. For patients who require high doses of steroids for long periods of time, immunosuppressive drugs such as azathioprine and cyclophosphamide may be used as steroid-sparing agents.

In addition to these immunomodulatory approaches, the optimal care of many SLE patients also involves assiduous treatment of hypertension, treatment of clotting diatheses, and other types of general therapeutic intervention.

TARSAL TUNNEL SYNDROME

ICD9 Code: 355.5

Definition: To enter the foot, the posterior tibial nerve must pass through the "tarsal tunnel," beneath a flexor retinaculum located just below the medial malleolus of the ankle. Compression of the nerve at this location may lead to local pain or numbness—tarsal tunnel syndrome. This is analogous to the carpal tunnel syndrome, which results from compression of the median nerve at the wrist.

Risk Factors: Local trauma (e.g., fracture), body habitus (e.g., valgus foot deformity), and repetitive use or injury are risk factors.

Demographics: Women are affected slightly more frequently than men.

Cardinal Findings: Patients typically present with numbness, burning pain, or paresthesias of the toes or the sole of the foot. Symptoms may be noted after a night's sleep or even awaken the patient. The diagnosis may be supported by a positive Tinel's test, in which repetitive tapping over the area of the flexor retinaculum (posterior to the medial malleolus) reproduces the symptoms.

Diagnostic Tests: Definitive diagnosis may be made by demonstration of prolonged motor and sensory latencies on electrodiagnostic testing (nerve conduction velocities; NCV).

Differential Diagnosis: Other peripheral neuropathies (e.g., those related to diabetes mellitus and alcoholism) are in the differential diagnosis. In those conditions, symptoms and findings at examination more commonly affect the entire foot, in the so-called stocking-glove pattern typical of diffuse neuropathies.

Therapy: Initial treatment may involve conservative measures, such as selecting optimal footwear or orthoses. Some physicians use injections of corticosteroids directly into the flexor retinaculum in an attempt to decrease local swelling and thereby relieve the compression. In patients who are refractory to conservative measures, the definitive therapy involves surgical decompression.

REFERENCES

Kuritz HM, Sokoloff TH. Tarsal tunnel syndrome. J Am Podiatry Assoc 1975;65:825–840.

TAKAYASU'S ARTERITIS

Synonyms: Aortic arch syndrome, pulseless disease, aortitis syndrome, occlusive thromboaortopathy

ICD9 Code: 446.7

Definition: Takayasu's arteritis is a large-vessel vasculitis of the aorta and its branches, resulting in vascular ischemia.

Etiology: Takayasu's arteritis is associated with HLA Bw52 in over 40% of afflicted individuals. Circulating anti-arterial antibodies have been investigated as putative etiologic agents.

Pathology: Granulomatous panarteritis results in concentric vascular narrowing. Lymphoplasmacytic cell infiltrates may be seen throughout the vessel wall but are often localized toward the outer aspects of the vessel.

Demographics: Takayasu's arteritis occurs worldwide, but most reports come from Japan, India, and China. It is rare in Caucasians (2.6 cases per million persons per year). It predominately affects women, usually in their reproductive years.

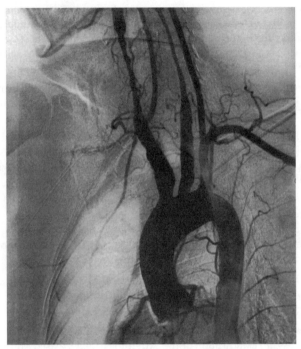

Figure 1. Schematic of subclavian angiogram showing stenosis. (From RM Gay, GV Ball. Vasculitis. In: Koopman WJ, ed. Arthritis and allied conditions: a textbook of rheumatology. 13th ed. Baltimore: Williams & Wilkins, 1997:1514, with permission.)

Cardinal Findings: Variations in presenting manifestations often result in significant diagnostic delays. Fever occurs in a minority of patients. Claudication, more common in the upper than lower extremities, results from ischemia of affected limbs. The subclavian (90%) vessels are a preferred site of involvement, but other large vessels including the aorta (65%), carotid (60%), renal (40%), and vertebral (35%) arteries may be involved as well. Pulselessness and pressure discrepancies between the two arms are common. A bruit over an affected artery helps identify an area of stenosis and is the most common clinical finding. The aortic arch may be more commonly affected in Japanese patients than in Americans. Pulmonary artery involvement occurs in up to 70% of patients, but frank pulmonary hypertension is much less common. Hypertension is present sometime during the disease course in 50% of patients and is often due to renal artery stenosis. CNS symptoms such as light headedness, dizziness, and visual disturbances are well reported by over 50% of patients. Musculoskeletal symptoms include chest wall pain, arthralgias, and myalgias and are seen in over 50% of patients. Only 40% (30% at disease onset) of patients have constitutional symptoms such as fever, weight loss, and malaise. Stroke due to vertebral or carotid ischemia or embolism has been described. Funduscopic findings of microaneurysms, venous dilation, and beading are noted early in the course of disease. Cardiac disease, including aortic regurgitation, angina, and pericarditis, is seen in almost 40% of cases. Skin lesions including erythema nodosum and hypersensitivity angiitis have been reported.

Uncommon Findings: Rare associations with other idiopathic inflammatory disorders such as inflammatory bowel disease and sarcoidosis have been reported.

Diagnostic Testing: The ESR is elevated in only about 30% of patients. However, the ESR is markedly increased in about 70% of patients with active disease. Vascular specimens at the time of surgical bypass reveal histologic evidence of active disease in about 40% of cases.

Imaging: Angiogram confirms a suspected vascular stenosis. Long-segment stenosis occurs almost four times more commonly than aneurysms. Magnetic resonance angiography (MRA) is gaining prominence for visualizing vasculature, particularly of the aortic arch. The chest radiograph may demonstrate a widened aortic root or irregularities in other segments of the aorta.

Keys to Diagnosis: Look for pulselessness of an extremity, often in young women of Asian descent. Aortography and angiograms of other large vessels is highly diagnostic.

Diagnosis Criteria: 1990 ACR Classification criteria include (*a*) age at onset 40 years or less; (*b*) claudication of the extremities; (*c*) decreased brachial artery pressure; (*d*) blood pressure difference of more than 10 mm Hg between arms; (*e*) bruit over the subclavian artery or aorta; and (*f*) arteriogram abnormality. Criteria for Takayasu arteritis are met if at least three of these six are present (sensitivity 90.5%, specificity 97.8%).

Therapy: High-dose corticosteroids should be given when active disease is diagnosed. Addition of methotrexate or cytotoxic therapy (such as cyclophosphamide) both for disease control and as a steroid-sparing agent may improve outcome and result in fewer steroid complications. Vascular bypass may be necessary if limb or organ ischemia appears threatening but is fraught with significant reocclusion problems.

Prognosis: The disease may be self-limiting in about 20% of cases. Approximately 25% of patients fail to achieve remission despite aggressive therapy. Half of the patients who respond to medical therapy later relapse. Arterial hypertension is an unfavorable prognostic indicator. Mortality is low (10–20%), but considerable morbidity is related to organ and limb infarction (stroke, myocardial infarction, and aortic dissection).

REFERENCES

Arend WP, Michel BA, Bloch DA, et al. The American College of Rheumatology 1990 criteria for the classification of Takayasu's arteritis. Arthritis Rheum 1990;33:1122–1128.
Kerr GS, Hallahan CW, Giordano J, et al. Takayasu arteritis. Ann Intern Med 1994;120:919–929.

TEMPORAL ARTERITIS

Synonyms: Giant cell arteritis (GCA), cranial arteritis

ICD9 Code: 446.5

Definition: Temporal arteritis (TA) is a large-vessel vasculitis preferentially affecting the superficial temporal artery and other branches of the external carotid artery system.

Etiology: The cause of TA is unknown. There is an association with HLA-DR4 and particular HLA-DRB1 alleles. These alleles are similar to those associated with rheumatoid arthritis but involve polymorphisms in the second rather than the third hypervariable region. Research has focused on the unexplained increased prevalence in Caucasian people of northern European origin and possible seasonal variation suggesting as yet undetermined environmental agents as precipitating factors.

Pathology: Biopsy of an involved large vessel shows a mononuclear cell infiltrate with intimal hyperplasia and occasional giant cells focused along the internal elastic lamina. Disruption of the internal elastic lamina is characteristic. Vasculitis often occurs in a "skip" pattern, which underscores the need for a suitably large biopsy specimen (≥ 3 cm in length) with careful cross-sectional and longitudinal histopathologic examination to minimize the number of false-negative results. The disease has a particular predilection for blood vessels that contain large quantities of elastic lamina. This may explain a low incidence of intracranial complications, since arteries lose their internal elastic lamina after passing through the dura matter.

Demographics: The prevalence of TA is highest in elderly Caucasians from northern Europe and in the north central United States. TA is very uncommon in non-Caucasians. Incidence increases with advancing age and varies from 15 to 94 cases per 100,000 in people over age 50. Women are afflicted twice as commonly as men.

Cardinal Findings: Onset may be abrupt or insidiously develop over weeks to months. Characteristically patients have profound constitutional symptoms with fever, weight loss, and occasional night sweats. Moderate-to-severe headache, particularly in the temporal or, less commonly, in the occipital area, is reported by over 90% of patients. Scalp tenderness is common, particularly in the temporal area. Headache may sometimes be reproduced by pressure over an affected artery. Visual symptoms of diplopia, blurred vision, or amaurosis fugax may antedate development of sudden unilateral blindness. Many patients describe a fullness or pressure sensation behind their eyes. Unfortunately, visual loss may be the presenting ophthalmologic symptom in some cases. Overall, 20 to 40% of patients experience vision loss. The most common cause of visual loss is ischemic optic neuropathy. Jaw claudication with prolonged chewing results from vascular insufficiency to the muscles of mastication. Over 60% of TA cases are accompanied by PMR. Indeed, PMR and TA may be varying manifestations of the same disorder, along a disease continuum. Seronegative synovitis may accompany TA with or without PMR. Tongue numbness or ulceration, cough, sore throat, dysphagia, hoarseness, and rare respiratory difficulties have all been described.

Uncommon Findings: Although the extracranial branches of the aorta supplying the eye and temporal area are preferentially affected, the aortic arch and subclavian vessels can be involved (10%) and lead to pulselessness and other complications. TA patients are at higher risk for thoracic aortic dissection and aortic valve insufficiency.

Complications: Neurologic complications appear uncommonly but may result from ischemia in the carotid or vertebral circulations. Transient ischemic attack or stroke has been reported in about 7% of cases. Peripheral neuropathies also have been reported.

Diagnostic Testing: Although biopsy-proven TA with normal ESR is well documented, a *markedly elevated* ESR is seen in well over 95% of cases. C-reactive protein (CRP) levels may be more sensitive to changes in disease activity and improvement with appropriate therapy. Anemia of chronic disease, decreased serum albumin, polyclonal gammopathy, and reactive thrombocytosis are also seen. Elevation in liver tests, particularly alkaline phosphatase, is common. Preliminary studies suggest a possible association of antiphospholipid antibodies with TA.

Biopsy/Imaging: A unilateral temporal artery biopsy is positive in about 80% of TA cases, and the sensitivity for diagnosis increases to 90% with biopsy of both sides. Provided the disease remains active, the positive predictive value of the biopsy is only modestly influenced by prior short-term corticosteroid. However, biopsy is best done as soon as possible when TA is strongly suspected. If pulselessness, extremity claudication, angina, or symptoms of cerebrovascular ischemia are present, selective angiograms may be indicated.

Keys to Diagnosis: Look for markedly elevated erythrocyte sedimentation rate accompanied by headaches, significant constitutional symptoms, and polymyalgia rheumatica.

Diagnostic Criteria: 1990 ACR classification criteria include (*a*) age at onset above 50 years; (*b*) new headache; (*c*) temporal artery tender to palpation, enlarged, or with decreased pulsation; (*d*) elevated erythrocyte sedimentation rate; or (*e*) abnormal temporal artery biopsy. The presence of any three carries a sensitivity of 93.5% and a specificity of 91.2%.

Differential Diagnosis: Other causes of headaches and visual disturbances include classic migraines and intracranial mass lesions. A markedly elevated ESR and fever may suggest occult malignancies (such as lymphoma, myeloma), chronic infections (including bacteria endocarditis), and other inflammatory disorders (other vasculitides). Takayasu's arteritis affects similar-sized vessels such as the subclavian arteries; however, it develops almost exclusively in young women.

Therapy: Because of the risk of visual loss, high-dose corticosteroid (prednisone 60 mg/day) should be initiated immediately if clinical suspicion is high. With appropriate treatment, the chance of subsequent blindness is less than 20%. Once the symptoms and signs have stabilized (usually within 1 month) and levels of acute-phase reactants have declined, the prednisone dose is tapered rapidly at first (5–10 mg every 2–4 weeks) and subsequently more slowly (1 mg every 1–2 weeks when below 10 mg/day). When weaning from corticosteroids, the patient's symptoms and ESR should be monitored closely. Limited data support the use of steroid-sparing agents, particularly oral methotrexate. NSAIDs may be added when the prednisone dose is below 10 mg, particularly for symptoms of PMR. Angioplasty or vascular bypass may be required if large vessel involvement is producing claudication or other potentially treatable complications.

Prognosis: Although most patients successfully taper and discontinue corticosteroids within 2 years of disease onset, the relapse rate in the first year exceeds 60%. As a result, the mean requirement for corticosteroids exceeds 5 years. Consequently, the most devastating long-term complications from TA commonly stem from corticosteroid-associated complications, particularly bone loss. Up to 60% of TA patients develop steroid toxicities, and steroid-associated fatalities may be as high as 21%.

REFERENCES

Hunder GH, Bloch DA, Michel BA, et al. The American College of Rheumatology 1990 criteria for the classification of giant cell arteritis. Arthritis Rheum 1990;33:1122–1128.

Huston KA, Hunder GH, Lie JT, et al. Temporal arteritis, a 25-year epidemiologic, clinical, and pathologic study. Ann Intern Med 1978;88:162–167.

Reich KA, Giansiracusa DF, Strongwater SL. Neurologic manifestations of giant cell arteritis. Am J Med 1990;89:67–72.

TUBERCULOUS ARTHRITIS

Synonyms: TB, consumption, Pott's disease

ICD9 Code: 711.4

Definition: Tuberculous arthritis is a subacute, or occasionally chronic, arthritis secondary to *Mycobacterium tuberculosis* infection.

Etiology: Tuberculosis (TB) spreads from pulmonary sites to peripheral joints hematogenously or via lymphatic channels. Peripheral joints are usually infected by contiguous spread from adjacent TB osteomyelitis. Spinal TB may originate from contiguous spread from the lungs or via blood or lymphatic routes. Because TB does not produce collagenase, joint destruction is slower than in bacterial arthritides.

Pathology: Synovial biopsy specimens may stain positively for the TB bacillus. Histologic findings include synovial proliferation, granulation tissue, and pannus.

Demographics: The prevalence of TB has declined considerably in the past 50 years, However, between 1985 to 1993 there was a resurgence of multidrug-resistant TB in the United States, associated with the rise in AIDS (with a relative risk for TB 500 times that of the general population) and an increase in TB among certain ethnic minorities and immigrants from underdeveloped countries. African Americans may be at higher TB risk owing to both genetic and socioeconomic factors. Osteoarticular TB is seen in 5% or less of all TB patients; 4- to 5-month delays in the diagnosis of osteoarticular TB are common in low-risk populations.

Cardinal Findings: Following an insidious onset, the diagnosis of TB arthritis is often suggested by a chronic monoarthritis (less commonly an oligoarthritis). Large weight-bearing joints may be preferentially affected in more endemic areas. Swollen joints may lack other manifestations of inflammation, such as warmth and erythema. Tuberculous spondylitis, or Pott's disease, frequently begins in a thoracic disc space. It accounts for about 50% of osteoarticular TB. Spinal lesions may lead to severe kyphosis due to vertebral destruction. Pulmonary disease is seldom active at the time of joint manifestations, although the chest radiograph remains abnormal in half of patients. Constitutional symptoms such as fever and weight loss are frequently present at the time of bone or joint disease.

Uncommon Findings: There are rare reports of tenosynovitis and fasciitis. Sacroiliac infection is present in about 7% of patients with skeletal TB. Poncet's syndrome describes a reactive polyarthritis of the hands and feet in patients with a current or past TB infection. Atypical mycobacteria may also cause arthritis or other musculoskeletal manifestations, particularly in patients with HIV disease.

Diagnostic Testing: Culture of *M. tuberculosis* from synovial fluid and/or synovial biopsy is positive in about 90% of cases. An acid-fast smear of synovial fluid alone has a yield of less than 10%. Improved culture techniques, such as use of radiometry, can detect organisms in a much shorter time. Synovial biopsy demonstrating noncaseating granulomas by histopathology is a less specific diagnostic option. CT-guided needle biopsy of spinal lesions may prove diagnostic. Nonspecific synovial fluid findings include neutrophilic pleocytosis (total white count is usually 10,000 to 20,000 cells/mm^3), elevated protein, and low synovial fluid glucose (detected in >50% of patients). Some 90% of people with osteoarticular disease exhibit a positive PPD, which is helpful as a general screening test for TB, provided the patient is not anergic.

Imaging: Radiographs of peripheral joints with late-stage TB arthritis may reveal destructive arthropathy without significant reactive bone formation.

Keys to Diagnosis: Look for a chronic monarthritis in an at-risk host, with acid-fast bacilli identified on joint fluid culture or synovial biopsy.

Differential Diagnosis: Fungal arthritis, inflammatory osteoarthritis, and pseudogout should be considered.

Therapy: Multidrug regimens for osteoarticular TB are usually the same as those for pulmonary TB; however, at least 6 to 9 months (3 months beyond negative culture in non-AIDS hosts and 6 months beyond negative cultures in AIDS patients) of treatment is required. Therapy is usually initiated with isoniazid (5 mg/kg, up to 300 mg/day), pyrazinamide (15–30 mg/kg, up to 2 g daily), and rifampin (10 mg/kg, up to 600 mg orally daily). Pyrazinamide can be discontinued after 8 weeks. If the incidence of multidrug resistance is below 4%, it is recommended that ethambutol (5–25 mg/kg) or streptomycin (15 mg/kg) be added until resistances are known. Treatment regimens are dictated by the resistance patterns in the community and the immune status of the host. Surgery may be necessary if extensive bone destruction has occurred or if the spinal cord is compromised in Pott's disease.

Prognosis: If there is minimal bone involvement, articular disease is successfully managed with drug therapy alone. Pott's disease may result in neurologic damage, and in older series, mortality was as high as 20%. More recent reports suggest almost 80% resolution of even severe disease with appropriate drug therapy.

REFERENCES

Centers for Disease Control and Prevention. Initial therapy for tuberculosis in the era of multi-drug resistance. Recommendations of the Advisory Council for Elimination of Tuberculosis. MMWR 1993;42(no. RR-7):1–7.

Hodgson S, Ormerod LP. Ten-year experience of bone and joint tuberculosis in Blackburn 1978–1987. J R Coll Surg Edinb 1990;35:259–262.

Mahowald ML, Messner RP. Arthritis due to mycobacteria, fungi, and parasites. In: Koopman WJ, ed. Arthritis and allied conditions: a textbook of rheumatology. 13th ed. Baltimore: Williams & Wilkins, 1997:2305–2320.

UVEITIS

Synonyms: Iritis, iridocyclitis, anterior uveitis, posterior uveitis, chorioretinitis

ICD9 Codes: Acute uveitis, 364.0; chronic uveitis, 364.1

Definition: Uveitis refers to any inflammatory disease that involves the uveal tract (or midportion of the eye, which includes the iris, ciliary body, and choroid layer). Between 20 and 40% of uveitis patients have an associated systemic disease. Anterior uveitis may involve the iris (iritis) or iris and ciliary body (iridocyclitis) and may be associated with HLA-B27 and inflammatory joint disease (e.g., ankylosing spondylitis, Reiter's syndrome, sarcoidosis). Posterior uveitis may involve the choroid (choroiditis), retina (retinitis), or vitreous near the macula and optic nerve. Posterior uveitis is commonly associated with infection. Sarcoidosis and Behçet's disease are unique conditions that may involve either the anterior or posterior chamber.

Etiology: Uveitis may be isolated and idiopathic or result from a variety of infectious or immunologic conditions (Table 1). An association is seen with HLA-B27 positivity in nearly 60% of acute anterior uveitis patients.

Table 1
Systemic Conditions Associated with Uveitis

Viral	HIV, herpes simplex, herpes zoster, CMV
Bacterial	Tuberculosis, leprosy, Lyme disease, syphilis, brucellosis
Parasitic	Toxoplasmosis, cysticercosis, amebiasis
Fungal	Histoplasmosis, coccidioidomycosis, candidiasis, aspergillosis, cryptococcus
Immunologic	Ankylosing spondylitis, Reiter's syndrome, psoriatic arthritis, Behçet's disease, Crohn's disease, ulcerative colitis, sarcoidosis, relapsing polychondritis, SLE, vitiligo, vasculitis, interstitial nephritis, multiple sclerosis, Sjögren's syndrome
Neoplastic (mistaken for uveitis)	Leukemia, lymphoma, retinoblastoma, retinitis pigmentosa

Pathology: Common findings include corneal edema, keratitic precipitates, and inflammatory changes in the anterior chamber. Posterior uveitis may show vitreal exudates, focal chorioretinal infiltrates, retinal vasculitis, or macular edema. Synechiae are fibrous scars (adhesions) that can be seen between the iris and lens or iris and cornea.

Demographics: Anterior uveitis is four times more prevalent than posterior uveitis. The incidence of anterior uveitis is 8.2 cases per 100,000 annually. Males and females are equally affected, unless the individual is HLA-B27(+), wherein males predominate.

Cardinal Findings: Acute anterior uveitis (AAU) usually has an acute onset, with deep eye pain, photophobia, and decreased visual acuity, with or without conjunctival injection. Corneal opacities (clouding) may be seen because of the inflammatory infiltrate in the anterior chamber. Synechiae may form between the lens and iris. Episodic or recurrent disease is not uncommon. Unilateral presentations are more common than bilateral. Bilateral uveitis has a greater association with systemic features and interstitial nephritis. Half of AAU patients are positive for HLA-B27. HLA-B27+ uveitis patients are more likely to have male predominance; younger onset; more synechiae; ocular complications and frequent association with a spondyloarthropathy (see p. 355). Chronic anterior uveitis is far less frequent and is seen in up to 20% of children with juvenile arthritis.

Posterior uveitis tends to have an insidious onset with less discomfort (rather than pain), decreased visual acuity, and floating spots, usually affecting both eyes.

Complications: Permanent visual loss is a grave complication that may result from precipitates on the cornea or lens, secondary glaucoma, obstructive synechiae, cataracts, or rarely vasculitis, vascular occlusion, or retinal infarction. Topical ocular steroid therapy may be complicated by increased intraocular pressure and cataracts.

Diagnostic Tests: No specific laboratory test can diagnose uveitis. Investigations are often necessary to identify an underlying disorder (e.g., CBC, creatinine, urinalysis, ANA, ESR, VDRL, PPD, HLA-B27).

Imaging: Imaging procedures are not necessary to diagnose uveitis. In those with low back pain, radiographs may disclose evidence of sacroiliitis. Chest radiographs may be helpful in the diagnosis of suspected systemic disorders such as tuberculosis, sarcoidosis, or lymphoma.

Keys to Diagnosis: Patients suspected of having uveitis should have a slit lamp examination by an ophthalmologist.

Differential Diagnosis: Conjunctivitis, episcleritis, scleritis, keratitis, and acute angle-closure glaucoma must be differentiated.

Therapy: Most patients respond well to topical corticosteroids and mydriatics (i.e., homoatropine hydrobromide 2% ophthalmic solution b.i.d.) that may retard development of synechiae. Prednisolone acetate 1% ophthalmic suspension is often given 2 gtt. every hour initially, then tapered to q.i.d. dosing. Chronic anterior uveitis may be more difficult to treat and may require systemic therapy. Posterior uveitis (not related to infection) may also require systemic therapy when vision is impaired. Infectious etiologies should be addressed with the appropriate antiinfective agent. Uveitis that is refractory to topical steroids may require systemic steroids, azathioprine, cyclosporine, chlorambucil, cyclophosphamide, or methotrexate.

REFERENCES

Rosenbaum JT. Uveitis: an internists view. Arch Intern Med 1989;149:1173–1176.
Tay-Dearney ML, Schwam BL, Lowder C, et al. Clinical features and associated systemic diseases of HLA-B27 uveitis. Am J Ophthalmol 1996;121:47–56.

WEGENER'S GRANULOMATOSIS

ICD9 Code: 446.4

Definition: Wegener's granulomatosis is a vasculitic syndrome associated with upper respiratory, pulmonary, and renal involvement. It is characterized histologically by necrotizing granulomatous vasculitis of small arteries and veins.

Etiology: Although it has long been suspected that Wegener's granulomatosis relates to exposure to some environmental agent, none has been implicated. There is no evidence of immune complex disease. There are no other associated risk factors nor any genetic predisposition. It is unknown if ANCA are pathogenic or epiphenomenal.

Pathology: Characteristic changes include granulomatous and vasculitic involvement of the upper and lower respiratory tract, sinuses, orbit, kidney, CNS, or heart. Vascular lesions involve small vessels with granuloma and multinucleated giant cells. Kidney lesions may present as pauciimmune rapidly progressive glomerulonephritis (GN), focal necrotizing GN, crescentic GN, and less commonly, diffuse proliferative GN or interstitial nephritis. Arteritis is seen in less than 8% of renal lesions. Vasculitis of the vasa nervorum is seen with mononeuritis multiplex.

Demographics: The mean age of onset is approximately 40 years, ranging from 8 to 80 years. Males are affected slightly more commonly than females. Wegener's granulomatosis is uncommon, with a prevalence of approximately 3 cases per 100,000 population. Nearly 97% of patients are Caucasian and 2% are African American.

Cardinal Findings: Wegener's patients may present with a variety of manifestations. The most common symptoms reflect upper and lower respiratory involvement (see Table 1). Patients may also exhibit constitutional symptoms, such as fever, weight loss, and malaise. Others have no or minimal symptoms and have their disease discovered on chest x-ray.

Although it can affect multiple organs, pulmonary, upper airway, and renal involvement are the most characteristic features. Approximately 25% of Wegener's granulomatosis patients have the classic triad of involvement in these three organ systems. Others have more-limited disease; about 20% have only upper and lower respiratory lesions, and about 17% each have renal involvement with either upper or lower respiratory involvement. The extent of lung and kidney disease usually determines therapy.

—*Upper Respiratory Tract:* Features include sinusitis, cough, rhinitis, nasal ulcers, serous otitis media, hearing loss, and rarely subglottic stenosis. Upper respiratory tract involvement in Wegener's granulomatosis is not typically life threatening. However, it can be a source of chronic and severe symptoms such as epistaxis, sinus tenderness, and purulent rhinorrhea. It can also destroy the nasal cartilage, leading to a "saddle nose" deformity. Many with Wegener's granulomatosis experience frequent bouts of infectious sinusitis, particularly with *Staphylococcus aureus.* Sinus symptoms related to infection may be quite difficult to distinguish from those related to a flare of vasculitis. There also may be a causal relationship between infection and disease relapse.

—*Pulmonary:* Findings include dyspnea, cough, hemoptysis, and pleurisy. Bilateral pulmonary infiltrates (often nodular) are seen in half of patients and may eventually cavitate.

—*Renal:* Kidney involvement almost always follows upper and lower respiratory tract disease and may manifest as proteinuria, hematuria, red cell casts, or renal insufficiency. Hypertension is rarely seen. Glomerulonephritis is seen in a minority of patients at the onset but eventually develops in nearly 85% of cases. The typical renal lesion of Wegener's granulomatosis is a focal and segmental glomerulonephritis. This may progress to a diffuse necrotizing crescentic glomerulonephritis and may be associated with rapid onset of renal failure. However, end-stage renal disease is seen in less than 10% of patients.

—*Ocular:* Nearly half of patients have ocular findings, including proptosis

Table 1
Organ System Involvement in Wegener's granulomatosis

Organ System	At Presentation (%)	Involvement Ever (%)
Lungs	71	95
Sinuses	67	90
Kidneys	15	85
Joints	44	67
Nasal	33	64
Ears	25	61
Eyes	16	58
Skin	15	45

(from retroorbital pseudotumor), conjunctivitis, dacryocystitis, scleritis, or cavernous sinus thrombosis.

Uncommon Findings: Less frequent manifestations of Wegener's granulomatosis include arthralgia (less commonly arthritis), cutaneous nodules, palpable purpura, granulomatous prostatitis, and parotitis. Mononeuritis multiplex is seen in less than 15% of patients. Other CNS findings include cranial neuropathy (II, V, VII, IX, XII) and polyneuropathy.

Complications: Complications may include saddle-nose deformity, hearing loss, labyrinthitis, tracheal obstruction, pulmonary cavitation, end-stage renal disease (<10%), visual loss, amenorrhea, and therapy-related infection. Cyclophosphamide therapy may result in hemorrhagic cystitis and an increased risk of bladder cancer.

Diagnostic Tests: Most patients exhibit a normochromic, normocytic anemia, leukocytosis without eosinophilia, elevated ESR, hypergammaglobulinemia, and normal complement levels.

—*ANCA:* A major advance in the treatment of patients with Wegener's granulomatosis was the description of antineutrophil cytoplasmic antibodies (ANCA; see p. 81). These antibodies bind to proteinase-3, a cytoplasmic enzyme. Depending upon disease activity, 50–90% of patients with Wegener's granulomatosis have positive cANCA tests. This test is relatively specific, as cANCA are uncommonly seen in other diseases. In the context of characteristic clinical findings, many physicians use the presence of cANCA as a diagnostic aid. The titer of cANCA may also vary with disease activity. A number of patients have a decreased cANCA titer or even disappearance of cANCA with successful therapy, and an increased titer with a flare of disease activity; however, the activity of Wegener's granulomatosis can not be determined solely by following cANCA titers.

Differential Diagnosis: Other pulmonary-renal syndromes, such as Goodpasture's syndrome, subacute bacterial endocarditis, and SLE are in the differential diagnosis. The upper respiratory involvement may resemble relapsing polychondritis and midline granuloma. Pulmonary manifestations of Wegener's granulomatosis mimic sarcoidosis or vasculitides (e.g., Churg-Strauss syndrome), granulomatous infectious processes (e.g., tuberculosis, histoplasmosis, blastomycosis), and neoplastic diseases (e.g., lymphomatoid granulomatosis, lymphoma).

Diagnosis: Wegener's granulomatosis may be diagnosed by several means. Histopathologic definition of granulomatous vasculitis on respiratory tract biopsy specimen establishes the diagnosis in the correct clinical setting. Pulmonary biopsy specimens should be obtained by open lung biopsy rather than transbronchially, as the latter has a lower diagnostic yield and may be associated with uncontrolled bleeding. Renal biopsy is seldom diagnostic or specific for Wegener's granulomatosis but may support the diagnosis depending on the other organ involvement. The American College of Rheumatology has formulated classification criteria that may help differentiate patients with Wegener's from those with other types of vasculitis (Table 2).

Therapy: Prior to the use of immunomodulatory drugs, Wegener's granulomatosis was usually a fatal disease with a mean survival of approximately 6 months and more than 80% 1-year mortality. Addition of prednisone prolonged the mean survival to approximately 1 year. Currently, the standard of care includes the use of cytotoxic drugs, particularly cyclophosphamide, and the long-term remission rate exceeds 90%. Therapy typically includes high-dose corticosteroids (e.g., 1 mg/kg/day of prednisone) in conjunction with cyclophosphamide at doses of 1 to 2 mg/kg/day. Intermittent "pulse" intravenous cyclophosphamide does not appear as efficacious as daily oral dosing. When the manifestations of disease are under control, the dose of prednisone may be tapered. In general, cyclophosphamide is continued for at least a year after the disease is quiescent. For patients not responding to, or intolerant of, therapy with cyclophosphamide, methotrexate has been used with some success. In anecdotal reports, trimethoprim/sulfamethoxazole was reported to have possi-

Table 2
1990 ACR Classification Criteria for Wegener's Granulomatosis

Criterion	Definition
1. Nasal/oral inflammation	Oral ulcers or purulent or bloody nasal discharge
2. Abnormal chest x-ray	Chest x-ray with nodules, cavities, or fixed infiltrates
3. Hematuria	Microhematuria (>5 RBC/hpf) or red cell casts
4. Granulomatous inflammation	Histologic changes on biopsy specimen showing granulomatous inflammation within the wall of an artery or in the perivascular area

A patient may be classified as having Wegener's granulomatosis if two or more criteria are present (sensitivity, 88.2%; specificity, 92%)

ble value in treating Wegener's, especially when limited to the upper respiratory tract. Long-term treatment with this antibiotic decreases relapse of disease activity slightly. However, this therapy should not be considered a substitute for immunomodulatory therapy in patients with active Wegener's granulomatosis.

Prognosis: Relapse is common in Wegener's granulomatosis; 45% or more of successfully treated patients experience a relapse; median time to relapse is 42 months. The chance of cure is uncertain. Thus all patients should be followed for relapse. The frequency of relapse and treatment exposure increases the risk of morbidity and mortality. Treatment-related morbidity may be significant and may include features related to corticosteroids (e.g., diabetes, fracture, osteonecrosis, cataracts) or cyclophosphamide (e.g., hair loss, hemorrhagic cystitis, bladder cancer, myelodysplasia). Death is usually related to renal disease, pulmonary disease, infection, or malignancy.

REFERENCES

Fauci AS, Haynes BF, Katz P, Wolff SM. Wegener's granulomatosis: prospective clinical and therapeutic experience with 85 patients for 21 years. Ann Intern Med 1983;98:76–85.

Hoffman GS. Advances in Wegener's granulomatosis. Hosp Pract 1995;April 15:29–36.

Hoffman GS, Kerr GS, Leavitt RY, et al. Wegener's granulomatosis: an analysis of 158 patients. Ann Intern Med 1992;116:488–498.

Leavitt RY, Fauci AS, Bloch DA, et al. The American College of Rheumatology 1990 criteria for the classification of Wegener's granulomatosis. Arthritis Rheum 1990;33:1101–1107.

Stegeman CA, Tervaert JWC, de Jong PE, Kallenberg CGM. Trimethoprim-sulfamethoxazole for the prevention of relapses of Wegener's granulomatosis. N Engl J Med 1996;335:16–20.

Talar-Williams C, Hijazi YM, Walther MM, et al. Cyclophosphamide-induced cystitis and bladder cancer in patients with Wegener granulomatosis. Ann Intern Med 1996;124:477–484.

WILSON'S DISEASE

Synonyms: Hepatolenticular degeneration

ICD9 Code: 275.1

Definition: Wilson's disease is a multisystem disorder caused by accumulation of copper in tissues.

Demographics: This unusual multisystem disorder is transmitted as an autosomal recessive gene and has an estimated prevalence of 1 in 30,000. Although manifestations may become apparent in childhood, about half of cases are not detected until after adolescence. It affects individuals between 6 and 40 years old.

Etiology: Manifestations are associated with an overabundance of copper that accumulates for unknown reasons, causing damage to target organs.

Cardinal Findings: Deposition of excess copper can be observed in the cornea as the characteristic Kayser-Fleischer rings, which are diagnostic. The most common symptoms are movement disorders (from basal ganglia deposition), jaundice or hepatic dysfunction, liver abnormalities, and renal tubular damage.

Musculoskeletal manifestations seen in 50% or fewer adults (rare in children) manifest as premature osteoarthritis with a polyarthropathy involving wrists, MCPs, knees, and spine. Knee effusion may be seen with associated chondromalacia patellae or chondrocalcinosis. Significant osteoporosis is present in about half of all patients. Joint abnormalities are generally not as severe as those seen in hemochromatosis.

Diagnostic Tests: Ceruloplasmin levels may be low, and there may be evidence of a renal tubular acidosis.

Imaging: Radiographic findings include joint space loss, marked osteophytes, subchondral cysts, and chondrocalcinosis.

Keys to Diagnosis: A diagnosis of Wilson's disease should be considered in any patient less than 40 years old who has persistent, unexplained liver abnormalities. The diagnosis is confirmed by measurement of low serum ceruloplasmin concentrations with either Kayser-Fleischer rings or increased copper in a liver biopsy sample.

Therapy: Wilson's disease is usually treated with penicillamine, which chelates copper. An initial dose of 1000 mg/day is recommended and may be later decreased to 750 mg/day. Probably, early effective treatment with penicillamine ameliorates the arthritic manifestations. Ironically, prolonged treatment with the relatively high doses of penicillamine which are required for effective control of excess copper can be associated with development of autoimmune phenomena such as a lupuslike syndrome or myasthenia.

WHIPPLE'S DISEASE

Synonyms: Intestinal lipodystrophy

ICD9 Code: 040.2

Definition: Whipple's disease is a multisystem infectious disorder characterized by inflammatory polyarthritis and small bowel colitis.

Etiology: Whipple's disease is due to infection with the gram-positive actinomycete, *Tropheryma whippelii*. Intestinal or lymph node biopsy specimens may disclose PAS-staining deposits in macrophages, and electron microscopy may show rod-shaped bacilli.

Demographics: Whipple's disease is most common in men (90%) above the age of 40 years.

Cardinal Findings: Diarrhea, steatorrhea, weight loss, fever, arthritis, serositis, and lymphadenopathy are seen. Arthralgia or arthritis frequently precedes the intestinal features. The inflammatory arthritis tends to be polyarticular, symmetric, and seronegative and may be chronic or transient.

Uncommon Findings: Iritis, vitritis, ocular palsy, and progressive encephalitis have been described.

Diagnostic Tests: The causative agent (*Tropheryma whippelii*) may be identified by PCR.

Keys to Diagnosis: A high index of suspicion is needed, especially in older men with seronegative RA-like polyarthritis, systemic features, and intestinal disease. Perform small bowel biopsy and a PCR test for the causative agent.

Therapy: Oral tetracycline (1 g/day) for 1 year is recommended.

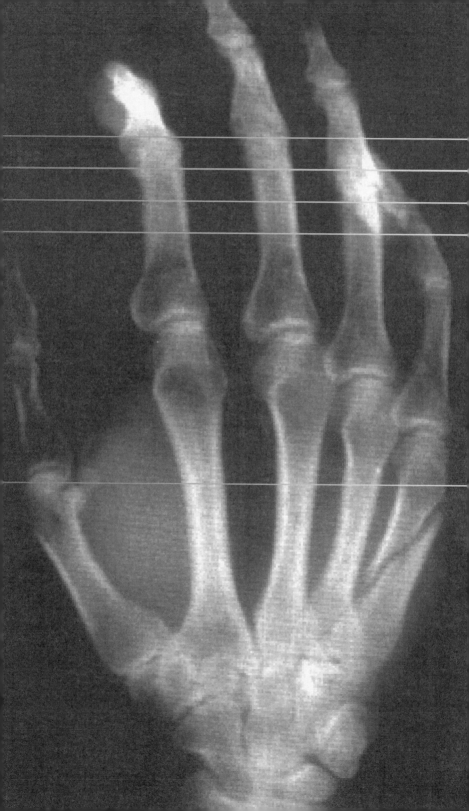

SECTION 3

PHARMACOPOEIA FOR THE RHEUMATIC DISEASES

This pharmacopoeia summarizes drugs commonly used in the treatment of patients with musculoskeletal diseases. The doses listed are provided as a guide for adult patients but need to be individualized according to clinical response and individual patients. Dose modifications may be required in particular patient populations such as the elderly and patients with impaired hepatic or renal function. The more common and clinically important adverse reactions and drug interactions are listed, but this information is not comprehensive.

Abbreviations (also see p. xi-xv)

ACE—angiotensin converting enzyme
CBC—complete blood count
CNS—central nervous system
CYP P450—cytochrome P450
DMARD—disease-modifying antirheumatic drug
FDA—Food and Drug Administration
g—gram
G6PD—glucose-6-phosphate dehydrogenase
GI—gastrointestinal
IM, IV—intramuscular, intravenous
IU—international units
LFT—liver function test
MAOI—monoamine oxidase inhibitors
μg—microgram
mg—milligram
ml—milliliter
NSAID—nonsteroidal antiinflammatory drug
OTC—over the counter
PDR—*Physicians' Desk Reference*
PO—by mouth
PRN—as needed
RA—rheumatoid arthritis
RDA—recommended daily allowance
SC—subcutaneous
SLE—systemic lupus erythematosus
WBC—white blood cells

Pregnancy Risk Category

The use of any drug in pregnancy represents a therapeutic decision reached after evaluating the potential risks and benefits to the mother and fetus. Drugs are classified into FDA-designated categories representing the risk of a particular drug being teratogenic. The pregnancy risk increases through categories A to D. X indicates drugs that are absolutely contraindicated in pregnancy. These categories are explained in the table below.

Category	Drug Effects on Fetus
A	Controlled studies show no risk to the fetus, and possibility of fetal harm appears remote
B	Either (a) animal studies have not demonstrated a fetal risk but there are no controlled studies in pregnant women or (b) animal studies have shown an adverse effect in pregnancy that was not confirmed in women in controlled studies
C	Either (a) animal studies demonstrate adverse effects on the fetus and there are no controlled studies in women or (b) studies in women and animals are not available
D	Positive evidence of human fetal risk but potential benefit may justify potential risk in certain circumstances
X	Contraindicated in women who are or may become pregnant

Cost of Medication

The following key is used to indicate the relative cost of medication to the patient. The relative scale used is not meant to indicate a specific monetary value but rather to portray the range of possible cost of treatment to the individual. Unless otherwise noted, the cost represents the average cost of generic medication using a median effective dose.

$ Inexpensive (even for those with limited financial resources)

$$ Affordable to most patients (cost concerns are limited with such a drug)

$$$ Expensive (less-expensive agents should be considered); agent may only be affordable when the cost of medication is subsidized by insurance programs

$$$$ Very expensive; cost limits use of this agent to those capable of affording the high price of medication or those with "liberal" prescription programs

$$$$$ Cost prohibitive! Should only be used if (a) the agent is absolutely indicated; (b) anticipated therapeutic benefits are sufficiently great; and (c) less-expensive therapeutic options have been exhausted or are contraindicated; often the cost of such agents is not covered by medical insurance programs

Pitfalls in Prescribing

The clinician should be careful to avoid the following common mistakes in prescribing:

1. *Prescribing a drug when no drug is needed.* Alternative, nondrug methods of symptom control may be the appropriate intervention.

2. *Prescribing no drug when a drug is indicated.* Therapeutic nihilism or therapeutic ignorance may deny patients effective and necessary treatment.

3. *Prescribing a poorly chosen drug for the disease.* A drug that is ineffective, expensive, and potentially harmful (e.g., methotrexate to treat gout) should be avoided. Also common is the mistake of choosing a drug that has similar efficacy but is more expensive or has more side effects than the treatment of choice.

4. *Prescribing a poorly chosen drug for the patient.* The patient is a major determinant of rational prescribing. Children, the elderly, pregnant or lactating women, patients with renal or liver disease, and patients receiving other drugs all require special consideration.

5. *Prescribing a drug incorrectly.* A correct drug for the patient and the illness may be chosen, but the drug may be prescribed incorrectly. The dose, dose interval, duration of therapy, and route of administration must be considered. An example of this is the prolonged use of high-dose corticosteroids in RA (which should be tapered as soon as possible).

6. *Not providing a patient with essential information.* This is particularly important in long-term therapy with potentially dangerous drugs (e.g., cyclophosphamide) and drugs that must be taken in a particular way (e.g., alendronate).

7. *Failing to monitor appropriately.* Many drugs are potentially toxic, and appropriate long-term monitoring is essential. Assessing the patient's clinical response and modifying therapy appropriately, in addition to laboratory monitoring, is important.

8. *Polypharmacy.* Many patients require long-term therapy with multiple drugs. Nonetheless, the requirement for ongoing medications should be thoughtfully reviewed.

9. *Illegibility.* Tragedies have occurred because of illegibility. Printing is preferable. Avoid abbreviations (e.g., MTX for methotrexate) when prescribing.

Therapeutic Aims

Primary aims in the treatment of musculoskeletal illness are

1. To relieve pain and stiffness
2. To maintain and restore function and strength
3. To maintain or improve the quality of life
4. If possible, to prevent recurrence or progression of disease

Formulation of a Therapeutic Plan

Treatment of the various musculoskeletal conditions depends on the diagnosis, the severity of disease, and the individual patient's response to different forms of therapy. All of these need to be evaluated before and during treatment. Treatment generally takes three major forms: (*a*) rehabilitation (including physical therapy, occupational therapy, splints); (*b*) drug therapy; and (*c*) surgery. A rational management plan is outlined below.

Key Steps in a Therapeutic Plan

Establish diagnosis

↓

Evaluate: disease severity, aggravating factors, modifiable contributors, functional status, psychosocial status, comorbidities

↓

Initiate treatment plan: patient education, appropriate physical and/or occupational therapy, appropriate drug or combination of drugs, surgery if indicated

↓

Monitor: monitor clinical status, complications, response to therapy, and toxicity from therapy

↓

Modify treatment plan: change therapy if unacceptable toxicity occurs or after an appropriate trial with inadequate efficacy; if response is acceptable, evaluate maintenance dosages or need for continued therapy

In some rheumatic diseases (e.g., osteoarthritis and fibromyalgia) the efficacy of drug therapy may be modest, and nondrug therapies play an important adjunctive role. Few rheumatic diseases are cured by treatment, and thus the therapeutic plan for an individual patient may change over time as the illness evolves. Optimal treatment of a particular condition may change over time as new data become available. A diagnostic consultation with a rheumatologist is more cost effective than ordering an extensive "rheumatology panel" of laboratory tests. Management of rheumatoid arthritis, systemic lupus erythematosus, dermato/polymyositis, and vasculitis is complex. Diagnostic and therapeutic issues may be clarified and complications or toxicities minimized by consulting a rheumatologist.

SPECIFIC AGENTS

ACETAMINOPHEN

Trade Names: Include *Acephen, Aceta, Apacet, Panadol, Tylenol*

Synonyms: Paracetamol

Drug Class: Analgesic/antipyretic

Preparations

Capsules: 325 mg, 500 mg ("Extra-Strength")

Tablets: 120 mg, 160 mg, 325 mg, 500 mg; 650 mg (Extended-Release)

Suppositories: 120 mg, 160 mg, 325 mg, 650 mg

Elixir: 120 mg/5 mL, 80 mg/5 mL, 160 mg/5 mL, 325 mg/5 mL

Dose: (Adults) 1–4 g/day in 3–4 divided doses. Do not exceed 4 g/day

Indications: Pain, musculoskeletal pain, headache, fever. In contrast to NSAIDs, acetaminophen does not cause GI ulceration.

Mechanism of Action: Uncertain; inhibits central prostaglandin synthesis

Contraindications: Hypersensitivity to acetaminophen

Precautions: Avoid concomitant alcohol. Use lower doses in liver disease. May cause severe hepatotoxicity in overdose.

Pregnancy Risk: B

Adverse Effects: Rarely causes allergy, rash, or agranulocytosis. Hepatotoxicity is rare at therapeutic doses. Overdose (usually >10 g/day) causes delayed (48–72 h) and potentially fatal hepatotoxicity. Controversial evidence links chronic use to increased risk of renal impairment.

Drug Interactions

Alcohol: Increases risk of hepatotoxicity

Warfarin: Acetaminophen (>2 g/day) may increase anticoagulant effect

Barbiturates, carbamazepine, hydantoins, sulfinpyrazone may increase hepatotoxicity of acetaminophen

Patient Instructions: Do not exceed prescribed dose. Do not take additional OTC or prescription medications that contain acetaminophen. Do not drink alcohol.

Clinical Pharmacology: Rapid complete oral absorption; 95% metabolized in the liver (mainly conjugation). Duration of action is 3–4 h. With overdose, a heptatotoxic metabolite accumulates.

Cost: $

ACETAMINOPHEN 1 OPIOID (CODEINE/ HYDROCODONE/OXYCODONE/ PROPOXYPHENE)

Trade Names

Acetaminophen + codeine: *Capital and Codeine, Phenaphen with Codeine, Tylenol with Codeine*

Acetaminophen + hydrocodone: *Anexsia, Cogesic, Dolacet, Hydrocet, Lortab , Lorcet, Lorcet Plus, Vicodin, Vicodin ES*

Acetaminophen + oxycodone: *Percocet, Roxicet, Roxilox, Tylox*

Acetaminophen + propoxyphene: *Darvocet N-50, Darvocet N-100*

Acetaminophen + pentazocine: *Talacen*

Drug Class: Analgesic/antipyretic with opioid analgesic

Preparations

Acetaminophen + codeine

Tablet: Acetaminophen with codeine #2, 300 mg acetaminophen/15 mg codeine; acetaminophen with codeine #3, 300/30 mg; acetaminophen with codeine #4, 300/60 mg

Capsule: Acetaminophen with codeine #2, 325 mg acetaminophen/15 mg codeine; acetaminophen with codeine #3, 325 mg/30 mg; acetaminophen with codeine #4, 325 mg/60 mg

Suspension: Acetaminophen with codeine, 120 mg/12 mg per 5 mL.

Acetaminophen + hydrocodone

Tablet: *Lortab 2.5/500* (2.5 mg hydrocodone/500 mg acetaminophen); *Lortab 5/500; Lortab 7.5/500; Lorcet Plus (7.5/650); Lorcet 10/650, Vicodin (5/500); Vicodin ES (7.5/750)*

Acetaminophen + oxycodone

Capsule: Acetaminophen 500 mg/oxycodone 5 mg (*Tylox*)

Tablet: Acetaminophen 325 mg/oxycodone 5 mg (*Percocet*)

Acetaminophen + propoxyphene: *Darvocet N-50* (50 mg propoxyphene and 325 mg of acetaminophen); *Darvocet N-100* (100/650)

Acetaminophen + pentazocine: *Talacen 25/650* (25 mg pentazocine and 650 mg acetaminophen)

Dose

Acetaminophen + codeine: Adult dose 1–2 tablets containing acetaminophen 300 mg + codeine 15 or 30 mg q 4–6 h PRN

Acetaminophen + hydrocodone: Adult dose 500–750 mg acetaminophen + 5–10 mg hydrocodone q 4–6 h PRN

Acetaminophen + oxycodone: Adult dose 1–2 tablets q 4–6 h PRN

Acetaminophen + propoxyphene: Adult dose 50–100 mg propoxyphene + 325–650 mg acetaminophen q 4 h PRN (maximum 600 mg propoxyphene/day)

Acetaminophen + pentazocine: Adult dose 1–2 tablet q 4 h PRN (not to exceed 600 mg pentazocine/day)

Indications: Pain unresponsive to nonopioid regimens. Most studies show little benefit over nonopioid regimens in chronic musculoskeletal pain.

Mechanism of Action: Acetaminophen (uncertain) inhibits central prostaglandin synthesis. Opioids bind to opioid receptors in CNS and modify pain perception.

Contraindications: Hypersensitivity reactions (commonly due to opioids, not acetaminophen); opioid or prescription drug abuse

Precautions: Concomitant alcohol use, liver disease, and fasting may increase the risk of acetaminophen hepatotoxicity. Use lower doses in liver disease (usually <2 g/day). Patient must avoid self-medication with OTC preparations that may also contain acetaminophen. Risk of psychologic and physical narcotic dependence should limit use. Avoid dose escalation. Limit dose and duration of therapy if possible. One physician should prescribe all opioids for a particular patient.

Pregnancy risk: C

Adverse Effects: Acetaminophen rarely causes allergy, rash, or agranulocytosis. Hepatotoxicity is rare at therapeutic doses. Overdose (usually >10 g/day) causes delayed (48–72 h) and potentially fatal hepatotoxicity. Controversial evidence links chronic use of acetaminophen to increased risk of renal impairment.

Opioid toxicity (common): GI intolerance, constipation, and dependence are seen with chronic use. Less common are allergy, confusion, dizziness, nervousness, insomnia, and respiratory depression.

Drug Interactions

Alcohol: Increases risk of hepatotoxicity

Warfarin: Acetaminophen (>2 g/day) may increase the anticoagulant effect

CNS depressants: Effects may be potentiated by opioids

Patient Instructions: Do not exceed prescribed dose. Do not take additional OTC or prescription medications that contain acetaminophen. Do not drink alcohol. May cause drowsiness and constipation. Contains a narcotic and is addictive. Only take for pain.

Comment: Opioid/narotic medications are seldom required in the treatment of inflammatory joint disease (i.e., RA, gout). In such conditions, control of inflammation usually controls the associated pain.

Clinical Pharmacology: Acetaminophen—oral absorption is rapid and complete. It is 95% metabolized in the liver (mainly conjugation). In overdose, a heptatotoxic metabolite accumulatzes.

Codeine is methylmorphine, and 10% is metabolized to morphine. Other opioids are modifications of the morphine molecule. Codeine undergoes hepatic metabolism and renal excretion.

Duration of action is 4–6 h.

Cost: $$

ALENDRONATE

Trade Names: *Fosamax*

Drug Class: Bisphosphonate

Preparations: 5-mg, 10-mg, 40-mg tablets

Dose/Administration

Osteoporosis: 5–10 mg PO daily

Paget's disease: 40 mg PO daily for 6 months. If disease relapses retreatment can be considered.

Indications: Treatment and prevention of osteoporosis; treatment of Paget's disease

Mechanism of Action: Localizes to areas of bone resorption and inhibits osteoclast activity without any effect on bone formation; increases bone mineral density and significantly reduces vertebral fracture rates. Does not induce osteomalacia.

Contraindications: Hypersensitivity to alendronate, hypocalcemia, esophageal stricture, or dysmotility. Not recommended for patients with severe renal insufficiency (creatinine clearance < 35 mL/min). Avoid use in patients who cannot stand or sit upright for 30 min after administration.

Precautions: If possible, avoid alendronate if esophageal problems or renal impairment are present. Ensure that patient understands how drug should be taken.

Pregnancy Risk: C

Adverse Effects: Headache, occasional mild GI disturbance (i.e., nausea, dyspepsia, dysphagia). Rarely, severe erosive esophagitis or rash are seen.

Drug Interactions: GI adverse events are increased in patients taking NSAIDs and more than 10 mg/day of alendronate.

Patient Instructions: Alendronate should be taken with a full glass of water on arising in the morning. Nothing other than water should be taken for at least 30 min after alendronate. Even coffee or fruit juice markedly reduce absorption. Delaying such intake for longer than 30 min (1–2 h if possible) maximizes absorption. After taking alendronate, the patient must remain upright to reduce risk of esophageal irritation. Any other medications must be taken at least 30 min after alendronate.

Comments: Supplemental calcium and vitamin D are usually coadministered.

Clinical Pharmacology: Oral bioavailability is very poor (<1%) and negligible if administered with or after food. It is 100% renally excreted and not metabolized. Terminal half-life exceeds 10 years, indicating localization and slow release from bone.

Cost: $$$$

REFERENCES

Delmas PD, Meunier PJ. The management of Paget's disease of bone. N Engl J Med 1997;336:558–566.

Jeel W, Barradell LB, McTavish D. Alendronate. A review of its pharmacological properties and therapeutic efficacy in postmenopausal osteoporosis. Drugs 1997;53:415–434.

Liberman UA, Weiss SR, Broll J, et al. Effect of alendronate on bone mineral density and the incidence of fractures in postmenopausal osteoporosis. N Engl J Med 1995;333:1437–1443.

ALLOPURINOL

Trade Names: *Lopurin, Zyloprim, Zurinol*

Drug Class: Xanthine oxidase inhibitor

Preparations: 100-mg, 300-mg tablets

Dose: Prophylaxis of gout: Initially use 100 mg daily, increased at 1- to 2-week intervals according to uric acid response. In the elderly use <50 mg/day initially.

Usual maintenance dose is 200–300 mg daily. Patients with severe hyperuricemia and tophi may require higher doses. Maximum recommended dose is 800 mg/day. Doses above 300 mg/day are given in divided doses.

In renal impairment, the dose is usually reduced to 25–200 mg/day (monitor closely for toxicity). If required in patients with renal failure, allopurinol dosage is modified according to creatinine clearance; for example, creatinine clearance 10 mL/min, give 100 mg every second day; 20 mL/min, 100 mg daily; 40 mL/min, 150 mg daily; and 60 mL/min, 200 mg daily.

Indications: Prophylaxis of gout, treatment of chronic gout, uric acid nephropathy, prophylaxis of renal calculi, used to treat extreme hyperuricemia (e.g., renal failure, chemotherapy, tumor lysis)

Mechanism of Action: Inhibits formation of uric acid by inhibiting xanthine oxidase; has no antiinflammatory activity

Contraindications: Prior hypersensitivity to allopurinol

Precautions: Reduce dose in the elderly, patients on diuretics, and patients with renal impairment. Concurrent azathioprine or mercaptopurine requires major dose reduction of the cytotoxic drug.

Pregnancy Risk: C

Monitoring: Monitor CBC and liver and renal function periodically, particularly in the first few months of treatment. Uric acid level guides the allopurinol dose. Aim to reduce uric acid concentration below 6 mg/dL and lower in tophaceous disease.

Adverse Effects

Common: Acute gout may occur with increased frequency after starting allopurinol, and thus it should not be initiated during an acute gouty attack. If allergic rash is mild and not associated with other features of allopurinol hypersensitivity syndrome, discontinue and reintroduce cautiously but discontinue if rash recurs.

Rarely: Allopurinol hypersensitivity syndrome (exfoliative dermatitis/erythema multiforme, renal failure, hepatic impairment, and vasculitis) is rare but may be fatal. Risk is increased in patients with impaired renal function or receiving diuretics. Desensitization has been tried in selected patients. Oxypurinol is sometimes tolerated by patients sensitive to allopurinol. Agranulocytosis and aplastic anemia are rare.

Drug Interactions

Azathioprine and mercaptopurine: Allopurinol decreases metabolism of these agents, leading to toxicity (bone marrow depression). If concurrent use cannot be avoided, the dose of azathioprine or mercaptopurine should be reduced to 25% of the usual dose and the CBC carefully monitored.

Warfarin: Anticoagulant effects potentiated

Cyclophosphamide: Increased potential for bone marrow suppression

Ampicillin/amoxicillin: Increased risk of rash

Thiazide diuretics: Increased risk of allopurinol toxicity

Theophylline: Increased theophylline levels

Chlorpropamide: Increased chlorpropamide serum half-life

Alcohol: Decreases effectiveness

Patient Instructions: This drug needs to be taken every day to *prevent* gout.

It has no effect on the symptoms of gout and will not help when your joints hurt. Discontinue drug and contact physician if rash develops. Do not drink alcohol.

Comments: Asymptomatic hyperuricemia should not routinely be treated. It is not necessary, especially when uric acid levels are below 11 mg/dL. Allopurinol is used primarily to lower the uric acid level in patients with recurrent attacks of acute gout (>1/year) or patients with tophaceous gout. Allopurinol is preferred over a uricosuric agent in patients with tophi, renal stones, and impaired renal function. Monitor serum uric acid and aim to decrease to 5–6 mg/dL. Failure to decrease uric acid often indicates poor compliance. Prevent acute attacks of gout with concurrent colchicine or NSAID treatment, particularly in first 3–6 months of therapy.

Clinical Pharmacology: Oral absorption is 90%; 70% is metabolized to the active metabolite, oxypurinol. Excretion is largely renal as oxypurinol, and accumulation occurs if renal function is impaired. Half-life of allopurinol is 2 h, and oxipurinol, 15 h. Reduction of uric acid is noted within days, and the level may normalize within weeks. If allopurinol is discontinued, uric acid concentrations return to pretreatment levels in weeks.

Cost: $

REFERENCES

Emmerson BT. The management of gout. N Engl J Med 1996;334:445–451.
Hande KR, Noone RM, Stone WJ. Severe allopurinol toxicity. Description and guidelines for prevention in patients with renal insufficiency. Am J Med 1984;76:47–56.

Ambien (see *Zolpidem*)

AMITRIPTYLINE

Trade Names: *Elavil, Endep, Enovil*

Drug Class: Tricyclic antidepressant

Preparations: 10, 25, 50, 75, 100, 150 mg tablets

Dose: Initially, 10 mg is taken 2 h before bedtime. Dose can be increased, if tolerated, to a maximum of 300 mg/day. Usual maintenance dose for fibromyalgia is 10–75 mg taken 2 h before bedtime.

Indications: Depression, fibromyalgia, insomnia; an adjunct for pain control (chronic or neuropathic); prophylaxis for migraines

Mechanism of Action: Increases synaptic concentrations of norepinephrine

Contraindications: Avoid in recovery period of myocardial infarction or if arrhythmias exist. Avoid for 14 days after patient has received an MAO inhibitor. Avoid in narrow-angle glaucoma.

Precautions: Escalate dose slowly. May cause drowsiness and affect ability to drive or operate machinery. Aggravates symptoms of prostatism and keratoconjunctivitis sicca. May precipitate acute glaucoma. High chronic doses should not be abruptly discontinued; use with caution in patients with a history of hyperthyroidism, renal or hepatic impairment, or cardiac conduction disturbances.

Pregnancy Risk: D

Adverse Effects

Common: Sedation and anticholinergic effects (dry eyes and mouth, blurred vision, constipation, difficulty with urination) are common; tolerance often occurs with continued use

Less common: Postural hypotension, restlessness, tremor, parkinsonian syndrome

Rarely: Agranulocytosis, hepatic dysfunction, alopecia, arrhythmias, breast enlargement

Drug Interactions

Alcohol and CNS depressants: Effect of tricyclic is potentiated

Cimetidine, methylphenidate: Inhibit metabolism of tricyclics; dose reduction (20–30%) may be required

MAOIs: Increased risk of hypertensive crises; deaths have been reported

Sympathomimetics: Tricyclics potentiate effect

Guanethidine: Amitriptyline prevents hypotensive effects

Warfarin: Prothrombin time may be prolonged

Patient Instructions: Avoid alcohol use. May cause drowsiness.

Clinical Pharmacology: Well absorbed, hepatic metabolism with renal excretion of metabolites; onset of antidepressant effects slow (2–4 weeks)

Cost: $

Amoxapine (*Asendin*; see *Appendix D*, p. 513)

Anaprox (see *Naproxen*)

Ansaid (see *Flurbiprofen*)

Antibiotics (see *Appendix E*, p. 515)

Antidepressants (see *Appendix D*, p. 513)

Aredia (see *Pamidronate*)

Aristocort (see *Corticosteroids, Intraarticular*)

Aristospan (see *Corticosteroids, Intraarticular*)

Arthropan (see *Choline Salicylate*)

Arthrotec (see *Diclofenac* and *Misoprostil*)

ARTIFICIAL TEARS

Trade Names

Artificial tears: *Liquifilm, Liquifilm Forte, Isopto Alkaline, Isopto Plain, Isopto Tears, Just Tears, Tears Naturelle, Tears Naturelle II*

Artificial tears preservative free: *Celluvisc, Hypotears PF Refresh, Tears Naturelle Free*

Ocular ointments: *Duratears, Lacrilube*

Ocular ointments preservative free: *Duolube, Refresh PM, Lacriserts*

Synonyms: Hydroxypropyl methylcellulose

Drug Class: Ophthalmic protectant

Preparations

Hydroxypropyl methylcellulose ophthalmic solution

0.3%: Bion Tears, Tears Naturelle, Tears Naturelle II, Tears Naturelle Free

0.4%: Artificial Tears, Nature's Tears

0.5%: Isopto Plain, Isopto Tears, Just Tears

0.8%: Ocucoat, Ocucoat PF

1%: Isopto Alkaline, Ultra Tears

Hydroxypropyl cellulose ocular system: *Lacrisert* 5-mg insert

Dose: 1 drop of a 0.3–1% tear solution applied topically to conjunctiva 3–4 times daily. In patients with keratoconjunctivitis sicca drops should be applied regularly even if no symptoms are present. Some patients require more frequent application (every 2 h). Hydroxypropyl cellulose 5-mg ophthalmic insert, use once or twice daily.

Indications: Dry eyes

Mechanism of Action: Promotes corneal wetting by stabilizing and thickening the tear film

Contraindications: Hypersensitivity

Precautions: Use preservative-free preparations if preservative causes irritation.

Pregnancy Risk: C

Adverse Effects: Blurring of vision; eye irritation

Drug Interactions: None

Patient Instructions: Tears may be used as often as required. Regular use rather than waiting until symptoms are present is best. Do not instill with contact lens in place unless preparation is designed for use with contact lenses. Always wash hands prior to administration. Never touch tip of dropper to the eye surface.

Clinical Pharmacology: No systemic effects after ocular administration

Cost: $

Ascriptin (see *Aspirin*)

ASPIRIN

Trade Names

Plain aspirin: *Bayer Aspirin, Empirin*

Buffered aspirin: *Ascriptin, Buffaprin, Buffasal, Buffinol, Bufferin, Alka-Seltzer*

Enteric coated aspirin: *Bayer Enteric, Ecotrin, Easprin, Genprin*

Extended-release aspirin: *8-Hour Bayer Timed Release, Measurin, Zorprin*

Synonyms: Acetylsalicylic acid, ASA

Drug Class: NSAID

Preparations

Chewable aspirin tablets: 81 mg

Tablets: 325 mg, 500 mg

Enteric coated tablets 165 mg, 325 mg, 500 mg, 650 mg, 975 mg

Timed/controlled-release tablets: 650 mg, 800 mg

Dose

Analgesic/antipyretic effect: 325–650 mg q 4–6 h (up to 4 g/day)

Antiinflammatory effect: 3.6–5.4 g/day in divided doses. In acute rheumatic fever, doses up to 7.8 g/day have been used, but dose-related toxicity is common.

Antithrombotic effect: 81–325 mg/day

Indications: Treatment of pain, inflammation, and pyrexia and as antithrombotic prophylaxis; used in RA, osteoarthritis, rheumatic fever, Still's disease, Kawasaki disease, and inflammatory conditions such as bursitis; used for antithrombotic effect in myocardial infarction, the anticardiolipin antibody syndrome, and transient/ischemic attacks

Mechanism of Action: Aspirin inhibits cyclooxygenase activity, decreasing formation of prostaglandins and thromboxane from arachidonic acid.

Contraindications: Hypersensitivity to aspirin (especially in those with asthma and nasal polyps), GI ulceration, hemorrhagic state, last trimester of pregnancy (may induce premature closure of ductus arteriosus), breast-feeding, children (risk of Reye's syndrome), and G6PD-deficiency (hemolysis).

Precautions: Fluid retention may aggravate heart failure and hypertension. Use with caution or avoid in patients at high risk of GI bleeding (i.e., prior GI bleeding, elderly, concurrent corticosteroid treatment). Administer with food. Use with caution in asthma, bleeding disorders, and hepatic or renal disease.

Monitoring: Monitor hematocrit, creatinine, and liver enzymes periodically (1 month after starting and then every 3–6 months). In patients at high risk of renal impairment (i.e., diuretics, receiving ACE inhibitors, edematous states, heart failure, renal failure, diabetes), monitor renal function more closely. Consider measuring salicylate levels if using high doses. Serum concentrations of 150–300 μg/mL are antiinflammatory. Salicylism (e.g., tinnitus) is common at levels above 200 μg/mL.

Pregnancy Risk: C (D in third trimester of pregnancy)

Adverse Effects

Common: GI irritation (dyspepsia, esophageal reflux, epigastric pain); dose-related side effects at concentrations above 200 μg/mL (tinnitus/deafness)

Less common: GI ulceration or hemorrhage, minor elevations of liver enzymes, hypersensitivity (asthma, urticaria, angioedema—particularly in patients with nasal polyps); acidosis with overdose and high serum concentrations (>400 μg/mL), especially in the elderly

Drug Interactions

Antacids: Decreased salicylate levels through increased elimination in alkaline urine

Anticoagulants: Activity of warfarin increased; increased hemorrhagic risk with other anticoagulants and thrombolytics

NSAIDs: Increased risk of GI side effects if aspirin is used with other NSAIDs

Methotrexate: May increase levels of methotrexate (however, with the doses of methotrexate used in RA, this is usually clinically insignificant); may potentiate methotrexate toxicity with high doses of MTX

Lithium: Increased lithium levels

Valproic acid: ASA may enhance toxicity of VPA

Probenecid: ASA may antagonize effects

Patient Instructions: Take with food. Discontinue and seek medical advice if unusual bleeding develops.

Comments: With high doses, metabolic pathways become saturated, and a small increase in dose can result in large increases in plasma concentrations. Enteric coated or delayed-release formulations of aspirin are better tolerated than regular aspirin.

Clinical Pharmacology: Rapidly and well absorbed after oral administration. Aspirin products are hydrolyzed to salicylate. There is hepatic metabolism and renal excretion of conjugated metabolites. Urinary pH alters elimination (alkaline urine increases elimination). Wide variation in plasma concentrations exists in individuals receiving the same dose. Half-life varies with dose (2–3 h with low doses, ≥20 h with high therapeutic doses). At high doses the elimination pathway is saturated, and a small increase in dose can lead to a large increase in serum concentration.

Cost: $

ASPIRIN 1 OPIOIDS (CODEINE/HYDRO-CODONE/OXYCODONE/PROPOXYPHENE)

Trade Names:

Aspirin + codeine: *Empirin with Codeine*

Aspirin + hydrocodone: *Azdone, Lortab ASA*

Aspirin + oxycodone: *Percodan, Roxiprin*

Aspirin + propoxyphene: *Darvon with A.S.A.*

Aspirin + pentazocine: *Talwin compound*

Drug Class: Analgesic/antiinflammatory with opioid analgesic

Preparations: Tablets

Aspirin + codeine: Aspirin with codeine #2, 325 mg aspirin/15 mg codeine;

Aspirin codeine #3, 325 mg/30 mg; Aspirin with codeine #4, 325 mg/60 mg

Aspirin + hydrocodone: 5 mg hydrocodone/500 mg aspirin

Aspirin + oxycodone: Aspirin 325 mg/oxycodone 4.5 mg (*Percodan*)

Aspirin + propoxyphene: 65 mg propoxyphene/325 mg of aspirin

Aspirin + pentazocine: 12.5 mg pentazocine/325 mg of aspirin

Dose

Aspirin + codeine: Adult dose, 1–2 tablets q 4 h PRN

Aspirin + hydrocodone: Adult dose, 1–2 tablets q 4–6 h PRN

Aspirin + oxycodone: Adult dose, 1 tablet q 4–6 h PRN

Aspirin + propoxyphene: Adult dose, 1 tablet q 4–6 h PRN

Aspirin + pentazocine: Adult dose, 2 caplets q 6–8 h PRN

Indications: Pain is unresponsive to nonopioid regimens. Most studies show little benefit over nonopioid regimens in chronic musculoskeletal pain.

Mechanism of Action: Aspirin inhibits prostaglandin synthesis. Opioids bind to opioid receptors in CNS and modify pain perception.

Contraindications: Hypersensitivity reactions to opioids or aspirin; opioid or prescription drug abuse

Precautions

Aspirin: Fluid retention may aggravate heart failure and hypertension. Consider misoprostol prophylaxis in patients at high risk of GI bleeding (prior GI bleeding, elderly, concurrent corticosteroid treatment). Administer with food. Use with caution in asthma, bleeding disorders, and hepatic or renal disease.

Opioids: Risk of psychologic and physical narcotic dependence should limit use. Avoid dose escalation. Limit dose and duration of therapy if possible. One physician should prescribe all opioids for a particular patient.

Pregnancy risk: C

Adverse Effects: (see Aspirin above). Opioid toxicity: (common) GI intolerance, constipation, dependence with chronic use; (less common) allergy, confusion, dizziness, nervousness, and insomnia

Drug Interactions: (see Aspirin above); effects of CNS depressants may be potentiated by opioids.

Patient Instructions: Do not exceed prescribed dose. Do not drink alcohol. May cause drowsiness or constipation. Contains a narcotic and is addictive. Only use for pain.

Clinical Pharmacology: See individual drugs

Cost: $$

AURANOFIN (ALSO SEE APPENDIX B, p. 509)

Trade Names: *Ridaura*

Synonyms: Oral gold

Drug Class: DMARD

Preparations: 3-mg capsules

Dose: (Adults) 6 mg PO daily as single or divided dose. If no response after 3 months, it can be increased to 9 mg/day (in 3 divided doses). If no response after a further 3 months, discontinue and consider an alternative DMARD.

Indications: Active RA, psoriatic arthritis, and other inflammatory arthritides

Mechanism of Action: Unknown; has several immunomodulatory effects, primarily affecting macrophages, including inhibition of phagocytosis

Contraindications: Hypersensitivity to gold; prior blood dyscrasias; severe renal impairment

Precautions: May exacerbate or cause exfoliative dermatitis. Use caution in hepatic or renal impairment.

Monitoring: CBC (WBC with differential, hemoglobin, and platelet count) and urinalysis before, 1–2 weeks after starting treatment, and then monthly. In patients who have tolerated auranofin well for 12 months or longer, the frequency of monitoring can often safely be decreased to every 2–3 months.

Discontinue use if significant rash, proteinuria, or decrease in blood elements develops.

Pregnancy Risk: C

Adverse Effects

Common: Diarrhea, rash, itching, mouth ulcers, proteinuria, conjunctivitis

Less common: Leukopenia, thrombocytopenia, agranulocytosis, aplastic anemia, hepatotoxicity, peripheral neuropathy, angioedema

Drug Interactions: Toxicity of other DMARDs (penicillamine, antimalarials, cytotoxic agents, immunosuppressants) may be increased if used in combination therapy.

Patient Instructions: Avoid sunlight as photosensitivity may occur. Regular monitoring of urine and blood count is required. Discontinue if rash develops. May take as long as 3 months for benefits to appear.

Comments: Onset of antirheumatic action is slow, over several months. Auranofin is most commonly used for patients with early and mild disease. Combination of auranofin with methotrexate did not increase efficacy but did increase side effects.

Clinical Pharmacology: Oral absorption is 25%. Renal excretion is the major route of elimination. Plasma half-life is 26 days.

Cost: $$$

REFERENCE

Williams HJ, Ward JR, Reading JC, et al. Comparison of Auranofin, methotrexate, and the combination of both in the treatment of rheumatoid arthritis. Arthritis Rheum 1992;35:259–269.

AZATHIOPRINE (ALSO SEE APPENDIX B, p. 509)

Trade Names: *Imuran*

Drug Class: Immunosuppressive, purine antagonist, DMARD

Preparations

Tablets: 50 mg, scored

Injection: 100 mg, reconstituted for IV use with 10 mL sterile water

Dose: Adult, 1–2.5 mg/kg/day (given once or twice daily)

Indications: Refractory RA; systemic lupus erythematosus; dermatomyositis/polymyositis; used as a "steroid-sparing" agent in a wide range of autoimmune disorders when the disease requires prolonged high doses of corticosteroids

Mechanism of Action: The active metabolite is 6-mercaptopurine, which is a purine analogue that interferes with purine synthesis and thus with DNA synthesis.

Contraindications: Hypersensitivity, concomitant allopurinol, lactation, or pregnancy

Precautions: Use caution in hepatic or renal impairment. If creatinine clearance is 10–50 mL/min, use 75% of usual dose; if below 10 mL/min, use 50% or less of usual dose. Azathioprine (AZA) is carcinogenic in animals and increases risk of malignancy, primarily lymphoma and leukemia, in humans.

Monitoring: CBC and platelet count every 1–2 weeks for the first 2 months or after a dose increase, then monthly on stable dose. Do LFTs every 1–3 months.

Pregnancy Risk: D

Adverse Effects

Common: Fever, chills, GI symptoms (vomiting, diarrhea, nausea), dose-related effects on bone marrow (thrombocytopenia, leukopenia)

Less common: Herpes zoster, hepatotoxicity, pancreatitis, pneumonitis, hypersensitivity, stomatitis, rash, secondary infection, increased risk of lymphoma/leukemia, hepatic venoocclusive disease

Drug Interactions

Allopurinol: Increased accumulation of 6-mercaptopurine and thus toxicity. Avoid concurrent treatment if possible; if necessary, reduce dose of AZA to 25% (or less) of usual dose and monitor frequently.

Immunosuppressants: Concurrent use with other immunosuppressants increases the risk of infection and long-term risk of malignancy.

Live vaccines: Replication of the attenuated virus may occur because of immunosuppression.

Patient Instructions: Use contraception to avoid pregnancy. Do not exceed prescribed dose. Regular monitoring of blood count is essential. Report to physician if persistent sore throat, unusual bleeding, bruises, or fatigue develops.

Comments: Rather than starting with a high maintenance dose, it is advisable to start at a low dose, usually 25–50 mg/day and increase by 25-mg increments at 1–2 week intervals. Onset of action is delayed, so reduce dose at first sign of a large or persistent ($<3,000/mm^3$) decrease in WBC or platelets ($<100,000/mm^3$). A genetic deficiency of the enzyme thiopurine methyltransferase occurs in 1/300 persons. This deficiency is associated with severe myelosuppression because of impaired metabolism of AZA. Testing for the enzyme deficiency is not generally available; thus starting at a low dose and monitoring response carefully is safest in all patients.

GI tolerability may improve with split (twice daily) dosing.

Response in RA may not occur for several months. AZA is not more effective than other DMARDs, but adverse effects are more common. Combination studies in RA show that methotrexate (MTX) plus AZA is more effective than AZA alone, but the MTX + AZA combination is not more effective than MTX alone and may have added toxicity. Uncontrolled studies suggest possible efficacy of MTX + AZA + antimalarial combination therapy. Combination therapy should not be undertaken routinely.

Clinical Pharmacology: AZA is well absorbed orally and largely biotransformed to 6-mercaptopurine and 6-thioinosinic acid; further metabolized by xanthine oxidase; renally excreted as metabolites. Half-life is 5 h (drug and active metabolites), but biologic effect and immunosuppressive action is prolonged.

Cost: $$$

REFERENCES

Kerstens PJ, Stolk JN, De Abreu RA, et al. Azathioprine-related bone marrow toxicity and low activities of purine enzymes in patients with rheumatoid arthritis. Arthritis Rheum 1995;38:142–145.

McCarty DJ, Harman JG, Grassanovich JL, et al. Combination drug therapy of seropositive rheumatoid arthritis. J Rheumatol 1995;22:1636–1645.

Willkens RF, Urowitz MB, Stablein DM, et al. Comparison of azathioprine, methotrexate, and the combination of both in the treatment of rheumatoid arthritis. Arthritis Rheum 1992;35:849–856.

Azulfidine (see *Sulfasalazine*)

Benemid (see *Probenecid*)

Bupropion (*Wellbutrin*; see *Appendix D*, p. 513)

Butazolidin (see *Phenylbutazone*)

Calcimar (see *Calcitonin*)

CALCITONIN

Trade Names

Injectable: *Calcimar* (salmon), *Cibacalcin* (human)

Nasal spray: *Miacalcin* (salmon)

Synonyms: Salmon calcitonin, human calcitonin

Drug Class: Hormone

Preparations

Salmon calcitonin: Injection 200 units/mL (2 mL), 100 units/mL (1 mL)

nasal spray 2 mL bottle, 200 IU/spray

Human calcitonin: Injection 0.5 mg/vial

Dose: Salmon calcitonin injection: Skin test 0.1 mL of a 10 IU/mL solution injected intradermally and observe for 15 min; appearance of more than mild erythema or a weal is a positive response, and the drug should not be used. Osteoporosis and Paget's disease use 50–100 IU qd or qod SC or IM. Hypercalcemia use 4 IU/kg every 12 h IM or SC (increase dose if necessary up to 8 IU/kg q 12 h). Salmon calcitonin nasal: One spray (200 IU) daily, use alternate nostrils. Human calcitonin: Paget's disease 0.5 mg/day SC initially. Dose required varies from 0.25–0.5 mg 2–3 times a week to 0.25–0.5 mg twice daily.

Indications

Injectable calcitonin: Treatment and prevention of osteoporosis, treatment of Paget's disease, and adjunctive treatment for hypercalcemia.

Nasal calcitonin: Osteoporosis

Mechanism of Action: Calcitonin inhibits osteoclastic bone resorption and promotes renal excretion of calcium.

Contraindications: Hypersensitivity to salmon protein

Precautions: Skin test prior to administering salmon calcitonin injection. Have epinephrine available to treat anaphylaxis. Skin testing should be considered prior to nasal calcitonin for patients with suspected sensitivity, but allergic reactions are less frequent than with the injectable form.

Monitoring: Serum electrolytes (especially calcium), alkaline phosphatase or 24-h urinary hydroxyproline concentrations or other bone turnover markers at 3- to 6-month intervals are useful for measuring response in Paget's disease. Repeated measurement of bone density at 1- to 2-year intervals may be useful as a guide to treatment of osteoporosis.

Pregnancy Risk: C

Adverse Effects

Common: Flushing, headache, nausea, diarrhea, injection site reaction

Less common: Chills, tingling, rash, hypersensitivity. Nasal calcitonin seldom causes the above systemic side effects, but rhinitis and nasal irritation are common.

Drug Interactions: None of significance

Patient Instructions: Teach patient injection technique. For nasal spray use alternate nostrils. Discontinue if nasal ulceration or bleeding occurs.

Comments: Antibody formation occurs more commonly to salmon calcitonin and 5 to 10% of patients may become resistant to treatment after long-term use. A decrease in both vertebral and hip fracture rate is not established with calcitonin. Thus, the decreased fracture rates shown with estrogens or alendronate make these, rather than calcitonin, the preferred drugs for osteoporosis. Adequate calcium (1000–1500 mg elemental calcium/day) and vitamin D (400 IU/day) intake is recommended when using calcitonin.

Clinical Pharmacology: Short half-life (1–2 h), rapid metabolism by kidneys. Absorption of nasal spray is poor (10–25%).

Cost: $$$$ ($200–300/month)

REFERENCES

Delmas PD, Meunier PJ. The management of Paget's disease of bone. N Engl J Med 1997;336:558–566.

Overgaard K, Hansen MA, Jensen SB, Christiansen C. Effect of salcalcitonin given intranasally on bone mass and fracture rate in established osteoporosis: a dose response study. Br Med J 1992;305:556–561.

Reginster JY. Calcitonin for prevention and treatment of osteoporosis. Am J Med 1993;95(5A):44S–47S.

Calcitriol (see *Vitamin D*)

CALCIUM SALTS

Trade Names

Calcium carbonate: *Alka-Mints, Calci-Chew, Caltrate, Os-Cal, Oyst-Cal 500, Rolaids Calcium Rich, Titralac, Tums, Tums E-X*

Calcium citrate: *Citracal*

Calcium glubionate: *Neo-Calglucon*

Calcium lactate: Generic

Calcium phosphate dibasic: Generic

Calcium phosphate tribasic: *Posture*

Drug Class: Calcium supplement

Preparations

Calcium carbonate: Tablets 500 mg, 650 mg, 667 mg, 1.25 g, 1.5 g; Tablets chewable 420 mg, 500 mg, 750 mg

Calcium citrate: Tablets 950 mg; effervescent tablets 2376 mg

Calcium glubionate: Syrup 1.8 g/5 mL

Calcium lactate: Tablets 325 mg, 650 mg

Calcium phosphate dibasic: Tablets 500 mg

Calcium phosphate tribasic: Tablets 300 mg, 600 mg

Dose: Prevention and treatment of osteoporosis in adults requires at least 1–1.5 g of elemental calcium/day, various salts contain

Calcium carbonate: 400 mg elemental calcium/g

Calcium citrate: 220 mg elemental calcium/g

Calcium glubionate: 64 mg elemental calcium/g

Calcium lactate: 130 mg elemental calcium/g

Calcium phosphate dibasic: 115 mg elemental calcium/g

Calcium phosphate tribasic: 400 mg elemental calcium/g

Indications: Prevention of osteoporosis, hypocalcemia

Mechanism of Action: Calcium supplement to prevent osteoporosis in patients with inadequate intake. Calcium in bone is in exchange with calcium in plasma, so bone stores are depleted if intake is inadequate.

Contraindications: Renal calculi, hypercalcemia, digoxin toxicity, or renal failure

Precautions: Use care in patients with arrhythmias.

Monitoring: Serum calcium before treatment and annually

Calcium Tablets and Costs

Drug	Elemental Calcium per Tablet (mg)	Tablets per Day[a]	Cost[b]
Calcium carbonate—average generic price	600	2	$2.12
Caltrate 600 (Lederle)	600	2	$6.03
Os-Cal 500 (SK Beecham)	500	2	$7.11
Tums 500 (SK Beecham)	500	2	$3.97
Calcium citrate—average generic price	200	5	$7.04
Citracal (Mission)			$10.31
Calcium gluconate—average generic price	60	17	$13.77
Calcium lactate—average generic price	84	12	$11.30
Calcium phosphate	600	2	$7.97
Posture-D (Whitehall)			

Reproduced with permission from the Medical Letter 1996;38:109.

[a] Needed to provide 1000–1200 mg elemental calcium daily.

[b] Cost to the pharmacist for a 30-day supply, according to wholesale price (AWP) listings in Drug Topics Red Book 1996 and November Update.

Pregnancy Risk: C, but problems are unlikely; used in pregnancy to supplement calcium intake

Adverse Effects

Common: Constipation, flatulence

Uncommon: Nausea, hypercalcemia, renal stones

Drug Interactions

Calcium channel antagonists: Doses of calcium that increase serum calcium concentrations may antagonize the effects of calcium channel antagonists.

Digoxin: Doses of calcium that increase serum calcium concentrations may increase risk of cardiac arrhythmias.

Iron supplements: Oral absorption is decreased if taken together.

Tetracyclines: Oral absorption is decreased if taken together.

Patient Instructions: Best taken with a large glass of water before or during a meal. Do not take calcium within 1–2 h of taking another medication (may impair absorption).

Comments: Most studies show that calcium and vitamin D do not increase bone density. In subjects with inadequate calcium intake, they may slow bone loss. Calcium and vitamin D supplements are therefore only part of the treatment of established osteoporosis (see p. 284).

Clinical Pharmacology: Poor absorption; 20% is eliminated renally and 80% appears in the stool. Vitamin D is required for absorption.

Cost: $ (see Table)

REFERENCES

Anonymous. Calcium supplements. Med Lett 1996;38:108–109.
Patel S. Current and potential future treatments for osteoporosis. Ann Rheum Dis 1996;55: 700–714.

Caltrate (see *Calcium*)

CAPSAICIN

Trade Names: *Zostrix, Capsin, Theragen, Trixaicin, Capsagel, Dolorac*

Drug Class: Topical analgesic

Preparations

Cream: 0.025% (45-g, 90-g tube); 0.075% (30-g, 60-g tube); 0.25% (30 g, 60 g)

Gel: 0.025% (15 g, 30 g)

Lotion: 0.025% (59 mL), 0.075% (59 mL)

Roll-on: 0.075% (60 mL)

Dose: Apply to affected area 3–4 times daily. Less frequent application is less effective.

Indications: Postherpetic neuralgia, RA, osteoarthritis, diabetic neuropathy, chronic neuralgic pain

Mechanism of Action: Depletes peripheral sensory neurons of substance P, a mediator of pain

Contraindications: Hypersensitivity to capsaicin

Precautions: Avoid contact with eyes, mucous membranes, genitalia, or open wounds. Wash hands immediately after applying.

Pregnancy Risk: C

Adverse Effects

Common: Transient sensation of burning when first applied diminishes with use.

Less common: Erythema

Drug Interactions: None

Patient Instructions: For external use only. Do not apply to broken skin. Wash hands after use or use gloves. Avoid contact with eyes. Regular use is required for effect. Effect is slow—clinical benefits may take weeks or months. Transient sensation of burning when first applied.

Comments: The transient burning that occurs in most patients initially has made it difficult to perform true double-blind studies to assess efficacy. In practice, few patients derive clinically useful benefit from capsaicin in the treatment of pain due to arthritis. Most suitable are patients with a few affected joints. The requirement for regular and frequent application and the slow onset of action over several weeks are disadvantages.

Clinical Pharmacology: Not known

Cost: $

REFERENCE

Zhang WY, Po ALW. The effectiveness of topically applied capsaicin. A meta-analysis. Eur J Clin Pharmacol 1994;46:517–522.

CARISOPRODOL

Trade Names: *Rela, Soma, Soprodol, Sodol, Soridol, Vanadol, Soma Compound*

Drug Class: Skeletal muscle relaxant

Preparations

Tablet: 350 mg

Compound tablet: Carisoprodol 200 mg and aspirin 325 mg

Dose: (Adults) 350 mg 2–4 times/day or 350 mg at night

Indications: Treatment of painful muscle spasm; useful in some patients with fibromyalgia

Mechanism of Action: Unknown; has a sedative effect and may modify pain perception

Contraindications: Hypersensitivity to carisoprodol; acute intermittent porphyria

Precautions: Use caution in renal or hepatic dysfunction.

Pregnancy Risk: C

Adverse Effects

Common: Drowsiness

Uncommon: Allergy, anaphylaxis, psychologic dependence and drug abuse, flushing, rash, nausea, fever, paradoxical stimulation, tremor, hematologic abnormalities

Drug Interactions

CNS depressants: Increased CNS depression

Increased toxicity: Alcohol, CNS depressants, phenothiazines, clindamycin, MAO inhibitors

Patient Instructions: Avoid alcohol. May cause drowsiness.

Comments: Nighttime sedative effect is sometimes useful in improving sleep and pain control in fibromyalgia.

Clinical Pharmacology: Rapid oral absorption, hepatic metabolism, renal excretion

Cost: $$

CHLORAMBUCIL

Trade Names: *Leukeran*

Drug Class: Alkylating agent

Preparations: 2-mg tablet

Dose: 0.05–0.2 mg/kg/day; usual dose range 4–8 mg/day, with dose adjusted according to WBC count

Indications: Immunosuppressant, usually as an alternative in patients who cannot tolerate cyclophosphamide

Mechanism of Action: Alkylation and cross-linking of DNA strands interfering with DNA replication

Contraindications: Hypersensitivity, bone marrow suppression

Precautions: Teratogenic, can cause severe immunosuppression, carcinogenic; caution in renal impairment

Monitoring: CBC, platelet count, serum uric acid, and LFTs 1–2 weeks after initiation, then every 4 weeks

Pregnancy Risk: D

Adverse Effects

Common: Myelosuppression, rash, GI intolerance, oral ulceration

Less common: Confusion, seizures, sterility, pulmonary fibrosis, liver necrosis, drug fever, secondary malignancy

Drug Interactions

Immunosuppressants: Concurrent use of chlorambucil increases risk of myelosuppression and infection.

Patient Instructions: Avoid live virus vaccines. Avoid pregnancy. Regular monitoring is required.

Comments: When possible, azathioprine and methotrexate are used in preference to alkylating agents because the risk of secondary neoplasms is lower.

Clinical Pharmacology: Well absorbed; food decreases absorption 20%. Half-life is 2 h; hepatic metabolism and renal excretion of metabolites

Cost: $$$

REFERENCE

Steinberg AD. Chlorambucil in the treatment of patients with immune-mediated rheumatic diseases. Arthritis Rheum 1993;36:325–328.

Chloroquine (see *Hydroxychloroquine*)

CHLORZOXAZONE

Trade Names: *Blanex, Flexaphen, Lobac, Paraflex, Parafon Forte, Skelex*

Drug Class: Skeletal muscle relaxant, centrally acting

Preparations: 500-mg caplet; 250-mg tablet

Dose: Usual dose, 250–500 mg 3–4 times a day; up to 750 mg 3–4 times/day

Indications: Relief of muscle spasm. Questionable efficacy and potentially serious adverse effects limit indications.

Mechanism of Action: Acts via spinal cord and subcortical regions to decrease muscle tone

Contraindications: Hypersensitivity to chlorzoxazone, impaired liver function

Monitoring: LFTs periodically with chronic use

Pregnancy Risk: C

Adverse Effects

Common: Drowsiness, lightheadedness, allergy, rash, nausea, cramps

Less common: Hematologic toxicity (aplastic anemia, leukopenia), unpredictable fatal hepatotoxicity

Drug Interactions: CNS depressants have increased effect.

Patient Instructions: May cause drowsiness. Avoid alcohol.

Clinical Pharmacology: Rapid absorption; hepatic metabolism and renal excretion of metabolites

Cost: $$

REFERENCE

Anonymous. Chlorzoxazone hepatotoxicity. Med Lett 1996;38:46.

CHOLINE MAGNESIUM TRISALICYLATE (ALSO SEE APPENDIX A, p. 507)

Trade Names: *Trilisate, Tricosal*

Drug Class: Nonacetylated salicylate, NSAID

Preparations

Liquid: 500 mg/5 mL

Tablets: 500 mg, 750 mg, 1000 mg

Dose: (Adult) 500 mg to 1.5 g, 2 or 3 times a day; usual maintenance dose 1–4.5 g/day

Indications: RA, osteoarthritis

Mechanism of Action: Weak inhibitor of prostaglandin synthesis

Contraindications: Hypersensitivity to salicylates

Precautions: Administer with food. Caution in asthma, bleeding disorders, and hepatic or renal disease.

Monitoring: Monitor hematocrit, creatinine, LFTs periodically (1 month after starting and then every 3–6 months). Periodically check serum magnesium with high-dose therapy or in the presence of impaired renal function.

Pregnancy Risk: C

Adverse Effects

Common: GI irritation (dyspepsia, reflux, epigastric pain)

Less common: GI ulceration or hemorrhage; minor elevations of liver enzymes; hypersensitivity (asthma, urticaria, angioedema—particularly in patients with nasal polyps). Cross-sensitivity occurs between NSAIDs, but hypersensitivity is less common with the nonacetylated salicylates. Dose-related side effects include tinnitus and deafness.

Drug Interactions

Antacids: Decreased salicylate levels because of increased elimination in alkaline urine

Anticoagulants: Activity of warfarin is increased

Patient Instructions: Take with food. Discontinue and seek medical advice if unusual bleeding occurs.

Comments: Magnesium may accumulate in patients with renal impairment. Serum salicylate concentrations of 150–300 μg/mL are antiinflammatory. Nonacetylated salicylates have little effect on platelet function and cause less GI toxicity than classical NSAIDs, which are more potent inhibitors of prostaglandin synthesis.

Clinical Pharmacology: Rapidly and well absorbed after oral administration; hepatic metabolism and renal excretion of conjugated metabolites. Urinary pH alters elimination (alkaline urine increases elimination). Wide variation in plasma concentrations occur in individuals receiving the same dose. Half-life varies with dose (2–3 h with low doses; 20 h or longer with high doses). At high doses, the salicylate elimination pathway is saturated, and a small increase in dose can lead to a large increase in serum concentrations.

Cost: $

REFERENCE

Anonymous. Drugs for rheumatoid arthritis. Med Lett 1991;33:65–70.

CHOLINE SALICYLATE

Trade Names: *Arthropan*

Drug Class: Nonacetylated salicylate, NSAID

Preparations: Liquid, 870 mg/5 mL

Dose: (Adult) 5–10 mL up to 4 times a day (870–1740 mg up to 4 times a day)

Indications: RA, osteoarthritis in patients who cannot swallow tablets

Mechanism of Action: Weak inhibitor of prostaglandin synthesis

Contraindications: Hypersensitivity to salicylates

Precautions: Administer with food. Caution in asthma, bleeding disorders, and hepatic or renal disease.

Monitoring: Monitor hematocrit, creatinine, liver enzymes periodically (1 month after starting and then every 12 months).

Pregnancy Risk: C

Adverse Effects

Common: GI irritation (dyspepsia, reflux, epigastric pain)

Less common: GI ulceration or hemorrhage; minor elevations of liver enzymes; hypersensitivity (asthma, urticaria, angioedema—particularly in patients with nasal polyps). Cross-sensitivity occurs between NSAIDs, but hypersensitivity is less common with the nonacetylated salicylates. Dose-related side effects include tinnitus and deafness.

Drug Interactions

Antacids: Salicylate levels are decreased through increased elimination in alkaline urine

Anticoagulants: Activity of warfarin is increased

Patient Instructions: Take with food. Discontinue and seek medical advice if unusual bleeding occurs.

Comments: Serum salicylate concentrations of 150–300 μg/mL are antiinflammatory. Nonacetylated salicylates have little effect on platelet function and cause less GI toxicity than classical NSAIDs, which are more potent inhibitors of prostaglandin synthesis.

Clinical Pharmacology: Rapidly and well absorbed after oral administration; hepatic metabolism and renal excretion of conjugated metabolites. Urinary pH alters elimination (alkaline urine increases elimination). Wide variation in plasma concentrations occur in individuals receiving the same dose. Half-life varies with dose (2–3 h with low doses; 20 h or longer with high doses). At high doses, the salicylate elimination pathway is saturated, and a small increase in dose can lead to a large increase in serum concentrations.

Cost: $

Cimetidine (*Tagamet*; see *Appendix C*)

CISAPRIDE

Trade Names: *Propulsid*

Drug Class: Gastric motility stimulant

Preparations

Tablet: 10 mg, 20 mg

Suspension: 1 mg/mL

Dose: 10 mg 15 min before meals and before bedtime; some patients may require up to 20 mg per dose.

Indications: Gastroparesis, gastroesophageal reflux disease, bowel hypomotility in scleroderma

Mechanism of Action: Local release of acetylcholine

Contraindications: Hypersensitivity to cisapride; mechanical bowel obstruction; concomitant therapy with drugs that inhibit CYP P450 (ketoconazole, fluconazole, itraconazole, miconazole, erythromycin, clarithromycin, trolandeomycin)

Precautions: Use caution if QT interval is prolonged (hypokalemia, hypomagnesemia, medications such as quinidine).

Pregnancy Risk: C

Adverse Effects

Common: Rash, abdominal cramps, diarrhea, flatulence

Less common: Ventricular arrhythmias (torsade des pointes) described in overdose and with concomitant use of drugs that inhibit metabolism (see contraindications listed above).

Drug Interactions: Concomitant therapy with drugs that inhibit CYP P450 3A (ketoconazole, fluconazole, itraconazole, miconazole, erythromycin, clarithromycin, trolandeomycin, warfarin, diazepam, cimetidine, ranitidine) increases concentrations of cisapride and have been associated with fatal arrhythmias.

Patient Instructions: Do not exceed dose.

Comments: The potentially fatal arrhythmias that may result from the interaction between cisapride and cytochrome P450 3A inhibitors require consideration when prescribing cisapride.

Clinical Pharmacology: Bioavailability 40%; metabolized to norcisapride and eliminated in urine; half-life 6–12 h

Cost: $$$$

REFERENCES

Klinkenberg-Knol EC, Festen HP, Meuwissen SE. Pharmacological management of gastro-esophageal reflux disease. Drugs 1995;49:695–710.
Sjogren RW. Gastrointestinal motility disorders in scleroderma. Arthritis Rheum 1994;37: 1265–1282.

Clinoril (see *Sulindac*)

CODEINE (ALSO SEE ACETAMINOPHEN + OPIOIDS)

Synonyms: Codeine sulfate, codeine phosphate

Drug Class: Narcotic analgesic

Preparations
Tablet: 15 mg, 30 mg, 60 mg
Oral solution: 15 mg/5 mL

Dose: 15–30 mg every 4–6 h (maximum dose should not exceed 360 mg/24 h)

Indications: Pain not controlled by nonopioid drugs

Mechanism of Action: Binds to opioid receptors in CNS

Contraindications: Hypersensitivity to codeine; substance abuse

Precautions: Use caution in patients with hypersensitivity to other opioids, respiratory disease, or renal or hepatic impairment. Decrease dose if hepatic or renal impairment.

Monitoring: Make sure drug is used to control pain.

Pregnancy Risk: C; D in high doses

Adverse Effects

Common: Drowsiness, constipation, dysphoria, nausea

Less common: Rash, CNS stimulation, insomnia, seizures

Drug Interactions: Increased toxicity occurs with other CNS depressants. Avoid with MAOIs.

Patient Instructions: Drug is metabolized to morphine and is addictive. Use only to control pain. Do not use with alcohol or other CNS depressants.

Comments: Patients with low CYP P450 2D6 activity have a genetic inability to form morphine from codeine and derive no therapeutic effect from the drug. Codeine is commonly administered as an acetaminophen/codeine combination (see Acetaminophen + Opioid).

Clinical Pharmacology: Oral absorption; hepatic metabolism to morphine; urinary elimination as metabolites

Cost: $$

REFERENCE

Cherny NI. Opioid analgesics. Comparative features and prescribing guidelines. Drugs 1996;51:713–737.

COLCHICINE

Drug Class: Antigout agent

Preparations

> Tablet: 0.5 mg, 0.6 mg
>
> Injection: 0.5 mg/mL

Dose

> Acute gout
>
> Oral: 0.5 or 0.6 mg every 1–2 h until pain is relieved, nausea/diarrhea develops, or maximum of 8 mg is administered
>
> IV: Initially, 1 or 2 mg slowly; then 0.5 mg at 6-h intervals until total of 2–4 mg is given; no further colchicine (any route) for 7 days (see comment)
>
> Prophylaxis of gout: 0.5 or 0.6 mg once or twice daily

Indications: Treatment of acute gout and prophylaxis of acute gout; also used in the treatment of familial Mediterranean fever and amyloidosis

Mechanism of Action: Decreases leukocyte migration and phagocytosis

Contraindications: Hypersensitivity to colchicine; serious renal or hepatic impairment

Precautions: Use caution in renal or hepatic impairment; dose reduction is required.

Pregnancy Risk: C

Adverse Effects

Common: Nausea, vomiting, GI cramps, diarrhea

Less common: Neuropathy, myopathy, rash, bone marrow suppression, hepatic damage, alopecia

Drug Interactions

> Cyclosporine: Increased risk of nephrotoxicity and myopathy
>
> Cimetidine, erythromycin, tolbutamide: Increased colchicine concentrations

Patient Instructions: Discontinue if nausea or vomiting occur.

Comments: In treatment of acute gout, colchicine is more effective if used early in the attack. *Intravenous use of colchicine has been associated with fatalities and should be avoided.* Depot corticosteroids (intramuscular or intraarticular) are safer and more effective than intravenous colchicine in patients in whom NSAIDs are contraindicated.

Clinical Pharmacology: Time to onset of action in gout is slow (6–12 h); peak effect 24–48 h following first oral dose; hepatic biotransformation and renal and hepatic elimination; high degree of tissue uptake, with only 10% of dose eliminated from the body in 24 h

Cost: $

REFERENCES

Emmerson BT. The management of gout. N Engl J Med 1996;334:445–451.
Moreland L, Ball GV. Colchicine and gout. Arthritis Rheum 1991;34:782–785.

CORTICOSTEROIDS

Trade Names

Oral

Prednisone: *Deltasone, Orasone*

Prednisolone: *Delta-Cortef*

Methylprednisolone: *Medrol*

Dexamethasone: *Decadron, Dexone*

Parenteral

Methylprednisolone sodium succinate: *Solu-Medrol*

Hydrocortisone: *Solu-Cortef*

Dexamethasone: *Decadron*

Intraarticular

Prednisolone terbutate suspension: *Hyldeltra T.B.A.*

Methylprednisolone acetate suspension: *DepoMedrol*

Triamcinolone acetonide suspension: *Kenalog*

Triamcinolone diacetate suspension: *Aristocort Forte*

Triamcinolone hexacetonide suspension: *Aristospan Intra-articular*

Drug Class: Glucocorticoid

Preparations

Oral

Prednisone: 1-mg, 2.5-mg, 5-mg, 10-mg, 20-mg, 50-mg tablet

Prednisolone: 2-mg, 4-mg, 8-mg, 16-mg, 24-mg tablet

Dexamethasone: 0.25-mg, 0.5-mg, 0.75-mg, 1-mg, 1.5-mg, 2-mg, 4-mg, 6-mg

Parenteral

Methylprednisolone sodium succinate injection: 40 mg, 125 mg, 500 mg, 1000 mg, 2000 mg

Hydrocortisone injection: 50 mg, 100 mg, 250 mg, 500 mg

Dexamethasone: 0.25 mg, 0.5 mg, 0.75 mg, 1 mg, 1.5 mg, 2 mg, 4 mg, 6 mg

Intraarticular

Methylprednisolone acetate suspension: 20 mg/mL, 40 mg/mL, 80 mg/mL

Prednisolone tebutate suspension: 20 mg/mL

Triamcinolone acetonide suspension: 10 mg/mL, 40 mg/mL

Triamcinolone diacetate suspension: 40 mg/mL

Triamcinolone hexacetonide suspension: 20 mg/mL

Dose: Varies according to the indication. For serious inflammatory disease, give 1 mg/kg/day of prednisone or equivalent initially and titrate down according to response. (Adult dose ranges from 5–80 mg/day in divided doses.)

Approximate equivalent doses for glucocorticoid efficacy: 0.75 mg dexamethasone = 4 mg methylprednisolone = 5 mg prednisone or prednisolone = 20 mg hydrocortisone. Intraarticular doses of depot steroid depend on the size of the joint (see p. 67).

Indications: Antiinflammatory or immunosuppressant therapy in a wide range of diseases including inflammatory arthritis, inflammatory muscle disease, vasculitis, SLE, and RA.

Mechanism of Action: A wide range of effects on numbers of inflammatory cells, their migration, and production of inflammatory mediators

Contraindications: Known hypersensitivity to a glucocorticoid preparation

Precautions: Use caution in diabetes, atherosclerosis, immunosuppression, hypertension, osteoporosis, infection, peptic ulcer, and cirrhosis.

Because of dose-related adverse effects, the minimum effective dose should be used. Following prolonged glucocorticoid therapy, acute adrenal insufficiency may occur if the glucocorticoid is discontinued abruptly. After discontinuation of glucocorticoid therapy, the hypothalamo-pituitary-adrenal axis may remain suppressed for up to a year, so supplementary doses of glucocorticoid are required during acute stress such as surgery.

Monitoring: Monitor for adverse effects with chronic therapy: potassium and glucose concentrations and bone density measurement (with chronic use).

Pregnancy Risk: C

Adverse Effects: Most are dose related. Almost all patients on high doses for more than a few weeks experience adverse effects, including cushingoid appearance, weight gain, skin fragility, bruising, edema, hypertension, diabetes, hypokalemia, atherosclerosis, cataracts, infection, insomnia, mood swings, psychosis, GI ulceration with NSAIDs, myopathy, osteoporosis, and fractures. Suppression of the hypothalamo-pituitary-adrenal axis and acute adrenal insufficiency may occur if therapy is discontinued suddenly or with severe physiologic stress (major surgery) after therapy has been discontinued.

Drug Interactions

Hepatic enzyme inducers (rifampin, phenytoin, phenobarbitone): Decreased effect of corticosteroids

Diuretics: Increased potassium depletion

Patient Instructions: Corticosteroids should not be discontinued suddenly. Prior to a procedure or surgery notify your surgeon or doctor that you are receiving corticosteroids. Watch your weight.

Comments: Marked leukocytosis and neutrophilia occur after even a single dose of glucocorticoid, and if the cause is not recognized, an unnecessary infection workup results.

Adverse effects are related to dose and duration of therapy. Once disease control has been established, high doses of steroids may be tapered relatively rapidly with 5–10 mg decrements at doses between 40 and 60 mg. Lower doses require a more gradual taper. Between 20 and 40 mg, taper in 5-mg decrements; between 10 and 20 mg, taper in 2.5-mg decrements, and below 10 mg, taper in 1-mg decrements. A common error is tapering high doses too slowly and low doses too fast, resulting in adverse effects and disease flare, respectively.

Triamcinolone hexacetonide is the least soluble intraarticular preparation and has the longest duration of action. Triamcinolone or other fluorinated corticosteroid preparations should not be used for injection of soft tissue or bursae, as marked atrophy of soft tissue may result. Methylprednisolone/prednisolone preparations can be used for such soft tissue injections.

Clinical Pharmacology: Prednisone is inactive until metabolized to prednisolone. Hepatic conversion is rapid and complete. Plasma half-life of prednisone/prednisolone is 3–4 h, but the biologic effect lasts 18–36 h.

Dexamethasone has almost no mineralocorticoid effect. It is more potent than prednisone/prednisolone but more difficult to titrate clinically.

Depot injections, either intraarticularly or intramuscularly, provide low plasma concentrations of steroid for 2–4 weeks.

Cost: $

REFERENCES

American College of Rheumatology Task Force on Osteoporosis Guidelines. Recommendations for the prevention and treatment of glucocorticoid-induced osteoporosis. Arthritis Rheum 1996;39:1791–1801.

McCarthy GM, McCarty DJ. Intrasynovial corticosteroid therapy. Bull Rheum Dis 1994;43:2–4.

Stein CM, Pincus T. Glucocorticoids. In: Kelley WN, Harris ED, Ruddy S, Sledge CB, eds. Textbook of rheumatology. 5th ed. Philadelphia: WB Saunders, 1997:787–803.

Cuprimine (see *Penicillamine*)

CYCLOBENZAPRINE

Trade Names: *Cycoflex, Flexeril*

Drug Class: Muscle relaxant

Preparations: 10-mg tablet

Dose: 20–40 mg /day in 2 divided doses (maximum dosing should not exceed 60 mg/day)

Indications: Muscle spasm, fibromyalgia

Mechanism of Action: Centrally acting skeletal muscle relaxant; related to tricyclic antidepressants

Contraindications: Hypersensitivity to cyclobenzaprine. Do not use within 14–21 days of an MAO inhibitor (MAOI).

Precautions: As for tricyclics—heart failure, arrhythmias, urinary obstruction

Pregnancy Risk: B

Adverse Effects

Common: Anticholinergic effects (dry mouth, difficulty urinating), drowsiness

Less common: Dizziness, blurred vision, weakness, allergy, GI symptoms, headache, confusion, arrhythmias

Drug Interactions

Tricyclic antidepressants: Additive toxicity

CNS depressants (alcohol, benzodiazepines): Increased effect

MAOIs: Hypertensive crisis

Patient Instructions: Causes drowsiness. May impair ability to drive.

Comments: Sedative effect is useful at night.

Clinical Pharmacology: Rapid complete oral absorption; hepatic metabolism and renal elimination of metabolites

Cost: $$

CYCLOPHOSPHAMIDE (ALSO SEE APPENDIX B)

Trade Names: *Cytoxan, Neosar*

Synonyms: CTX, CYT

Drug Class: Cancer chemotherapeutic; alkylating agent

Preparations

Tablet: 25 mg, 50 mg

Powder for injection: 100 mg, 200 mg, 500 mg, 1 g, 2 g

Dose: Varies according to indication and patient response

Oral dose: 50–100 mg/m^2/day, or 1–3 mg/kg/day

IV infusion: "Pulse" dose of 500–1000 mg/m^2 repeated every 21–28 days

Adjust dose according to clinical response and WBC nadir and recovery. In SLE nephritis, after 6–12 months of monthly infusions, the frequency of infusions may be gradually decreased to every 3 months.

Indications: Vasculitis, rheumatoid vasculitis, systemic lupus erythematosus with organ involvement, polymyositis/dermatomyositis refractory to treatment

Mechanism of Action: Interferes with DNA synthesis by alkylating and cross-linking DNA strands

Contraindications: Hypersensitivity to cyclophosphamide

Precautions: Bone marrow suppression, active infection, decrease dose in renal/hepatic impairment

Monitoring: Frequent monitoring of CBC and platelets is required. Nadir of WBC occurs 10–14 days after a single dose. A WBC nadir of 3000/mm^3 is used as a target.

With chronic use, monitor urinalysis for blood. During and after long-term oral use, monitor for bladder cancer with urinalysis, cytology, and (if needed) cystoscopy.

Pregnancy Risk: D.

Adverse Effects: Dose and duration dependent; myelosuppression (WBC more than platelets), infections (usual bacterial and viral infections and opportunistic organisms). Hemorrhagic cystitis is more common with daily oral regimens. Gonadal suppression and permanent infertility occur. Risk of ovarian failure is greater with oral regimes and increases in frequency with increased age of female patients. GI symptoms increase with dose. Pulmonary fibrosis, rashes, hypersensitivity, and fluid retention occur. Long-term risk of secondary malignancy—bladder, lymphoma, leukemia, and skin cancers exists.

Drug Inteïractions

Allopurinol: Increases myelosuppression of cyclophosphamide

Thiazide diuretics: May cause prolonged leukopenia

Immunosuppressants: Concurrent therapy increases risk of myelosuppression and infection

Digoxin: Cyclophosphamide may decrease serum digoxin levels

Patient Instructions: Take as a single dose in the morning and drink lots of liquids to keep urine dilute. Empty bladder frequently. Report blood in urine. Avoid live virus vaccines. Regular follow-up is essential. Report any significant fever.

Comments: Life-threatening complications may occur with cyclophosphamide treatment. Titrate dose according to WBC. Oral regimens are preferred by many for vasculitis, and the less toxic monthly IV regimen is preferred for SLE. Duration of cyclophosphamide therapy is empirical, but after disease remission, the frequency of infusions can often be decreased to every 3 months. Premedicate with antiemetic regimen and continue antiemetic prophylaxis for 24–48 h.

Mesna (see Mesna) intravenously initially and then orally may be used with IV regimens to protect against hemorrhagic cystitis.

Clinical Pharmacology: Good rapid oral absorption; hepatic metabolism to several active metabolites including 4-hydroxycyclophosphamide. Plasma half-life is 2–10 h. Metabolites are eliminated in the urine. Acrolein is the urinary metabolite thought to cause hemorrhagic cystitis.

Cost: $$$$

REFERENCES

Fraiser LH, Kanekal S, Kehrer JP. Cyclophosphamide toxicity—characterizing and avoiding the problem. Drugs 1991;42:781–795.
Steinberg AD, Gourley M. Cyclophosphamide in lupus nephritis. J Rheumatol 1995;22:1812–1815.

CYCLOSPORINE (ALSO SEE APPENDIX B, p. 509)

Trade Names: *Sandimmune, Neoral*

Synonyms: Cyclosporin, cyclosporin A, CyA, CSA

Drug Class: Immunosuppressant, DMARD

Preparations

>Soft gelatin capsule: 25 mg, 50 mg, 100 mg
>
>Oral liquid: 100 mg/mL
>
>Injection: 50 mg/mL

Dose: Starting dose in autoimmune disease is 2.5 mg/kg/day orally in divided doses. Calculate dose according to approximate ideal body weight in obese patients. After 8–12 weeks the dose may be increased monthly by 0.5 mg/kg/day to maximum of 4 mg/kg/day. The risk of renal disease increases above 4 mg/kg/day. Few patients with RA tolerate doses above 5 mg/kg. Minimum effective dose is between 2–3 mg/kg/day. The dose of the two preparations available (Neoral and Sandimmune) is similar. However, if switching from Sandimmune to Neoral, lower doses of Neoral may be required.

Indications: RA refractory to standard DMARD treatment; also approved for use in psoriasis; anecdotal reports of efficacy in psoriatic arthritis, SLE, myositis, Behçet's syndrome, and pyoderma gangrenosum

Mechanism of Action: Inhibits production of IL-2, immunomodulator

Contraindications: Hypersensitivity to cyclosporine, immunodeficiency, renal failure.

Precautions: Avoid if past or present malignancy, uncontrolled hypertension, or renal or hepatic dysfunction.

Monitoring: Monitor BP and creatinine every 2 weeks for first 2–3 months and then monthly if stable. If creatinine rises by more than 30% above baseline values, reduce dose of cyclosporine by 0.5 mg/kg/day and check again in a week. Continue dose reduction until the creatinine concentration is back within 30% of baseline. Elevations of creatinine level, (>30% of baseline) *even if within the normal range*, require action. Monitor potassium and uric acid levels, and hepatic enzymes every 1–3 months. Monitoring of cyclosporine levels is only necessary if there are concerns with compliance, absorption, or toxicity.

Pregnancy Risk: C

Adverse Effects

Common: Hypertension, increased creatinine, hirsutism, nausea, cramps, tremor, gingival hypertrophy, hyperkalemia, hypomagnesemia, hyperuricemia

Less common: Seizures, headache, muscle cramps, allergy, myositis, pancreatitis, infection, lymphoma

Drug Interactions

Increased concentrations of cyclosporine: Grapefruit juice, azithromycin, clarithromycin, erythromycin, ketoconazole, fluconazole, itraconazole, diltiazem, verapamil, nicardipine

Decreased cyclosporine concentrations: Rifampicin, phenytoin, phenobarbital, carbamazepine, isoniazid

K^+-Sparing diuretics: Hyperkalemia

Lovastatin: Increased risk of myopathy, rhabdomyolysis, acute renal failure

Nephrotoxic drugs: Increased nephrotoxicity

Patient Instructions: Avoid sunlight (skin cancer). Regular blood monitoring is required.

Comments: *Neoral* is a newer microemulsion formulation of cyclosporine that gives a more favorable pharmacokinetic profile with higher peak levels and less inter- and intraindividual variability in levels. Data in transplantation suggest that efficacy and toxicity of Neoral and Sandimmune are similar. There are few data comparing the two formulations in RA.

There is limited long-term safety data for cyclosporine in RA. Cyclosporine as a single agent in RA is no more effective than other available drugs. The combination of methotrexate and cyclosporine is more effective than methotrexate alone, but limited safety data exist for this combination.

The use of NSAIDs is permitted in RA patients taking cyclosporine, and in many studies they have been used together. However, NSAIDs may be stopped if renal function declines while taking cyclosporine. Monitoring blood levels of cyclosporine is a poor predictor of efficacy and toxicity in autoimmune disease and is seldom indicated (e.g., assessing compliance, absorption, drug interaction).

Clinical Pharmacology: Cyclosporine is variably and erratically absorbed. The Neoral formulation has more predictable bioavailability. Hepatic metabolism is by CYP P450 3A enzymes, which is the source of the multiple drug interactions with cyclosporine. Renal excretion of metabolites.

Cost: $$$$

REFERENCES

Panayi G, Tugwell P. The use of cyclosporin A in rheumatoid arthritis: conclusions of an international review. Br J Rheumatol 1994;33:967–969.
Stein CM. Cyclosporine in the treatment of rheumatoid arthritis. Bull Rheum Dis 1995;44:1–4.

Cytotec (see *Misoprostol*)

Cytoxan (see *Cyclophosphamide*)

DANAZOL

Trade Names: *Danocrine*

Drug Class: Attenuated androgen—gonadotropin inhibitor

Preparations: 50-mg, 100-mg, 200-mg capsules

Dose: Hereditary angioedema, 400–600 mg/day in 2 or 3 divided doses

Indications: Hereditary angioedema prophylaxis, fibrocystic breast disease, endometriosis, SLE, or ITP with refractory thrombocytopenia

Mechanism of Action: Prevents attacks of angioedema by increasing concentrations of C1 esterase inhibitor and thus C4; suppresses ovarian production of pituitary gonadotropins and ovarian hormone production; has weak androgenic effects

Contraindications: Hypersensitivity, pregnancy, significant renal or hepatic impairment, undiagnosed vaginal bleeding, androgen-dependent tumors

Precautions: Thromboembolic disease, hepatic or renal dysfunction, seizure disorders, migraines, cardiac disease

Pregnancy Risk: X

Adverse Effects

Common: Androgenic effects—hirsutism, irregular menstrual cycles, intercycle menstrual bleeding, weight gain; fluid retention

Less common: Cholestatic jaundice or liver dysfunction, pancreatitis, leukopenia, thrombocytopenia, rashes, benign intracranial hypertension

Drug Interactions

Warfarin: Increased anticoagulant effect

Carbamazepine: Increased carbamazepine concentrations

Insulin: Danazol may decrease insulin requirements.

Patient Instructions: Nonhormonal contraception is recommended. Avoid sunlight because of photosensitivity.

Clinical Pharmacology: Hepatic metabolism and renal excretion; half-life 4–6 h

Cost: $$$$

Danocrine (see *Danazol*)

DANTROLENE SODIUM

Trade Names: *Dantrium*

Synonyms: Dantrolene

Drug Class: Antispasticity agent

Preparations

Capsules: 25 mg, 50 mg, 100 mg

Injection: 20 mg powder for injection

Dose: Orally, initially 25 mg/day, increased at weekly intervals to a maximum of 100 mg 2–4 times a day

Indications: Muscle spasticity associated with upper motor neuron lesions; prevention and treatment of malignant hyperthermia

Mechanism of Action: Acts on the sarcoplasmic reticulum of muscle to inhibit release of calcium

Contraindications: Hepatic dysfunction

Precautions: Use caution if cardiac or pulmonary function is impaired.

Monitoring: LFTs before and at intervals during therapy

Pregnancy Risk: C

Adverse Effects

Common: Drowsiness, dizziness, fatigue, rash, GI symptoms such as diarrhea, cramps, and vomiting

Less common: Pleural or pericardial effusion, seizures, respiratory depression, speech and visual disturbances, hepatotoxicity (especially in women over 30 taking estrogens). Hepatotoxicity may occasionally be fatal.

Drug Interactions

Hepatotoxic medications: Increased risk of hepatotoxicity

Estrogens: Increased hepatotoxicity

CNS depressant effects: Additive depressant effect

Additional drug interactions: MAO inhibitors, phenothiazines, clindamycin, verapamil, warfarin, clofibrate, and tolbutamide

Patient Instructions: Avoid alcohol and CNS depressants. May cause drowsiness.

Comments: Baclofen is usually tried first.

Clinical Pharmacology: Poor absorption from GI tract; hepatic metabolism; half-life, 9 h

Cost: $$$$

DAPSONE

Trade Names: *Avlosulfon*

Drug Class: Sulfone bacteriostatic

Preparations: 25-mg, 100-mg tablets

Dose: 50 mg/day initially, increased by 25- to 50-mg increments up to 200 mg/day

Indications: Skin lesions of systemic or discoid lupus erythematosus, urticarial vasculitis, and pyoderma gangrenosum; has been used in relapsing polychondritis and RA. Nonrheumatologic uses include leprosy, malaria, prophylaxis of *Pneumocystis carinii,* and dermatitis herpetiformis.

Mechanism of Action: Immunomodulatory mechanism unknown; has sulfonamide-like action competing for *p*-aminobenzoic acid (PABA) and preventing bacterial synthesis of folic acid

Contraindications: Hypersensitivity to dapsone

Precautions: Use caution in patients allergic to sulfonamides, G6PD deficiency, and severe anemia.

Monitoring: Determine G6PD status before treatment of patients from ethnic groups at greater risk. Monitor CBC in all patients initially weekly, then monthly, and then every 2–3 months. Monitor LFTs at intervals.

Pregnancy Risk: C

Adverse Effects

Common: Rash, dose-related hemolysis, and methemoglobinemia

Less common: GI intolerance, leukopenia, agranulocytosis, exfoliative dermatitis, hepatitis, cholestatic jaundice

Drug Interactions

Rifampin: Decreased effect of dapsone

Folic acid antagonists (trimethoprim, sulfonamides): Increased toxicity

Patient Instructions: Regular blood monitoring is required. May cause photosensitivity.

Comments: The incidence of hemolytic anemia can be reduced by using concomitant antioxidant therapy (vitamin E or C).

Clinical Pharmacology: Well absorbed; acetylated in the liver. Acetylator phenotype (slow or fast) does not affect clinical use. CYP P450–mediated hydroxylation; renal elimination of metabolites; half-life, 30 h

Cost: $$

Darvocet (see *Acetaminophen + Opioid*)
Daypro (see *Oxaprozin*)

Demerol (see *Meperidine*)
Depen (see *Penicillamine*)
DepoMedrol (see *Corticosteroids, Intraarticular*)
Desyrel (see *Trazodone*)
Dexamethasone (see *Corticosteroids*)

DICLOFENAC (SEE APPENDIX A)

Trade Names: *Cataflam* (immediate release), *Voltaren* (enteric coated, extended release), *Voltaren XR, Arthrotec* (diclofenac + misoprostil)

Drug Class: NSAID

Preparations

> Tablet: 25 mg, 50 mg, 75 mg. Diclofenac/misoprostil 50 mg/200 mcg or 75 mg/200 mcg.

> Sustained-release tablet (XR): 100 mg

Dose: 100–200 mg/day in 2–4 divided doses (100 mg/day of sustained release)

Indications: RA, JRA, osteoarthritis, ankylosing spondylitis, spondylarthropathy, gout, pain

Mechanism of Action: Inhibition of cyclooxygenase activity thus decreasing formation of prostaglandins and thromboxane from arachidonic acid; may decrease neutrophil function

Contraindications: Hypersensitivity to NSAIDs, GI ulceration, hemorrhagic state, and last trimester of pregnancy (risk of premature closure of ductus arteriosus)

Precautions: Fluid retention may aggravate heart failure and hypertension. Use with caution or avoid with patients at high risk of GI bleeding (i.e., prior GI bleeding, elderly, concurrent corticosteroid treatment). Administer with food. Caution in asthma, bleeding disorders, and GI, hepatic, or renal disease.

Monitoring: Monitor hematocrit, creatinine, liver enzymes periodically (1 month after starting and then every 3–6 months). In patients at high risk of renal impairment (diuretics, receiving ACE inhibitors, edematous states, heart failure, renal failure, diabetes), monitor renal function more closely after starting treatment.

Pregnancy Risk: *Arthrotec*-category X. Category B, but category D in third trimester

Adverse Effects

Common: GI irritation (dyspepsia, reflux, epigastric pain), rash, fluid retention

Less common: GI ulceration, hemorrhage, or gastric outlet obstruction; hepatitis with elevations of liver enzymes; hypersensitivity (anaphylaxis, asthma, urticaria, angioedema—particularly in patients with nasal polyps, exfoliative dermatitis); hematologic toxicity (agranulocytosis, anemia, leukopenia, thrombocytopenia); renal toxicity (interstitial nephritis, proteinuria, nephrotic syndrome, acute renal failure, hypertension, hyperkalemia); CNS toxicity (drowsiness, insomnia, nervousness)

Drug Interactions

Anticoagulants: Increased hemorrhagic risk with other anticoagulants and thrombolytics

NSAIDs: Increased risk of GI side effects if combinations of NSAIDs used

Methotrexate: Increased levels of methotrexate with many NSAIDs, but with the MTX doses used in RA, usually not of clinical importance

Cyclosporine: May increase diclofenac levels and increase risk of nephrotoxicity.

Diuretics: Decreased effects of thiazides and furosemide; increased renal toxicity with diuretics; increased risk of hyperkalemia with K^+-sparing diuretics

Lithium: Increased lithium levels

Antihypertensive agents: Antihypertensive effect reduced

Patient Instructions: Take with food. Discontinue and seek medical advice if unusual bleeding occurs.

Comments: Diclofenac, like other NSAIDs, may cause hepatitis. Periodic monitoring of LFTs is required.

Clinical Pharmacology: Well absorbed after oral administration; hepatic metabolism and renal excretion of metabolites; half-life, 2–3 h

Cost: $$$

Didronel (see *Etidronate*)

DIFLUNISAL

Trade Names: *Dolobid*

Drug Class: NSAID

Preparations: 250-mg, 500-mg tablet

Dose: 500–1500 mg/day in 2–3 divided doses

Indications: RA, osteoarthritis, pain

Mechanism of Action: Inhibition of cyclooxygenase activity, thus decreasing formation of prostaglandins and thromboxane from arachidonic acid; may decrease neutrophil function

Contraindications: Hypersensitivity to NSAIDs, GI ulceration, hemorrhagic state, and last trimester of pregnancy (increased risk of premature closure of ductus arteriosus)

Precautions: Fluid retention may aggravate heart failure and hypertension. Use with caution or avoid in patients at high risk of GI bleeding (i.e., prior GI bleeding, elderly, concurrent corticosteroid treatment). Administer with food. Use caution in asthma, bleeding disorders, and GI, hepatic, or renal disease.

Monitoring: Monitor hematocrit, creatinine, liver enzymes periodically (1 month after starting and then every 3–6 months). In patients at high risk of renal impairment (diuretics, receiving ACE inhibitors, edematous states, heart failure, renal failure, diabetes), monitor renal function more closely (every 1–2 weeks) when starting treatment.

Pregnancy Risk: C; D in third trimester

Adverse Effects

Common: GI irritation (dyspepsia, reflux, epigastric pain), rash, fluid retention, headache

Less common: GI ulceration, hemorrhage or gastric outlet obstruction; elevations of liver enzymes; hypersensitivity (anaphylaxis, asthma, urticaria, angioedema—particularly in patients with nasal polyps, exfoliative dermatitis); hematologic toxicity (agranulocytosis, anemia, leukopenia, thrombocytopenia); renal toxicity (interstitial nephritis, proteinuria, nephrotic syndrome, acute renal failure, hypertension, hyperkalemia); CNS toxicity (drowsiness, insomnia, nervousness)

Drug Interactions

Anticoagulants: Activity of warfarin increased; increased hemorrhagic risk with other anticoagulants and thrombolytics

NSAIDs: Increased risk of GI side effects if combinations of NSAIDs are used

Methotrexate: Increased levels of methotrexate with many NSAIDs, but with the MTX doses used in RA, usually not of clinical importance

Diuretics: Decreased effects of thiazides and furosemide; increased renal toxicity with diuretics; increased risk of hyperkalemia with K^+-sparing diuretics

Lithium: Increased lithium levels

Patient Instructions: Take with food. Discontinue and seek medical advice if unusual bleeding develops.

Clinical Pharmacology: Well absorbed after oral administration; hepatic metabolism and renal excretion of metabolites; half-life, 8–12 h

Cost: $$$

Disalcid (see *Salsalate*)

DMARDs/SAARDs/SMARDs (see *Appendix B*)

Dolobid (see *Diflunisal*)

Doxepin (*Sinequan*; see *Appendix D*)

Doxycycline (see *Tetracycline*)

Duragesic (see *Fentanyl*)

Easprin (see *Aspirin*)

Ecotrin (see *Aspirin*)

EDROPHONIUM CHLORIDE

Trade Names: *Tensilon, Enlon, Reversol*

Drug Class: Short-acting cholinesterase inhibitor

Preparations: Injection, 10 mg/mL (1 mL)

Dose: Diagnostic test for myasthenia gravis—2 mg IV over 15–30 seconds; then, if no response is seen, 8 mg 45 seconds later

Indications: Diagnostic test for myasthenia gravis; used to differentiate cholinergic crisis from myasthenic crisis

Mechanism of Action: Increases acetylcholine concentrations by inhibiting its breakdown by acetylcholinesterase

Contraindications: Hypersensitivity to edrophonium or sulfites; GI or GU obstruction

Precautions: May worsen weakness if this is due to overtreatment (cholinergic crisis); IV atropine must be available to treat cholinergic symptoms. Use with caution in patients with asthma or those receiving cardiac glycosides.

Monitoring: Must be administered under medical supervision with resuscitation facilities on hand.

Pregnancy Risk: C

Adverse Effects

Common: Cholinergic symptoms—nausea, vomiting, cramps, diarrhea, salivation, sweating, small pupils, lacrimation

Less common: Bradycardia, seizures, hypersensitivity, bronchospasm, laryngospasm

Drug Interactions: Anticholinesterases neostigmine and physostigmine show increased effect.

Clinical Pharmacology: Onset of action within 60 seconds; duration of effect, 10 min.

Cost: $$$

Elavil (see *Amitriptyline*)
Equagesic (see *Meprobamate* and *Aspirin*)

ETIDRONATE

Trade Names: *Didronel*

Synonyms: Disodium etidronate, sodium etidronate

Drug Class: Bisphosphonate

Preparations

Tablets: 200 mg, 400 mg

Injection: 50 mg/mL (6 mL)

Dose

Paget's disease: 5 mg/kg/day orally for up to 6 months

Osteoporosis: 400 mg for 14 days every 3 months. Calcium (1 g/day) and vitamin D (400 U/day) supplementation is usual.

Indications: Paget's disease, hypercalcemia of malignancy, heterotropic calcification after hip replacement, osteoporosis

Mechanism of Action: Adsorbs onto hydroxyapatite crystals and blocks their aggregation and growth

Contraindications: Hypersensitivity to bisphosphonates; severe renal impairment; osteomalacia; Paget's disease with lytic lesions that have a risk of fracture

Precautions: Reduce dose in mild renal impairment.

Monitoring: In Paget's disease, alkaline phosphatase and urinary hydroxyproline are monitored as measures of response to treatment.

Pregnancy Risk: B

Adverse Effects

Common: Nausea, diarrhea, metallic taste

Less common: Increased bone pain in Paget's, osteomalacia with increased risk of fractures, constipation, hypocalcemia, hypersensitivity, seizures

Drug Interactions

Antacids: Decreased bioavailability of etidronate

Calcium: If taken together, decreased bioavailability of etidronate

Patient Instructions: Take on an empty stomach (2 h before meals). Supplement calcium and vitamin D intake.

Comments: Alendronate is FDA approved for treatment of osteoporosis; etidronate is not. The newer bisphosphonates are less likely to cause osteomalacia than etidronate, are more potent, and are generally favored above etidronate. The role of etidronate in osteoporosis is minor, and it is usually reserved for patients who have esophageal disease that precludes use of alendronate.

Clinical Pharmacology: Absorption 1–5%; no metabolism; renal excretion. Half of absorbed dose is eliminated in 24 h; the rest binds to calcium phosphate surfaces and is eliminated over months to years.

Cost: $$$

REFERENCES

Delmas PD, Meunier PJ. The management of Paget's disease of bone. N Engl J Med 1997;336:558–566.
Patel S. Current and potential future treatments for osteoporosis. Ann Rheum Dis 1996;55: 700–714.

ETODOLAC (ALSO SEE APPENDIX A, p. 507)

Trade Names: *Lodine, Lodine XL*

Synonyms: Etodolic acid

Drug Class: NSAID

Preparations

Capsule: 200 mg, 300 mg

Tablet: 400 mg, 500 mg

Tablet extended release (XL): 400 mg, 500 mg, 600 mg

Dose: 200–400 mg 2 or 3 times a day; maximum daily dose 20 mg/kg for patient weighing less than 60 kg. Extended release.

Indications: Osteoarthritis, pain, RA

Mechanism of Action: Inhibition of cyclooxygenase activity, thus decreasing formation of prostaglandins and thromboxane from arachidonic acid; may decrease neutrophil function

Contraindications: Hypersensitivity to NSAIDs, GI ulceration, hemorrhagic state, and last trimester of pregnancy (risk of premature closure of ductus arteriosus)

Precautions: Fluid retention may aggravate heart failure and hypertension. Use with caution or avoid in patients at high risk of GI bleeding (i.e., prior GI bleeding, elderly, concurrent corticosteroid treatment). Administer with food. Use caution in asthma, bleeding disorders, and GI, hepatic, or renal disease.

Monitoring: Monitor hematocrit, creatinine, liver enzymes periodically (1 month after starting and then every 3–6 months). In patients at high risk of renal impairment (receiving diuretics or ACE inhibitors, edematous states, heart failure, renal failure, diabetes), monitor renal function closely (every 1–2 weeks) when starting treatment.

Pregnancy Risk: C; D in third trimester

Adverse Effects

Common: GI irritation (dyspepsia, reflux, epigastric pain); rash; fluid retention; headache; dizziness

Less common: GI ulceration, hemorrhage, or gastric outlet obstruction; elevations of liver enzymes; hypersensitivity (anaphylaxis, asthma, urticaria, angioedema—particularly in patients with nasal polyps, exfoliative dermatitis); hematologic toxicity (agranulocytosis, anemia, leukopenia, thrombocytopenia); renal toxicity (interstitial nephritis, proteinuria, nephrotic syndrome, acute renal failure, hypertension, hyperkalemia); CNS toxicity (drowsiness, insomnia, nervousness)

Drug Interactions

Anticoagulants: Activity of warfarin increased; increased hemorrhagic risk with other anticoagulants and thrombolytics

NSAIDs: Increased risk of GI side effects if combinations of NSAIDs are used

Methotrexate: Increased levels of methotrexate with many NSAIDs, but with the MTX doses used in RA, usually not of clinical importance

Diuretics: Decreased effects of thiazides and furosemide; increased renal toxicity with diuretics; increased risk of hyperkalemia with K^+-sparing diuretics

Lithium: Increased lithium levels

Patient Instructions: Take with food. Discontinue and seek medical advice if unusual bleeding develops.

Clinical Pharmacology: Well absorbed after oral administration; hepatic metabolism and renal excretion of metabolites; half-life, 7 h

Cost: $$$

ETRETINATE

Trade Names: *Tegison*

Drug Class: Retinoid

Preparations: 10-mg, 25-mg capsule

Dose: Starting dose, 0.75–1 mg/kg/day in divided doses; maintenance dose, 0.5–0.75 mg/kg/day

Indications: Refractory psoriasis—anecdotal use in psoriatic arthritis and Reiter's syndrome

Mechanism of Action: Unknown

Contraindications: Pregnancy; women who plan further pregnancies; unreliable contraception

Precautions: Do not use in women of childbearing age unless they are capable of complying with contraceptive requirements. Effective contraception must be used for 1 month before starting therapy and continued during therapy. Perform pregnancy test before starting treatment. Duration of the teratogenic effect of the drug is unknown but is at least 2 years; therefore, patients must not become pregnant or donate blood after discontinuing therapy.

Monitoring: Monitor blood lipids and LFTs at intervals.

Pregnancy Risk: X, highly teratogenic

Adverse Effects

Common: Fatigue, headache, bone and joint pain, hyperlipidemia

Less common: Gout, hepatitis, mouth ulcers, pseudotumor cerebri

Drug Interactions

Vitamin A: Increased toxicity

Methotrexate: Increased risk of hepatotoxicity

Patient Instructions: Do not become pregnant during or after taking this drug. Use contraceptive measures during and after stopping drug. Do not donate blood while or after taking this drug. Do not take vitamin A.

Comments: The possibility of teratogenic effects during and after discontinuing therapy restrict the use of this drug. Often used in combination with other agents in the treatment of psoriasis.

Clinical Pharmacology: Absorption is increased by milk and high-fat meals. Hepatic first-pass metabolism to acitretin, an active metabolite; half-life is 80–175 days.

Cost: $$$

REFERENCE

Orfanos CE, Zouboulis CC, Almond-Roesler B, et al. Current use and future potential role of retinoids in dermatology. Drugs 1997;53:358–388.

Famotidine (*Pepcid*; see *Appendix C*)

Feldene (see *Piroxicam*)

FENOPROFEN (ALSO SEE APPENDIX A)

Trade Names: *Nalfon*

Synonyms: Fenoprofen calcium

Drug Class: NSAID

Preparations

Capsule: 200 mg, 300 mg

Tablet: 600 mg

Dose: 300–600 mg 3–4 times a day; maximum dose not to exceed 3.2 g/day

Indications: Osteoarthritis, pain, RA

Mechanism of Action: Inhibition of cyclooxygenase activity, thus decreasing formation of prostaglandins and thromboxane from arachidonic acid; may decrease neutrophil function

Contraindications: Hypersensitivity to NSAIDs, GI ulceration, hemorrhagic state, and last trimester of pregnancy (risk of premature closure of ductus arteriosus)

Precautions: Fluid retention may aggravate heart failure and hypertension. Use with caution or avoid in patients at high risk of GI bleeding (i.e., prior GI bleeding, elderly, concurrent corticosteroid treatment). Administer with food. Use caution in asthma, bleeding disorders, and GI, hepatic, or renal disease.

Monitoring: Monitor hematocrit, creatinine, liver enzymes periodically (1 month after starting and then every 3–6 months). In patients at high risk of renal impairment (receiving diuretics or ACE inhibitors, edematous states, heart failure, renal failure, diabetes), monitor renal function closely (every 1–2 weeks) when starting treatment.

Pregnancy Risk: B; D in third trimester

Adverse Effects

Common: GI irritation (dyspepsia, reflux, epigastric pain), rash, fluid retention, headache, dizziness

Less common: GI ulceration, hemorrhage, or gastric outlet obstruction; elevations of liver enzymes; hypersensitivity (anaphylaxis, asthma, urticaria, angioedema—particularly in patients with nasal polyps, exfoliative dermatitis); hematologic toxicity (agranulocytosis, anemia, leukopenia, thrombocytopenia);

renal toxicity (interstitial nephritis, proteinuria, nephrotic syndrome, acute renal failure, hypertension, hyperkalemia); CNS toxicity (drowsiness, insomnia, nervousness)

Drug Interactions

Anticoagulants: Activity of warfarin increased; increased hemorrhagic risk with other anticoagulants and thrombolytics

NSAIDs: Increased risk of GI side effects if combinations of NSAIDs used

Methotrexate: Increased levels of methotrexate with many NSAIDs, but with the MTX doses used in RA, usually not of clinical importance

Diuretics: Decreased effects of thiazides and furosemide; increased renal toxicity with diuretics; increased risk of hyperkalemia with K^+-sparing diuretics

Lithium: Increased lithium levels; increases toxicity of phenytoin, sulfonamide, sulfonylureas

Patient Instructions: Take with food. Discontinue and seek medical advice if unusual bleeding occurs. Do not crush tablets.

Clinical Pharmacology: Well absorbed after oral administration; hepatic metabolism and renal excretion of metabolites; half-life, 3 h

Cost: $$

FENTANYL

Trade Names: *Duragesic, Sublimaze*

Drug Class: opioid analgesic

Preparations

Injection: 0.05 mg/mL (2 mL, 5 mL, 10 mL, 20 mL, 50 mL)

Lozenge: 200 μg, 300 μg, 400 μg

Transdermal system: 25 μg/h (10 cm^2), 50 μg/h (20 cm^2), 75 μg/h (30 cm^2), 100 μg/h (40 cm^2)

Dose: Adult pain control, initially use transdermal 25 μg/h system and titrate according to response. Most patients require application every 72 h. Apply to dry, nonhairy skin on trunk or upper arms.

Indications: Chronic intractable pain; sedation for procedures

Mechanism of Action: Binds to opioid receptors in CNS.

Contraindications: Hypersensitivity to fentanyl, substance abuse

Precautions: Use caution in patients with hypersensitivity to other opioids, respiratory disease, or renal or hepatic impairment. Decrease dose if hepatic or renal impairment.

Monitoring: Ensure that drug is used to control pain.

Pregnancy Risk: B (D in high doses)

Adverse Effects

Common: Drowsiness, constipation, dysphoria, nausea, hypotension, brady-cardia

Less common: CNS stimulation, insomnia, seizures, respiratory depression, dependence, itching, hives

Drug Interactions

CNS depressants: Increased toxicity

MAO inhibitors: Risk of hypertensive crisis

Patient Instructions: Drug is addictive. Use only to control pain. Do not use with alcohol or other CNS depressants.

Comments: Respiratory depressant effect may last longer than analgesic effect. Absorption from patch increases in patients with fever. Patch is suitable for continuous pain, but slow onset of action makes it unsuitable for immediate pain control.

Clinical Pharmacology: Slow absorption from transdermal preparation; hepatic metabolism and urinary elimination as metabolites. After application of a new dose, evaluate analgesic effect after 24 h.

Cost: $$$$

REFERENCES

Cherny NI. Opioid analgesics. Comparative features and prescribing guidelines. Drugs 1996;51:713–737.
Jeal W, Benfield P. Transdermal fentanyl. A review of its pharmacological properties and therapeutic efficacy in pain control. Drugs 1997;53:109–138.

Ferrous Sulfate, Ferrous Gluconate (see *Iron Preparations*)

Flexeril (see *Cyclobenzaprine*)

FLURBIPROFEN

Trade Names: *Ansaid*

Drug Class: NSAID

Preparations: 50-mg, 100-mg tablet

Dose: 200–400 mg/day in 2–4 divided doses

Indications: Osteoarthritis, pain, RA

Mechanism of Action: Inhibition of cyclooxygenase activity, thus decreasing formation of prostaglandins and thromboxane from arachidonic acid; may decrease neutrophil function

Contraindications: Hypersensitivity to NSAIDs, GI ulceration, hemorrhagic state, and last trimester of pregnancy (risk of premature closure of ductus arteriosus).

Precautions: Fluid retention may aggravate heart failure and hypertension. Use misoprostol prophylaxis in patients at high risk of GI bleeding (i.e., prior GI bleeding, elderly, concurrent corticosteroid treatment). Administer with food. Use caution in asthma, bleeding disorders, and GI, hepatic, or renal disease.

Monitoring: Monitor hematocrit, creatinine, liver enzymes periodically (1 month after starting and then every 3–6 months). In patients at high risk of renal impairment (receiving diuretics or ACE inhibitors, edematous states, heart failure, renal failure, diabetes), monitor renal function closely (every 1–2 weeks) when starting treatment.

Pregnancy Risk: C; D in third trimester

Adverse Effects

Common: GI irritation (dyspepsia, reflux, epigastric pain), rash, fluid retention, headache, dizziness

Less common: GI ulceration, hemorrhage, or gastric outlet obstruction; elevations of liver enzymes; hypersensitivity (anaphylaxis, asthma, urticaria, angioedema—particularly in patients with nasal polyps, exfoliative dermatitis); hematologic toxicity (agranulocytosis, anemia, leukopenia, thrombocytopenia); renal toxicity (interstitial nephritis, proteinuria, nephrotic syndrome, acute renal failure, hypertension, hyperkalemia); CNS toxicity (drowsiness, insomnia, nervousness)

Drug Interactions

Anticoagulants: Activity of warfarin increased; increased hemorrhagic risk with other anticoagulants and thrombolytics

NSAIDs: Increased risk of GI side effects if combinations of NSAIDs are used

Methotrexate: Increased levels of methotrexate with many NSAIDs, but with the doses of MTX used in RA, usually not of clinical importance

Diuretics: Decreased effects of thiazides and furosemide; increased renal toxicity with diuretics; increased risk of hyperkalemia with K^+-sparing diuretics

Lithium: Increased lithium levels

Patient Instructions: Take with food. Discontinue and seek medical advice if unusual bleeding develops.

Clinical Pharmacology: Well absorbed after oral administration; renal elimination; half-life, 4 h

Cost: $$

Fluoxetine (*Prozac*; see *Appendix D*)

FOLIC ACID

Trade Names: *Folvite*

Synonyms: Folate, pteroylglutamic acid

Drug Class: Vitamin

Preparations

Tablet: 0.1 mg, 0.4 mg, 0.8 mg, 1 mg

Injection: 5 mg/mL, 10 mg/mL

Dose: Prophylaxis of methotrexate adverse effects 1–2 mg/day

Indications: Used to prevent adverse effects due to methotrexate (oral ulcers, GI intolerance, hematologic)

Mechanism of Action: May inhibit effects of methotrexate in certain cells; does not affect methotrexate control of RA

Contraindications: Vitamin B_{12} deficiency. Folate may obscure the diagnosis of pernicious anemia. Neurologic deficit may progress while anemia improves.

Precautions: If patient is macrocytic, check vitamin B_{12} level before folate supplementation.

Pregnancy Risk: A

Adverse Effects

Uncommon: Flushing, rash

Comments: Patients treated with methotrexate should usually receive folic acid. Recent evidence suggests elevated homocysteine levels are a risk factor for coronary heart disease (CHD). Folic acid lowers homocysteine levels.

Cost: $

REFERENCE

Dijkmans BA. Folate supplementation and methotrexate. Br J Rheumatol 1995;34:1172–1174.

FOLINIC ACID

Trade Names: *Wellcovorin*

Synonyms: Leucovorin calcium, citrovorum factor, tetrahydrofolate

Drug Class: Vitamin

Preparations

> Injection: 3 mg/mL
>
> Powder for injection: 25–50 mg, 100 mg, 350 mg
>
> Tablet: 5 mg, 15 mg, 25 mg

Dose: After high-dose methotrexate, inadvertent overdose, or prolonged methotrexate concentrations in renal failure patients, use folinic acid 10 mg/m^2 IV every 6 h for 72 h until MTX concentrations fall below 1×10^{-8} M. Extremely high concentrations of MTX may require higher doses of folinic acid. (Dosing graphs are available to further delineate dose.) With routine methotrexate use, 5 mg of folinic acid is given post-dose to lessen side effects.

Indications: MTX toxicity

Mechanism of Action: Replaces the folinic acid whose synthesis is inhibited by MTX

Monitoring: In MTX overdose, measurement of MTX concentrations is a useful guide to therapy.

Pregnancy Risk: C

Comments: Folinic acid has been used to prevent minor adverse effects due to MTX, but the data supporting the use of folic acid are stronger, folic acid is cheaper, and there is concern that folinic acid may antagonize the antiinflammatory effects of MTX.

Cost: $$$

REFERENCE

Dijkmans BA. Folate supplementation and methotrexate. Br J Rheumatol 1995;34:1172–1174.

Fosamax (see *Alendronate*)

GAMMA GLOBULIN

Trade Names: *Gamimune, Gammagard, Iveegam, Polygam, Sandoglobulin*

Synonyms: Intravenous immune globulin, IVIG

Drug Class: Immunoglobulin

Preparations

> Gamimune: 10 mL, 50 mL, 100 mL (50 mg/mL) + 100 mg/mL
>
> Gammagard and Polygam: 0.5 g, 2.5 g, 5 g, 10 g

Iveegam: 0.5 g, 1 g, 2.5 g, 5 g

Sandoglobulin: 1 g, 3 g, 6 g

Dose

Administered intravenously at the rate specified by the manufacturers' instructions; generally start at a slow rate 0.5–1 mL/min and increase.

Primary immunodeficiencies: 200–400 mg/kg every 4 weeks

Kawasaki disease: 2 g/kg in one dose, or 800 mg/kg/day for 2 days, or 400 mg/kg/day for 4 days. Concomitant aspirin therapy is indicated.

Chronic ITP: 400 mg/kg/day for 5 days or 1 g/kg/day for 1–2 days; repeated at 10- to 21-day intervals according to platelet count

Inflammatory myositis: 1 g/kg/day for 2 days once a month

Other autoimmune disease: 400 mg–1 g/kg for 1 or 2 days a month or 400 mg/kg/day for 4 days

Indications: Primary immunodeficiencies associated with hypogammaglobulinemia or agammaglobulinemia; also used in idiopathic thrombocytopenic purpura, Kawasaki disease, Guillain-Barré syndrome, chronic inflammatory demyelinating polyneuropathy. Uncontrolled reports suggest efficacy in autoimmune disease refractory to other treatment.

Mechanism of Action: In primary immunodeficiencies, IVIG replaces IgG; in autoimmune disease, mechanism unknown. Theories include blockade of Fc receptors, T cell inhibition, and solubilization of immune complexes.

Contraindications: Hypersensitivity to immune globulin. In patients with profound IgA deficiency (serum IgA < 5 mg/dL), many IVIG products containing larger amounts of IgA are contraindicated as they may cause anaphylactic reactions.

Precautions: Patients with profound IgA deficiency may develop anaphylactic reactions. If IVIG is required in these patients, use an IgA-deficient preparation (Gammagard, Polygam).

Monitoring: For autoimmune disease, IVIG is usually administered in hospital on an outpatient basis, with monitoring of vital signs.

Pregnancy Risk: C

Adverse Effects

Common: Flushing, tachycardia, chills, dyspnea—all usually respond to slowing the rate of infusion

Less common: Hypotension, anaphylaxis, aseptic meningitis. Transmission of viral infection is uncommon. In the past, rare cases of transmission of hepatitis C have occurred with inadequately treated preparations.

Drug Interactions: May interfere with the action of live virus vaccines

Comments: Prepared from pooled plasma. Few controlled trials exist to guide appropriate use of IVIG in the rheumatic diseases.

Cost: $$$$$

REFERENCES

Dalakas MC, Illa I, Dambrosia JM, et al. A controlled trial of high dose intravenous immuno-globulin infusion as treatment for dermatomyositis. N Engl J Med 1993;329:1993–2000.
Dwyer JM. Manipulating the immune system with immune globulin. N Engl J Med 1992;326:107–116.
Prieur AM. Intravenous immunoglobulins in Stills disease: still controversial, still unproven. J Rheumatol 1996;23:797–800.

GOLD—INJECTABLE PREPARATIONS

Trade Names: Aurothioglucose, *Solganal;* gold sodium thiomalate, *Aurolate, Myochrysine* (no longer available)

Drug Class: DMARD

Preparations

>Aurothioglucose: 50 mg/mL (10 mL)

>Gold sodium thiomalate: 10 mg/mL, 25 mg/mL, 50 mg/mL

Dose: 10 mg IM test dose first week, 25 mg IM next week, and 50 mg/week IM thereafter until response or a cumulative dose of 1 g. Once response is obtained, decrease frequency of injections to every 2 weeks for 2 months, then decrease frequency and maintain on 50 mg IM every 3–4 weeks. Most patients receive a maintenance dose of 50 mg monthly (q 4 weeks).

Indications: RA, JRA, psoriatic arthritis

Mechanism of Action: Unknown; probably interferes with normal macro-phage function

Contraindications: Hypersensitivity to gold, severe renal or hepatic disease, blood dyscrasias

Precautions: Regular monitoring is required. Administer first few doses under medical supervision with facilities to treat anaphylaxis.

Monitoring: Perform baseline CBC, creatinine, and LFTs. Check CBC, platelets, and urinalysis before each injection and LFTs periodically. Discontinue gold if there is a rapid fall in any blood parameter or if WBC is below 4000, granulocytes below 1500, or platelets below 100,000. If mild rash occurs, decrease frequency of injections. If severe rash occurs, discontinue. If there is persistent proteinuria (>300 mg/24 h), discontinue.

Pregnancy Risk: C

Adverse Effects

Common: Rash, itching, painful mouth ulcers, altered taste, proteinuria

Less common: Anaphylaxis, exfoliative dermatitis, glomerulonephritis, nephrotic syndrome, blue/black skin discoloration ("chyrsiasis"). Blood dyscrasias (aplastic anemia, agranulocytosis, thrombocytopenia) should be looked for as they may be severe, precipitous, and fatal. Hepatotoxicity, pulmonary fibrosis, and peripheral neuropathy are uncommon. Gold sodium thiomalate preparations have uncommonly been associated with a nitritoid reaction (flushing, sweating, and dizziness) after the injection.

Drug Interactions: Potentially increased toxicity with other DMARDs

Patient Instructions: Frequent monitoring is essential. Do not become pregnant. Notify physician of rash and mouth sores.

Comments: Onset of response is slow (6–12 weeks). If no response by 24 weeks, consider stopping. If there is a poor response after 1 g total dose, discontinue. A minority of RA patients respond very well to IM gold and tolerate it long term. Less than 20% of patients initiating gold therapy will still be receiving it 3–5 years later. Toxicity is common.

Clinical Pharmacology: Injectable gold is only given IM. Absorption is slow and erratic. Most is renally excreted. Plasma half-life is about 30 days, but gold is present in tissues months to years later.

Cost: $$ (Medication is relatively inexpensive, but the cost of weekly administration and laboratory work increases the total cost.)

REFERENCE

American College of Rheumatology Ad Hoc Committee on Clinical Guidelines. Guidelines for monitoring drug therapy in rheumatoid arthritis. Arthritis Rheum 1996;5:723–731.

Gold—Oral Preparation (see *Auranofin*)
Hydeltra (see *Corticosteroids, Intraarticular*)
Hydrocodone (see *Acetaminophen + Opioids*)
Hydrocortisone (see *Corticosteroids*)

HYDROXYCHLOROQUINE AND CHLOROQUINE PHOSPHATE

Trade Names: Hydroxychloroquine, *Plaquenil;* chloroquine, *Aralen*

Drug Class: Antimalarial, DMARD

Preparations

Hydroxychloroquine: 200-mg tablets (base 155 mg)

Chloroquine: 250-mg tablets (150-mg base), 500-mg tablets (300-mg base)

Dose

Hydroxychloroquine: 5–6 mg/kg lean body weight. The usual initial dose is 400 mg/day (once daily or in divided doses). The dose may be reduced to 200–300 mg/day once a clinical response is achieved.

Chloroquine: Up to 4 mg/kg lean body weight; usually 250 mg daily

Indications: RA, SLE, discoid LE, palindromic rheumatism, psoriatic arthritis. In RA, it is used as a single agent for mild or early disease. With more severe disease, it may be used in combination with other DMARD regimens. In SLE, it is particularly useful for skin and joint manifestations; generally not felt to be effective in controlling renal, CNS, or hematologic manifestations of SLE.

Hydroxychloroquine is the preferred antimalarial, as it is less toxic to the eye. Chloroquine is sometimes tolerated by patients who do not tolerate hydroxychloroquine.

Mechanism of Action: Unknown; theories include interference with macrophage presentation of antigen to T cells

Contraindications: Hypersensitivity to hydroxychloroquine, chloroquine, or 4-aminoquinolines

Precautions: Use caution in hepatic disease, psoriasis, and porphyria. Rare reports suggest that antimalarials may exacerbate psoriasis, but they are often safely used to treat psoriatic arthritis.

Monitoring: Ophthalmologic (retinal and visual field) testing should be performed at baseline or soon after drug initiation and then every 6 months. Risks of retinal toxicity with hydroxychloroquine increase with a cumulative dose above 800 g, age above 70 years, daily dose above 6.0 mg/kg, and impaired hepatic or renal function.

Pregnancy Risk: C

Adverse Effects

Common: GI irritation, headache, rash, itch, blurred vision due to ciliary muscle dysfunction

Less common: Yellow/orange is more common than blue/black discoloration of skin; also uncommon are reversible corneal opacities, irreversible retinal toxicity, neuromyopathy, blood dyscrasias, ototoxicity, emotional changes, and hemolysis with G6PD deficiency.

Drug Interactions: Penicillamine: increased toxicity

Comments: Retinal toxicity is very rare, and some maintain it almost never occurs with a hydroxychloroquine dose of 6.5 mg/kg/day or less. When it does occur, retinal toxicity occurs after many years of use, is slow in onset, and is irreversible. Baseline ophthalmologic monitoring can be deferred until the patient has been on the drug for a few months and seems likely to continue on it.

Clinical Pharmacology: Good oral absorption, may be taken with food, partial hepatic metabolism and renal elimination; extensive tissue deposition with tissue concentrations 300 times that of plasma. Only 10% of a dose is excreted in 24 h, and hydroxychloroquine remains in tissues for months.

Cost: $$$

REFERENCES

Maksymowych W, Russel AS. Antimalarials in rheumatology: efficacy and safety. Semin Arthritis Rheum 1987;16:206–221.
Wallace D. Antimalarial agents and lupus. Rheum Dis Clin North Am 1994;20:243–263.

IBUPROFEN

Trade Names: *Advil* (OTC), *Genpril, Ibuprin, Motrin, Nuprin* (OTC), *Rufen*

Drug Class: NSAID

Preparations

Tablet: 300 mg, 400 mg, 600 mg, 800 mg

Suspension (oral): 100 mg/5 mL

Drops: 40 mg/mL

OTC: 200 mg

Chewable tablets: 50 mg, 100 mg

Dose: 400–800 mg 3–4 times a day; maximum of 3.2 g/day

Indications: RA, JRA, osteoarthritis, ankylosing spondylitis, gout, pain

Mechanism of Action: Inhibition of cyclooxygenase activity, thus decreasing formation of prostaglandins and thromboxane from arachidonic acid; may decrease neutrophil function

Contraindications: Hypersensitivity to NSAIDs, GI ulceration, renal failure, hemorrhagic state, and last trimester of pregnancy (risk of premature closure of ductus arteriosus)

Precautions: Fluid retention may aggravate heart failure and hypertension. Use with caution or avoid in patients at high risk of GI bleeding (i.e., prior GI bleeding, elderly, concurrent corticosteroid treatment). Administer with food. Also use with caution in asthma, bleeding disorders, GI, cardiac, hepatic, or renal disease.

Monitoring: Monitor hematocrit, creatinine, liver enzymes periodically (1 month after starting and then every 3–6 months). In patients at high risk of renal impairment (receiving diuretics or ACE inhibitors, edematous states, heart failure, renal failure, diabetes), monitor renal function closely (every 1–2 weeks) when starting treatment.

Pregnancy Risk: B (but D in third trimester)

Adverse Effects

Common: GI irritation (dyspepsia, reflux, epigastric pain), rash, fluid retention

Less common: GI ulceration, hemorrhage, or gastric outlet obstruction; hepatitis with elevations of liver enzymes; hypersensitivity (anaphylaxis, asthma, urticaria, angioedema—particularly in patients with nasal polyps, exfoliative dermatitis, rash); hematologic toxicity (agranulocytosis, anemia, leukopenia, thrombocytopenia); renal toxicity (interstitial nephritis, proteinuria, nephrotic syndrome, acute renal failure, hypertension, hyperkalemia); CNS toxicity (headache, drowsiness, insomnia, nervousness); aseptic meningitis, particularly in SLE

Drug Interactions

Anticoagulants: Increased hemorrhagic risk with anticoagulants and thrombolytics

NSAIDs: Increased risk of GI side effects if combinations of NSAIDs are used

Methotrexate: Increased levels of methotrexate may be seen with NSAID use, but with the low doses of MTX used in RA, this is usually not of clinical importance

Diuretics: Decreased effects of thiazides and furosemide; increases renal toxicity with diuretics; increases risk of hyperkalemia with K^+-sparing diuretics

Lithium: Increased lithium levels

Antihypertensive agents: Effect reduced

Patient Instructions: Take with food. Discontinue and seek medical advice if fainting, vomiting of blood, or unusual bleeding develops.

Comments: Ibuprofen may have less GI toxicity than other NSAIDs, but this may be because of the comparatively low doses of ibuprofen included in these analyses.

Clinical Pharmacology: Well absorbed after oral administration; hepatic metabolism and renal excretion of metabolites; half-life, 2–4 h

Cost: $

Imipramine (*Tofranil*; see *Appendix D*)

Imuran (see *Azathioprine*)

Indocin (see *Indomethacin*)

INDOMETHACIN

Trade Names: *Indocin, Indocin-SR, Indameth, Indochron ER*

Drug Class: NSAID

Preparations

Capsule: 25 mg, 50 mg

Capsule, sustained release: 75 mg

Suspension oral: 25 mg/5 mL

Suppository: 50 mg

Dose

25–50 mg orally or rectally 2–3 times a day (1–2 mg/kg/day); maximum, 200 mg/day

Sustained-release capsule (75 mg) administered 1–2 times/day

Indications: RA, JRA, osteoarthritis, ankylosing spondylitis, gout, pain

Mechanism of Action: Inhibition of cyclooxygenase activity, thus decreasing formation of prostaglandins and thromboxane from arachidonic acid; may decrease neutrophil function

Contraindications: Hypersensitivity to NSAIDs, GI ulceration, renal failure, hemorrhagic state, and last trimester of pregnancy (risk of premature closure of ductus arteriosus)

Precautions: Fluid retention may aggravate heart failure and hypertension. Use with caution or avoid in patients at high risk of GI bleeding (i.e., prior GI bleeding, elderly, concurrent corticosteroid treatment). Administer with food. Also use with caution in asthma, bleeding disorders, and GI, cardiac, hepatic, or renal disease.

Monitoring: Monitor hematocrit, creatinine, liver enzymes periodically (1 month after starting and then every 3–6 months). In patients at high risk of renal impairment (receiving diuretics or ACE inhibitors, edematous states, heart failure, renal failure, diabetes), monitor renal function closely (every 1–2 weeks) when starting treatment.

Pregnancy Risk: B (but D in third trimester)

Adverse Effects

Common: GI irritation (dyspepsia, reflux, epigastric pain), rash, fluid retention

Less common: GI ulceration, hemorrhage, or gastric outlet obstruction; hepatitis with elevations of liver enzymes; hypersensitivity (anaphylaxis, asthma, urticaria, angioedema—particularly in patients with nasal polyps, exfoliative dermatitis); hematologic toxicity (agranulocytosis, anemia, leukopenia, thrombocytopenia); renal toxicity (interstitial nephritis, proteinuria, nephrotic syndrome, acute renal failure, hypertension, hyperkalemia); CNS toxicity (headache, drowsiness, insomnia, nervousness)

Drug Interactions

Anticoagulants: Increased hemorrhagic risk with anticoagulants and thrombolytics

NSAIDs: Increased risk of GI side effects if combinations of NSAIDs are used

Methotrexate: increased levels of methotrexate may be seen with NSAID use, but with the low MTX doses used in RA, this is usually not of clinical importance

Diuretics: Decreased effects of thiazides and furosemide; increased renal toxicity with diuretics; increased risk of hyperkalemia with K^+-sparing diuretics

Lithium: Increased lithium levels

Antihypertensive agents: Effect reduced

Patient Instructions: Take with food. Discontinue and seek medical advice if fainting, vomiting of blood, or unusual bleeding develops. Do not crush or break extended-release product.

Comments: Indomethacin may be more likely to cause CNS side effects (headaches, somnolence, cognitive dysfunction), particularly in the elderly.

Clinical Pharmacology: Well absorbed after oral administration; hepatic metabolism and renal excretion of metabolites; half-life, 4–5 h

Cost: $

Intravenous Immunoglobulin (IVIG) (see *Gamma Globulin*)

IRON PREPARATIONS (ORAL)

Trade Names: Ferrous fumarate: *Femiron, Feostat, Ferro-Sequels, Fumasorb, Fumerin*
Ferrous gluconate: *Fergon, Ferralet, Simron*
Ferrous sulfate: *Feosol, Feratab, Fer-iron, Slow FE*

Drug Class: Antianemia agent (iron supplement)

Preparations

Ferrous fumarate (elemental iron 33%)

Tablets: 63 mg (*Femiron*), 195 mg (*Fumerin*), 200 mg (*Fumasorb*), 300 mg, 325 mg

Chewable tablets: 100 mg (*Feostat*)

Oral suspension: 100 mg/5 mL (*Feostat*)

Ferrous gluconate (elemental iron 11.6%)

Capsules : 86 mg (*Simiron*), 325 mg (generic)

Tablet: 300 mg, 320 mg, 325 mg

Elixir: 300 mg/5 mL (*Fergon*)

Ferrous sulfate (elemental iron 20%)

Tablets: 195 mg, 300 mg, 325 mg

Extended-release tablets: 525 mg (*Fero-Gradumet*)

Extended-release capsules: 150 mg, 250 mg

Oral solution: 125 mg/mL

Enteric coated tablets: 300 mg, 325 mg

Ferrous sulfate dried preparations (elemental iron 32%)

Capsules: 159 mg (*Feosol*), 190 mg (*Fer-In-Sol*)

Tablets: 200 mg (*Feosol*)

Extended-release tablets: 160 mg (*Slow Fe*)

Dose

Treatment of iron deficiency anemia : 60–100 mg of *elemental* iron twice daily

Prophylaxis of iron deficiency: 60–100 mg of *elemental* iron daily

Indications: Prevention and treatment of iron deficiency anemia

Mechanism of Action: Replaces deficient iron stores

Contraindications: Hypersensitivity to iron preparations; hemochromatosis

Precautions: Tablets/capsules may be corrosive to the bowel. In patients with dysphagia, liquid preparations are preferred.

Monitoring: Hemoglobin and reticulocyte count to monitor response

Pregnancy Risk: A; oral iron preparations are often required in pregnancy

Adverse Effects

Common: GI cramps, nausea, constipation, dark stools

Less common: Diarrhea, GI ulceration

Drug Interactions

Tetracyclines: Decreased absorption of tetracycline and iron

Antacids: Decreased iron absorption

Penicillamine: Decreased absorption of iron and penicillamine

Fluoroquinolones: Decreased absorption of antibiotic

Patient Instructions: Take regularly. May cause blackish/dark green stools or guaiac-positive tests for occult blood. Keep out of reach of children.

Comments: Many patients with inflammatory rheumatic disease have a hypochromic microcytic anemia that is not due to iron deficiency but due to chronic disease. This anemia does not respond to iron therapy. Failure of an iron deficiency anemia to respond to oral therapy usually signals an incorrect diagnosis or poor compliance. Once the hemoglobin concentration has been corrected, continue prophylactic doses of iron for 3–6 months to load body iron stores.

Clinical Pharmacology: Oral absorption of iron is increased to 30% in iron deficiency anemia. Absorption is decreased by gastrectomy and achlorhydria. Absorbed iron is stored in the body and is eliminated in small amounts by cellular shedding. After starting treatment, onset of reticulocytosis is rapid (3–5 days), and hemoglobin increases within 2–4 weeks.

Cost: $

IRON DEXTRAN (PARENTERAL)

Trade Names: *InFed, Dexferrum*

Drug Class: Antianemia agent (iron supplement)

Preparations: Injection, 50 mg/mL (2 mL, 10 mL)

Dose: Test dose 0.5 mL IV or IM. Observe for at least 1 h before administering dose. Calculate dose by referring to the treatment nomogram in the package insert. Alternatively, the dose may be calculated by the formula

Dose (mL) = 0.0476 × wt (kg) × (normal hemoglobin − observed hemoglobin) + (1 mL/5 kg [up to a maximum of 14 mL])

Entire dose may be administered IV. IV injection must be slow. Dilute in 250–1000 mL normal saline and infuse over 1–6 h. Infuse very slowly initially, and observe for allergy or anaphylaxis. IM regimen requires daily IM injections (maximum at one site is 2 mL).

Indications: Treatment of iron deficiency anemia in patients unable to take oral medication

Mechanism of Action: Replaces deficient iron stores

Contraindications: Hypersensitivity to iron preparations; hemochromatosis

Precautions: Administer under medical supervision with facilities available to treat anaphylaxis. Administer test dose first. If administered by IM injection must be by a deep IM injection, using a Z-track technique, in the upper outer quadrant of the buttock (not in upper arm).

Monitoring: Monitor for allergy/anaphylaxis during administration. Use hemoglobin and reticulocyte count to monitor response.

Pregnancy Risk: C

Adverse Effects

Common: Dizziness, fever, sweating, nausea, vomiting, metallic taste, discolored urine, staining skin at site of injection, leukocytosis

Less common: Anaphylaxis, cardiovascular collapse, urticaria. Onset of arthralgia, sweating, urticaria, and dizziness may be delayed 1–2 days after administration.

Cost: $$$ (includes cost of administration)

Kenalog (see *Corticosteroids, Intraarticular*)

KETOPROFEN

Trade Names: *Orudis, Oruvail* (sustained release), *Orudis KT* (OTC), *Actron* (OTC)

Drug Class: NSAID

Preparations

Capsule: 25 mg, 50 mg, 75 mg

Capsule, sustained release: 100 mg, 200 mg

OTC: 12.5 mg

Dose: 50–75 mg 3–4 times a day; maximum 300 mg/day. Sustained release, 200 mg once daily

Indications: RA, osteoarthritis, ankylosing spondylitis, pain

Mechanism of Action: Inhibition of cyclooxygenase activity, thus decreasing formation of prostaglandins and thromboxane from arachidonic acid; may decrease neutrophil function

Contraindications: Hypersensitivity to NSAIDs, GI ulceration, renal failure, hemorrhagic state, and last trimester of pregnancy (risk of premature closure of ductus arteriosus)

Precautions: Fluid retention may aggravate heart failure and hypertension. Use with caution or avoid in patients at high risk of GI bleeding (i.e., prior GI bleeding, elderly, concurrent corticosteroid treatment). Administer with food. Also use with caution in asthma, bleeding disorders, and GI, cardiac, hepatic, or renal disease.

Monitoring: Monitor hematocrit, creatinine, liver enzymes periodically (1 month after starting and then every 3–6 months). In patients at high risk of renal impairment (receiving diuretics or ACE inhibitors, edematous states, heart failure, renal failure, diabetes), monitor renal function closely (every 1–2 weeks) when starting treatment.

Pregnancy Risk: B (but D in third trimester)

Adverse Effects

Common: GI irritation (dyspepsia, reflux, epigastric pain), rash, fluid retention

Less common: GI ulceration, hemorrhage, or gastric outlet obstruction; hepatitis with elevations of liver enzymes; hypersensitivity (anaphylaxis, asthma, urticaria, angioedema—particularly in patients with nasal polyps, exfoliative dermatitis); hematologic toxicity (agranulocytosis, anemia, leukopenia, thrombocytopenia); renal toxicity (interstitial nephritis, proteinuria, nephrotic syndrome, acute renal failure, hypertension, hyperkalemia); CNS toxicity (headache, drowsiness, insomnia, nervousness)

Drug Interactions

Anticoagulants: Increased hemorrhagic risk with anticoagulants and thrombolytics

NSAIDs: Increased risk of GI side effects if combinations of NSAIDs are used

Methotrexate: Increased levels of methotrexate may be seen with NSAID use, but with the low doses of MTX used in RA, this is usually not of clinical importance.

Diuretics: Decreased effects of thiazides and furosemide; increased renal toxicity with diuretics; increased risk of hyperkalemia with K^+-sparing diuretics

Lithium: Increased lithium levels

Antihypertensive agents: Effect reduced

Patient Instructions: Take with food. Discontinue and seek medical advice if fainting, vomiting of blood, or unusual bleeding develops.

Clinical Pharmacology: Well absorbed after oral administration; hepatic metabolism and renal excretion of metabolites. Half-life is 1–4 h.

Cost: $$

KETOROLAC

Trade Names: *Toradol*

Drug Class: NSAID

Preparations

Tablet: 10 mg

Injection: 15 mg/mL (1 mL), 30 mg/mL (1 mL, 2 mL)

Dose

Tablet: 10 mg 3–4 times a day; maximum 40 mg/day; maximum 5 days administration

Injection: 30 mg then 15–30 mg every 6 h as needed for 5 days maximum

Indications: Short-term management of acute pain

Mechanism of Action: Inhibition of cyclooxygenase activity, thus decreasing formation of prostaglandins and thromboxane from arachidonic acid; may decrease neutrophil function

Contraindications: Hypersensitivity to NSAIDs, GI ulceration, renal failure, hemorrhagic state, and last trimester of pregnancy (risk of premature closure of ductus arteriosus)

Precautions: Fluid retention may aggravate heart failure and hypertension. Use with caution or avoid in patients at high risk of GI bleeding (i.e., prior GI bleeding, elderly, concurrent corticosteroid treatment). Administer with food. Also use with caution in asthma, bleeding disorders, and GI, cardiac, hepatic, or renal disease.

Monitoring: Monitor hematocrit, creatinine during use and 2–4 weeks after.

Pregnancy Risk: B (D in third trimester)

Adverse Effects

Common: GI irritation (dyspepsia, reflux, epigastric pain), rash, fluid retention

Less common: GI ulceration, hemorrhage, or gastric outlet obstruction; hepatitis with elevations of liver enzymes; hypersensitivity (anaphylaxis, asthma, urticaria, angioedema—particularly in patients with nasal polyps, exfoliative dermatitis, rash); hematologic toxicity (agranulocytosis, anemia, leukopenia, thrombocytopenia); renal toxicity (interstitial nephritis, proteinuria, flank pain, acute renal failure, hypertension, hyperkalemia); CNS toxicity (headache, drowsiness, insomnia, nervousness)

Drug Interactions

Anticoagulants: Increased hemorrhagic risk with anticoagulants and thrombolytics

NSAIDs: Increased risk of GI side effects if combinations of NSAIDs are used

Methotrexate: Increased levels of MTX may be seen with NSAID use, but with the low MTX doses used in RA, this is usually not of clinical importance.

Diuretics: Decreased effects of thiazides and furosemide; increased renal toxicity with diuretics; increased risk of hyperkalemia with K^+-sparing diuretics

Lithium: Increased lithium levels

Antihypertensive agents: Effect reduced

Patient Instructions: Take with food. Discontinue and seek medical advice if fainting, vomiting of blood, or unusual bleeding develop.

Comments: Only use for short-term control of pain.

Clinical Pharmacology: Well absorbed after oral administration; hepatic metabolism; renal excretion of 60% of drug unchanged. Half-life of 2–8 h is increased in elderly persons.

Cost: $$$

REFERENCE

Gillis JC, Brogden RN. Ketorolac. A re-appraisal of its pharmacodynamic and pharmacokinetic properties and therapeutic use in pain management. Drugs 1997;53:139–188.

Lansoprazole (*Prevacid*; see *Appendix C*)

Lodine (see *Etodolac*)

Lortab (see *Acetaminophen + Opioids*)

Magnesium Choline Salicylate (see *Choline Magnesium Salicylate*)

Maprotilene (*Ludiomil*; see *Appendix D*)

MECLOFENAMATE SODIUM

Trade Names: *Meclomen*

Drug Class: NSAID

Preparations: 50-mg, 100-mg capsule

Dose: 200–400 mg/day in 3–4 divided doses

Indications: RA, osteoarthritis, inflammatory arthritis, pain

Mechanism of Action: Inhibition of cyclooxygenase activity, thus decreasing formation of prostaglandins and thromboxane from arachidonic acid; may decrease neutrophil function

Contraindications: Hypersensitivity to NSAIDs, GI ulceration, renal failure, hemorrhagic state, and last trimester of pregnancy (risk of premature closure of ductus arteriosus)

Precautions: Fluid retention may aggravate heart failure and hypertension. Use with caution or avoid in patients at high risk of GI bleeding (i.e., prior GI bleeding, elderly, concurrent corticosteroid treatment). Administer with food. Also use with caution in asthma, bleeding disorders, and GI, cardiac, hepatic, or renal disease.

Monitoring: Monitor hematocrit, creatinine, liver enzymes periodically (1 month after starting and then every 3–6 months). In patients at high risk of NSAID-induced renal failure (heart failure, receiving diuretics or ACE inhibitors, elderly, and impaired renal function), monitor renal function carefully, weekly initially for 2–4 weeks, then every 1–3 months.

Pregnancy Risk: B (but D in third trimester)

Adverse Effects

Common: GI irritation (dyspepsia, reflux, epigastric pain), diarrhea, rash, fluid retention, dizziness

Less common: GI ulceration, hemorrhage, or gastric outlet obstruction; hepatitis with elevations of liver enzymes; hypersensitivity (anaphylaxis, asthma, urticaria, angioedema—particularly in patients with nasal polyps, exfoliative dermatitis); hematologic toxicity (agranulocytosis, anemia, leukopenia, thrombocytopenia); renal toxicity (interstitial nephritis, proteinuria, nephrotic syndrome, acute renal failure, hypertension, hyperkalemia); CNS toxicity (headache, drowsiness, insomnia, nervousness)

Drug Interactions

Anticoagulants: Increased hemorrhagic risk with anticoagulants and thrombolytics

NSAIDs: Increased risk of GI side effects if combinations of NSAIDs are used

Methotrexate: NSAIDs may increase MTX levels, but with MTX doses used in RA, this is usually not of clinical importance.

Diuretics: Decreased effects of thiazides and furosemide; increased renal toxicity with diuretics; increased risk of hyperkalemia with K^+-sparing diuretics

Lithium: Increased lithium levels

Antihypertensive agents: Hypotensive effect reduced

Patient Instructions: Take with food. Discontinue and seek medical advice if fainting, vomiting of blood, or unusual bleeding develops.

Clinical Pharmacology: Well absorbed after oral administration; hepatic metabolism and renal excretion of metabolites; analgesic effect lasts 4–6 h.

Cost: $$

Meclomen (see *Meclofenamate Sodium*)

MEPERIDINE

Trade Names: *Demerol*

Synonyms: Meperidine hydrochloride, pethidine

Drug Class: Narcotic analgesic, opioid

Preparations

> Tablets: 50 mg, 100 mg
>
> Syrup: 50 mg/5 mL (500 mL)
>
> Injection: 10 mg/mL, 50 mg/mL, 100 mg/mL

Dose: Oral, IM, IV, or SC: 50–150 mg/dose every 3–4 h (50–75 mg of meperidine is roughly equivalent to 10 mg of morphine). The oral dose is less potent than the IM dose.

Indications: Pain not controlled by nonopioid drugs. Morphine is generally preferred. Do not use to treat chronic pain.

Mechanism of Action: Binds to opioid receptors in CNS

Contraindications: Hypersensitivity to meperidine; substance abuse; patients receiving MAOIs in the previous 14 days; renal failure

Precautions: Use caution in patients with hypersensitivity to other opioids, seizure disorder, respiratory disease, renal or hepatic impairment. Decrease dose if hepatic or renal impairment. The metabolite normeperidine accumulates in patients with impaired renal function and causes CNS stimulation and seizures. Meperidine is not suitable for chronic use. Use the lowest dose necessary to control pain. Escalate dose only with uncontrolled pain.

Monitoring: Monitor blood pressure and respiration if used parenterally.

Pregnancy Risk: B; D in high doses

Adverse Effects

Common: Drowsiness, constipation, dysphoria, nausea, hypotension

Less common: Rash, CNS stimulation, insomnia, twitchiness, seizures, respiratory depression, dependence, histamine release

Drug Interactions

> CNS depressants: Increased toxicity
>
> MAO inhibitors: Avoid because risk of hypertensive crisis
>
> Serotonin uptake inhibitors: Avoid fluoxetine and other drugs of this class because of increased effect of meperidine
>
> Cimetidine: Increased meperidine levels

Patient Instructions: Drug is a narcotic and is addictive. Use only to control pain. Do not use with alcohol or other CNS depressants.

Comments: Meperidine offers little advantage over morphine and has a worse adverse-effect profile, particularly the increased risk of seizures due to normeperidine. Meperidine is often given IM along with IM hydroxyzine (Vistaril, 25–50 mg) to decrease nausea.

Clinical Pharmacology: Onset of action within 10 minutes, duration of effect is 2–4 h; hepatic metabolism; urinary elimination as metabolites. Half-life of meperidine is 3–4 h, but half-life of the toxic metabolite, normeperidine, is 15–30 h and depends on renal function.

Cost: $

MEPROBAMATE AND ASPIRIN

Trade Names: *Equagesic*

Drug Class: Analgesic (ASA) combined with anxiolytic (meprobamate)

Preparations: 200 mg meprobamate + 325 mg aspirin

Dose: 1–2 tablets 3–4 times a day as needed

Indications: Pain with anxiety, tension headache, muscle spasm

Mechanism of Action: Combination of an NSAID and CNS depressant acting through unknown mechanisms

Contraindications: Hypersensitivity to meprobamate or aspirin

Precautions: Same as for aspirin (see Aspirin). Meprobamate may result in physical or psychologic dependence and abuse. Use the lowest dose necessary to control pain. Escalate dose only with uncontrolled pain.

Monitoring: Monitor for continued need for drug, physical dependence, or abuse. Perform CBC periodically.

Pregnancy Risk: D

Adverse Effects: Aspirin (see aspirin), meprobamate

Common: Drowsiness, dizziness, rash, diarrhea

Less common: Edema, paradoxical excitement, confusion, purpura, thrombocytopenia, leukopenia, renal failure

Drug Interactions: Same as Aspirin (see Aspirin)

CNS depressants: Increased effect of meprobamate

Patient Instructions: May cause drowsiness. Avoid with alcohol. Risk of GI bleeding exists.

Comments: The use of meprobamate is largely obsolete as its side effect profile is worse than that seen with the benzodiazepines.

Clinical Pharmacology: Same as Aspirin (see Aspirin)
Meprobamate: Hepatic metabolism, renal elimination. Half-life is 10 h.

Cost: $$

MESNA

Trade Names: *Mesnex*

Drug Class: Thiol compound

Preparations: 100 mg/mL (2 mL, 4 mL, 10 mL)

Dose

IV: Administer mesna to a total of 60–200% of the cyclophosphamide dose (mg for mg) divided into several doses, given 15 min prior to cyclophosphamide and 3, 6, 9 and 12 h after cyclophosphamide. For IV infusions, mesna is diluted in normal saline (concentration 1–20 mg/mL) or D5W and administered over 15–30 min.

Oral: Administer mesna equivalent to 40% of the cyclophosphamide dose (mg for mg) for first dose before cyclophosphamide and 2 doses at 3- to 4-h intervals after cyclophosphamide (total dose, 120% of cyclophosphamide dose). For oral administration, the injectable form can be diluted in carbonated drinks or apple or orange juice. IV mesna is recommended over oral therapy.

Indications: Prophylaxis of hemorrhagic cystitis due to cyclophosphamide or ifosfamide

Mechanism of Action: Binds and detoxifies with urotoxic metabolites such as acrolein (seen with cyclophosphamide therapy)

Contraindications: Hypersensitivity to mesna

Pregnancy Risk: B

Adverse Effects

Common: Bad taste, headache, diarrhea, nausea, musculoskeletal pain

Uncommon: Allergic rash, hives

Comments: Most rheumatologists prefer IV cyclophosphamide (CTX) protocols to the oral form, as there is less hemorrhagic cystitis. Thus mesna prophylaxis is largely reserved for patients experiencing hemorrhagic cystitis with IV or oral CTX therapy.

Clinical Pharmacology: Peak plasma levels 2–3 h after oral administration; rapidly oxidized in the blood to mesna disulfide; excreted by glomerular filtration. Half-life of mesna disulfide is 1.2 h.

Cost: $$$

METHOCARBAMOL

Trade Names: *Delaxin, Marbaxin, Robaxin, Robomol*

Drug Class: Skeletal muscle relaxant

Preparations

Tablet: 500 mg, 750 mg

Injection: 100 mg/mL (10 mL)

Dose

Oral: 4 g/day in 3–6 divided doses (the IV preparation is rarely indicated in the treatment of musculoskeletal disorders)

Indications: Treatment of painful muscle spasm; useful in some patients with fibromyalgia

Mechanism of Action: Reduces spinal nerve traffic to skeletal muscle

Contraindications: Hypersensitivity to methocarbamol; renal impairment

Precautions: Use caution in hepatic and renal dysfunction and patients with seizures. Avoid extravasation of IV solution, which is hypertonic.

Pregnancy Risk: C

Adverse Effects

Common: Drowsiness; dizziness—although methocarbamol is less sedating than other muscle relaxants

Uncommon: Allergy, flushing, rash, nausea, leukopenia. Urine may turn dark when left to stand.

Drug Interactions

CNS depressants: increased CNS depression

Patient Instructions: Avoid alcohol. May cause drowsiness.

Comments: Nighttime sedative effect is sometimes useful in improving sleep in fibromyalgia.

Clinical Pharmacology: Rapid oral absorption; hepatic metabolism; renal excretion. Half-life is 1–2 h.

Cost: $$

METHOTREXATE

Trade Names: *Folex, Rheumatrex*

Synonyms: MTX

Drug Class: Antimetabolite and cytotoxic (at high doses); DMARD, antiinflammatory (at low doses)

Preparations

Tablets: 2.5 mg; dose packs of 4 cards (with either 2, 3, 4, 5, or 6 tablets each); one card is taken on the same day each week.

Injection: 25 mg/mL (2 mL vial)

Dose: MTX is typically initiated in a dose of 7.5–10 mg once a week (all taken on the same day). Start elderly patients with 5 mg/week. Most patients start on oral tablets. Dose may be increased after 6–8 weeks if clinical benefit is not achieved. If necessary, increase dose by 2.5 mg (1 tablet) every 4–8 weeks up to 15 mg/week. Higher doses are occasionally used in RA (up to 20 or 25 mg/week), based on limited evidence of incremental efficacy. Doses of 20–25 mg/week may be necessary to control cutaneous psoriasis or inflammatory muscle disease.

If nausea, diarrhea, or mucositis occurs, the clinician has several options: (*a*) lower the dose or temporarily suspend therapy (for 1–2 weeks); (*b*) divide the total weekly dose and administer 2 doses at 12-h intervals; (*c*) premedicate with antiemetics (e.g., promethazine); or (*d*) switch to weekly IM or SC injections for an improved side effect profile and more reliable absorption (patients can be taught to self-administer weekly SC injections).

The injectable form is 80–90% cheaper than the tablets and is the preferred alternative for those of limited financial resources. The injectable (parenteral) form may be administered IM, SC, or orally (diluted in water or fruit juice). Patients must be taught how to draw up the proper amount of parenteral MTX accurately and that 0.1 mL of the parenteral form equals 2.5 mg (or 1 tablet) of MTX.

All patients should receive concomitant folate (1 mg daily) to lessen the incidence of toxicity.

Indications: RA, psoriasis, psoriatic arthritis, JRA, inflammatory myositis, maintenance in vasculitis (after control achieved with cyclophosphamide), SLE, Reiter's syndrome, inflammatory arthritis

Mechanism of Action: The cytotoxic action is based on inhibition of dihydrofolate reductase by MTX, but this does not appear to be the mechanism of action with the doses typically used in rheumatic diseases. Thus, concomitant folate administration will not negate the clinical effects of MTX. Postulated mechanisms underlying its antiinflammatory effects include inhibition of methylation reactions and increased adenosine release.

Contraindications: Hypersensitivity to MTX, liver disease, alcoholism, pregnancy, or renal impairment. Most rheumatologists avoid use in patients with marked leukopenia, HIV, or severe hepatitis B or hepatitis C infection.

Precautions: The patient must understand the risks and benefits of treatment and the requirement for monitoring. Pregnant women must not receive MTX. Contraceptive methods should be reviewed and strongly advised (in both men and women) before starting, during MTX therapy, and for 1–3 months after discontinuing MTX. Patients should wait at least 3 months after discontinuing MTX before becoming pregnant.

MTX toxicity may be more common in those with renal impairment, Down's syndrome, or folate deficiency and those receiving high-dose aspirin (4–6 g/day).

Monitoring

Baseline: CBC, platelets, LFTs, creatinine, CXR (within the last year). Check for hepatitis B and C infection; if at risk, exclude HIV infection.

Maintenance: CBC and creatinine 2 weeks after initiating treatment; then CBC, LFTs (including albumin, AST, ALT), and creatinine every 4 weeks until efficacy and stable dose are achieved. Patients on a stable dose with no prior WBC or LFT abnormalities may have the laboratory testing interval gradually increased to every 6–8 weeks. Dose reduction is indicated for minor increases in liver enzymes. Inquire if the patient is receiving other hepatotoxic agents (e.g., alcohol, NSAIDs). If minor elevations persist, a liver biopsy or discontinuation of MTX should be considered. CXR should only be repeated if there is a suspicion of MTX pneumonitis or if it is otherwise indicated. Detailed guidelines on monitoring MTX use in RA have been established and are outlined in the table below.

Recommendations for Monitoring for Hepatic Safety in Rheumatoid Arthritis (RA) Patients Receiving Methotrexate (MTX)

A. Baseline
  1. Tests for all patients
     a. Liver blood tests (aspartate aminotransferase [AST], alanine aminotransferase [ALT], alkaline phosphatase, albumin, bilirubin), hepatitis B and C serologic studies
     b. Other standard tests, including complete blood cell count and serum creatinine determination
  2. Pretreatment liver biopsy (Menghini suction-type needle) only for patients with
     a. Prior excessive alcohol consumption
     b. Persistently abnormal baseline AST values
     c. Chronic hepatitis B or C infection
B. Monitor AST, ALT, albumin at 4- to 8-week intervals
C. Perform liver biopsy if
  1. Five of 9 determinations of AST within a given 12-month interval (6 of 12 if tests are performed monthly) are abnormal (i.e., above the upper limit of normal)
  2. Serum albumin level falls below the normal range (in the setting of well-controlled RA)
D. If results of liver biopsy are
  1. Roenigk grade I, II, or IIIA, resume MTX and monitor as in B, C1, and C2 above
  2. Roenigk grade IIIB or IV, discontinue MTX
E. Discontinue MTX in patients with persistent liver test abnormalities as defined in C1 and C2 above who refuse liver biopsy

---

Reproduced with permission from Kremer JM, Alarcon GS, Lightfoot RW, et al. Arthritis Rheum 1994;37: 316–328.

Pregnancy Risk: X (teratogen). Ensure that women are not pregnant before starting treatment, ensure reliable contraception during treatment, and avoid conception for 3 months after discontinuing MTX.

Adverse Effects

Common: Oral ulcers, postdose (1–2 days) nausea or diarrhea

Less common: Worsening of rheumatoid nodules (MTX nodulosis), fatigue, somnolence, photosensitivity, reversible hair fall, vomiting

Uncommon: Pneumonitis ("methotrexate lung"), impotence, elevated uric acid level, bone marrow suppression (primarily leukopenia or pancytopenia), osteoporosis (with chronic high-dose MTX), increased risk of infection, irreversible hepatic fibrosis, lymphoma (sometimes reversible on stopping MTX)

Drug Interactions

Trimethoprim/sulfamethoxazole: Increased marrow toxicity of methotrexate

Immunosuppressants: Additive toxicities

NSAIDs: Minor increases in methotrexate levels (seldom of clinical significance)

Probenecid: increase risk of methotrexate toxicity

Patient Instructions: Take methotrexate only once a week. Never increase the dose by yourself. Do not become pregnant. Do not drink alcohol. Avoid prolonged exposure to direct sunlight.

Comments: MTX has become the most widely used first-line drug for treatment of RA in the United States, primarily because of its ease of use, relatively rapid onset of action (4–8 weeks), and durable responses. Approximately 40–50% of patients are still taking it after 5 years. Folic acid supplementation (1 mg/day) decreases side effects and is used routinely by many rheumatologists.

Preliminary studies of MTX used in combination with cyclosporine and also in combination with sulfasalazine and hydroxychloroquine suggest increased benefit in patients not controlled on MTX alone.

MTX is not a first-line drug in the treatment of vasculitis but has been used after control is achieved with cyclophosphamide in conditions such as Wegener's granulomatosis. Similarly, in SLE and inflammatory myositis, methotrexate has been used as a steroid-sparing agent.

Clinical Pharmacology: Most administered MTX is eliminated unchanged in urine. Some is metabolized in the liver to 7-hydroxymethotrexate. Plasma half-life is 20 h. Intracellular MTX may form polyglutamates, which increase the biologic effect and toxicity of MTX beyond that expected from the plasma half-life. Cellular toxicity is related to concentration, but more importantly, to duration of exposure.

Cost: Parenteral form $; oral tablets $$$

REFERENCES

American College of Rheumatology ad hoc Committee on Clinical Guidelines. Guidelines for monitoring drug therapy in rheumatoid arthritis. Arthritis Rheum 1996;39:723–731.

Bannwarth B, Labat L, Moride Y, Schaeverbeke T. Methotrexate in rheumatoid arthritis. An update. Drugs 1994;47:25–50.

Cronstein BN. Molecular therapeutics. Methotrexate and its mechanism of action. Arthritis Rheum 1996;39:1951–1960.

Kremer JM, Alarcon GS, Lightfoot RW, et al. Methotrexate for rheumatoid arthritis: suggested guidelines for monitoring liver toxicity. Arthritis Rheum 1994;37:316–328.

Miacalcin (see *Calcitonin*)

MINOCYCLINE

Trade Names: *Minocin, Dynacin*

Synonyms: Minocycline hydrochloride

Drug Class: Tetracycline antibiotic

Preparations

>Capsule: 50 mg, 100 mg

>Injection: 100 mg

>Suspension: 50 mg/5 mL (60 mL)

Dose: Effective dose in RA is 200 mg/day (100 mg b.i.d.)

Indications: RA (see PDR for infectious indications and doses)

Mechanism of Action: Unknown; RA effects are probably related to down-regulation of intraarticular metalloproteinases rather than antibacterial effects

Contraindications: Hypersensitivity to minocycline; children less than 9 years old; pregnancy

Precautions: Renal impairment

Pregnancy Risk: D

Adverse Effects

Common: Diarrhea, nausea, photosensitivity, discoloration of teeth in children

Less common: Rash, increased intracranial pressure, pericarditis, dysphagia, enterocolitis, drug-induced lupus.

Drug Interactions: Antacids: Decreased absorption of minocycline
Oral contraceptive: Decreased contraceptive efficacy

Patient Instructions: Avoid sunlight. Do not take with antacids or milk.

Comments: Clinical effect in RA is small but statistically measurable. May be most suitable for patients with mild disease. May be used as an adjunctive agent in combination with other antirheumatic therapies (e.g., NSAIDs, DMARDs) in those not responding to conventional regimens.

Clinical Pharmacology: Well absorbed after oral administration; renal elimination. Half-life is 15 h.

Cost: $$$

REFERENCE

Tilley BC, Alarcon GS, Heyse SP, et al. Minocycline in rheumatoid arthritis. A 48-week, double blind, placebo-controlled trial. Ann Intern Med 1995;122:81–89.

MISOPROSTOL

Trade Names: *Cytotec, Arthrotec* (misoprostil + declofenac)

Synonyms: Synthetic prostaglandin E_1

Drug Class: Synthetic prostaglandin, protects against NSAID gastropathy

Preparations: 100-mcg, 200-mcg tablets

Dose: Prophylaxis of NSAID-induced gastropathy 100–200 μg 4 times a day. Efficacy best demonstrated for 200 μg 4 times a day, but lower doses (200 μg b.i.d. or 100 μg q.i.d.) are better tolerated and may be nearly as effective.

Indications: Prevention of NSAID-induced gastropathy (see Comments)

Mechanism of Action: Substitutes for endogenous prostaglandins (necessary to stimulate gastric mucus and bicarbonate secretion) whose synthesis is inhibited by NSAIDs

Contraindications: Hypersensitivity to misoprostol, pregnancy

Precautions: Safety in children is not established. Ensure that women are not pregnant before starting treatment, and ensure reliable contraception while receiving misoprostol.

Pregnancy Risk: X (abortifacient)

Adverse Effects

Common: Diarrhea, abdominal cramps

Less common: Headaches, vaginal bleeding, miscarriage

Patient Instructions: Do not consider becoming or become pregnant while on misoprostol. May cause diarrhea. Take with food.

Comments: Misoprostol reduces serious GI complications due to NSAIDs by 40%. Prophylactic therapy should be considered in patients at high risk of NSAID-induced GI complications (previous GI bleeding, previous peptic ulcer, elderly, combination NSAID and corticosteroid therapy) if therapy with an

NSAID is necessary. Prophylaxis in unselected NSAID users is not cost-effective. Misoprostol does not prevent GI pain (indigestion, dyspepsia) associated with NSAID use.

Clinical Pharmacology: Rapidly absorbed and metabolized to the free acid. Plasma concentrations are highest within 30 min of dosing. Half-life is 20–40 min. Dose reduction is not required in patients with renal impairment.

Cost: $$$

REFERENCES

Levine JS. Misoprostol and nonsteroidal anti-inflammatory drugs: a tale of effects, outcomes and costs [Editorial]. Ann Intern Med 1995;123:309–310.

Silverstein FE, Graham DY, Senior JR, et al. Misoprostol reduces serious gastrointestinal complications in patients with rheumatoid arthritis receiving nonsteroidal anti-inflammatory drugs. A randomized, double-blind, placebo-controlled trial. Ann Intern Med 1995;123:241–249.

Walt RP. Misoprostol for the treatment of peptic ulcer and antiinflammatory drug-induced gastroduodenal ulceration. N Engl J Med 1992;327:1575–1580.

Motrin (see *Ibuprofen*)

Myochrysine (see *Gold*)

NABUMETONE

Trade Names: *Relafen*

Drug Class: NSAID

Preparations: 500-mg, 750-mg tablet

Dose: 1000 mg/day in a single or divided doses. Dose may be increased to 1500–2000 mg/day in divided doses.

Indications: RA, osteoarthritis, analgesia

Mechanism of Action: Inhibition of cyclooxygenase activity, thus decreasing formation of prostaglandins and thromboxane from arachidonic acid; may decrease neutrophil function

Contraindications: Hypersensitivity to NSAIDs, GI ulceration, renal failure, hemorrhagic state, and last trimester of pregnancy (increased risk of premature closure of ductus arteriosus)

Precautions: Fluid retention may aggravate heart failure and hypertension. Use with caution or avoid in patients at high risk of GI bleeding (i.e., prior GI bleeding, elderly, concurrent corticosteroid treatment). Administer with food. Also use with caution in asthma, bleeding disorders, and GI, cardiac, hepatic, or renal disease.

Monitoring: Monitor hematocrit, creatinine, liver enzymes periodically (1 month after starting and then every 3–6 months). In patients at high risk of renal impairment (receiving diuretics or ACE inhibitors, edematous states, heart failure, renal failure, diabetes), monitor renal function closely (every 1–2 weeks) when starting treatment.

Pregnancy Risk: C (D in third trimester)

Adverse Effects

Common: GI irritation (dyspepsia, reflux, epigastric pain), rash, dizziness, fluid retention

Less common: GI ulceration, hemorrhage, or gastric outlet obstruction; hepatitis with elevations of liver enzymes; hypersensitivity (anaphylaxis, asthma, urticaria, angioedema—particularly in patients with nasal polyps, exfoliative dermatitis, rash); hematologic toxicity (agranulocytosis, anemia, leukopenia, thrombocytopenia); renal toxicity (interstitial nephritis, proteinuria, acute renal failure, hypertension, hyperkalemia); CNS toxicity (headache, drowsiness, insomnia, nervousness)

Drug Interactions

Anticoagulants: Increased hemorrhagic risk with anticoagulants and thrombolytics

NSAIDs: Increased risk of GI side effects if combinations of NSAIDs are used

Methotrexate: increased levels of MTX may be seen with NSAID use, but with the low doses of MTX used in RA, this is usually not of clinical importance

Diuretics: Decreased effects of thiazides and furosemide; increased renal toxicity with diuretics; increased risk of hyperkalemia with K^+-sparing diuretics

Lithium: Increased lithium levels described with many NSAIDs

Antihypertensive agents: Effect reduced

Patient Instructions: Take with food. Discontinue and seek medical advice if fainting or vomiting blood or if unusual bleeding develops.

Comments: Some data suggest that nabumetone may have less GI toxicity than other commonly used NSAIDs.

Clinical Pharmacology: Well absorbed after oral administration. Nabumetone is an inactive prodrug that is metabolized to the 6-methoxy-2-naphthyl acetic acid. Hepatic metabolism. Half-life is 20–30 h (even longer in the elderly).

Cost: $$$

Nalfon (see *Fenoprofen*)
Naprosyn (see *Naproxen*)

NAPROXEN

Trade Names: *Aleve* (OTC), *Anaprox, EC-Naprosyn, Naprelan, Naprosyn*

Synonyms: Naproxen sodium

Drug Class: NSAID

Preparations

Tablet: 250 mg, 375 mg, 500 mg

Tablet (enteric coated [EC]): 375 mg, 500 mg

Tablet, as sodium (Anaprox): 275 mg (250 mg base), 550 mg (500 mg base).

OTC: 220 mg (200 mg base)

Oral suspension: 125 mg/5 mL

Dose: 500–1000 mg/day in 2 divided doses

Indications: RA, osteoarthritis, ankylosing spondylitis, gout, JRA, pain

Mechanism of Action: Inhibition of cyclooxygenase activity, thus decreasing formation of prostaglandins and thromboxane from arachidonic acid; may decrease neutrophil function

Contraindications: Hypersensitivity to NSAIDs, GI ulceration, renal failure, hemorrhagic state, and last trimester of pregnancy (increased risk of premature closure of ductus arteriosus)

Precautions: Fluid retention may aggravate heart failure and hypertension. Use with caution or avoid in patients at high risk of GI bleeding (i.e., prior GI bleeding, elderly, concurrent corticosteroid treatment). Administer with food. Also use with caution in asthma, bleeding disorders, and GI, cardiac, hepatic, or renal disease.

Monitoring: Monitor hematocrit, creatinine, liver enzymes periodically (1 month after starting and then every 3–6 months). In patients at high risk of renal impairment (receiving ACE inhibitors or diuretics, edematous states, heart failure, renal failure, diabetes), monitor renal function closely (every 1–2 weeks) when starting treatment.

Pregnancy Risk: B (D in third trimester)

Adverse Effects

Common: GI irritation (dyspepsia, reflux, epigastric pain), rash, dizziness, fluid retention

Less common: GI ulceration, hemorrhage, or gastric outlet obstruction; hepatitis with elevations of liver enzymes; hypersensitivity (anaphylaxis, asthma, urticaria, angioedema—particularly in patients with nasal polyps, exfoliative dermatitis, rash); hematologic toxicity (agranulocytosis, anemia, leukopenia, thrombocytopenia); renal toxicity (interstitial nephritis, proteinuria, acute renal failure, hypertension, hyperkalemia); CNS toxicity (headache, drowsiness, insomnia, nervousness); photosensitivity, pseudoporphyria

Drug Interactions

Anticoagulants: Increased hemorrhagic risk with anticoagulants and thrombolytics

NSAIDs: Increased risk of GI side effects if combinations of NSAIDs are used

Methotrexate: Increased levels of MTX may be seen with NSAID use, but with the low doses of MTX used in RA, this is usually not of clinical importance

Diuretics: Decreased effects of thiazides and furosemide; increased renal toxicity with diuretics; increased risk of hyperkalemia with K^+-sparing diuretics

Lithium: Increased lithium levels described with many NSAIDs

Antihypertensive agents: Effect reduced

Patient Instructions: Take with food. Discontinue and seek medical advice if fainting, vomiting of blood, or unusual bleeding develops.

Clinical Pharmacology: Well absorbed after oral administration; hepatic metabolism; renal elimination. Half-life is 13 h.

Cost: OTC (low dose) $; generic $$

Neoral (see *Cyclosporine*)

NITROGLYCERIN OINTMENT

Trade Names: *Nitro-Bid Ointment, Nitrol Ointment*

Synonyms: Nitropaste, NTG, glyceryl trinitrate

Drug Class: Nitro vasodilator

Preparations: 2% ointment

Dose: For angina use 2–5 cm (15–30 mg) applied to skin 2–3 times daily. For digital ulcers, smaller amounts are applied to the fingertips.

Indications: Severe Raynaud's syndrome with digital ulceration

Mechanism of Action: Nitric oxide donor. Nitric oxide acts through cyclic GMP to relax vascular smooth muscle.

Contraindications: Hypersensitivity to nitroglycerin

Pregnancy Risk: C

Adverse Effects

Common: Flushing, headache, dizziness, rash

Comments: Use small amounts on tips of fingers. Efficacy is uncertain.

Clinical Pharmacology: Systemic absorption occurs transdermally, and this preparation is used to treat angina. Duration of action is 2–12 h.

Cost: $

Nizatidine (*Axid*; see *Appendix C*)
Norflex (see *Orphenadrine*)

NORTRIPTYLINE

Trade Names: *Aventyl Hydrochloride, Pamelor*

Drug Class: Antidepressant

Preparations

Capsule: 10 mg, 25 mg, 50 mg, 75 mg

Oral solution: 10 mg/5 mL

Dose

Depression (adults): 25 mg 3–4 times a day (up to 150 mg/day)

Fibromyalgia: Initiate with 10–25 mg at bedtime, can often be given as a single 10- to 75-mg dose at night.

Indications: Depression, chronic pain, fibromyalgia

Mechanism of Action: Increases synaptic concentrations of neurotransmitters such as norepinephrine and serotonin by blocking their reuptake.

Contraindications: Hypersensitivity to tricyclic antidepressants, narrow-angle glaucoma, urinary retention, pregnancy

Precautions: Use caution in cardiac disease, renal or hepatic impairment, hyperthyroidism

Monitoring: Blood pressure and pulse at scheduled visits

Pregnancy Risk: D

Adverse Effects

Common: Dizziness, drowsiness, anticholinergic effects (dry mouth, constipation, urinary retention, blurred vision), weight gain

Less common: Postural hypotension, arrhythmias, confusion, parkinsonism, tremor, anxiety, seizures, hepatitis, hematologic abnormalities, worsening of psychosis in schizophrenics

Overdose signs: Confusion, restlessness, agitation, vomiting, fever, rigidity, hyperreflexia, abnormal ECG, hypotension, seizures, respiratory depression

Drug Interactions

CNS depressants: Additive action
MAOIs: Hypertensive crisis, fever, hyperpyrexia, tachycardia
Warfarin: Increase in anticoagulation effect
Sympathomimetics: Potentiates effects of norepinephrine and epinephrine
Cimetidine: Reduces metabolism

Patient Instructions: Avoid alcohol. May cause drowsiness. May discolor urine. Dry mouth often improves after a few weeks.

Clinical Pharmacology: Hepatic metabolism; eliminated largely as metabolites in the urine. Half-life is 30 h.

Cost: $$

Nonsteroidal Antiinflammatory Drugs (NSAIDs) (see individual drugs and *Appendix A*)

Omeprazole (*Prilosec*; see *Appendix C*)

Ophthalmic Solutions (see *Artificial Tears*)

ORPHENADRINE CITRATE

Trade Names: *Norflex*

Drug Class: Muscle relaxant

Preparations

> Tablet: 100 mg
>
> Sustained-release tablet: 100 mg

Dose: 100 mg twice daily

Indications: Treatment of muscle spasm

Mechanism of Action: Central atropine-like action is thought to induce skeletal muscle relaxation.

Contraindications: Hypersensitivity to orphenadrine; myasthenia gravis, bowel obstruction, glaucoma

Precautions: Use caution with cardiac arrhythmias.

Pregnancy Risk: C

Adverse Effects

Common: Drowsiness, blurred vision

Less common: Tachycardia, rash, anticholinergic effects, nausea, constipation, flushing

Drug Interactions

Anticholinergics: Additive anticholinergic effects

Patient Instructions: May cause drowsiness. Avoid alcohol.

Clinical Pharmacology: Hepatic metabolism and renal excretion. Half-life is 14–16 h.

Cost: $$$

Orudis (see *Ketoprofen*)
Oruvail (see *Ketoprofen*)
Oscal (see *Calcium*)

OXAPROZIN

Trade Names: *Daypro*

Drug Class: NSAID

Preparations: 600-mg tablet

Dose: 600–1200 mg/day once daily. Do not exceed maximum dose of 1800 mg/day or 26 mg/kg (whichever is lower).

Indications: RA, osteoarthritis, pain

Mechanism of Action: Inhibition of cyclooxygenase activity, thus decreasing formation of prostaglandins and thromboxane from arachidonic acid; may decrease neutrophil function

Contraindications: Hypersensitivity to NSAIDs, GI ulceration, renal failure, hemorrhagic state, and last trimester of pregnancy (risk of premature closure of ductus arteriosus)

Precautions: Fluid retention may aggravate heart failure and hypertension. Use with caution or avoid in patients at high risk of GI bleeding (i.e., prior GI bleeding, elderly, concurrent corticosteroid treatment). Administer with food. Also use with caution in asthma, bleeding disorders, and GI, cardiac, hepatic, or renal disease.

Monitoring: Monitor hematocrit, creatinine, liver enzymes periodically (1 month after starting and then every 3–6 months). In patients at high risk of renal impairment (diuretics, edematous states, heart failure, renal failure, diabetes), monitor renal function closely (every 1–2 weeks) when starting treatment.

Pregnancy Risk: C (D in third trimester)

Adverse Effects

Common: GI irritation (dyspepsia, cramps, epigastric pain), rash, dizziness, fluid retention

Less common: GI ulceration, hemorrhage, or gastric outlet obstruction; hepatitis with elevations of liver enzymes; hypersensitivity (anaphylaxis, asthma, urticaria, angioedema—particularly in patients with nasal polyps, exfoliative dermatitis, rash); rash; hematologic toxicity (agranulocytosis, anemia, leukopenia, thrombocytopenia); renal toxicity (interstitial nephritis, proteinuria, acute renal failure, hypertension, hyperkalemia); CNS toxicity (headache, drowsiness, insomnia, nervousness)

Drug Interactions

Anticoagulants: Increased hemorrhagic risk with anticoagulants and thrombolytics

NSAIDs: Increased risk of GI side effects if combinations of NSAIDs are used

Methotrexate: Increased levels of MTX may be seen with NSAID use, but with the low doses of MTX used in RA, this is usually not of clinical importance

Diuretics: Decreased effects of thiazides and furosemide; increased renal toxicity with diuretics; increased risk of hyperkalemia with K^+-sparing diuretics

Lithium: Increased lithium levels described with many NSAIDs

Antihypertensive agents: Effect reduced

Patient Instructions: Take with food. Discontinue and seek medical advice if fainting, vomiting of blood, or unusual bleeding develops.

Clinical Pharmacology: Well absorbed after oral administration. Half-life is 40–50 h.

Cost: $$$

OXYCODONE

Trade Names: *Roxicodone, Oxycontin, Oxyir*

Drug Class: Narcotic analgesic

Preparations

Tablet: 5 mg

Tablet (controlled release): 10, 20,40, 80 mg

Oral suspension: 5 mg/5 mL

Dose: 5–10 mg 3–4 times a day; may divide and convert total dose to q12h sustained release.

Indications: Pain not controlled by nonopioid drugs

Mechanism of Action: Binds to opioid receptors in CNS

Contraindications: Hypersensitivity to oxycodone; substance abuse

Precautions: Use caution in patients with hypersensitivity to other opioids, respiratory disease, or renal or hepatic impairment. Decrease dose if hepatic or renal impairment.

Monitoring: Use the lowest dose necessary to control pain. Escalate dose only with uncontrolled pain.

Pregnancy Risk: D

Adverse Effects

Common: Drowsiness, dizziness, constipation, dysphoria, nausea

Less common: rash, CNS stimulation, insomnia, hypotension

Drug Interactions: Increased toxicity with other CNS depressants. Avoid with MAOIs.

Patient Instructions: Drug is addictive. Use only to control pain. Do not use with alcohol or other CNS depressants.

Comments: 30 mg oxycodone by mouth is equivalent in opioid effect to 10 mg of morphine IM.

Clinical Pharmacology: Oral absorption and hepatic metabolism; urinary elimination as metabolites. Half-life is 3 h. Duration of effect is 3–4 h.

Cost: $$

Oxycodone and Acetaminophen (see *Acetaminophen + Opioids*)

Oxycodone and Aspirin (see *Aspirin + Opioids*)

Pamelor (see *Nortriptyline* and *Appendix D*)

PAMIDRONATE

Trade Names: *Aredia*

Drug Class: Bisphosphonate

Preparations: Powder for injection: 30 mg, 60 mg, 90 mg

Dose

Paget's disease: 60 mg as a single IV infusion over 4–24 h or 30 mg over 4 h for 3 days.

Hypercalcemia of malignancy: 60–90 mg as a slow infusion over 4–24 h, may need to be repeated at 2- to 3-week intervals

Indications: Hypercalcemia of malignancy, Paget's disease

Mechanism of Action: Localizes to areas of bone resorption and inhibits osteoclast activity

Contraindications: Hypersensitivity to pamidronate or other bisphosphonates

Precautions: Use caution in renal impairment.

Monitoring: Monitor serum electrolytes periodically.

Pregnancy Risk: C

Adverse Effects

Common: Fever, hypocalcemia, hypokalemia, hypomagnesemia, nausea, diarrhea, bone pain, dyspnea, thrombophlebitis at infusion site

Less common: Rash, hypersensitivity, leukopenia

Drug Interactions

Diuretics: Increased risk of electrolyte abnormalities

Comments: Alendronate is more commonly used for the treatment of Paget's disease. Supplemental calcium and vitamin D are usually administered when bisphosphonates are used to treat Paget's disease.

Clinical Pharmacology: Oral bioavailability is very poor; renal excretion. Plasma half-life is short (2–3 h) but bone half-life is 1 year, indicating localization and release from bone.

Cost: $$

REFERENCES

Delmas PD, Meunier PJ. The management of Paget's disease of bone. N Engl J Med 1997;336: 558–566.
Fitton A, McTavish D. Pamidronate: a review of its pharmacological properties and therapeutic efficacy in resorptive bone diseases. Drugs 1991;41:289–318.

Parafon Forte (see *Chlorzoxazone*)
Paroxetine (*Paxil*; see *Appendix D*)

PENICILLAMINE

Trade Names: *Cuprimine, Depen*

Synonyms: D-Penicillamine, β,β-dimethylcysteine

Drug Class: Chelating agent, DMARD

Preparations

> Capsule: 125 mg, 250 mg
>
> Tablet: 250 mg

Dose: Rheumatoid arthritis, use 125 mg daily initially. Increase by 125-mg increments at 1- to 3-month intervals until usual maintenance dose of 375–750 mg/day is reached. Do not exceed maximum dose of 1.5 g/day.

Indications: RA, Felty's syndrome, scleroderma, primary biliary cirrhosis, Wilson's disease, cystinuria, lead poisoning

Mechanism of Action: In RA, mechanism is unknown, but may be related to inhibition of T cell function.

Contraindications: Hypersensitivity to penicillamine

Precautions: Cross-sensitivity to penicillin is possible. Penicillamine has a high frequency of adverse effects, and most patients experience an adverse drug reaction.

Monitoring: CBC, differential, platelets, and urinalysis (for protein) should initially be done within 1–2 weeks, and then monthly until therapeutic effect and a stable dose is achieved. The frequency of laboratory testing may be changed to every 8–12 weeks if the laboratory indices remain stable on repetitive testing.

Pregnancy Risk: D

Adverse Effects

Common: Rash, hives, itching, altered ("metallic") taste, proteinuria

Less common: Fever, hematologic toxicity (agranulocytosis, thrombocytopenia, leukopenia, aplastic anemia), glomerulonephritis, myasthenia gravis, Goodpasture's syndrome, optic neuritis, hepatitis, lymphadenopathy, drug-induced lupus, pemphigus, inflammatory myositis

Drug Interactions: Antacids/iron/food: Significantly decreased absorption of penicillamine

Patient Instructions: Take on an empty stomach. Altered taste may occur. Regular laboratory monitoring is required. Do not become pregnant.

Comments: Penicillamine has largely been replaced by MTX for the treatment of RA but is still useful in the occasional patient who cannot tolerate MTX or other agents (i.e., gold, hydroxychloroquine). Most patients who take penicillamine for RA discontinue it within 1–2 years for lack of efficacy or toxicity. Data supporting the benefits of penicillamine in scleroderma are largely based on retrospective studies, and its efficacy for this indication remains unproven. Beneficial effects may be seen in skin thickness scores.

Clinical Pharmacology: Absorption is 50%. Half-life is 2–3 h. Elimination is primarily renal as unchanged drug.

Cost: $$$

REFERENCE

Taylor HG, Samanta A. Penicillamine in rheumatoid arthritis. A problem of toxicity. Drug Safety 1992;7:46–53.

Percocet (see *Acetaminophen + Codeine*)

Percodan (see *Aspirin + Codeine*)

PHENYLBUTAZONE

Trade Names: *Butazolidin, Butazone*

Drug Class: NSAID

Preparations: 100-mg tablet

Dose: 100 mg 3–4 times a day

Indications: Ankylosing spondylitis refractory to other NSAIDs

Mechanism of Action: Inhibition of cyclooxygenase activity, thus decreasing formation of prostaglandins and thromboxane from arachidonic acid; may decrease neutrophil function

Contraindications: Hypersensitivity to NSAIDs, GI ulceration, renal failure, hemorrhagic state, and last trimester of pregnancy (risk of premature closure of ductus arteriosus)

Precautions: Fluid retention may aggravate heart failure and hypertension. Use with caution or avoid in patients at high risk of GI bleeding (i.e., prior GI bleeding, elderly, concurrent corticosteroid treatment). Administer with food. Also use with caution in asthma, bleeding disorders, and GI, cardiac, hepatic, or renal disease. Phenylbutazone is rarely used, because of hematologic toxicity, and should only be used in ankylosing spondylitis patients when other NSAIDs have failed to control active disease. The drug should not be given to elderly persons, as they are at greatest risk for hematologic toxicity.

Monitoring: Monitor CBC, creatinine, liver enzymes periodically (1 month after starting and then every 2–4 months). In patients at high risk of renal impairment (diuretics, edematous states, heart failure, renal failure, and diabetes), monitor renal function closely (every 1–2 weeks) when starting treatment.

Pregnancy Risk: C (D in third trimester)

Adverse Effects

Common: GI irritation (dyspepsia, reflux, epigastric pain), rash, dizziness, fluid retention

Less common: GI ulceration, hemorrhage, or gastric outlet obstruction; hepatitis with elevations of liver enzymes; hypersensitivity (anaphylaxis, asthma, urticaria, angioedema—particularly in patients with nasal polyps, exfoliative dermatitis, rash); hematologic toxicity (agranulocytosis, anemia, leukopenia, thrombocytopenia); renal toxicity (interstitial nephritis, proteinuria, acute renal failure, hypertension, hyperkalemia); CNS toxicity (headache, drowsiness, insomnia, nervousness)

Drug Interactions

> Anticoagulants: Increased hemorrhagic risk with anticoagulants and thrombolytics

> NSAIDs: Increased risk of GI side effects if combinations of NSAIDs are used. May potentiate effects of sulfonylureas; may increase serum concentration of Phenylin

> Methotrexate: Increased levels of MTX may be seen with NSAID use, but with the low doses of MTX used in RA, this is usually not of clinical importance.

> Diuretics: Decreased effects of thiazides and furosemide; increased renal toxicity with diuretics; increased risk of hyperkalemia with K^+-sparing diuretics

> Lithium: Increased lithium levels described with many NSAIDs

> Antihypertensive agents: Effect reduced

Patient Instructions: Take with food. Discontinue and seek medical advice if fainting, vomiting of blood, unusual bleeding, bruising, or infection develops. Frequent monitoring of blood tests is required with chronic use.

Comments: Phenylbutazone is no longer widely available commercially. For reasons that are unclear, it may be effective in patients with ankylosing spondylitis who have not responded to other NSAIDs. Its use should be restricted to rheumatologists. The potential risks and benefits must be evaluated with the patient before prescribing phenylbutazone.

Clinical Pharmacology: Rapid absorption; hepatic metabolism; renal elimination. Half-life is 50–100 h.

Cost: N/A

PIROXICAM

Trade Names: *Feldene*

Drug Class: NSAID

Preparations: 10-mg, 20-mg capsule

Dose: 10–20 mg/day as a single dose

Indications: RA, osteoarthritis, ankylosing spondylitis, analgesia

Mechanism of Action: Inhibition of cyclooxygenase activity, thus decreasing formation of prostaglandins and thromboxane from arachidonic acid; may decrease neutrophil function

Contraindications: Hypersensitivity to NSAIDs, GI ulceration, renal failure, hemorrhagic state, and last trimester of pregnancy (increased risk of premature closure of ductus arteriosus)

Precautions: Fluid retention may aggravate heart failure and hypertension. Use with caution or avoid in patients at high risk of GI bleeding (i.e., prior GI bleeding, elderly, concurrent corticosteroid treatment). Administer with food. Also use with caution in asthma, bleeding disorders, and GI, cardiac, hepatic, or renal disease.

Monitoring: Monitor hematocrit, creatinine, liver enzymes periodically (1 month after starting and then every 3–6 months). In patients at high risk of renal impairment (receiving ACE inhibitors or diuretics, in edematous states, or with heart failure, renal failure, diabetes), monitor renal function closely (every 1–2 weeks) when starting treatment.

Pregnancy Risk: B (D in third trimester)

Adverse Effects

Common: GI irritation (dyspepsia, reflux, epigastric pain), rash, dizziness, fluid retention

Less common: GI ulceration, hemorrhage, or gastric outlet obstruction; hepatitis with elevations of liver enzymes; hypersensitivity (anaphylaxis, asthma, urticaria, angioedema—particularly in patients with nasal polyps, exfoliative dermatitis, rash); hematologic toxicity (agranulocytosis, anemia, leukopenia, thrombocytopenia); renal toxicity (interstitial nephritis, proteinuria, acute renal failure, hypertension, hyperkalemia); CNS toxicity (headache, drowsiness, insomnia, nervousness)

Drug Interactions

Anticoagulants: Increased hemorrhagic risk with anticoagulants and thrombolytics

NSAIDs: Increased risk of GI side effects if combinations of NSAIDs are used

Methotrexate: Increased levels of MTX may be seen with NSAID use, but with the low doses of MTX used in RA, this is usually not of clinical importance.

Diuretics: Decreased effects of thiazides and furosemide; increased renal toxicity with diuretics; increased risk of hyperkalemia with K^+-sparing diuretics

Lithium: Increased lithium levels described with many NSAIDs

Antihypertensive agents: Effect reduced

Patient Instructions: Take with food. Discontinue and seek medical advice if fainting, vomiting of blood, or unusual bleeding develops.

Clinical Pharmacology: Well absorbed after oral administration. The drug undergoes hepatic metabolism and renal elimination. Half-life is 50 h.

Cost: $$

Plaquenil (see *Hydroxychloroquine*)
Plasmapheresis (see *Chapter 3.3*, p. 503)
Prednisolone (see *Corticosteroids*)
Prednisone (see *Corticosteroids*)

PROBENECID

Trade Names: *Benemid, Probalan*

Drug Class: Uricosuric

Preparations: 500-mg tablet

Dose: Initially, 250 mg twice a day for the first week, then increased to 500 mg twice a day and, if needed, up to a maintenance dose of 1–3 g/day in divided doses

Indications: Hyperuricemia associated with gout in patients who excrete less than 800 mg of urate in a 24-h urine collection, have normal renal function and no tophi, and no history of renal calculi.

Mechanism of Action: Inhibits renal tubular reabsorption of uric acid

Contraindications: Hypersensitivity to probenecid, renal impairment, nephrolithiasis. Do not administer to patient with either acute gout or chronic tophaceous gout.

Precautions: Use caution with peptic ulcer. Inhibits excretion of penicillins, and toxic levels may accumulate in patients with impaired renal function.

Monitoring: Monitor uric acid periodically

Pregnancy Risk: B

Adverse Effects

Common: Nausea, vomiting, headache

Less common: Rash, itch, allergy, precipitation of an acute attack of gout, leukopenia, aplastic anemia, urate nephropathy, nephrotic syndrome

Drug Interactions

Salicylates (high dose): Antagonize uricosuric effect

β-Lactams (penicillins, cephalosporins): Increased plasma levels of antibiotics

Methotrexate: Increased MTX toxicity

Antivirals: Reduced excretion of acyclovir and zidovudine

Patient Instructions: Drink plenty of fluids. Avoid aspirin or other salicylates (may antagonize the uricosuric effect).

Comments: To prevent acute attacks of gout, chronic colchicine or NSAID therapy is coadministered for the first 3–12 months of probenecid therapy. In patients with tophi or renal stones, allopurinol is preferred.

Clinical Pharmacology: Rapid, complete absorption; hepatic metabolism and renal excretion. Half-life is 6–12 h

Cost: $

REFERENCE

Emmerson BT. The management of gout. N Engl J Med 1996;334:445–451.

Propulsid (see *Cisapride*)
Ranitidine (*Zantac*; see *Appendix C*)
Refresh (see *Artificial Tears*)
Relafen (see *Nabumetone*)
Rheumatrex (see *Methotrexate*)
Ridaura (see *Auranofin*)
Robaxin (see *Methocarbamol*)
Rocaltrol (see *Vitamin D*)

SALSALATE

Trade Names: *Argesic-SA, Disalcid, Salflex*

Synonyms: Disalicylic acid, salicylsalicylic acid

Drug Class: Nonacetylated salicylate, NSAID

Preparations

Capsule: 500 mg

Tablet: 500 mg, 750 mg

Dose: (Adult) 3 g/day in 2 or 3 divided doses

Indications: RA, osteoarthritis, pain

Mechanism of Action: Weak inhibitor of prostaglandin synthesis

Contraindications: Hypersensitivity to salicylates

Precautions: Administer with food. Caution in asthma, bleeding disorders, anticoagulant use, or hepatic or renal disease.

Monitoring: Monitor hematocrit, creatinine, liver enzymes periodically (1 month after starting and then every 3–6 months). Serum salicylate levels may be assayed periodically if necessary.

Pregnancy Risk: C

Adverse Effects

Common: GI irritation (dyspepsia, reflux, epigastric pain)

Less common: GI ulceration or hemorrhage; minor elevations of liver enzymes; hypersensitivity (asthma, urticaria, angioedema—particularly in patients with nasal polyps); cross-sensitivity occurs between NSAIDs, but hypersensitivity is less common with the nonacetylated salicylates; dose-related side effects include tinnitus and deafness

Drug Interactions

Antacids: Decreased salicylate levels through increased elimination in alkaline urine

Anticoagulants: Activity of warfarin increased

Uricosurics: Decreased uricosuric effect

Patient Instructions: Take with food. Discontinue and seek medical advice if fainting, vomiting of blood, or unusual bleeding develops.

Comments: Nonacetylated salicylates have little effect on platelet function and cause less GI toxicity than classical NSAIDs, which are more potent inhibitors of prostaglandin synthesis. In practice, the antiinflammatory effect of salsalate is less than that of classical NSAIDs.

Clinical Pharmacology: Rapidly and well absorbed after oral administration; hepatic metabolism and renal excretion of conjugated metabolites. Urinary pH alters elimination (alkaline urine increases elimination). Wide variation in plasma concentrations in individuals receiving the same dose. Half-life varies with dose (2–3 h with low doses, 20 h or more with high doses). At high doses, the salicylate elimination pathway is saturated, and a small increase in dose can lead to a large increase in serum concentrations.

Cost: $

REFERENCE

Anonymous. Drugs for rheumatoid arthritis. Med Lett 1991;33:65–70.

Sandimmune (see *Cyclosporine*)

Sertraline (*Zoloft*; see *Appendix D*)

Solganol (see *Gold*)

Soma (see *Carisoprodol*)

Sucralfate (*Carafate*; see *Appendix C*)

SULFASALAZINE

Trade Names: *Azulfidine, Azulfidine EN-tabs*

Synonyms: Salazopyrin; 5-aminosalicylic acid (5-ASA) plus sulfapyridine

Drug Class: Sulfonamide/salicylate congener

Preparations

> Tablet: 500 mg
>
> Tablet enteric coated: 500 mg
>
> Oral suspension: 250 mg/5 mL

Dose: In rheumatic diseases, 2–3 g/day in 2 or 3 divided doses. Initial dose of 500 mg daily is increased by 500-mg increments weekly as tolerated. Usual maintenance dose is 2–3 g/day. Higher doses may be associated with greater GI toxicity.

Indications: RA, JRA, Reiter's syndrome, ankylosing spondylitis, psoriatic arthritis, inflammatory bowel disease

Mechanism of Action: Unknown. The sulfonamide component is thought to be more active in the treatment of rheumatic diseases than the 5-ASA component.

Contraindications: Hypersensitivity to sulfonamides or salicylates, porphyria, GI/GU obstruction

Precautions: Use caution in impaired renal function; may cause hemolysis in G6PD deficiency; blood deprivation

Monitoring: Hematologic adverse effects are most likely in the first 6 months. CBC every 2–3 weeks for first 3 months, then gradually decrease frequency to every 3 months. Periodic LFTs (3- to 6-month intervals) should be done.

Pregnancy Risk: B (D at term)

Adverse Effects

Common: GI side effects (nausea, vomiting, diarrhea, cramps), rash, itch, dizziness, headache

Less common: Reversible oligospermia, neutropenia, aplastic anemia, agranulocytosis, hemolysis, Stevens-Johnson syndrome, photosensitivity, SLE-like syndrome, nephrotic syndrome, orange-yellow discoloration of urine

Drug Interactions

Warfarin: Increased anticoagulant effect

Methotrexate: Increased MTX toxicity (see Comments)

Patient Instructions: May cause orange-yellow discoloration of skin, urine, and contact lenses. Beware of photosensitive reactions to prolonged sunlight exposure.

Comments: GI intolerance is often prominent when starting treatment. Thus, start with a low dose and work up. Some evidence indicates that the enteric coated tablets are better tolerated. Efficacy in RA appears similar to that of MTX, but there may be more minor side effects and less serious toxicity. Widely used in Europe as a first-line DMARD for RA; more recently, used in combination with MTX and hydroxychloroquine in RA patients not responding to MTX alone. Efficacy in ankylosing spondylitis, Reiter's syndrome, and psoriatic arthritis is variable and probably greatest in those with peripheral arthropathy (rather than axial disease alone). It may cause folate deficiency (consider supplementation with folate, 1 mg/day).

Clinical Pharmacology: Sulfasalazine is poorly absorbed, and the azo bond joining 5-ASA and sulfapyridine is broken by bacteria in the colon. Approximately 15–30% is absorbed; hepatic metabolism; renal excretion. Half-life is 6–10 h. Slow acetylators have higher sulfapyridine blood levels and perhaps more minor side effects, but acetylator status need not be routinely determined.

Cost: Generic, $$; enteric coated, $$$

REFERENCES

O'Dell JR, Haire CE, Erikson N, et al. Treatment of rheumatoid arthritis with methotrexate alone, sulfasalazine and hydroxychloroquine, or a combination of all three medications. N Engl J Med 1996;334:1287–1291.

Rains CP, Noble S, Faulds D. Sulfasalazine. A review of its pharmacological properties and therapeutic efficacy in the treatment of rheumatoid arthritis. Drugs 1995;50:137–156.

SULFINPYRAZONE

Trade Names: *Anturane*

Drug Class: Uricosuric

Preparations

Tablet: 100 mg

Capsule: 200 mg

Dose: 100–200 mg twice a day. Maximum daily dose is 800 mg.

Indications: Hyperuricemia associated with gout in patients who excrete 800 mg or less of urate/24 h, have normal renal function, no tophi, and no renal calculi

Mechanism of Action: Decreases renal reabsorption of filtered uric acid

Contraindications: Hypersensitivity to sulfinpyrazone, renal failure, gouty nephropathy, bone marrow depression, hyperuricemia of cancer, or chemotherapy

Precautions: Caution with renal impairment, peptic ulcer disease

Monitoring: Monitor uric acid periodically.

Pregnancy Risk: C

Adverse Effects

Common: Nausea, vomiting, cramps

Less common: Rash, dizziness, anemia, leukopenia, hepatitis, nephrotic syndrome

Drug Interactions

Salicylates: Decreased uricosuric effect

Theophylline: Decreased theophylline levels

Verapamil: Decreased verapamil levels

Anticoagulants: Effect of warfarin enhanced

Antidiabetics: Sulfonylurea effects enhanced

Patient Instructions: Drink plenty of fluids and take with food. Avoid large doses of aspirin or other salicylates.

Clinical Pharmacology: Well absorbed; hepatic metabolism and renal excretion. Half-life is 4 h.

Cost: $$

SULINDAC

Trade Names: *Clinoril*

Drug Class: NSAID

Preparations: 150-mg, 200-mg tablet

Dose: 150–200 mg twice a day

Indications: RA, osteoarthritis, gout, ankylosing spondylitis, analgesia

Mechanism of Action: Inhibition of cyclooxygenase activity, thus decreasing formation of prostaglandins and thromboxane from arachidonic acid; may decrease neutrophil function

Contraindications: Hypersensitivity to NSAIDs, GI ulceration, renal failure, hemorrhagic state, and last trimester of pregnancy (increased risk of premature closure of ductus arteriosus)

Precautions: Fluid retention may aggravate heart failure and hypertension. Use with caution or avoid in patients at high risk of GI bleeding (i.e., prior GI bleeding, elderly, concurrent corticosteroid treatment). Administer with food. Also use with caution in asthma, bleeding disorders, and GI, cardiac, hepatic, or renal disease.

Monitoring: Monitor hematocrit, creatinine, liver enzymes periodically (1 month after starting and then every 3–6 months). In patients at high risk of renal impairment (receiving ACE inhibitors or diuretics, edematous states, heart failure, renal failure, diabetes), monitor renal function closely (every 1–2 weeks) when starting treatment.

Pregnancy Risk: B (D in third trimester)

Adverse Effects

Common: GI irritation (dyspepsia, reflux, epigastric pain), rash, dizziness, fluid retention

Less common: GI ulceration, hemorrhage, or gastric outlet obstruction; hepatitis with elevations of liver enzymes; hypersensitivity (anaphylaxis, asthma, urticaria, angioedema—particularly in patients with nasal polyps, exfoliative dermatitis, rash); hematologic toxicity (agranulocytosis, anemia, leukopenia, thrombocytopenia); renal toxicity (interstitial nephritis, proteinuria, acute renal failure, hypertension, hyperkalemia); CNS toxicity (headache, drowsiness, insomnia, nervousness)

Drug Interactions

Anticoagulants: Increased hemorrhagic risk with anticoagulants and thrombolytics

NSAIDs: Increased risk of GI side effects if combinations of NSAIDs are used

Methotrexate: Increased levels of MTX may be seen with NSAID use, but with the low doses of MTX used in RA, this is usually not of clinical importance.

Diuretics: Decreased effects of thiazides and furosemide; increased renal toxicity with diuretics; increased risk of hyperkalemia with K^+-sparing diuretics

Lithium: Increased lithium levels described with many NSAIDs

Antihypertensive agents: Effect reduced

Patient Instructions: Take with food. Discontinue and seek medical advice if fainting, vomiting of blood, or unusual bleeding develops.

Comments: Sulindac may be safer than other NSAIDs in patients at high risk for renal impairment. Such benefits may only apply for short-term use (<6 weeks), and claims that sulindac is "renal-sparing" are based on limited and controversial evidence.

Clinical Pharmacology: Well absorbed after oral administration, sulindac is a prodrug. After ingestion, there is hepatic metabolism to an active sulfide metabolite, which later undergoes renal elimination. Half-life of parent drug is 7 h and of metabolite is 18 h.

Cost: Generic, $$

Talacen (see *Acetaminophen + Opioids*)
Tears, Artificial (see *Artificial Tears*)
Tegison (see *Etretinate*)
Tensilon (see *Edrophonium*)

TETRACYCLINES (ALSO SEE MINOCYCLINE)

Trade Names

   Tetracycline: *Achromycin, Tetracyn*

   Doxycycline: *Doxy, Vibramycin*

Synonyms: Tetracycline hydrochloride, doxycycline monohydrate

Drug Class: Antibiotic

Preparations

   Tetracycline

      Capsule and tablets: 100 mg, 250 mg, 500 mg

      Syrup: 125 mg/5 mL

   Doxycycline

      Capsule: 50 mg, 100 mg

      Syrup: 50 mg/5 mL

      Tablet: 50 mg, 100 mg

Dose

   Tetracycline: 250–500 mg every 6 h

   Doxycycline: 100 mg once or twice a day

Indications: Bacterial infections due to susceptible organisms, *Chlamydia, Rickettsia, Mycoplasma,* and *Borrelia burgdorferi*

Mechanism of Action: Inhibits bacterial protein synthesis

Contraindications: Hypersensitivity to tetracyclines; pregnancy. In children, staining of tooth enamel occurs.

Precautions: Hepatic or renal impairment

Pregnancy Risk: D

Adverse Effects

Common: Photosensitivity, nausea, diarrhea

Less common: Rash, hepatotoxicity, increased intracranial pressure, *Candida* superinfection

Drug Interactions: Decreased absorption with calcium, milk, food, antacids

Patient Instructions: Take 1 hour before or 2 hours after meals. Do not take with antacids.

Comments: Doxycycline is only 25% renally excreted and does not accumulate significantly in renal impairment.

Clinical Pharmacology: Half-life of tetracycline is 10 h and of doxycycline is 12–24 h.

Cost: $

Tolectin (see *Tolmetin*)

TOLMETIN

Trade Names: *Tolectin*

Synonyms: Tolmetin sodium

Drug Class: NSAID

Preparations: 200-mg, 400-mg, 600-mg tablet

Dose: 600–1800 mg daily in 3 or 4 divided doses

Indications: RA, osteoarthritis, gout, ankylosing spondylitis, analgesia

Mechanism of Action: Inhibition of cyclooxygenase activity, thus decreasing formation of prostaglandins and thromboxane from arachidonic acid; may decrease neutrophil function

Contraindications: Hypersensitivity to NSAIDs, GI ulceration, renal failure, hemorrhagic state, and last trimester of pregnancy (increased risk of premature closure of ductus arteriosus)

Precautions: Fluid retention may aggravate heart failure and hypertension. Use with caution or avoid in patients at high risk of GI bleeding (i.e., prior GI bleeding, elderly, concurrent corticosteroid treatment). Administer with food. Also use with caution in asthma, bleeding disorders, and GI, cardiac, hepatic, or renal disease.

Monitoring: Monitor hematocrit, creatinine, liver enzymes periodically (1 month after starting and then every 3–6 months). In patients at high risk of renal impairment (receiving ACE inhibitors or diuretics, edematous states, heart failure, renal failure, diabetes), monitor renal function closely (every 1–2 weeks) when starting treatment.

Pregnancy Risk: B (D in third trimester)

Adverse Effects

Common: GI irritation (dyspepsia, reflux, epigastric pain), rash, dizziness, fluid retention

Less common: GI ulceration, hemorrhage, or gastric outlet obstruction; hepatitis with elevations of liver enzymes; hypersensitivity (anaphylaxis, asthma, urticaria, angioedema—particularly in patients with nasal polyps, exfoliative dermatitis, rash); hematologic toxicity (agranulocytosis, anemia, leukopenia, thrombocytopenia); renal toxicity (interstitial nephritis, proteinuria, acute renal failure, hypertension, hyperkalemia); CNS toxicity (headache, drowsiness, insomnia, nervousness)

Drug Interactions

Anticoagulants: Increased hemorrhagic risk with anticoagulants and thrombolytics

NSAIDs: Increased risk of GI side effects if combinations of NSAIDs are used

Methotrexate: Increased levels of MTX may be seen with NSAID use, but with the low doses of MTX used in RA, this is usually not of clinical importance.

Diuretics: Decreased effects of thiazides and furosemide; increased renal toxicity with diuretics; increased risk of hyperkalemia with K^+-sparing diuretics

Lithium: Increased lithium levels described with many NSAIDs

Antihypertensive agents: Effect reduced

Patient Instructions: Take with food. Discontinue and seek medical advice if fainting, vomiting of blood, or unusual bleeding develops.

Clinical Pharmacology: Well absorbed after oral administration; hepatic metabolism and renal elimination; half-life of 2–5 h

Cost: $$

Toradol (see *Ketorolac*)

TRAMADOL

Trade Names: *Ultram*

Drug Class: Opioid analgesic

Preparations: 50-mg tablet

Dose: (Adults) 50–100 mg every 4–6 h (not to exceed 400 mg/day)

Indications: Pain not controlled by nonopioid analgesics

Mechanism of Action: Binds to μ opioid receptors; inhibits uptake of norepinephrine and serotonin

Contraindications: Hypersensitivity to tramadol or opioids; drug abuse

Precautions: Seizure risk is increased in patients also receiving tricyclic antidepressants and structurally related drugs (cyclobenzaprine, promethazine), MAOIs, selective serotonin reuptake inhibitors. Renal and hepatic impairment decreases clearance of tramadol.

Monitoring: Use the lowest dose necessary to control pain. Escalate dose only with uncontrolled pain.

Pregnancy Risk: C

Adverse Effects

Common: Dizziness, nausea, constipation, headache, sleepiness, itch

Less common: Respiratory depression, seizures, dependence, increased hepatic enzymes

Drug Interactions

Antidepressants: Increased seizure risk

Quinidine: Increased tramadol concentrations

Carbamazepine: Decreased tramadol concentrations

Patient Instructions: Drug is addictive and must only be used to control pain. Do not drink alcohol. May cause drowsiness.

Comments: Efficacy seems similar to that of other weak opioids. It is thought to have less potential for abuse, but data regarding long-term administration are limited.

Clinical Pharmacology: Bioavailability 70%; hepatic metabolism by CYP P450 2D6 to M1 metabolite. Half-life is 5 h.

Cost: $$$

REFERENCE

Dayer P, Collart L, Desmeules J. The pharmacology of tramadol. Drugs 1994;47(Suppl 1):3–7.

TRAZODONE

Trade Names: *Desyrel*

Drug Class: Antidepressant

Preparations: 50-mg, 100-mg, 150-mg, 300-mg tablet

Dose

Depression: Initially 150 mg/day in 3 divided doses, increase dose by 50 mg/day every week, if needed, to maximum of 600 mg/day.

Fibromyalgia: As a sleep aid, the usual starting dose is 25–50 mg nightly. This can be increased by 50 mg per week (up to 150 mg) until maximum improvement in sleep is achieved without causing morning somnolence.

Indications: Treatment of depression or sleep disturbance in fibromyalgia

Mechanism of Action: Inhibits presynaptic uptake of norepinephrine and serotonin

Contraindications: Hypersensitivity to trazodone

Precautions: Sedating but little anticholinergic effect. Concomitant MAOI therapy is potentially dangerous. Allow a 14-day washout between trazodone and MAOI therapy. Use caution in cardiac, renal, and hepatic disease.

Monitoring: Plasma levels are not routinely measured and may not correlate with efficacy.

Pregnancy Risk: C

Adverse Effects

Common: Sedation, nausea, bad taste, dry mouth, dizziness, weight gain

Less common: Weakness, diarrhea, constipation, nightmares

Uncommon: Rash, orthostatic symptoms (tachycardia, postural dizziness), arrhythmias, heart block, agitation, seizures, extrapyramidal effects, priapism, urinary retention

Drug Interactions

CNS depressants: Increased CNS depression

Phenytoin: Increased phenytoin levels reported

Increased toxicity: MAOI

Patient Instructions: May cause drowsiness. Avoid alcohol. Keep medication away from children.

Comments: Maximum effect may be delayed for 4 weeks. Sometimes used for sedative effect to correct sleep disorders caused by SSRIs (selective serotonin reuptake inhibitors).

Clinical Pharmacology: Well absorbed; 90% protein bound; hepatic metabolism with half-life of 5–9 h

Cost: $

Tricyclic Antidepressants (see *Appendix D*)
Trilisate (see *Choline Magnesium Salicylate*)
Tums (see *Calcium*)
Tylenol (see *Acetaminophen*)
Tylenol #3 (see *Acetaminophen + Opioids*)
Tylox (see *Acetaminophen + Opioids*)
Ultram (see *Tramadol*)
Venflaxine (*Effexor,* see *Appendix D*)
Vicodin (see *Acetaminophen + Opioids*)

VITAMIN D (ERGOCALCIFEROL, CALCITRIOL)

Trade Names: Ergocalciferol, *Calciferol;* calcitriol, *Rocaltrol*

Synonyms: Ergocalciferol, vitamin D_2; calcitriol, 1,25-dihydroxycholecalciferol

Drug Class: Vitamin

Preparations

> Ergocalciferol: capsule 50,000 units (1.25 mg), multiple OTC preparations containing 400 units/tablet
>
> Calcitriol: 0.25-μg, 0.5-μg capsule

Dose

> Ergocalciferol: Dietary supplement/prevention of osteoporosis, 400 units/day; treatment of osteomalacia, 1000–5000 units/day.
>
> Calcitriol: Renal failure, individualize dose to maintain serum calcium level; usual dose, 0.25 μg daily or alternate days. Higher doses may be required.

Indications: Most often used as a dietary supplement with calcium to ensure adequate intake of calcium and vitamin D in the prophylaxis and treatment of osteoporosis. Vitamin D is also used to treat rickets/osteomalacia, and calcitriol is used to treat hypocalcemia associated with renal failure.

Mechanism of Action: Promotes absorption of calcium from GI tract and stimulates calcium reabsorption from the renal tubule

Contraindications: Hypercalcemia, vitamin D toxicity

Precautions: Adequate calcium intake required. Avoid hypercalcemia.

Monitoring: With dietary supplementation using doses in the range of the RDA (400 u/day) of vitamin D_2, serum calcium may be monitored occasionally. With higher doses of vitamin D or use of the more potent calcitriol or alphacidol preparations, close monitoring of serum calcium level is prudent.

Pregnancy Risk: A, but D in doses above recommended daily allowance

Adverse Effects: Doses of vitamin D_2 in the RDA range have minimal side effects. The more potent calcitriol or alphacidol preparations have more often been associated with hypercalcemia, hypercalciuria, and renal stones.

With any vitamin D preparation, dose-related hypercalcemia may occur, resulting in weakness, anorexia, polyuria, thirst, constipation, nausea, myalgia, irritability, and psychosis.

Drug Interactions: Increased serum calcium with thiazide diuretics

Comments: The effect of vitamin D preparations on osteoporosis is controversial. Generally, vitamin D is supplemented in the treatment and prophylaxis of osteoporosis in doses that ensure a daily intake that meets the RDA. The risk/benefit balance of using a more potent vitamin D preparation such as calcitriol or alphacidol in osteoporosis is controversial, and they are not widely used for this purpose.

Clinical Pharmacology: Cholecalciferol (vitamin D_3) and ergocalciferol (vitamin D_2) are activated in the liver to calcifediol (25-hydroxycholecalciferol) and then in the kidneys to calcitriol (1,25-dihydroxycholecalciferol). Vitamin D is fat soluble and is stored in the liver and fat; thus, effects are prolonged for weeks or months.

Cost: $$$

REFERENCE

Orcel P. Calcium and vitamin D in the prevention and treatment of osteoporosis. J Clin Rheumatol 1997;3:S52–S56.

Voltaren (see *Diclofenac*)

ZOLPIDEM

Trade Names: *Ambien*

Drug Class: Sedative-hypnotic

Preparations: 5-mg, 10-mg tablet

Dose: Usual dose, 5–10 mg before bedtime (elderly use 5 mg)

Indications: Treatment of insomnia

Mechanism of Action: Not a benzodiazepine but binds to the benzodiazepine 1 subtype of the γ-aminobutyric acid (GABA) receptor

Contraindications: Hypersensitivity to zolpidem

Precautions: May cause impaired cognitive and motor performance, particularly in the elderly. There is decreased elimination with impaired hepatic function; decrease dose to 5 mg in such patients. It may exacerbate sleep apnea.

Pregnancy Risk: B

Adverse Effects

Common: Headache, drowsiness

Less common: Confusion, falls, amnesia, allergy, paradoxical agitation

Drug Interactions: CNS depressants have increased effect

Patient Instructions: Causes drowsiness. Avoid alcohol. Keep away from children.

Comments: Limit use to short periods of time.

Clinical Pharmacology: Rapid absorption; 70% first-pass extraction; 90% protein bound; hepatic metabolism to inactive metabolites. Half-life is 2–4 h.

Cost: $$$

REFERENCE

Kupfer DJ, Reynolds CF. Management of insomnia. N Engl J Med 1997;336:341–346.

Zorprin (see *Aspirin*)
Zostrix (see *Capsaicin*)
Zyloprim (see *Allopurinol*)

INDICATIONS FOR SURGERY

Orthopaedic surgical procedures can dramatically improve the quality of life for patients with various types of arthritis. Progress in the development of surgical interventions has been among the most important advances in the care of arthritis patients during the past century.

Types of Surgery

Commonly available types of orthopaedic procedures include: 1) *synovectomy* or *tenosynovectomy* (i.e., removing synovial tissue from joints or tendons); 2) ligament or *tendon reconstruction* (e.g., repair of torn or fraying tendons); 3) *osteotomy* (cutting of bone to optimize mechanics); 4) *arthrodesis* (intentional fusion of joints); or 5) *arthroplasty* (joint replacement surgery).

Joint replacement surgery has been particularly useful for severe arthritis of the hip and knee joints. Many patients can have successful results for 10 to 20 years or more after surgery; therefore, joint replacement is often the preferred procedure for the hips or knees. Other joints that may be considered for joint replacement include the metacarpophalangeal, shoulder, and first carpometacarpal joints. Osteotomy is a more limited procedure than joint replacement. It may be useful in certain instances (e.g., unilateral knee osteoarthritis) where realignment may optimize joint mechanics and thereby improve pain and function. Arthrodesis is considered for joints for which the results of joint replacement have not been so promising (e.g., wrists, ankles). It should be noted that repeated attempts at replacing the same joint are often more difficult and less successful than the first procedure.

Indications: The main indications for joint surgery include: 1) intractable or refractory pain and 2) significant functional limitation. When considering referring patients to an orthopaedic surgeon, it should be clear that either the pain and/or the impairment in functional status are directly related to damage to, or destruction of, the affected joint. For example, a person with advanced degenerative changes on x-ray, who experiences severe pain both with activity and at rest, should be considered a potential candidate for surgical intervention. On the other hand, if a patient has severe pain but no evidence of joint damage, other etiologies for the pain should be considered (e.g., neuropathic pain, fibromyalgia, etc). In addition, before undertaking surgery, other interventions should be tried. For example, simple analgesics are the first step in managing pain, and assist devices can help optimize functional status.

Tenosynovectomy and tendon or ligament repairs are generally less extensive surgical procedures than joint replacement. Indications for these procedures include: 1) rupture or impending rupture and 2) severe, refractory localized synovitis.

Contraindications: Contraindications to joint surgery include active infection
and uncontrolled bleeding diathesis. Because postoperative rehabilitation is crucial to a good outcome following joint replacement, many of the relative contraindications to this surgery include conditions that could interfere with rehabilitation potential (e.g., decreased mobility unrelated to the involved joint,
morbid obesity, lack of motivation, severe comorbid diseases). Younger age is
also a relative contraindication to joint replacement surgery because: 1) patients
who are extremely physically active following joint replacement may experience failure of the prosthesis sooner than those with normal activity, and 2) repeat procedures are often associated with a poorer outcome.

Complications: The risk of an infected prosthesis following joint replacement
is $\leq 2\%$.

Cost: The cost of total joint arthroplasty (hip or knee) is usually between
\$25,000–35,000.

CHAPTER 3.3

PLASMAPHERESIS

Indications: Plasmapheresis can be effective in a number of rheumatologic and immunologic disorders, including Goodpasture's syndrome, myasthenia gravis, Guillain-Barré syndrome, hyperviscosity syndrome (e.g., with Waldenström's macroglobulinemia), cryoglobulinemia (particularly with renal involvement), thrombotic thrombocytopenic purpura (TTP), idiopathic demyelinating polyneuropathy, rapidly progressive glomerulonephritis (RPGN), and refractory autoimmune hemolytic anemia or posttransfusion purpura. In addition to TTP, plasmapheresis may be of benefit in other disorders associated with microangiopathic hemolytic anemia, including hemolytic-uremic syndrome (HUS), SLE presenting with TTP-like features, and DIC. Plasmapheresis may be of benefit in other conditions, e.g., SLE with transverse myelitis or other CNS or PNS manifestations. However, the evidence is anecdotal at best. For SLE nephritis, several studies showed that in unselected groups of patients, plasmapheresis is of no benefit. Whether plasmapheresis is indicated in certain instances, for example SLE nephritis with a rapidly deteriorating course, in conjunction with high-dose cyclophosphamide, is still controversial. Plasmapheresis is not indicated in rheumatoid arthritis or dermatomyositis/polymyositis.

Mechanisms of Action: Plasmapheresis nonspecifically removes plasma constituents, including immunoglobulins and other plasma proteins. Removal of particular antibodies or immune complexes presumably underlies its effect in most diseases. In TTP, some of the benefit also derives from infusion of normal plasma.

Comments: There are few adequate controlled trials in rheumatic diseases. Plasmapheresis should usually be used in conjunction with immunosuppressive therapy to prevent rebound increase in antibody production. Evidence suggests little benefit in RA or polymyositis/dermatomyositis. Plasmapheresis alone has no benefit in lupus nephritis, but plasmapheresis with pulse cyclophosphamide has anecdotally been beneficial.

Cost: \$\$\$\$\$. An important consideration in the use of plasmapheresis is its cost, which runs upward of several thousand dollars for a treatment. While generally well tolerated, it may also be associated transiently with hypocalcemia and bleeding diathesis.

REFERENCES

Campion EW. Desperate diseases and plasmapheresis. N Engl J Med 1992;326:1425–1428.
Euler HH, Schroeder JO, Harten P, et al. Treatment-free remission in severe systemic lupus erythematosus following synchronization of plasmapheresis with subsequent pulse cyclophosphamide. Arthritis Rheum 1994;37:1784–1794.

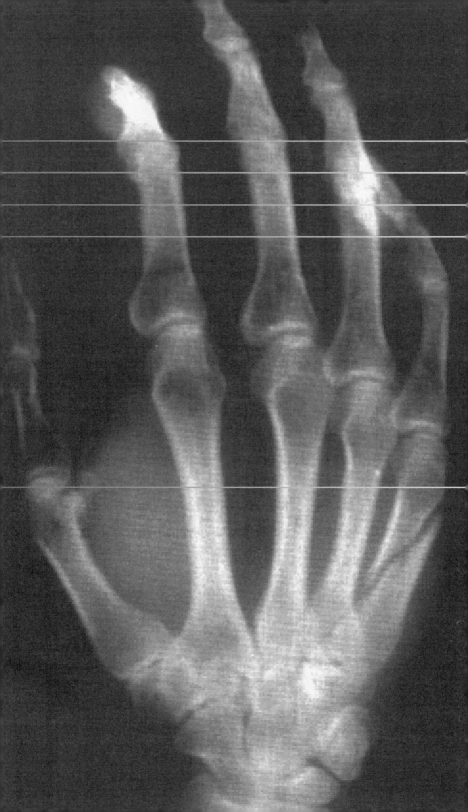

APPENDICES

APPENDIX A

COMPARISON OF NONSTEROIDAL ANTIINFLAMMATORY DRUGS

Generic Name	Trade Name(s)	Pill Strength (mg)	Daily Frequency	Total Daily Dose (range)	Other Preparations
Very cheap (generic form, $0.30/day)					
Aspirin	Ecotrin, Easprin, Bufferin	325, 500, 650, 975	3–4	(2000–6000 mg)	Suppository, enteric-coated
Ibuprofen	Motrin	200, 400, 600, 800	2–4	(1200–3200 mg)	Suspension
Indomethacin	Indocin	25, 50	3–4	(75–200 mg)	Suspension, suppository
Cheap (generic form, $0.30–0.75/day)					
Choline Mg salicylate	Trilisate	500, 750, 1000	3–4	(2000–4000 mg)	Suspension
Indomethacin-SR	Indocin-SR	75	1–2	(75–150 mg)	—
Naproxen	Naprosyn, Naprelan	250, 375, 500	2–3	(500–1500 mg)	Liquid, enteric-coated
Piroxicam	Feldene	10,20	1–2	(10–20 mg)	—
Salsalate	Disalcid	500,750	2–3	(2000–4500 mg)	—
Sulindac	Clinoril	150,200	1–2	(200–400 mg)	—
Tolmetin	Tolectin	200,400, 600	3–4	(1200–1800 mg)	—
Expensive ($$$ 1.00–2.50/day)					
Diclofenac	Voltaren, Cataflam	50, 75	2–4	(150–225 mg)	Suppository, ophthalmic sol'n
Diflunisal	Dolobid	250,500	2–3	(1000–1500 mg)	—
Etodolac	Lodine	200,300 400,500	2–4	(600–1200 mg)	—
	Lodine XL	400,500, 600	1–2	(800–1200 mg)	—
Fenoprofen	Nalfon	200,300, 600	3–4	(1200–3200 mg)	—
Flurbiprofen	Ansaid	50, 100	2–4	(200–400 mg)	Ophthalmic sol'n
Ketoprofen	Orudis	25,50,75	2–3	(150–300 mg)	—
Ketoprofen-SR	Oruvail	100,150,200	1	(100–200 mg)	—
Ketorolac	Toradol	10	1–4	(10–40 mg)	Parenteral
Meclofenamate	Meclomen	50,100	3–4	(300–400 mg)	—
Nabumetone	Relafen	500,750	1–2	(1000–2000 mg)	—
Oxaprozin	Daypro	600	1–2	(1200–1800)	—

SECOND-LINE DRUGS FOR THE TREATMENT OF RHEUMATOID ARTHRITIS

Drug	Mechanisms of Action	Common Adverse Effects	Usual Dosing Regimens
Disease-Modifying Antirheumatic Drugs (DMARDs)			
Injectable gold -aurothioglucose -gold sodium thiomalate	-Inhibits macrophage function -Inhibits angiogenesis -Inhibits protein kinase C	-Mucocutaneous eruptions -Proteinuria -Thrombocytopenia	50 mg i.m./week to a total dose of 1000 mg; then 50 mg i.m. q. 2–4 weeks
Oral gold	-Inhibits macrophage function	-Diarrhea	3 mg p.o., b.i.d.
-auranofin	-Inhibits PMN function	-Mucocutaneous eruptions	
Antimalarials	-Inhibits cytokine secretion	-Rash	400 mg p.o., q.d.
-Hydroxychloroquine	-Inhibits lysosomal enzymes -Inhibits macrophage function	-Visual disturbance	
D-Penicillamine	-Inhibits helper T cell function -Inhibits angiogenesis	-Mucocutaneous eruptions -Proteinuria -Thrombocytopenia	500–1000 mg p.o., q.d.
Sulfasalazine	-Inhibits B cell responses -Inhibits angiogenesis	-Nausea, abdominal pain, diarrhea -Rash	1000 mg p.o., b.i.d. or t.i.d.
Methotrexate	-Dihydrofolate reductase inhibitor -Antiinflammatory via induction of adenosine release -Inhibits chemotaxis	-Mucocutaneous eruptions -Bone marrow suppression -Nausea, diarrhea -Hepatic abnormalities	7.5–20 mg, p.o., per week (may also be administered parenterally)
Systemic immunosuppressives			
Cyclosporine	-Inhibits synthesis of IL-2 and other T cell cytokines	-Hypertension -Renal insufficiency -Hirsutism	2.5–4 mg/kg p.o., q.d.
Azathioprine	-Inhibits DNA synthesis and	-Bone marrow suppression	1–2 mg/kg p.o., q.d.

(continued)

Drug	Mechanisms of Action	Common Adverse Effects	Usual Dosing Regimens
	cellular proliferation	-Nausea -Hepatic abnormalities	
Cyclophosphamide	-Crosslinks DNA and inhibits cellular proliferation	-Nausea, emesis	1–2 mg/kg p.o., q.d.
		-Bone marrow suppression -Ovarian failure -Hemorrhagic cystitis -↑ Risk of cancer	

DRUGS USED TO TREAT PEPTIC ULCER DISEASE

Drug	Dose
H_2-receptor antagonists	
Cimetidine (Tagamet)	400 mg twice daily
Famotidine (Pepcid)	20 mg twice daily
Nizatidine (Axid)	150 mg twice daily
Ranitidine (Zantac)	150 mg twice daily
Proton-pump inhibitors	
Lansoprazole (Prevacid)	30 mg once daily
Omeprazole (Prilosec)	20 mg once daily
Miscellaneous Drugs	
Misoprostol (Cytotec)	200 μg four times/day
Sucralfate (Carafate)	1 g four times/day

Note: H_2-receptor antagonists are often used in lower doses for maintenance after ulcer healing. H_2-receptor antagonists and proton-pump inhibitors are most often used to treat peptic ulcers and reflux esophagitis. Cimetidine inhibits cytochrome P450 drug metabolism, and clinically important interactions occur with warfarin, theophylline, phenytoin, quinidine, and propranolol. Omeprazole is particularly useful in reflux esophagitis associated with scleroderma. Misoprostol (see p. 470) and omeprazole are most often used to prevent NSAID-related GI complications.

COMPARISON OF COMMON ANTIDEPRESSANTS

Drug	Daily Dose Range[a] (mg/day)	Anticholinergic	Drowsiness	Arrhythmias
First-generation anti- depressants (tricyclics)				
Amitriptyline (Elavil)	75–300	++++	++++	+++
Doxepin (Sinequan)	75–300	++++	++++	++
Imipramine (Tofranil)	75–200	+++	+++	++
Nortriptyline (Pamelor)	50–100	++	+	+++
Second-generation antidepressants				
Amoxapine (Asendin)	100–400	++	++	++
Maprotilene (Ludiomil)	100–225	++	+++	++
Trazodone (Desyrel)	150–400	0/+	++++	+
Bupropion (Wellbutrin)	200–450	0/+	0	+
Third-generation antidepressants				
Selective serotonin-reuptake inhibitors (SSRIs)				
Fluoxetine (Prozac)	10–40	0	0	0
Paroxetine (Paxil)	20–50	0/+	0/+	0
Sertraline (Zoloft)	50–150	0	0	0
Norepinephrine/serotonin reuptake inhibitors				
Venlafaxine (Effexor)	75–225	+	+	+

[a] Usual dose ranges for depression are expressed as total daily dose. For many drugs, this is administered in 2 or 3 divided doses. Initial doses and doses for other indications (e.g., insomnia, pain control) may be much lower than maintenance doses for depression. Monoamine oxidase inhibitors (MAOIs) are not included and should only be prescribed by experts in the treatment of depression.

APPENDIX E

ANTIBIOTICS FOR SEPTIC ARTHRITIS

Below is a population-oriented listing of common pathogens that cause bacterial arthritis and recommended empirical antibacterial therapy. In areas where the prevalence of methicillin-resistant *Staphylococcus aureus* is high, drugs such as vancomycin or teicoplanin must be considered instead of nafcillin. Streptococci mainly include group A β-hemolytic streptococcus (*Streptococcus pyogenes*), other streptococcal groups, and infrequently *Streptococcus pneumoniae*.

Patient Population	Likely Pathogens	Antibacterial Selection	Daily Dosage	Doses/ Day
Neonates	*Staphylococcus aureus* Enterobacteriaceae Group B streptococci	Nafcillin **and** cefotaxime or gentamicin	100 mg/kg 150 mg/kg 7.5 mg/kg	4 3 3
Children under 5 years	*S. aureus* *Haemophilus influenzae* type b Streptococci	Nafcillin **or** cefuroxime	150 mg/kg 150 mg/kg	4 3
Children 5 years or older	*S. aureus* Streptococci	Nafcillin	150 mg/kg	4
Adolescents and adults with possible STD contact	*Neisseria gonorrhoeae* *S. aureus*	Ceftriaxone **or** cefotaxime	1–2 g 3–6 g	1 3
Adults unlikely to have STD[a]	*S. aureus* Streptococci Enterobacteriaceae	Nafcillin **and** cefotaxime or gentamicin	6–12 g 3–6 g 5 mg/kg	6 3 3
Adults with joint prosthesis or infection following procedure/ surgery	*Staphylococcus epidermidis* *S. aureus* Streptococci Gram-negative bacilli including *Pseudomonas* spp.	Vancomycin **and** ceftazidime or aztreonam or ciprofloxacin or gentamicin	2 g 3–6 g 3–6 g 800 mg 5 mg/kg	2 3 3 2 3

From Hamed KA, Tam JY, Prober CG. Pharmacokinetic optimization of the treatment of septic arthritis. Clin Pharmacokinet 1996;31:156–163. With permission.

[a] STD, sexually transmitted disease.

COMPARISON OF INFECTIOUS ARTHROPATHIES

Bacterial Arthritis

	Staphylococcal	Gonococcal	Gram-negative
Pattern	Acute monoarticular	Acute monoarticular or migratory polyarticular with tenosynovitis	Acute monoarticular
Demographics	All ages	Sexually active young adults	IV drug abuse; very young or very old
Synovial fluid	WBC > 50,000	WBC > 50,000	WBC > 50,000
Cultures	Usually positive	Usually negative	Usually positive
Treatment	Nafcillin (± rifampin) or vancomycin	Ceftriaxone	Aminoglycoside + semisynthetic penicillin or 3rd-generation cephalosporin
Outcome	Inversely correlated with age	Generally good	Generally good, poor in elderly

Nonbacterial Arthritis

	Viral	Fungal	Mycobacterial
Pattern	Acute polyarticular	Chronic monoarticular	Chronic monoarticular
Demographics	All ages	Immunocompromised host	All ages
Synovial fluid	WBC <20,000	Variable WBC	WBC 10,000–20,000
Cultures	Usually negative	Usually negative	Usually negative; requires biopsy
Treatment	Symptomatic	Amphotericin B (± 5-fluorocytosine)	INH, rifampin, and pyrazinamide
Outcome	Self-limited with preserved joint	Mixed; deformity possible	Mixed; destructive bone changes are possible

COMPARISON OF CRYSTALLINE ARTHROPATHIES

Crystal Type	Associations	Microscopy	Skeletal Radiography
Monosodium urate (MSU)	• Acute gout	Negatively birefringent, needle-shaped crystals	Punched-out lesions with sclerotic borders; normal mineralization
	• Chronic tophaceous gout • Urate nephropathy • Urolithiasis		
Calcium pyrophosphate dihydrate (CPPD)	• Acute psuedo-gout • Chondrocalcinosis • Chronic CPPD arthro-pathy	Positively birefringent rhomboidal or rod-shaped crystals	Chondrocalcinosis (linear calcification of fibrocartilage; e.g., menisci of knee, symphysis pubis)
Basic calcium phosphate (BCP)	• Calcific periarthritis • Milwaukee shoulder/knee syndrome • Acute BCP arthritis	Below detection threshold of light microscopy; scanning electron microscopy reveals spheroidal aggregates. Large deposits visualized as calcifications in periarticular structures	
Cholesterol	• Xanthomas • Cholesterol tophi • Chronic synovial effusions	Highly birefringent, large, flat, rectangular plates, with notched corners	None

DERMATOMAL MAPS

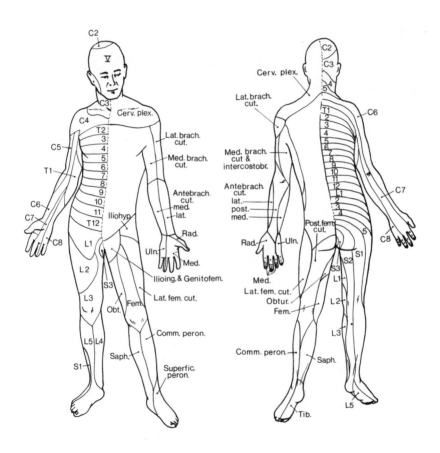

(From Gilroy J, Holliday PL. Basic neurology. New York: Macmillan, 1982. With permission.)

VASCULITIS: CLASSIFICATION AND COMPARISONS[a]

Diagnosis (by vessel size)	Demographic Features	Local Findings	Systemic Findings	Diagnostic Test(s)[b]	Treatment
Small vessel vasculitis Leukocytoclastic (hypersensitivity) vasculitis	M = F; all ages can be affected	Palpable purpura; superficial erosions, bullae, urticaria	Associated with HSP, cryoglobulinemia, RA, SLE, PAN, Wegener's, Churg-Strauss, PBC, ulcerative colitis, drugs, infection (gonococcus, meningococcus, staphylococcus, SBE, HBV, HCV, CMV, EBV), neoplasia (Hodgkin's, lymphoma, leukemia, myeloma)	Skin Bx is diagnostic	Treat underlying disorder; seldom requires the use of steroids, colchicine, or dapsone
Henoch-Schönlein purpura	M = F; children (2–11 years), adults (30–70 years)	Palpable purpura of the lower extremities and buttocks; diarrhea, cramping, intussusception	Renal failure, arthralgia, arthritis, fever	IgA deposition on skin, GI or renal Bx	Self-limiting in most and will only require supportive care; steroids are not effective and are reserved for CNS, testicular, intestinal, or joint disease

(continued)

Diagnosis (by vessel size)	Demographic Features	Local Findings	Systemic Findings	Diagnostic Test(s)[b]	Treatment
Hypocomplementemic urticarial vasculitis	F > M; usually young adults (range, 20–60 years)	Recurrent or chronic urticaria, palpable purpura	Arthralgias, arthritis, abdominal pain, N/V, fever, lymphadenopathy	Dx by skin Bx; low C3, C4, CH50; ↑ ESR, RF negative, some have low-titer ANA	Most are treated with NSAIDs or prednisone; hydroxy-chloroquine or cytotoxic therapy is seldom needed
Microscopic polyangiitis	M > F; middle-aged and elderly adults (range, 40–60 years)	Palpable purpura, hemoptysis, abdominal pain, hematochezia, neuropathy, crescentic GN	Arthralgia, myalgia, fever	Dx by tissue Bx; 40% cANCA +; 60% pANCA +; ↑ ESR	↑ Dose prednisone and CTX
Small and medium-size vasculitis					
Wegener's granulomatosis	M > F; middle-aged and elderly Caucasians	Sinusitis, otitis media, cough, hemoptysis, dyspnea, proteinuria, hematuria, renal failure	Fever, weight loss, malaise, arthralgia, mononeuritis multiplex, polyneuropathy	Dx by tissue (nasal, pul-monary, renal) Bx (granulo-matous vasculitis), 90% cANCA+, ↑ ESR	CTX + prednisone; SMX/TMP for localized disease
Polyarteritis nodosa	M > F (2:1); age 40–60 years	Renal failure, proteinuria, mononeuritis multiplex, abdominal pain, GI hemorrhage,	Hypertension, fever, malaise, weight loss, arthralgias, myalgias, back pain	Dx by angiogram or tissue (nerve, muscle, testicle, kidney)	↑ Dose prednisone and CTX or azathioprine

		bowel infarction, livedo reticularis, skin ulcers		Bx; ↑ ESR, leukocytosis, anemia, low C4 or C3, hepatitis B or C positive in some	↑ Dose prednisone
Churg-Strauss angiitis (allergic angiitis)	M > F; middle-aged adults (range 15–70 years)	Asthma, pulmonary infiltrates, rhinitis, cardiac (CHF) involvement	Arthralgia, fever, mononeuritis multiplex	Eosinophilia; necrotizing vasculitis with eosinophils and granuloma, 70% pANCA+	↑ Dose prednisone; some may require oral or IV CTX
Rheumatoid vasculitis	M > F, with longstanding, severe, seropositive RA	Splinter hemorrhages, skin ulcers, peripheral neuropathy, palpable purpura, visceral arteritis	Weight loss, splenomegaly, nodules	Dx by tissue (skin, rectal, nerve) Bx or angiogram; ↑ titer RF, ↑ ESR, low C3 or C4, anemia	↑ Dose prednisone
Large vessel vasculitis Giant cell arteritis	F > M; elderly (>60 years) Caucasians	Headache, diplopia, blindness, scalp tenderness, jaw claudication	PMR symptoms (girdle muscle pain and stiffness), fever, weight loss	Extreme ↑ ESR; temporal artery Bx positive 80–90% of patients	↑ Dose prednisone
Takayasu arteritis	>90% F; young/ middle-aged adults; common	Arm claudication, bruits, pulselessness and pressure	Hypertension, arthralgias, myalgias, fever, weight loss	Dx by angiogram; ↑ ESR in 70%	↑ Dose prednisone; may require

(continued)

Diagnosis (by vessel size)	Demographic Features	Local Findings	Systemic Findings	Diagnostic Test(s)[b]	Treatment
	in Japan, China, India; rare in whites	difference			MTX or CTX in resistant patients
Primary CNS angiitis	M > F; adults 20–60 years	Headache, confusion, cognitive dysfunction, seizure, cranial neuropathy	Uncommon: arthralgia, myalgia, fever	Dx by angiogram or lepto-meningeal Bx; ↑ ESR	↑ Dose prednisone ± CTX

[a] Abbreviations: M, male; F, female; HSP, Henoch-Schönlein purpura; RA, rheumatoid arthritis; SLE, systemic lupus erythematosus, PAN, polyarteritis nodosa; PBC, primary biliary cirrhosis; SBE, subacute bacterial endocarditis; HBV, hepatitis B virus; HCV, hepatitis C virus;. CMV, cytomegalovirus; EBV, Epstein Barr virus; Bx, biopsy; GI, gastrointestinal; N/V, nausea and vomiting; ESR, erythrocyte sedimentation rate; RF, rheumatoid factor; ANA, antinuclear antibody; Dx, diagnosis; CTX, cyclophosphamide; MTX, methotrexate; SMX/TMP, sulfamethoxazole-trimethoprim; CHF, congestive heart failure; IV, intravenous; PMR, polymyalgia rheumatica.

[b] List of those tests most helpful in establishing the diagnosis.

Index

Page numbers followed by "f" denote figures; page numbers followed by "t" denote tables.

Vision loss
  in temporal arteritis, 375
Vitamin D (ergocalciferol, Calcitriol),
    497–499
Vitamin K deficiency
  hemophilia *versus,* 228
Vocational counseling
  in psoriatic arthritis, 309
Voltaren. *See* Diclofenac
von Willebrand's disease
  hemophilia *versus,* 228

Waldenström's macroglobulinemia
  immunoglobulin M in, 123
Wasserman test. *See* Rapid plasma reagin
    (RPR) test
Weakness. *See* Muscle weakness
Weber-Christian disease, 290, 290t. *See also*
    Panniculitis
  erythema nodosum *versus,* 203
Wedge-shaped deformities
  in osteoporosis, 284
Wegener's granulomatosis, 381–385,
    524
  biopsy in, 54
  Churg-Strauss angiitis *versus,* 187
  classification criteria for
    ACR, 384–385
  complications of, 383
  cytoplasmic antineutrophil cytoplasmic
    antibody in, 81–82
  demographics in, 53–54
  disease association with, 53, 54
  morbidity in
    treatment-related, 385
  organ system involvement in, 382–383,
    383t
  relapsing polychondritis *versus,*
    321
Weight-bearing exercise
  for osteoporosis, 285
Westergren method, of erythrocyte sedi-
    mentation rate, 76
Whipple's disease, 386–387. *See* Entero-
    pathic arthritis
White blood cells (WBCs)
  abnormalities in, 95, 96t–97t

Wilson's disease, 385–386
  arthritis of joints and spine in, 45
  musculoskeletal manifestations of, 386
Wissler-Fanconi syndrome. *See* Adult-onset
    Still's disease (AOSD)
Wrist and hand
  ganglion cysts and, 215–216
  pain in, 23–26
    anatomic considerations in, 23
    articular abnormalities and clinical
      correlates, 23–25, 24f
    diagnostic testing in, 25–26
    differential diagnosis of, 25t
    imaging in, 26
    sites of involvement and disease asso-
      ciations, 23, 24f
  radiographic views for, 135
Wrist drop
  in carpal tunnel syndrome, 179
  in peripheral neuropathy, 267
  splints for, 334
Wrist (radiocarpal joint)
  arthrocentesis and corticosteroid injec-
    tion of, 70, 71f
  materials and doses for, 67t, 70
  sites/entry angle in, 70, 71f
  tenosynovitis of, 270

Xanthomatosis
  normocholesterolemic. *See* Multicentric
    reticulohistiocytosis
    (MRH)
Xerophthalmia. *See* Dry eyes (xeroph-
    thalmia)
Xerostomia. *See* Dry mouth
    (xerostomia)
X-ray. *See* Radiography

Young adults
  bacterial arthritis in, 164, 165, 515t
  infectious mononucleosis in, 198
  knee pain in, 34

Zolpidem, 499–500
Zorprin. *See* Aspirin
Zostrix. *See* Capsaicin
Zyloprim. *See* Allopurinol